Nanoformulations in Human Health

Sushama Talegaonkar • Mahendra Rai
Editors

Nanoformulations in Human Health

Challenges and Approaches

Springer

Editors
Sushama Talegaonkar
Department of Pharmaceutics
Delhi Pharmaceutical Science
and Research University
New Delhi, India

Mahendra Rai
Department of Biotechnology
Sant Gadge Baba Amravati University
Amravati, Maharashtra, India

ISBN 978-3-030-41857-1 ISBN 978-3-030-41858-8 (eBook)
https://doi.org/10.1007/978-3-030-41858-8

This Springer imprint is published by the registered company Springer Nature Switzerland AG
The registered company address is: Gewerbestrasse 11, 6330 Cham, Switzerland

Foreword

In the era of the Fourth Industrial Revolution, several technologies are poised to bring swift changes in the approach and the living style of mankind. Nanotechnology is one of such fields that has multifaceted applications in healthcare ranging from medicines, surgical materials to devices and even means to prevent diseases. Initially, nanotechnology was looked upon for novel and targeted drug delivery systems, but now it is used for precision medicine for prevention of disease through appropriate medical gazette.

The book entitled *Nanoformulations in Human Health: Challenges and Approaches* edited by Dr. Sushama Talegaonkar and Dr. Mahendra Rai focusses on the application of nanoformulations in human healthcare. The authors have dedicated years in the field of nanomedicine and have carried out original research work achieving numerous milestones in their professional journey. They have helped many students and scholars in this field. This book reflects dedication, hard work, and collaborative efforts of the authors. I congratulate the authors and contributors for ensemble of in-depth information in simple language. I am sure that the book will prove to be useful to healthcare specialists including researchers, scholars, and academicians.

This book provides comprehensive information of nanomedicine with special emphasis on drug targeting, theranostics, chronic disorders, and topical afflictions. There is a specific emphasis on preformulation of active pharmaceutical ingredients, advantages of nanoformulations over conventional therapy, and formulation, characterization, and application of various nanocarriers. Parts have been dedicated entirely on various routes of drug delivery like ocular, topical, and nose-to-brain targeting along with elaborate chapters covering diseases like glaucoma, epilepsy, colonic ailments, candidiasis, neuropathic pain, respiratory disorders, tuberculosis, and cancer.

R. K. Goyal
Vice-Chancellor, DPSRU, New Delhi, India

Preface

Nanotechnology, i.e., the science of nanosized agents, is one of the fastest-growing fields which is on its way of giving breakthroughs to the healthcare industry. Nano-agents usually are in the size range of 1–100 nm. Owing to their extremely small size and majorly large surface area, they possess distinct special characteristics which enable them to do wonders in biomedical applications. Characteristics like ability to cross the cell membrane and increased reactivity make them more useful than conventional therapy. Particularly in biomedical sciences, nanotechnology can be used for therapy and diagnostics. In addition to their therapeutic properties, they are more commonly used to carry the therapeutic agents to the diseased site in the body, thus achieving targeted therapy. Delivery of drugs through a nano-agent directly to the target site also results in a decrease of the required dose of the active agent. More recently, the application of nanotechnology has been explored for monitoring the progress and success of therapy inside the body. Many countries are now investing in developing nanotechnology for healthcare applications. For instance, the first generation of cancer drugs delivered via nanoparticles has already been approved by the US Food and Drug Administration (FDA).

However, nanoformulation for healthcare is also a topic of hot debate as this minute size also brings the concern of toxicity. Though regardless of the varying opinions, the research and development have actively been going on to take nanotechnology to the commercial level to be used for the benefits of the health of humans.

The main goal of the book titled *Nanoformulations in Human Health: Challenges and Approaches* is to serve as a complete reference guide to understand the role of nanotechnology in the healthcare system and as a ready reference for all aspects related to the theme. The book is intended to provide a multidisciplinary approach signifying the role of nanosizing in the treatment of various challenging diseases. It is planned to highlight the pathophysiology of disease with special emphasis on various targets, receptors, biomarkers, and transporters associated with the disease. Young researchers/scientists who plan to initiate research in this important field would find this book extremely relevant and handy. Each chapter of this book will be immensely useful to identify the new targets for drug delivery systems and drug discovery. This book is a true amalgamation of the experience and expertise of all the contributors in the field of nanotechnology especially in designing novel nanoformulations in the treatment of various challenging diseases. It is an exhaustive compilation of the multifaceted arena of nanoformulations in the healthcare system.

This book includes six parts concerning nanoformulations: Part I includes emerging trends and challenges in the area; Part II describes their role in drug targeting; Part III incorporates applications in ocular diseases; Part IV deliberates role in topical diseases; Part V discusses their role in natural therapeutics delivery; and finally, Part VI focuses on other applications such as in respiratory diseases, tuberculosis, and cancer.

The book would cater to the needs of postgraduate students of pharmacy, nanotechnology, and biotechnology, medical students, and researchers. In addition, the book will also be very useful for the pharmaceutical industries, regulatory bodies, pharmacy, medical institutes, etc. involved in research and development activities related to drug discovery, newer treatment modalities, and technology.

New Delhi, India — Sushama Talegaonkar
Amravati, Maharashtra, India — Mahendra Rai

Contents

Contributors

Ashish Kumar Agrawal Department of Pharmaceutical Engineering & Technology, Indian Institute of Technology (Banaras Hindu University), IIT (BHU), Varanasi, UP, India

Waseem Ali University Institute of Pharmaceutical Sciences, Panjab University, Chandigarh, India

Rajendra Awasthi Amity Institute of Pharmacy, Amity University, Noida, Uttar Pradesh, India

Janmejai Bag Department of Life Science, NIT Rourkela, Rourkela, Odisha, India

Meenakshi Bajpai Institute of Pharmaceutical Research, GLA University, Mathura, India

Nagendra Bhuwane University Institute of Pharmacy, Pandit Ravishankar Shukla University, Raipur, Chhattisgarh, India

Costica Caizer West University of Timisoara, Faculty of Physics, Timisoara, Romania

Isabela Simona Caizer "Victor Babes" University of Medicine and Pharmacy, Faculty of Pharmacy, Timisoara, Romania

Apala Chakraborty Department of Pharmaceutical Technology, Jadavpur University, Kolkata, India

Samrat Chakraborty Department of Pharmaceutical Technology, Jadavpur University, Kolkata, India

Dinesh Kumar Chellapan Department of Life Sciences, School of Pharmacy, International Medical University, Kuala Lumpur, Malaysia

Ishwari Choudhary University Institute of Pharmacy, Pandit Ravishankar Shukla University, Raipur, Chhattisgarh, India

Dorina Elena Coricovac "Victor Babes" University of Medicine and Pharmacy, Faculty of Pharmacy, Department of Toxicology and Drug Industry, Timisoara, Romania

Shweta Dang Department of Biotechnology, Jaypee Institute of Information Technology, Noida, UP, India

Cristina Dehelean "Victor Babes" University of Medicine and Pharmacy, Faculty of Pharmacy, Department of Toxicology and Drug Industry, Timisoara, Romania

Surbhi Dhawan (DST INSPIRE fellow) Department of Pharmaceutical Sciences, Maharshi Dayanand University, Rohtak, Haryana, India

Kamal Dua Centenary Institute, Royal Prince Alfred Hospital, Camperdown, NSW, Australia

Priority Research Centre for Healthy Lungs, Hunter Medical Research Institute (HMRI) & School of Biomedical Sciences and Pharmacy, University of Newcastle, Callaghan, NSW, Australia

Discipline of Pharmacy, Graduate School of Health, University of Technology Sydney, Ultimo, NSW, Australia

School of Pharmaceutical Sciences, Shoolini University, Bajhol, Sultanpur, Solan, Himachal Pradesh, India

Ishaan Duggal University Institute of Pharmaceutical Sciences, Panjab University, Chandigarh, India

Harish Dureja Department of Pharmaceutical Sciences, Maharshi Dayanand University, Rohtak, India

Iman Ehsan Department of Pharmaceutical Technology, Jadavpur University, Kolkata, India

Reema Gabrani Department of Biotechnology, Jaypee Institute of Information Technology, Noida, UP, India

Honey Goel University Institute of Pharmaceutical Sciences and Research, Baba Farid University of Health Sciences, Faridkot, Punjab, India

Gaurav Gupta School of Pharmaceutical Sciences, Jaipur National University, Jaipur, India

Swati Gupta Amity Institute of Pharmacy, Amity University Uttar Pradesh, Noida, India

Philip M. Hansbro School of Life Sciences, University of Technology Sydney, Sydney, NSW, Australia

Centenary Institute, Royal Prince Alfred Hospital, Camperdown, NSW, Australia

Priority Research Centre for Healthy Lungs, Hunter Medical Research Institute (HMRI) & School of Biomedical Sciences and Pharmacy, University of Newcastle, Callaghan, NSW, Australia

Josef Jampílek Department of Analytical Chemistry, Faculty of Natural Sciences, Comenius University, Bratislava, Slovakia

Vandita Kakkar University Institute of Pharmaceutical Sciences, Panjab University, Chandigarh, India

Pallavee Kapoor Department of Biotechnology, Jaypee Institute of Information Technology, Noida, UP, India

Shubham Khot Department of Pharmaceutics, Institute of Pharmacy, Nirma University, Ahmedabad, Gujarat, India

Seema Kohli Department of Pharmaceutical Sciences, Kalaniketan Government Polytechnic College, Jabalpur, Madhya Pradesh, India

Katarína Kráľová Institute of Chemistry, Faculty of Natural Sciences, Comenius University, Bratislava, Slovakia

Leena Kumari Department of Pharmaceutical Technology, Jadavpur University, Kolkata, India

Shalini Kumari Institute of Pharmaceutical Research, GLA University, Mathura, India

Manoj Kumar F&D, Health Kart, Gurgaon, India

Pooja Lamba Department of Pharmaceutical Sciences, Guru Jambheshwar University of Science and Technology, Hisar, Haryana, India

Priyanka Maurya Department of Pharmaceutical Sciences, Babasaheb Bhimrao Ambedkar University, Lucknow, India

Meenu Mehta School of Pharmaceutical Sciences, Lovely Professional University, Phagwara, Punjab, India

Harshita Mishra Department of Pharmaceutics, Delhi Pharmaceutical Sciences Research University, New Delhi, India

Monalisa Mishra Department of Life Science, NIT Rourkela, Rourkela, Odisha, India

Nidhi Mishra Department of Pharmaceutical Sciences, Babasaheb Bhimrao Ambedkar University, Lucknow, India

Srishti Mittal Department of Biotechnology, Jaypee Institute of Information Technology, Noida, UP, India

Alankar Mukherjee Department of Pharmaceutical Technology, Jadavpur University, Kolkata, India

Biswajit Mukherjee Center for Advanced Research in Pharmaceutical Sciences, Department of Pharmaceutical Technology, Jadavpur University, Kolkata (Calcutta), India

Sanju Nanda Department of Pharmaceutical Sciences, Maharshi Dayanand University, Rohtak, Haryana, India

Priyanka Narula University Institute of Pharmaceutical Sciences, Panjab University, Chandigarh, India

Kuldeep Nigam Department of Biotechnology, Jaypee Institute of Information Technology, Noida, UP, India

Raquibun Nisha Department of Pharmaceutical Sciences, Babasaheb Bhimrao Ambedkar University, Lucknow, India

Sanjeev Paikra Department of Life Science, NIT Rourkela, Rourkela, Odisha, India

Parijat Pandey Shri Baba Mastnath Institute of Pharmaceutical Sciences and Research, Baba Mastnath University, Rohtak, India

Vikas Pandey Department of Pharmaceutics, Guru Ramdas Khalsa, Institute of Science and Technology (Pharmacy), Jabalpur, Madhya Pradesh, India

Krishna Kumar Patel Department of Pharmaceutical Engineering & Technology, Indian Institute of Technology (Banaras Hindu University), IIT (BHU), Varanasi, UP, India

Mayur M. Patel Department of Pharmaceutics, Institute of Pharmacy, Nirma University, Ahmedabad, Gujarat, India

Kamla Pathak Pharmacy College Saifai, Uttar Pradesh University of Medical Sciences, Etawah, India

Priya Prasad University Institute of Pharmaceutical Sciences, Panjab University, Chandigarh, India

Parteek Prasher Department of Chemistry, University of Petroleum and Energy Studies, Dehradun, India

Pratishtha Amity Institute of Pharmacy, Amity University Uttar Pradesh, Noida, India

Mahendra Rai Department of Biotechnology, SGB Amravati University, Amravati, Maharashtra, India

Shweta Ramkar University Institute of Pharmacy, Pandit Ravishankar Shukla University, Raipur, Chhattisgarh, India

Vikas Rana Department of Pharmaceutical Sciences and Drug Research, Punjabi University, Patiala, India

Rekha Rao Department of Pharmaceutical Sciences, Guru Jambheshwar University of Science and Technology, Hisar, Haryana, India

Shruti U. Rawal Department of Pharmaceutics, Institute of Pharmacy, Nirma University, Ahmedabad, Gujarat, India

Purnam Hoshe Ruba Department of Biotechnology, Jaypee Institute of Information Technology, Noida, UP, India

Abhishek K. Sah Department of Pharmacy, Shri G. S. Institute of Technology & Science, Indore, Madhya Pradesh, India

Komal Saini University Institute of Pharmaceutical Sciences, Panjab University, Chandigarh, India

Megha Saini University Institute of Pharmaceutical Sciences, Panjab University, Chandigarh, India

Shubhini A. Saraf Department of Pharmaceutical Sciences, Babasaheb Bhimrao Ambedkar University, Lucknow, India

Shounak Sarkhel Department of Pharmaceutical Technology, Jadavpur University, Kolkata, India

Amita Sarwal University Institute of Pharmaceutical Sciences, Panjab University, Chandigarh, India

Saurabh Satija School of Pharmaceutical Sciences, Lovely Professional University, Phagwara, Punjab, India

Huma Shafi Institute of Pharmaceutical Research, GLA University, Mathura, India

Pragya Sharma Department of Pharmaceutical Sciences, Maharshi Dayanand University, Rohtak, Haryana, India

Radhika Sharma Department of Pharmaceutical Sciences and Drug Research, Punjabi University, Patiala, India

Sachin Sharma University Institute of Pharmaceutical Sciences, Panjab University, Chandigarh, India

Shivani Sharma Department of Pharmaceutical Sciences and Drug Research, Punjabi University, Patiala, India

Shakti Shukla Priority Research Centre for Healthy Lungs, Hunter Medical Research Institute (HMRI) & School of Biomedical Sciences and Pharmacy, University of Newcastle, Callaghan, NSW, Australia

Lubna Siddiqui Department of Pharmaceutics, School of Pharmaceutical Education and Research, Jamia Hamdard, New Delhi, India

Gurpreet Singh University Institute of Pharmaceutical Sciences, Panjab University, Chandigarh, India

Samipta Singh Department of Pharmaceutical Sciences, Babasaheb Bhimrao Ambedkar University, Lucknow, India

Sanjay Singh Department of Pharmaceutical Engineering & Technology, Indian Institute of Technology (Banaras Hindu University), IIT (BHU), Varanasi, UP, India

Babasaheb Bhimrao Ambedkar University, Lucknow, UP, India

Vanshika Singh Department of Biotechnology, Jaypee Institute of Information Technology, Noida, UP, India

Gautam Singhvi Department of Pharmacy, Birla Institute of Technology and Science (BITS), Pilani, India

Richu Singla Department of Microbiology, Viral Research Diagnostic Laboratory (VRDL), Guru Gobind Singh Medical College and Hospital, Baba Farid University of Health Sciences, Faridkot, India

C. Soica "Victor Babes" University of Medicine and Pharmacy, Faculty of Pharmacy, Timisoara, Romania

Samridhi Srivastava Amity Institute of Pharmacy, Amity University Uttar Pradesh, Noida, India

Preeti K. Suresh University Institute of Pharmacy, Pandit Ravishankar Shukla University, Raipur, Chhattisgarh, India

Sushama Talegaonkar Department of Pharmaceutics, Delhi Pharmaceutical Sciences and Research University (DPSRU), New Delhi, India

Ashok K. Tiwary Department of Pharmaceutical Sciences and Drug Research, Punjabi University, Patiala, India

Varsha Department of Pharmaceutical Sciences, Guru Jambheshwar University of Science and Technology, Hisar, Haryana, India

Ridhima Wadhwa Faculty of Life Sciences and Biotechnology, South Asian University, New Delhi, India

Part I

Emerging Trends and Challenges in Nanoformulations

Nanoformulations: Opportunities and Challenges

1

Lubna Siddiqui, Harshita Mishra, Sushama Talegaonkar, and Mahendra Rai

Abstract

Nanotechnology has revolutionized each aspect of healthcare along with other associated sciences. Drug-loaded nanocarriers and nanocrystalline active ingredients have overcome various challenges faced by conventional therapy like limited bioavailability, multiple drug resistance, poor patient compliance, adverse drug reactions, particularly untoward effects of chemotherapy, etc. Nanosized systems have proven to be a boon for cosmetic industry too. Now safe, efficient, customer-friendly and long-lasting cosmetics are available in the market. Nanotechnology has also made it possible to combine therapy and diagnostics together into theranostics. This chapter introduces various advantages, achievements and applications of nanoformulations, not only in the field of healthcare but also in diagnostics and cosmetics.

L. Siddiqui
Department of Pharmaceutics, School of Pharmaceutical Education and Research, Jamia Hamdard, New Delhi, India

H. Mishra · S. Talegaonkar (✉)
Department of Pharmaceutics, Delhi Pharmaceutical Sciences Research University, New Delhi, India

M. Rai
Department of Biotechnology, SGB Amravati University, Amravati, Maharashtra, India

Keywords

Nanoformulations · Healthcare · Multidrug resistance · Theranostics · Toxicity concerns

1.1 Nanoformulations as a Promising Strategy

Nanoformulations have gained immense popularity in almost every aspect of scientific fields. The surface chemistry, reactivity and other properties of nanosized materials widely differ from their macro/micro counterparts. Thus, they find application in engineering sciences, biomedical sciences, cosmetology, environmental sciences, etc. (Martin 1994) (Table 1.1 and Fig. 1.1).

Healthcare has received great benefits over a period of time by nanotechnology. Various shortcomings and challenges presented by conventional therapy have been overcome by nanotechnology. New chemical entity having exceptional therapeutic efficacy can face challenge during formulation development and clinical application due to adverse physicochemical aspects like poor solubility (Talegaonkar et al. 2013). Nanonization of drug improves its solubility, in turn enhancing its bioavailability and permeability. Nanoformulations like nanocrystals, nanoparticles, nanoemulsions and micellar encapsulation greatly improve solubility of drug (Chen et al. 2011). Chen et al. (2012) observed

S. Talegaonkar, M. Rai (eds.), *Nanoformulations in Human Health*,
https://doi.org/10.1007/978-3-030-41858-8_1

Table 1.1 Marketed nanoformulations used in healthcare, cosmetics and theranostics

Marketed name	Nanoformulation	Drug	Indication
Rapamune (Wyeth Pharmaceuticals)	Nanocrystalline drug	Sirolimus	Immunosuppressant to prevent organ rejection
DepoCyt® (Pacira Pharmaceuticals)	Liposomes	Cytarabine	Malignant lymphomatous meningitis
Myocet® (Teva Pharma)	Liposomes	Doxorubicin	Metastatic breast cancer
Emend® (Merck)	Nanocrystal dispersion	Aprepitant	Emesis
Eligard® (Tolmar)	PLGH nanoparticles (DL-lactide/glycolide)	Leuprolide acetate	Advanced prostate cancer
Opaxio® (Cell Therapeutics, Inc.)	Polyglutamate solid nanoparticles	Paclitaxel	Glioblastoma
Abraxane® (Celgene)	Serum albumin nanoparticles	Paclitaxel	Metastatic breast cancer
Dermosome (Croda)	Liposomes	Soy lecithin phospholipids	Skin moisturizer
Lumessence Eye Cream (Aubrey Organics)	Liposomes	Phospholipids, wheat and oat proteins	Wrinkles and fine lines removal
Identik Masque Floral Repair (Identik)	Niosomes	Punica granatum seed extract	Hair damage prevention
Allure Parfum Bottle (Chanel)	Solid lipid nanoparticles	Mandarin orange, rose de mai and vanilla	Perfume
Swiss Cellular White Illuminating Eye Essence (La prairie)	Nanostructured lipid carriers	Whitening and DNA repair complex	Under-eye dark patches and pigmentation
Tony Moly Nano Gold BB Cream SPF 50 PA+++ (Tony Moly)	Nanoparticles	Gold	Skin whitening, UV protection and anti-wrinkle
Ferumoxytol, Feraheme® (AMAG Pharmaceuticals)	Nanoparticles	Superparamagnetic iron oxide	Imaging
Feridex (Eiken Chemical Co., Ltd)	Nanoparticles	Superparamagnetic iron oxide with dextran coating	MRI imaging
Netspot (Medscape)	Lyophilized powder	Gallium Ga-68 dotatate	Radioactive diagnostic agent used in PET/CT scan

marked improvement in the solubility and bioavailability of methotrexate on nanonization by solution-enhanced dispersion by supercritical CO_2 (SEDS) (Chen et al. 2012).

Drug resistance is another drawback encountered by conventional therapy. Antibiotic resistance and multidrug resistance in cancer are known to cost lives (Negi et al. 2014a, b). The efficacy of conventional treatment fades off due to mechanisms like increased drug efflux, enzyme inactivation, DNA mutations/alterations, reduced sensitivity of targets, etc. (Gillet and Gottesman 2010). Imatinib mesylate has immense potential in treating colon cancer, but P-gp overexpression causes efflux of drug leading to reduced efficacy (Fig. 1.2). Negi et al. (2015) reported development of imatinib mesylate-loaded liposomes decorated with hyaluronan for overcoming the multidrug resistance observed in colon cancer (Negi et al. 2015).

Targeted therapy achieved by nanoformulations is a boon for healthcare as it improves overall efficacy of therapy and reduces untoward effects on normal cells (Torchilin 2000). Targeting can be passive or active. In case of passive targeting, particle size and surface chemistry play an important role. Maeda and Matsumura demonstrated enhanced permeability and retention (EPR) phenomenon in murine solid tumours. Tumours are usually associated with leaky vascu-

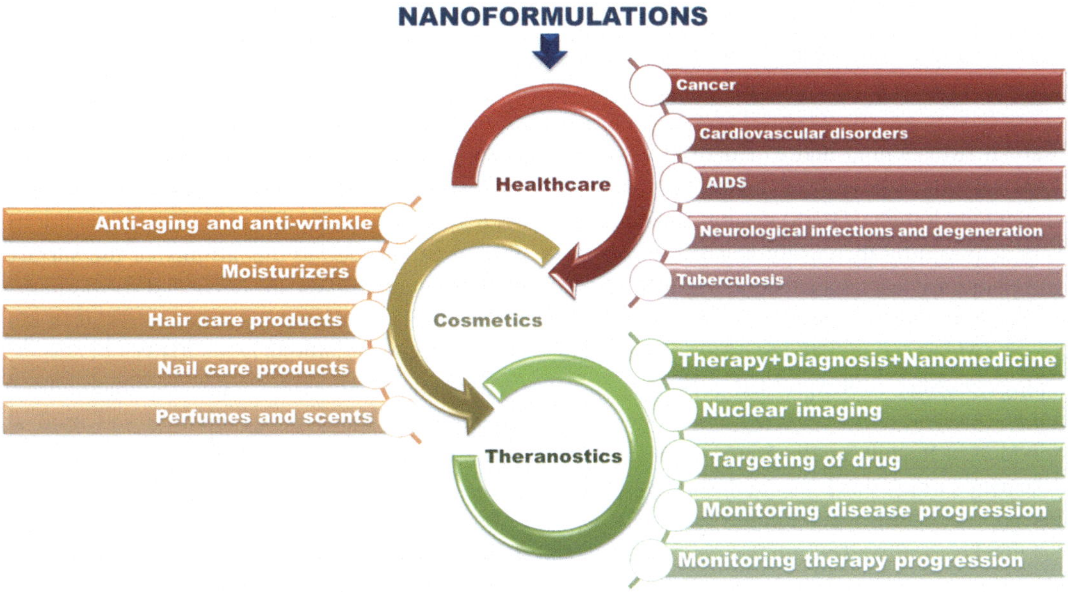

Fig. 1.1 Applications of nanoformulations in various fields

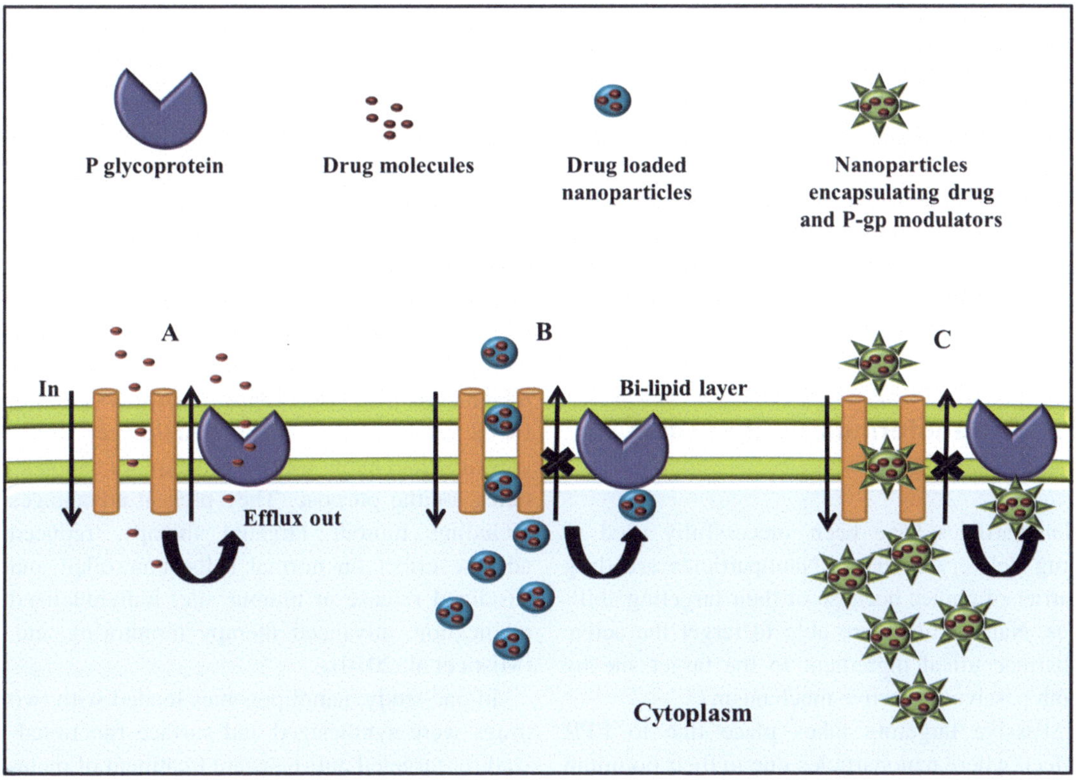

Fig. 1.2 Role of nanoformulations in drug resistance. (**a**) P-glycoprotein (P-gp) acts as efflux pump which forces the drug out of cell leading to reduced drug concentration and drug resistance. (**b**) Nanoparticles mask the drug from P-gp, thus preventing drug efflux and leading to improved efficacy of therapy. (**c**) Various P-gp modulators can also be incorporated along with drug in nanoformulations to prevent drug efflux

lature and poor lymphatic drainage; thus, a 70-fold increase in permeation and accumulation of nanocarriers in the microenvironment of tumour having size between 10 and 400 nm was observed (Matsumura and Maeda 1986; Maeda and Matsumura 1989). Passive targeting of drugs to reticuloendothelial (RES) system can be effectively achieved by increasing negative charge or hydrophobicity of nanocarriers, as it leads to opsonisation, thus increased clearance by macrophages (Alexis et al. 2008a). Active targeting employs various overexpressed receptors, proteins and enzymes at the targeted site. Monoclonal antibodies or ligands are decorated on the surface of the nanocarriers that binds to the targeted cells. This approach offers advantages like increased drug uptake, improved circulation time, increased drug efficiency and reduced untoward effect on normal cells (Siddiqui et al. 2018; Yasukawa et al. 2000).

Another highlight of nanoformulations is theranostics, where single nanocarrier exerts therapeutic effect while acting as diagnostic agents. It includes functionalization of drug-loaded nanocarriers with MRI contrast agents, fluorescence materials and agents capable of nuclear imaging, so that diagnosis can be carried out alongside therapy (Kelkar and Reineke 2011). Thus, nanotechnology is a promising strategy to overcome the hurdles and shortcomings of conventional therapy.

1.2 Nanoformulations as Drug Carrier

Nanoparticles have been successfully used as drug delivery systems. Nanoparticles are drug carrier of choice because of their targeting abilities. Nanoparticles are able to target the active pharmaceutical ingredient to the target site by both passive and active mechanism.

Passive targeting takes place due to EPR effect, where nanoparticles due to their optimum size enter the diseased cells which have loose vasculature. Nanoparticles are then retained inside the cells. Nanoparticles then release their drug payload resulting in drug action at the target site (Patel and Patel 2019).

Targeting ability of drug-carrying nanoparticles can be further increased by binding a ligand to the surface of the nanoparticles. The ligand possesses a specific affinity towards the receptors overexpressed by the diseased tissues (but not by normal cells). Due to this affinity of the surface ligand, nanoparticles are navigated to the target site where they release the drugs to result in targeted therapy (Friedman et al. 2013).

Example, Abraxane are commercialized nanoparticles made up of albumin and used as drug carrier for the anticancer drug paclitaxel.

1.2.1 Nanoformulations in Major Diseases

Nanoformulations have proven to be a boon in treating various life-threatening diseases. Nanocarriers can overcome the drawbacks of conventional therapy including untoward effects on normal cells, high dose size and dosing frequency, reduced patient compliance, longevity of treatment, non-selective targeting, lack of personalized medication, etc. (Barst et al. 1996).

Treatment and management of dreadful disease like cancer went up a notch on introduction of nanocarriers (Alexis et al. 2008b). Cancer is supposedly the most extensively researched area, definitely because of its deadly and difficult-to-treat nature. Since oncologists are always looking for newer and more effective anticancer strategies, it is inevitable for them to explore nanoparticles for the purpose. They present advantages including tumour targeted therapy, reduced adverse effect on normal cells, controlled and sustained release at tumour site, individualized medication, advanced therapy monitoring, etc. (Misra et al. 2010).

In one study, nanoliposomes loaded with two drugs were synthesized and surface functionalized for targeted anti-resistant treatment of melanoma. The nanoformulation displayed successful overcoming of resistance in aggressive melanoma cells, thus displaying the potential of nanoformulations in targeted treatment of resistant and deadly cancers (Mishra et al. 2019).

Employing nanocarriers have not only improved the target specificity of anticancer agents like doxorubicin (Doxil), erlotinib (Tarceva) and irinotecan (Onivyde) but also reduced toxicity on normal cells along with dose reduction (Gmeiner and Ghosh 2014). Researchers have developed a combination therapy where radiotherapy was combined with drug-loaded nanocarriers for treating cancer. Combination therapy of lipid nanoparticles loaded with cyclopamine was administered with polymeric micelles labelled with lutetium-177 which led to marked reduction in tumour volume when compared with monotherapy (Mi et al. 2016).

Initially research on nanocarriers focused on cancer therapy, but now it has spanned its wings to curb other diseases too. Magnetic imaging of macrophages in atherosclerosis has been made possible with the introduction of paramagnetic iron nanoparticles (Iverson et al. 2008). Researcher have also achieved liver targeting of atorvastatin with reduced hepatotoxicity by active targeting of drug through glycyrrhetinic acid-modified chitosan nanoparticles (Rohilla et al. 2016). Similarly pharmacokinetic and pharmacodynamics properties of anti-tubercular drugs have been modified by nanomedicines for overall improvement of safety and efficacy of treatment. Studies showed marked reduction in dosing frequency from 45 days to merely 15 days when aerosolized alginate nanoparticles loaded with isoniazid, rifampicin and pyrazinamide were administered through inhalation (Zahoor et al. 2005).

Brain targeting was once a far-fetched goal of researchers due to the presence of blood-brain barrier, which acts as ironclad gates between the brain and systemic circulation. But with advancement of nanoformulations, various molecules including drugs have been able to reach the environment of brain (Kanwar et al. 2012). Treatment and symptomatic relief of neurodegenerative diseases like Parkinsonism and Alzheimer's are now possible. In one such study, transferrin antibody OX26 was attached to the surface of tempol-loaded poly-(lactide-co-glycolide) nanoparticles for active delivery of reactive oxygen species scavenger for the prevention of neurodegeneration (Carroll et al. 2010). Intranasal administration of didanosine-loaded chitosan nanoparticles showed marked improvement in drug concentration in brain tissues and thus can be used to combat retroviruses in the brain as observed in case of AIDS (Al-Ghananeem et al. 2010).

1.2.2 Bioimaging with Nanoformulations

Nanoparticles are also used for the imaging of biological tissues (known as bioimaging). Significance of bioimaging lies in the diagnosis of diseases and monitoring of therapy. Nanoparticles can be used for early detection of diseases as dangerous as breast cancer. This application of nanoparticles can be owed to their better contrasting properties. Nanoparticles are preferred as imaging agents also because they have longer retention time in vivo and can be modified to target a specific tissue as well as to enhance their imaging abilities (Singh and Nalwa 2011).

Recently, Chang et al. prepared nanoparticles of graphene oxide for dual modal imaging. These nanoparticles were less toxic and accumulated in tumour by EPR effect (Chang et al. 2020). Another recent report documents the synthesis of liposomes coated with three different polyfluorenes to obtain blue, green and red fluorescent particles. Experiments with mammalian cells demonstrated the ability of nanoparticles to highlight and visualize cells with different colours, thus proving the potential of these nanoparticles in imaging (Rubio-Camacho et al. 2019).

1.2.3 Nanoformulations in Theranostics

Strategic combination of therapy with diagnostic aids is termed as theranostics. Various nanosized formulations have been developed in recent times that serve the purpose of both therapy and diagnosis in single unit dose (Kelkar and Reineke 2011). Theranostics employs techniques at molecular and genetic level catering specific needs of the individual. It curbs the long practice of one medicine for all. It helps in identifying the specific subgroup of diseases encountered in an individual and helps to identify genetic makeup behind the same, thus ensuring optimum safety and efficacy of the treatment along with monitoring of the progression of therapy in combating diseases (Lim et al. 2014). The most common example of theranostics is the use of iodine-131 therapy for the diagnosis and treatment of thyroid cancer. It is a well-established treatment accepted worldwide (Feine et al. 1996). Positron emission tomography (PET) scan employing the use of positron emitter Ga-68 octreotate has gained immense popularity in recent years for the treatment and diagnosis of various somatostatin-expressing tumours like neuroendocrine tumours (Hofman et al. 2012).

Metal nanoparticles having inherent anticancer activity have become a choice of nanotool in theranostics. Due to their unique physical and chemical properties like photoluminescence or supermagnetism, they support various imaging techniques, and due to their potential of producing superoxides in vivo, they pose cytotoxic effects on cancer cells. And due to highly reactive surfaces, active targeting to cancer cells of metal nanoparticles like iron, gold, zinc oxide, etc. can be easily achieved (Sharma et al. 2015). Luminescent nanocrystals made up of semiconductors having size range of 5–50 nm are known as quantum dots. Their high surface-to-volume ratio makes them an excellent theranostic tool (Ho and Leong 2010).

1.2.4 Nanoformulations in Cosmetics

Nanotechnology not only plays an important role in healthcare, but recently nanonization has expanded its aegis in the field of cosmetics also. Researchers and manufacturers utilize nanosized excipients and ingredients to achieve improved dermal penetration, UV protection, texture and products having long-lasting effects (Raj et al. 2012). Liposomes consisting of phosphatidylcholine, phospholipids and cholesterol are used in various formulations like lipsticks, deodorant, cold creams, moisturizing cream, anti-ageing creams and sunscreen (Kaul et al. 2018). Another such product based on nanocarriers encapsulating vitamins A, C and K was NanoSerum launched in Brazil by *O Boticário* as anti-ageing and skin whitening serum (Melo et al. 2015). Gold and silver nanoparticles are also used as nanopigments in lipsticks. Nanosized gold has red colour and nanosilver has yellow colour; thus, they are used as colouring pigments in cosmetics in place of synthetic dyes as they are safe and non-toxic. Similarly titanium dioxide nanoparticles are used in skin whitening products as they disperse uniformly giving natural fair look (Nanda et al. 2016).

1.3 Major Challenges of Nanoformulation

It is quite uncommon that something offers only outstanding advantages and has no limitations or unwanted side effects. Nanoformulations are no exception. They have greatly and positively impacted health industry in the last couple of decades; however, even after a remarkable progress, they still face a few challenges.

Maniam et al. have broadly classified the challenges of nanoformulations in three broad categories, namely, scale-up production, biological barriers and safety concerns (Maniam et al. 2018).

The successful use of nanoformulations demands their synthesis at large scale so that a bigger section of health industry may get benefits. Although several new technologies for the synthesis have been developed, their scale-up still remains a challenge in most of the cases. Scaling up requires highly trained labour and expensive chemicals. Running costs increase drastically, which may affect the risk-to-benefit ratio of the nanoformulations (Tighe et al. 2013).

Safety concerns associated with the nanoformulations are the biggest challenge for the scientists who are aiming at successful use of nanocarriers for better management of diseases with nanoformulations. Nanosize, which on one hand has emerged as a boon for therapeutic sector, also poses safety challenges due to nonspecific interactions with the body cells.

Another challenge faced by nanoformulations is the desired residence time in the systemic circulation. Macrophages recognize nanoforms in circulation as foreign particles and rapidly remove them from the bloodstream. This problem however can be managed to some extent by giving a hydrophilic surface to the nanoformulation (Maniam et al. 2018).

1.4 Regulatory Hurdles for Nanoformulation

Even if some nanoformulation successfully overcomes the above-mentioned challenges, stringent regulatory check may create the bottleneck towards marketing. In US market, currently there are eight nanoformulations (liposomes and nanoparticles) approved by FDA. Despite the fact that they are doing a great business, there are no generic equivalents present of any of them. Reason for this is regulatory requirements.

The two important requirements of FDA for the approval of generic nanoformulations are (i) demonstrating bioequivalence and (ii) fulfilling FDA requirements for parenteral administration.

Demonstrating bioequivalence for other routes of administration is comparatively easier and can be shown by plasma concentration data. However, for parenteral administration, tissue distribution needs to be demonstrated. Also, data in healthy volunteers is not acceptable by FDA as it may differ from actual diseased tissues; and invasive procedures in diseased volunteers are restricted by ethical reasons (Burgess et al. 2010). Before introducing products in the market, stringent clinical trials are carried out on each product to establish not only its efficacy but its safety too (Table 1.2).

In addition to short-term studies to analyse the immediate effect, long-term studies are also needed to assess the effects of degraded nanoparticles on the body. The length of the study required depends upon the rate of degradation and excretion of the material from the body. This long study period adds to the cost of the product, affecting its cost efficiency (Skotland et al. 2014).

1.5 Toxicity: The Major Concern

Along with a commendable growth and vast application of nanomaterials, toxicity still remains a major concern that scientists and healthcare professionals are dealing with. Though enough in vitro data is collected for every nanomaterial developed, the correlation of in vitro data with in vivo is challenging. This adversely affects the commercial potential of the nanoformulations (Hofmann-Amtenbrink et al. 2015).

The reason of worthy applications of nanoformulations is their nanosize; however, the reason of their toxicity is also their nanosize.

Due to their nanosize, they are preferentially taken up by the reticuloendothelial system (RES). Thus, accumulation and toxicity of nanoparticles in the liver and kidney remain a cause of concern. Another reason of toxicity can be immunological reaction of body towards nanoformulations (Szebeni 2014).

The issue of toxicity is however being tried to be addressed by different approaches such as choosing more biocompatible material. For example, lipids are safer than metals, and thus lipid nanoparticles are supposed to be less toxic than metallic nanoparticles. Uptake by RES can be minimized by giving the nanoparticles a hydrophilic surface by coating with some hydrophilic polymer such as polyethylene glycol (PEG) or hyaluronic acid (HA).

Another approach that can be used is active targeting which enables accumulation of nanoformulation at the target site and minimum interaction with normal body cells (Mishra et al. 2019). Toxicity due to accumulation of nanoparticles is not only a cause of concern on administration, but long-term exposure to the skin or accidental inhalation of nanoparticles during manufacturing, evaluation, packaging, storage and transportation by personnel is also plausible.

Table 1.2 Nanoformulations under various clinical trials for application in healthcare, cosmetics and theranostics

Nanoformulation	Drug	Indication	Clinical trial (phase)
Promitil pegylated liposomes	Mitomycin-C	Cancer	I
Sonazid liposomes	F- butane	Contrast material	I/IV
Cerulean nanoparticles	Camptothecin	Colon cancer and other solid tumours	II
RadProtect (Iron and PEG micelles)	Amifostine	Acute radiation syndrome	I
Polymer-drug conjugate	Paclitaxel and polyglutamic acide	Non-small cell lung cancer	III
Gold Colloids	Recombinant human tumour necrosis factor (rhTNF)	Solid tumours	I
Silica nanoparticles with PEG coating	NIR fluorophore and radiolabelled ^{124}I	Imaging of tumours	I
Nano gold	–	Recovering skin damaged by chemicals	0

Metallic nanoparticles or nanocarriers loaded with chemotherapeutic agents or immunotherapeutics can be disastrous when not handled with care.

So to keep nanoformulations in India under strict vigilance, guidelines on "Evaluation of Nanopharmaceuticals in India" have been released in October 2019. These guidelines have been jointly documented by the Department of Biotechnology (DBT), Ministry of Science and Technology, Ministry of Health and Family Welfare, Indian Council of Medical Research (ICMR) and Central Drugs Standard Control Organization (CDSCO) to streamline the quality, safety, efficacy and regulatory aspects of nanoformulations in India.

Revolution in combating toxicity issues of nanoformulations has also been brought about by environmentally sustainable form of nanotechnology addressed by various terms like "green nanotechnology" or "green nanomedicine". This field is basically an amalgamation of wonders of nanotechnology with the environment-friendly attributes of green chemistry. The idea is to use and promote methods and materials that support sustenance of nature (Rawat et al. 2015). Abolishing the use of harmful organic solvents and synthetic polymers, promoting one-pot synthesis and fabrication of polymeric nanocomposites, nanometals, etc. are some of the means by which nanoformulations can be made environment friendly throughout their lifecycle (Nath and Banerjee 2013).

Basically, toxicity of nanoformulations is a complex aspect governed by several factors. Moreover, risk-to-benefit ratio should be considered to make a wise decision whether nanoparticles are to be used or not.

1.6 Conclusion

Nanoformulations deserve all the attention that they have gained in the last few decades. Extensive research is going on to make the best possible use of dynamic nanoparticles. From drug delivery to bioimaging, nanoparticles have proven their potential in the entire sphere of biomedical field. The properties of nanoparticles such as inherent ability of passive targeting to the ability of being desirably modified make them suitable to be used in a range of diseases. Even the diseases as deadly as cancer have been better managed with the help of various types of nanoparticles.

However, nanoparticles possess their share of limitations also. Due to their nanosize, non-specific interactions with cells and toxicity towards living cells always remain a cause of concern for scientists. Regulatory hurdles are another set of challenges that nanoparticles face. Due to risk of toxicity, regulatory bodies impose strict regulations on approval and use of nanoparticles.

Nonetheless, nanoparticles have ushered a new era of therapeutics and are taking the treatment strategies towards more positive outcomes. However, insights into the details are needed to get a better picture of the status of nanoparticles in the field of therapeutics.

References

Alexis F, Pridgen E, Molnar LK, Farokhzad OC (2008a) Factors affecting the clearance and biodistribution of polymeric nanoparticles. Mol Pharm 5(4): 505–515

Alexis F, Rhee J-W, Richie JP, Radovic-Moreno AF, Langer R, Farokhzad OC (2008b) New frontiers in nanotechnology for cancer treatment. Elsevier, Urol Oncol pp 74–85

Al-Ghananeem AM, Saeed H, Florence R, Yokel RA, Malkawi AH (2010) Intranasal drug delivery of didanosine-loaded chitosan nanoparticles for brain targeting; an attractive route against infections caused by AIDS viruses. J Drug Target 18(5):381–388

Barst RJ, Rubin LJ, Long WA, McGoon MD, Rich S, Badesch DB et al (1996) A comparison of continuous intravenous epoprostenol (prostacyclin) with conventional therapy for primary pulmonary hypertension. N Engl J Med 334(5):296–301

Burgess P, Hutt PB, Farokhzad OC, Langer R, Minick S, Zale S (2010) On firm ground: IP protection of therapeutic nanoparticles. Nat Biotechnol 28(12):1267–1270

Carroll RT, Bhatia D, Geldenhuys W, Bhatia R, Miladore N, Bishayee A et al (2010) Brain-targeted delivery of Tempol-loaded nanoparticles for neurological disorders. J Drug Target 18(9):665–674

Chang X, Zhang M, Wang C, Zhang J, Wu H, Yang S (2020) Graphene oxide/BaHoF5/PEG nanocomposite for dual-modal imaging and heat shock protein inhibitor-sensitized tumor photothermal therapy. Carbon 158:372–385

Chen H, Khemtong C, Yang X, Chang X, Gao J (2011) Nanonization strategies for poorly water-soluble drugs. Drug Discov Today 16(7–8):354–360

Chen A-Z, Li L, Wang S-B, Zhao C, Liu Y-G, Wang G-Y et al (2012) Nanonization of methotrexate by solution-enhanced dispersion by supercritical CO2. J Supercrit Fluids 67:7–13

Feine U, Lietzenmayer R, Hanke J-P, Held J, Wöhrle H, Müller-Schauenburg W (1996) Fluorine-18-FDG and iodine-131-iodide uptake in thyroid cancer. J Nucl Med 37(9):1468–1472

Friedman AD, Claypool SE, Liu R (2013) The smart targeting of nanoparticles. Curr Pharm Des 19(35):6315–6329

Gillet J-P, Gottesman MM (2010) Mechanisms of multidrug resistance in cancer. In: Multi-drug resistance in cancer. Springer, Methods Mol Biol pp 47–76

Gmeiner WH, Ghosh S (2014) Nanotechnology for cancer treatment. Nanotechnol Rev 3(2):111–122

Ho Y-P, Leong KW (2010) Quantum dot-based theranostics. Nanoscale 2(1):60–68

Hofman MS, Kong G, Neels OC, Eu P, Hong E, Hicks RJ (2012) High management impact of Ga-68 DOTATATE (GaTate) PET/CT for imaging neuroendocrine and other somatostatin expressing tumours. J Med Imaging Radiat Oncol 56(1):40–47

Hofmann-Amtenbrink M, Grainger DW, Hofmann H (2015) Nanoparticles in medicine: current challenges facing inorganic nanoparticle toxicity assessments and standardizations. Nanomedicine Nanotechnol Biol Med 11(7):1689–1694

Iverson N, Plourde N, Chnari E, Nackman GB, Moghe PV (2008) Convergence of nanotechnology and cardiovascular medicine. BioDrugs 22(1):1–10

Kanwar JR, Sun X, Punj V, Sriramoju B, Mohan RR, Zhou S-F et al (2012) Nanoparticles in the treatment and diagnosis of neurological disorders: untamed dragon with fire power to heal. Nanomedicine Nanotechnol Biol Med 8(4):399–414

Kaul S, Gulati N, Verma D, Mukherjee S, Nagaich U (2018) Role of nanotechnology in cosmeceuticals: a review of recent advances [Internet]. J Pharm 2018:1

Kelkar SS, Reineke TM (2011) Theranostics: combining imaging and therapy. Bioconjug Chem 22(10):1879–1903

Lim E-K, Kim T, Paik S, Haam S, Huh Y-M, Lee K (2014) Nanomaterials for theranostics: recent advances and future challenges. Chem Rev 115(1):327–394

Maeda H, Matsumura Y (1989) Tumoritropic and lymphotropic principles of macromolecular drugs. Crit Rev Ther Drug Carrier Syst 6(3):193–210

Maniam G, Mai C-W, Zulkefeli M, Dufès C, Tan DM-Y, Fu J-Y (2018) Challenges and opportunities of nanotechnology as delivery platform for tocotrienols in cancer therapy. Front Pharmacol 26:9

Martin CR (1994) Nanomaterials: a membrane-based synthetic approach. Science 266(5193):1961–1966

Matsumura Y, Maeda H (1986) A new concept for macromolecular therapeutics in cancer chemotherapy: mechanism of tumoritropic accumulation of proteins and the antitumor agent smancs. Cancer Res 46(12 Part 1):6387–6392

Melo A, Amadeu MS, Lancellotti M, de Hollanda LM, Machado D, Melo A et al (2015) The role of nanomaterials in cosmetics: national and international legislative aspects. Quím Nova 38(4):599–603

Mi Y, Shao Z, Vang J, Kaidar-Person O, Wang AZ (2016) Application of nanotechnology to cancer radiotherapy. Cancer Nanotechnol 7(1):11

Mishra H, Mishra PK, Iqbal Z, Jaggi M, Madaan A, Bhuyan K et al (2019) Co-delivery of eugenol and dacarbazine by hyaluronic acid-coated liposomes for targeted inhibition of survivin in treatment of resistant metastatic melanoma. Pharmaceutics 11(4):163

Misra R, Acharya S, Sahoo SK (2010) Cancer nanotechnology: application of nanotechnology in cancer therapy. Drug Discov Today 15(19–20):842–850

Nanda S, Nanda A, Lohan S, Kaur R, Singh B (2016) Nanocosmetics: performance enhancement and safety assurance. In: Grumezescu AM (ed.) Nanobiomaterials in galenic formulations and cosmetics. William Andrew: Elsevier, pp 47–67

Nath D, Banerjee P (2013) Green nanotechnology–a new hope for medical biology. Environ Toxicol Pharmacol 36(3):997–1014

Negi LM, Talegaonkar S, Jaggi M, Verma AK, Verma R, Dobhal S et al (2014a) Surface engineered nanostructured lipid carriers for targeting MDR tumor: part I. synthesis, characterization and in vitro investigation. Colloids Surf B Biointerfaces 123:600–609

Negi LM, Talegaonkar S, Jaggi M, Verma AK, Verma R, Dobhal S et al (2014b) Surface engineered nanostructured lipid carriers for targeting MDR tumor: part II. In vivo biodistribution, pharmacodynamic and hematological toxicity studies. Colloids Surf B Biointerfaces 123:610–615

Negi LM, Jaggi M, Joshi V, Ronodip K, Talegaonkar S (2015) Hyaluronan coated liposomes as the intravenous platform for delivery of imatinib mesylate in MDR colon cancer. Int J Biol Macromol 73:222–235

Patel JK, Patel AP (2019) Passive targeting of nanoparticles to cancer. In: Pathak YV (ed) Surface modification of nanoparticles for targeted drug delivery. Springer International Publishing, Cham, pp 125–143

Raj S, Jose S, Sumod US, Sabitha M (2012) Nanotechnology in cosmetics: opportunities and challenges. J Pharm Bioallied Sci 4(3):186–193

Rawat P, Manglani K, Gupta S, Vohora D, Ahmad FJ, Talegaonkar S (2015) Design and development of bioceramic based functionalized PLGA nanoparticles of risedronate for bone targeting: in-vitro characterization and pharmacodynamic evaluation. Pharm Res 32(10):3149–3158

Rohilla R, Garg T, Bariwal J, Goyal AK, Rath G (2016) Development, optimization and characterization of glycyrrhetinic acid–chitosan nanoparticles of atorvastatin for liver targeting. Drug Deliv 23(7):2290–2297

Rubio-Camacho M, Alacid Y, Mallavia R, Martínez-Tomé MJ, Mateo CR (2019) Polyfluorene-based multicolor fluorescent nanoparticles activated by temperature for bioimaging and drug delivery. Nano 9(10):1485

Sharma H, Mishra PK, Talegaonkar S, Vaidya B (2015) Metal nanoparticles: a theranostic nanotool against cancer. Drug Discov Today 20(9):1143–1151

Siddiqui L, Mishra H, Mishra PK, Iqbal Z, Talegaonkar S (2018) Novel 4-in-1 strategy to combat colon cancer, drug resistance and cancer relapse utilizing functionalized bioinspiring lignin nanoparticle. Med Hypotheses 121:10–14

Singh R, Nalwa HS (2011) Medical applications of nanoparticles in biological imaging, cell labeling, antimicrobial agents, and anticancer nanodrugs. J Biomed Nanotechnol 7(4):489–503

Skotland T, Iversen T-G, Sandvig K (2014) Development of nanoparticles for clinical use. Nanomedicine 9(9):1295–1299

Szebeni J (2014) Complement activation-related pseudoallergy: a stress reaction in blood triggered by nanomedicines and biologicals. Mol Immunol 61(2):163–173

Talegaonkar S, Ahmad Z, Tariq M, Khan Z, Negi L, Khan A et al (2013) Emerging trends in oral bioavailability enhancement. Int J Drug Regul Aff 1(2):20–38

Tighe CJ, Cabrera RQ, Gruar RI, Darr JA (2013) Scale up production of nanoparticles: continuous supercritical water synthesis of Ce–Zn oxides. Ind Eng Chem Res 52(16):5522–5528

Torchilin VP (2000) Drug targeting. Eur J Pharm Sci 11:S81–S91

Yasukawa T, Kimura H, Tabata Y, Miyamoto H, Honda Y, Ikada Y et al (2000) Active drug targeting with immunoconjugates to choroidal neovascularization. Curr Eye Res 21(6):952–961

Zahoor A, Sharma S, Khuller G (2005) Inhalable alginate nanoparticles as antitubercular drug carriers against experimental tuberculosis. Int J Antimicrob Agents 26(4):298–303

Nanoformulations in Human Health Conditions: The Paradigm Shift

2

Vikas Pandey and Seema Kohli

Abstract

Salient features like strapping targeted drug delivery, improvisation in efficacy and safety profiles, extraordinary distinctiveness in physicochemical properties, etc. made nanopharmaceuticals immensely popular among formulators over the past few years. Nanoformulations, which are legacy of applications of nanotechnology, concern the use of specifically engineered materials to fabricate new therapeutic and diagnostic techniques. Exceptional physicochemical properties make nanoformulations more powerful in combating serious concerns that were associated with conventional formulation systems. Improved nanocarriers like nanoliposomes, nanoparticles, dendrimers, quantum dots, nanoemulsions and nanosuspensions came up with great control over controlled drug delivery, thus consistently emerging as most promising technology in this era. Nanotechnology presents a wide range of quality from diagnostic applications in early detection of diseases such as cancer to prolonged lowering of blood glucose levels in hyperglycaemia. Additionally, nanoformulation system has also gained success in the management of diseases by incorporating both imaging and therapeutic competence. A comprehensive assessment of each nanoformulation is necessary to enhance our current gamut in nanopharmaceuticals. With this aim, this chapter delivers a cursory detail on major nanopharmaceutical formulation systems and their roles in various medical conditions.

Keywords

Nanoparticles · Nanoemulsions · Cancer · Diabetes · Nanosuspensions · Quantum dots · Arthritis · Dendrimers · Nanoliposomes

2.1 Introduction

In this modern era, rapidity to achieve goals, unhealthy lifestyle and infested food became a part of our life. Apart from these three, there are enormous concealed factors that play a significant role in evolving innumerable critical medical conditions. Out of 57 million deaths across the world in 2017, more than 50% occurred due to severe prevailing diseases (Kruk et al. 2018). Diseases like ischaemic heart disease, heart

V. Pandey
Department of Pharmaceutics, Guru Ramdas Khalsa Institute of Science and Technology (Pharmacy), Jabalpur, Madhya Pradesh, India

S. Kohli (✉)
Department of Pharmaceutical Sciences, Kalaniketan Polytechnic College, Jabalpur, Madhya Pradesh, India

S. Talegaonkar, M. Rai (eds.), *Nanoformulations in Human Health*,
https://doi.org/10.1007/978-3-030-41858-8_2

stroke and cancer were the leaders that accounted for approximately 16 million deaths. In addition, these diseases retain their top position in the list since the last two decades (Prabhakaran et al. 2018). According to the latest reports of the World Health Organization (WHO), chronic obstructive pulmonary disease claimed more than 2.9 million lives in 2018, whereas lung cancer caused 2 million deaths (WHO 2018). On one side, diabetes prevalence increased from 20% (1980) to 60% (2016), and on another side, death ratio due to dementia grew rapidly (more than 50%) within just 10 years.

The cause of death statistics consistently assists healthcare authorities to examine and concentrate on taking serious measures. In order to combat these life-taking critical medical conditions, pharmaceutical sector has always played a significant role. In the voyage of unremitting progress and development, pharmaceutical sector has come up with diversified array of potential tools and formulation systems, which is well-equipped to have strong conflict with these diseases. This chapter aims to explore the various roles of impending novel formulations developed over the past few years and also exemplifies their promising modality towards a brighter future.

Over pastone decade, because of potential attributes, Nanotechnology has gained immense attraction in pharmaceutical arena. The word "nano" which means one billionth of a metre has revolutionized the pharmaceutical arena in several aspects. Over the past few years, nanotechnology has also gained significant interest in reconnoitring the concealed boulevards of medical sciences. Ranging from imaging, sensing, gene delivery to implanting artificial structures, nanotechnology flourished everywhere (Nasimi and Haidari 2013). Along with this, the several new chemical entities are nanosystems of polymers, metals or ceramics, which are proficient enough to contest with critical medical conditions like cancer (Zhao et al. 2018).

Applications of nanotechnology in therapeutic management, monitoring, finding and getting control over diseases are fundamentally denoted as "nanomedicine system". Applications of nanotechnology in pharmaceutical seem to be an epitome of recent technology, but actually it comes from the past decades back. Liposomes, today's chief pharmaceutical player, come from family of lipid vesicles, introduced in 1965 (Bangham et al. 1965); macromolecules having controlled-release polymer system were first introduced in 1976 (Langer and Folkman 1976); the first quantum dot bioconjugate was mentioned in 1994 (Bruchez et al. 1998; Chan and Nie 1998). Several novel targeted nanoparticle-based approaches have emerged, which are significantly contributing in early diagnosis of medical conditions like atherosclerosis and cardiovascular pathology at cellular and molecular level, which represents upcoming endeavours of theranostics (Nakhlband et al. 2018).

Nanotechnology-based potential markers and accurate devices significantly improved patient management, compliance, overall quality life and reduction in mortality rates due to medical conditions like Alzheimer's disease and cancer. The distinctive characteristics and efficacy of nanoformulations provide various useful attributes like size similarity with biomolecules like proteins and polynucleic acids.

2.1.1 Nanopharmaceuticals: An Emerging Potential

On the basis of significant advancement in nanoscale technology, the National Institute of Health (NIH) instigated a federal government programme in 2000 named "National Nanotechnology Initiative" (NNI). This programme is launched with the motive to accelerate research and development on grounds of nanoscience. Further, centralization of this programme facilitated consistent development of nanopharmaceuticals, which had placed a great impression on health science. Clubbing and implementing nanotechnology with medicine is the key intention behind this perception. Pharmaceutical scientists and formulators successfully acquired nanoscience technology with the help of which they succeed in developing various nanopharmaceuticals. Transforming conventional dosage forms into novel new nanosized design comes into trend and also emerged as potential partner of pharmaceutical research. Colloidal systems transformed into nanosystems, colloidal drug delivery systems emerged as nano-drug delivery systems and much more (Babu et al. 2014).

Approximately more than 50 years ago, colloidal systems were developed and utilized for biomedical research, and attempts for their applicability in drug delivery were started 40 years ago (Bangham et al. 1965; Marty et al. 1978). For example, encapsulation of anthracyclines into liposomes was done in the 1970s (Forssen and Tökès 1981); further, in the 1980s, three US-based companies (Vestar in Pasadena, CA, USA; The Liposome Company in Princeton, NJ, USA; and Liposome Technology Inc., in Menlo Park, CA, USA) were in firm competition with each other for production of liposome anthracycline formulations. Nanosized liposome formulation got its first breakthrough in 1995 after USFDA approval of Doxil®, the very first approved nanoformulations (Barenholz 2012). From then on, nanopharmaceuticals are continuously evolving, and there are also two basic criteria that have been set for considering upcoming formulations as "nano": first, the dosage form must be fabricated with the help of nano-engineering technology; second, nanomaterial utilized in formulation of dosage form must either have therapeutic potential or convene superfluous and distinctive properties to the active therapeutic agent.

2.2 Nanoemulsions (NEs) as a Multifunctional Tool in Various Medical Conditions

NEs are kinetically stable disperse systems having a mean droplet size in the range of 50–200 nm (Fig. 2.1). Often they are also termed as ultrafine emulsions or mini-emulsions. The significant feature that differentiates NEs from microemulsion is that NEs are thermodynamically unstable since Gibbs free energy (ΔG) change is more than zero upon formation of NEs (Gupta et al. 2016). More than 40% of catastrophes in the series of formulation and development of therapeutic agents occur due to pitiable biopharmaceutical properties and poor solubility or we can say low permeability (Kotta et al. 2012).

Along with high kinetic stability, small droplet size, optical transparency and superior practical applications made NEs popular among formulation scientists. In addition, there are several other features like enhanced solubilization capacity, decreased intersubject variations on grounds of gastrointestinal fluid volume and longer shelf life, safety in terms of toxicity and ease

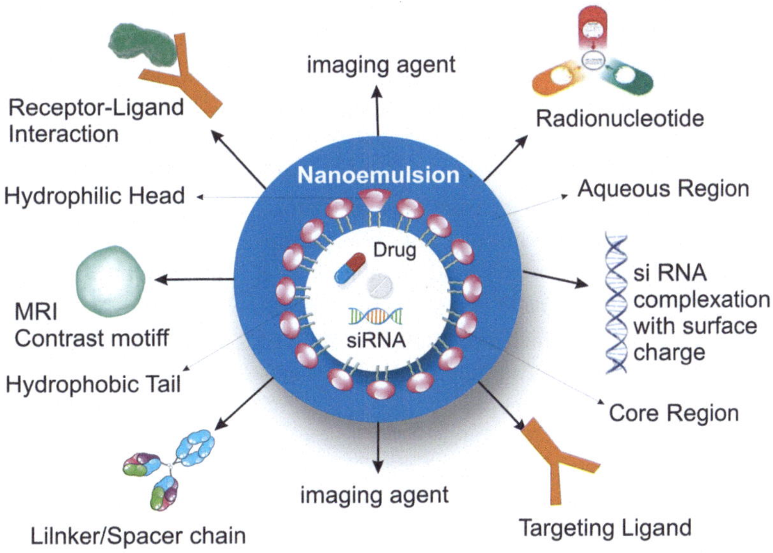

Fig. 2.1 A schematic diagram of nanoemulsion (oil in water) along with its multifunctional capabilities

in large-scale production which presented NEs as a potential tool in addressing bioavailability issues associated with poorly aqueous soluble therapeutic agents.

2.2.1 NEs in Cancer Therapy

Medications (chemotherapy agents) used in the treatment of cancer suffer from the drawback of unsuitability of long-term usage because of associated side effects such as carnage of red blood cells, hair follicles, gut epithelia, lymphatic cells and bone marrow (Mahto 2017). On the other hand, potential therapeutic agents suffer from low solubility issues. This creates a two-sided jeopardy situation for formulators while fabricating drug delivery systems which could specifically target cancer cells. During the era of combating various issues associated with drug development process, NEs came up as a potential tool in targeting delivery of drugs to specific sites. NEs provide an adjunct feature of loading the drug in its core, which prevents it from getting degraded, and eventual increment in the circulation time. Enhanced circulation time affords NEs high permeability and increased retention (EPR effect), due to which NEs can stay up to longer periods of time at malfunctioning vasculatures like tumours (Jaiswal et al. 2015). In another study, Shanmugapriya and team formulated astaxanthin and alpha-tocopherol with sodium caseinate-loaded NEs and exploited in vitro their antitumour potential. Results revealed reduced apoptosis morphology in cancer cells that inhibits cell death (Shanmugapriya et al. 2019).

NEs consist of lipids as their basic component; these lipids come from various natural sources like soya bean oil, egg yolk phospholipids, etc. and have rich fatty acid content such as omega-3 and omega-6 and essential vitamins like vitamins E and K, which eventually makes NEs as potential carriers for targeted delivery of several chemotherapeutic agents.

2.2.1.1 Nanoemulsion-Based Drug Delivery to Cancer Cells: The Active and Passive Targeting

Several exploratory findings revealed that even large structure-based proteins and peptides can also be successfully delivered at both targets i.e. systemic as well locally with the help of NEs. Findings of these reports fruitfully assisted in the development of cellular and humoral antigen-specific immune responsive based vaccines. Further, these vaccines were successfully delivered to immunostimulatory CpG along with gastric cancer-based antigen MG7. Results revealed marked improvement in controlling tumour growth in mice treated with NE-based vaccine loaded with MG7 and cpG and that cancer was generated in mice by MG7-expressing cancer cell; this exploratory study proved that NE can be fruitfully utilized in vaccine delivery. In another study, Ge et al. (2009) explored the potential of NEs in targeting melanoma in the form of vaccine; firstly they fabricated heat-shock protein 70 and staphylococcal enterotoxin A in capsules and then targeted melanoma cells. The vaccine triggered inhibition of tumour-specific immunity against melanoma-associated antigens in mice. Animals were consistently administered with subcutaneous NE-based vaccine of heat-shock protein 70 and staphylococcal enterotoxin A, which perfectly reduced tumour growth (Ge et al. 2009).

The absence of distinct lymphatic system allows tumours to remain for a longer period of time in contrast to normal tissues (Binnewies et al. 2018). The rationale behind is the compression of lymphatic vessels by large-sized tumours, which results in its collapse and the complete discharge of lymph. This process obstructs the effectual allowance of macromolecules collected in solid tumour tissues. This amalgamation of increased vascular permeability and deprived lymphatic damage is collectively known as enhanced permeability and retention (EPR) effect. This EPR effect emerged as a potential tool in formulation and development of anticancer drug delivery systems along with significant assistance in molecular imaging, micelles and protein-polymer conjugates (Kim and Park 2017a). Passive targeting works by using this EPR effect.

In active targeting by NE formulations, objective ligands were loaded onto NEs which target tumoured organ, tissue or cells (Muhamad et al. 2018). The major contrasting advantage of active targeting is that it particularly reaches to a specific site and delivers drug after binding with cancer cell receptors. Another benefit is that NEs offer a wide variety of ligands (targeting and imaging both) to be attached to them (Din et al. 2017). NEs loaded with targeting ligands specifically bind to cells through ligand-receptor interaction and release drugs inside the cells. Active targeting is more in demand in cancer therapy because it prevents chances of damage to healthy tissues from harmful drugs.

2.2.1.2 Multifunctionalization of Nanoemulsions

NEs bear multiple capabilities of carrying and assimilating various agents used in targeting, imaging and therapeutic action, and this feature is more favourable for multifunctionalization which results in a proficient treatment option for various medical conditions. Multifunctionalization of NE provides ease of delivering more than two therapeutic agents in a single shot, e.g. gene silencing and drug delivery. Further, imaging agents can also be combined with drugs to have more specific targeting. In comparison with conventional nano- or microparticles, multifunctional NEs can assimilate various important properties within their core or surface in order to exhibit the utmost desired therapeutic effect (Fig. 2.1). NEs have also gained popularity by delivering the drug through stimuli-responsive elements on target and timed basis. A summary of reported multifunctional capabilities of NE system is presented in Table 2.1.

2.2.2 Nanoemulsions as an Essential Tool in the Enhancement of Oral Bioavailability of Poorly Aqueous Soluble Anti-diabetics

Diabetes is a global prevailing metabolic disorder progressing with rocketing speed worldwide. In order to combat this serious concern, more than 40 active therapeutic agents have been discerned so far, out of which more than 90% suffer from poor solubility issues and poor bioavailability. Further, to overcome solubility concerns, various techniques have been explored like nanoparticle, liposome and solid dispersions, melt granulation, hot melt extrusion, etc., out of which lipid-based formulations especially NE system have gained immense popularity among formulation scientists. The rationale behind NEs being the right choice is that, in contrast to all other techniques, it presents numerous advantages like greater solubilization capacity, instant onset of action, minimal intersubject variability, longer shelf life, ease of large-scale production and freedom of usage of large number of excipients (Jaiswal et al. 2015).

Over the past few several years, anti-diabetic molecules suffering from poor solubility issues have been exploited by formulating them in NE system. In an exploratory finding by Akhtar et al., prandial glucose regulator repaglinide was taken as target molecule and used to enhance its solubility and bioavailability. Repaglinide was loaded into NE fabricated with the help of Sefsol-218, Tween 80 and Transcutol. Results of the study showed marked improvement in in vitro release, i.e. > 98.22%, and marked enhancement in hypoglycaemic activity (Akhtar et al. 2016). In a recent study, Espinoza and team explored the potential of pioglitazone in skin inflammatory diseases by fabricating them in the form of NE; results showed substantial increment in anti-inflammatory activity by decreasing the expression of inflammatory cytokines IL-6, IL-1β and

Table 2.1 Summary of multifunctional capabilities of NEs and SNEDDS in enhancing the potential of various therapeutic agents

Therapeutic/imaging agent	Targeting ligand/ complexing agent/ modified dosage forms	Imaging agent/excipient and technique utilized	Perusal/outcome	Reference
Olaparib	–	PARPi-FL	Utilized imaging agent showed delineated subcutaneous xenografts of small cell lung cancer which proved to be an effective imaging agent	Gonzales et al. (2018)
Amyl acetate	–	A3E1S; lactic acid, propionic acid, amyl acetate, toluene and butanone	First, of its kind, the study reported the ability of nanoemulsion formulation to attract and influence the activity of fruit flies D. melanogaster	Krittika et al. (2019)
Cisplatin	Endothelial growth factor receptor	Gadolinium	Persistent blood platinum and gadolinium levels with nanoemulsions in nu/nu mice and extension of survival time of ovarian cancer-induced mice	Ganta et al. (2015)
Docetaxel	Stearylamine	DiIC18(5) oil (1,1′-dioctadecyl-3,3,3′,3′-tetramethylindodicarbocyanine perchlorate)	Significant inhibition in tumour growth (55.62 ± 5.41%, 54.27 ± 4.85% and 80.01 ± 2.74%) in solid tumours induced in C57BL/6 mice	Muzammil et al. (2016)
Paclitaxel	Hyaluronan	–	Inhibition in tumour growth along with a marked reduction in toxicity in tumour-transplanted mice	Kim and Park (2017b)
Oxaliplatin and 5-fluorouracil	Nα-deoxycholyl-l-lysyl-methylester	–	Marked enhancement in oral bioavailability (> 9.19- and 1.39) and maximal inhibition in tumour growth (73.9%, 48.5% and 38.1%) in colorectal adenocarcinoma cell (CT26)-bearing mouse model	Pangeni et al. (2016)
Piplartine	–	–	1.5-fold increase in oral bioavailability and significant improvement in antitumour activity	Fofaria et al. (2016)
Library of 12 plain NEs for multispectral optoacoustic tomography	–	NE-IRDye QC1, NE-IR780, NE-ICG, NE-DYQ700, NE-Cy7.5	NEs proved as potential optoacoustic sonophores in non-invasive imaging of tumours	Roberts et al. (2018)

C6 ceramide and tributyrin	Chitosan	–	Prolonged localization of drug in mammillary tissue through NE formulation in contrast to the normal solution	Migotto et al. (2018)
Chlorpromazine	Liquid SNEDDS	Captex, Tween 85 and ethanol	Long-chain triglyceride (LCT14) showed a 1.5-fold increased elimination half-life ($p < 0.01$), up to six-fold increased oral bioavailability, and 1.7-fold decreased plasma clearance rate ($p < 0.01$) compared to a drug suspension	Baloch et al. (2019)
Cilostazol	Solid SNEDDS powder	Peceol (oil), Tween 20 (surfactant) and Labrasol (cosurfactant); spray-drying	1.2-fold higher oral bioavailability than the drug powder and marketed product	Mustapha et al. (2016)
Olmesartan medoxomil	Solid SNEDDS powder	Capryol 90, Cremophor RH40 and Transcutol HP	Significant enhancement in C_{max} and AUC (1.72 and 2.77 fold) in contrast to a marketed product	Nasr et al. (2016)
Vitamin K1	Liquisolid tablets	Soybean lecithin and glycocholic acid (surfactant) and Transcutol HP (cosurfactant); liquisolid technology for solidification and direct compression for tableting	Remarkable increment in mean C_{max} and AUC from SNEDDS tablets	Tong et al. (2018)
Sertraline	Tablets	Labrafil M2125, Lauroglycol 90 and Maisine; solid adsorption	Six- and fivefold increased absorption from SNEDDS tablets	Rahman and Mujahid (2018)
Cinnarizine	Pellets	Oleic acid, Imwitor308 and Cremophor El; fluid bed coating	Formulation self-nanoemulsifying pellets maintained >85% of Cinnarizine in solution, even at pH 6.8; this has proven solubilization benefits	Shahba et al. (2017)

TNF-α. The suggested study proved pioglitazone as a potential alternative in treatment of inflammatory skin diseases such as rosacea, atopic dermatitis or psoriasis (Espinoza et al. 2019).

2.2.3 Self-Nanoemulsifying Drug Delivery Systems (SNEDDS): An Emerging Potential in Combating Various Medical Conditions

In combating various formulation issues especially poor aqueous solubility, along with NEs, self-nanoemulsifying drug delivery systems (SNEDDS) have appeared as another potential lipid-based drug delivery system. SNEDDS are basically isotropic mixtures of oil, surfactant and cosurfactant which upon agitation form ultrafine NE (droplet <100 nm) (Shahba et al. 2012). Some silent features of SNEDDS make them markedly distinguished from other formulation options:

1. Decreased droplet size and increased surface area make SNEDDS easily acceptable by in vivo environment, which can be further integrated into micellar form which easily passes through the intestinal lumen.
2. The capability of accelerating lipid fluidity of enterocytes and membranes and reduction in efflux pumps makes SNEDDS a good choice in improvising oral bioavailability.
3. Reduction in cytopchrome-P450 metabolism in gut enterocytes.
4. Protection against first-pass metabolism, thereby increasing half-life.
5. Enhanced lymphatic transport.
6. Ease of large-scale production, increased patient compliance, long-term stability, easy conversion to solid dosage form and dose reduction.

SNEDDS is actually an advanced version of its precursor, i.e. self-microemulsifying drug delivery system (SMEDDS), consisting smaller sized globule. After the commercial success of SMEDDS in the form of "Sandimmune Neoral", various SNEDDS products are now ready to hit the market soon. Easy conversion of liquid SNEDDS into solid form by various techniques like spray-drying, melt granulation and adsorption makes SNEDDS more patient compliable. Accordingly over the past few years, various exploratory findings have been reported presenting SNEDDS in various dosage forms, a summary of which is presented in Table 2.1.

2.3 Nanoparticles as Promising Carrier over the Past One Decade

Nanotechnology is a new technology that is knocking at the door. It has wider applications and is the central focus for many technologies to converge and open a large number of applications. It deals with things smaller than 100 nanometres in size. Nanos means dwarf. This technology is concerned with material science and its applications at the nanometre scale (one billionth of a metre). A nanoparticle is a microscopic particle whose size is measured in nanometres. It is defined as a particle with at least one dimension less than 100 nm. Nanoparticles are often referred to as clusters. Nanospheres, nanorods and nanocups are few shapes that have been developed.

The properties of many conventional materials change when formed from nanoparticles. This is typical because nanoparticles have a greater surface area per weight than larger particles which causes them to be more reactive to some other molecules.

Nanotechnology has attained a promising role in the area of drug delivery as drug carriers and in early diagnosis of disease. Liposomal and nanoparticle formulation technologies are coming up in a big way in drug market. Nanoparticles consist of three layers: the surface layer, the shell layer and the core. The surface layer usually consists of a variety of molecules such as metal ion, surfactants and polymers. Nanoparticles may contain a single material or may be consisted of a combination of several materials. Nanoparticles can exist as suspensions, colloids or dispersed aerosols depending on their chemical and electromagnetic properties. Nanoparticles can be tailor-made for their size and surface properties for entrapment of drugs. The nanostructures have the ability to enter cells that typically internalize materials below 100 nm. When incorporated materials are produced from nanoparticles in the 1–100 nm size range instead of bigger microparticles, they have a large surface area for the same volume, smaller pore size, improved solubility and different structural properties. This can improve both the diffusion and degradation properties of loaded drug.

Nanoparticles prepared using biodegradable polymers such as gelatin, other proteins and polysaccharides function as effective drug delivery devices for the controlled delivery of drugs. The nano approach also reduces the side effects and improves the efficacy of the drug along with improved patient compliance and convenience (Gupta and Nguyen 2014; Shinde et al. 2019).

Initially, the nanoparticles were developed as carriers for vaccines and anticancer drug targeting. Simultaneously investigations were conducted for CNS and ophthalmic and oral drug delivery. Some of the applications of NPs have been detailed here.

2.3.1 Targeting Tuberculosis with Nanoparticles

Tuberculosis (TB) is caused by bacteria (*Mycobacterium tuberculosis*) that mostly affect the lungs. TB is an airborne disease. When people with lung TB cough, sneeze or spit, they drive the TB germs into the air. And simply a few germs can cause infection. The WHO confers that about one-quarter of the world's population has latent TB. Latent TB implies that people have been infected by TB bacteria but cannot transmit the disease. When a person suffers from active TB disease, the symptoms (such as cough, fever, night sweats or weight loss) may be feeble for many months and can be ignored by the patient. This can lead to delays in seeking care and results in transmission of the bacteria to others.

The foremost problems linked with treatment of TB are long duration of treatment and continuous and recurrent multiple drug dosing that results in poor compliance of patients to drug therapy. This finally contributes to the recurrence of the disease and the development of multidrug-resistant (MDR) tuberculosis (Gladwin et al. 1998). This reinforces the need to develop new and effective anti-TB drug delivery system to overcome the problem of drug resistance, shorten the treatment course and promote better compliance (Nasiruddin et al. 2017). The nanoparticles of three major anti-TB drugs were prepared by the solvent evaporation technique using PLG for oral administration. It was verified that drug levels were maintained above the least inhibitory concentration (MIC90) in mice after a single oral administration of drug-loaded PLG NPs for 6 to 9 days in the plasma as compared to free drugs that were vacated from plasma within 12–24 hours following the oral administration (Pandey et al. 2004). Lectin-conjugated PLG nanoparticles of these drugs also presented promising results on oral administration. Pandey et al. (2005) also studied the injectable routes of drug delivery of these drugs in nanoform. A single subcutaneous injection of PLG nanoparticles loaded with RMP, INH and PZA resulted in sustained therapeutic drug levels in plasma for 32 days and in the lungs or spleen for 36 days. In another study, the researcher studied the coinfection of monocyte-derived macrophages (MDMs) with HIV and avirulent *M. tuberculosis* strain (H37Rv) in the presence of gallium nanoparticles. Results depicted significant growth inhibition of both HIV and *M. tuberculosis* within MDMs for up to 15 days after loading the cells with gallium nanoparticles (Choi et al. 2019).

2.3.2 Nanoparticles in Cancer Therapy: The State of the Art

Cancer is one of the leading causes of death worldwide. In spite of voluminous research and innovations, the current treatment is limited to surgery, radiotherapy and chemotherapy. The letdown of this treatment is linked with associated adverse effects like drug resistance and toxicity issues. Copious investigations have shown that both tissue and cell distribution profiles of anticancer drugs can be controlled by their entrapment in nanoparticles. The advancement in novel nanomaterials and nanocarriers has resulted in value-added drug delivery in cancer.

The foremost objective in employing nanocarriers is to protect the drug from rapid degradation after systemic delivery and letting it reach the targeted tumour site at desired therapeutic concentrations. This would also avoid the entry of drugs to other normal cell sites, thus reducing the side effects. The prudent design of NPs performs a critical role in drug action as the various characters of nanoparticles guide the pharmacokinetics, internalization and safety of the drugs.

Gradisher and team studied the albumin-bound paclitaxel nanoparticles for the treatment of breast cancer. Similar studies were carried out with albumin nanoparticles loaded with osteonectin for breast, prostate and lung cancer (Gradishar et al. 2005). Sultana and co-workers prepared and evaluated poly(isohexyl cyanoacrylate) nanoparticles with doxorubicin for hepatocellular carcinoma (Sultana et al. 2012). Gelatin nanoparticles have been extensively used for the delivery of anticancer drugs including cytarabine, methotrexate, camptothecin, curcumin, resveratrol, paclitaxel, cisplatin and noscapine with the objective of improving the cancer therapy by targeted delivery of drugs (Aslan et al. 2013). In another study, Yan and team explored combined monomodal photodynamic therapy (PDT) or photothermal therapy (PTT) approach by making upconversion-polymer hybrid nanoparticles with surface-loaded chlorin e6 photosensitizer as basis for antitumour activation. Results showed that the combination enhanced primary tumour elimination and presented antitumor immunity against disseminated tumours. The authors also found that synergistic phototherapy can elicit robust systemic and humoral antitumor immune responses. When combined with immune checkpoint blockades, it inhibited tumour relapse and metastasis as well as prolonged the survival of tumour-bearing mice in two types of tumour metastasis models (Yan et al. 2019).

2.3.3 Nanoparticles in Ocular Delivery: The Story Behind

Countless efforts have been made to improve and enhance the ocular delivery of drugs. The corneal barrier and poor retention time of the drug in the ocular cavity lead to bioavailability issues. These can be overcome by employing nanotechnology approaches. The drug-loaded nanoparticles increase the residence time, decrease the toxicity and enhance the penetration of the drug to deeper tissues. Lipid-based nanoparticles are the most appropriate and biocompatible for ocular delivery. They also produce bioadhesion that increases the residence time of the drug in the cavity. Gene delivery to the retina is being made possible by making use of lipid nanoparticles. Antibiotics (tobramycin, chloramphenicol, levofloxacin), antifungal agents (itraconazole, ketoconazole) and antiviral agents (acyclovir) when loaded in lipid nanoparticles showed improved action. Some anti-inflammatory drugs, mostly NSAIDs such as diclofenac, ibuprofen, flurbiprofen and indomethacin, when entrapped in lipid nanoparticles exhibited better performance. Antioxidants baicalin, quercetin and epigallocatechin have been observed for ocular therapy through lipid nanoparticles. These antioxidants in LN were proven to be biocompatible with corneal cells and also showed upgraded corneal permeation. Timolol, pilocarpine and methazolamide in LN presented promising results in glaucoma therapy. *Calendula officinalis* extract loaded in nanoparticles was found to have noteworthy corneal wound-healing effect (Zhou et al. 2013). In another study, a researcher formulated timolol maleate-loaded polymeric nanoparticles of flaxseed gum and chitosan and examined their potential in ocular delivery in rabbits. Results depicted enhanced corneal penetration of drug in contrast to marketed eye drops; along with this, formulated nanoparticles also reduced the intraocular pressure in rabbits for prolonged period when compared to conventional eye drops (Mittal and Kaur 2019).

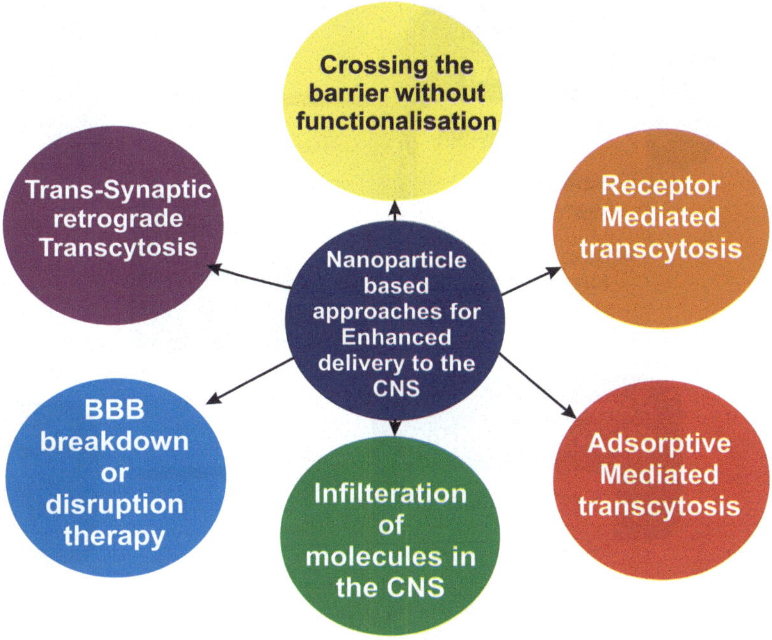

Fig. 2.2 Strategies of drug delivery to the brain

2.3.4 Nanoparticles in Targeting the Central Nervous System (CNS)

CNS disorders have always been a gigantic challenge for scientists and researchers. The blood-brain barrier (BBB) is the key hindrance in the delivery of drugs to the CNS because of its selectively permeable and lipoidal nature and restricted pore size (Pardridge 2012).

Alzheimer's and Parkinson's diseases are among the two most common neurodegenerative diseases. Nanoparticles coated with different polymers are competent to overcome the BBB issues and improve the efficacy of drugs in CNS disorders (Silva 2008). Kuplennik and team fabricated nanoparticles from highly hydrophobic poly(ethylene glycol)-b-poly(ε-caprolactone) (PEG-b-PCL) block copolymer functionalized with an amine moiety in the edge of the PEG block by a simple nanoprecipitation method, loaded with folate. Developed PEG blocks further conjugated the targeting ligand FRα. Results depicted that conjugation of FRα-FA complex to the NP surface promotes higher accumulation in the brain, highlighting the promise of FRα-FA-modified NPs to serve as a platform for the targeting of active molecules to the CNS from the systemic circulation (Kuplennik et al. 2019).

NPs allows the delivery of various drugs to the CNS, particularly to the brain. Such drugs include anticancer agents (taxol), analgesics, anti-Alzheimer's drugs, anti-Parkinson's agents (levodopa), protease inhibitors and anti-epileptic drug molecules (Fig. 2.2).

2.3.5 Nanoparticles in Wound Healing

Wound healing is a forced response to various types of stimuli that affects the skin or any organ. In the case of tissue or skin injury, a sequential process of events occurs which eventually results in the rebuilding of normal tissue (Pastar et al. 2014). Wound healing is a typical process comprising haemostasis, inflammation, proliferation and remodelling. A schematic presentation of these activities is presented in Fig. 2.3.

The wound care management is a strong area of research and seeks attention of researchers. It depends on effective dressing material. There are definite factors that impede the wound healing process: poor blood supply, diminished

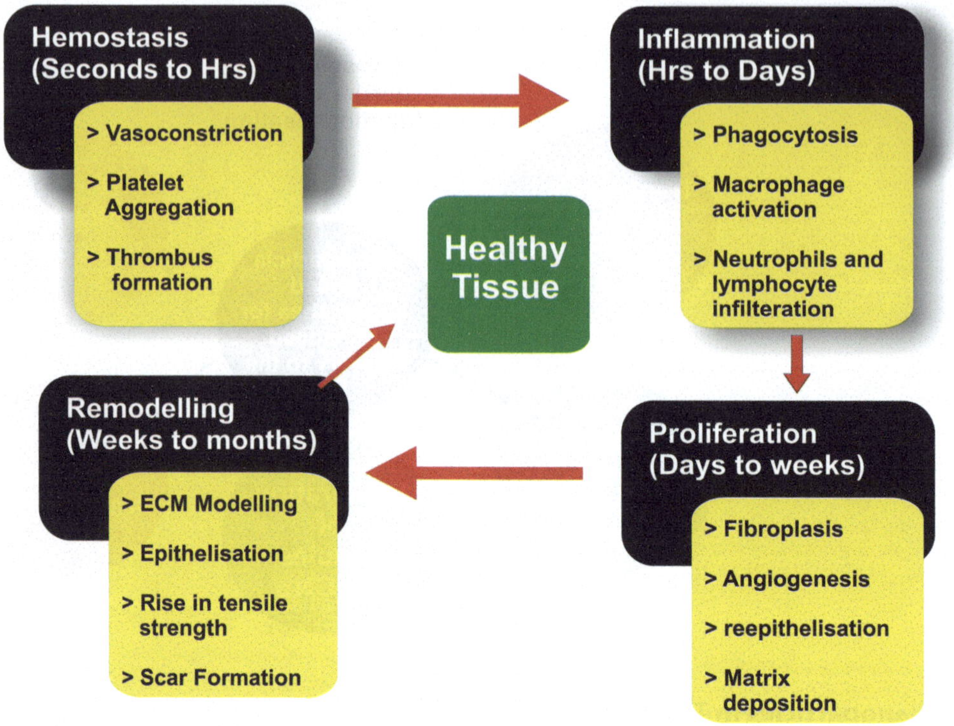

Fig. 2.3 Sequential events in normal wound healing process

venous drainage, wound dehiscence, presence of foreign bodies and reduced macrophage action. The commonly used wound healing materials aim to increase the blood clotting, absorb the exudates and hasten the healing process and also moisten the wound environment. These wound healing materials also incorporate bioactive agents to fasten the process. Nanoparticles present superlative approach in enhancing the wound-healing process. NPs allow for the external delivery of substances that are produced at the site of injury, for instance, NO (nitrous oxide). In slow healing, the release of NO is lowered. So to improve that, nanoparticles are employed.

A wide range of studies is dedicated to the use of nanosilver for wound healing. Metal nanoparticles such as aurum (Au), palladium (Pd) and platinum (Pt) are considered to function as antioxidants due to their strong catalytic activity (Fig. 2.4). There is some research aimed at the use of zinc oxide (ZnO) for regeneration and wound healing. Selenium in nanoform is another promising regenerative medicine (Rajendran et al. 2018).

2.3.6 Nanoparticles for Oral Gene Delivery

Oral delivery of drugs is often very challenging owing to the presence of acidic pH in the stomach and the enzymes such as pepsin that causes the degradation of proteins. This results in poor bioavailability of the drug. Nucleic acids are also used as drugs either as a vaccine or in gene therapy form. Oral gene delivery faces similar bioavailability issues. Nanoparticles are the solution to these problems. The nanoparticles may partially protect the loaded drug and improve cellular uptake by endocytosis. A number of polymers or lipids have been employed for the preparation of these nanoparticles. Leong and team reported the preparation of chitosan-DNA nanoparticles by coacervation technique (Leong et al. 1998). Kaul and Aimiji were the first to develop type B

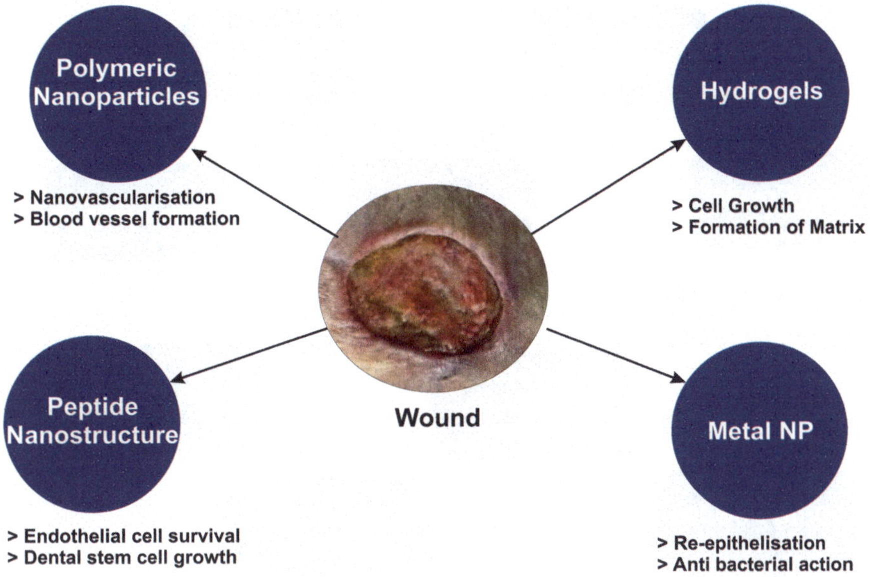

Fig. 2.4 Various approaches for wound healing

gelatin nanoparticles as non-condensing gene delivery system for oral gene therapy (Kaul and Amiji 2002).

Nanoparticles have an expanded role in the delivery of antimicrobial and anti-leishmaniasis drugs also. Owing to the limitation of chapter length, these are not detailed here.

2.4 Nanosuspension in Pharmaceuticals

Nanotechnology-based approaches can be applied to resolve the solubility issues related to numerous chemical entities in aqueous as well as lipid media. Nanosuspensions are submicron colloidal dispersions of nanosized particles stabilized by using surfactants. The liquid media could be aqueous or non-aqueous. The particle size in nanosuspensions is less than a micron ranging between 200 and 600 nm. The nanosuspensions by virtue of nanosized particles enjoy the attributes of large surface area that improves the solubility of the drug in the media and subsequently enhances the bioavailability of the drug. The reduced particle size renders the possibility of IV administration of poorly water-soluble drugs without blocking the blood capillaries. This formulation features high drug loading capacity, low cost and reduced side effects. Nanosuspensions formulated by employing steric polymers like polyethylene glycol (PEG) have enticed great attention. They have been found to have particles in the size range of 10–100 nm. These nanoparticles are able to accumulate in targeted areas such as cancer tissues with least destruction to normal healthy cells (Patel and Agrawal 2011).

The pluses of nanosuspensions are:

- The dose of the drug can be reduced.
- Solubility and bioavailability can be improved.
- Low-cost factor.
- High drug loading is possible.
- Drug targeting is feasible.
- Stability, both physical and chemical, of the drug is enhanced.

Nanosuspensions are generally prepared by two approaches, that is, bottom-up technology and top-down technology. In bottom-up method, the drug powder is made into nanoparticle by techniques like precipitation, melt emulsification and microemulsion, while in top-down method, larger particles are disintegrated into nanoparticles by using milling and homogenization

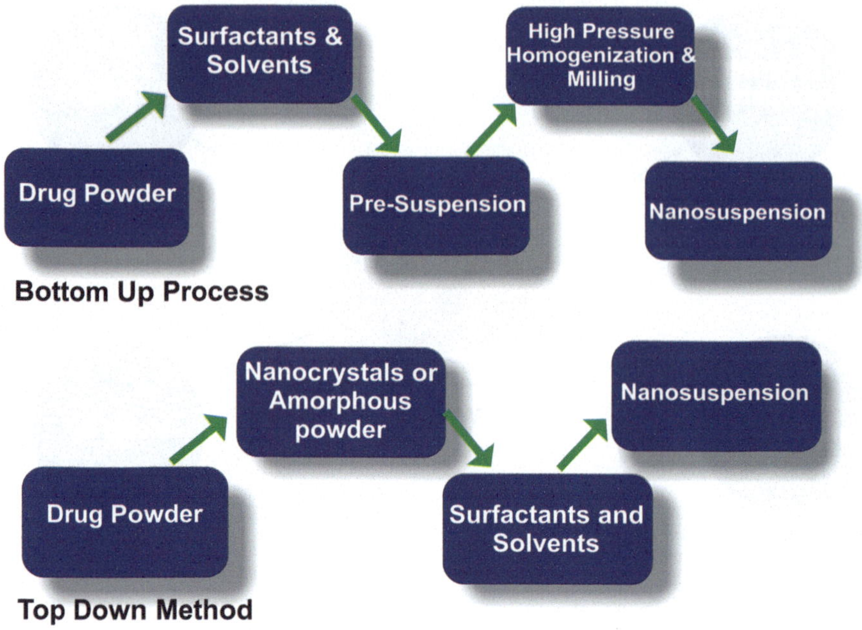

Fig. 2.5 The two popular approaches for formulation of nanosuspensions

techniques (Deoli 2012). The two methods are summarized in Fig. 2.5.

2.4.1 Nanosuspensions in Bioavailability Enhancement of Poorly Soluble Drugs

The Biopharmaceutics Classification System (BCS) categorizes the drug into four classes on the basis of solubility and permeability characteristics. According to BCS, class I comprises molecules with high solubility and high permeability; class II includes molecules with low solubility and high permeability; class III includes drugs with high solubility and low permeability; and class IV includes drug molecules with low solubility and low permeability.

As per the above categorization, class I drugs are free from any bioavailability issues, while the other classes present a problem in oral absorption. Finally, the bioavailability snags develop with drug molecules. To resolve these problems, various approaches are adopted based on the properties of drug excipients used. These approaches are precisely presented as:

Conventional techniques

- Modification of media of drug like change in solvent, co-solvent, mixture of solvents, pH and used surfactants
- Making of complexes with cyclodextrin and lipid formulation
- Solid-state modification, for example, solid dispersions and solid melts, and size reduction like micronization and particle engineering
- Salt formation

Novel techniques

- Nanotechnology drug delivery methods: nanoparticles, nanosponges, nanocrystals, vesicles, etc.

The conventional techniques have limited utility to drugs. Vesicular systems suffers from a big disadvatage and i.e their compatibility with limtied number of drug molecules (Leone and Cavalli 2015; Chingunpituk 2007). The development of nanosuspension has evolved as a novel

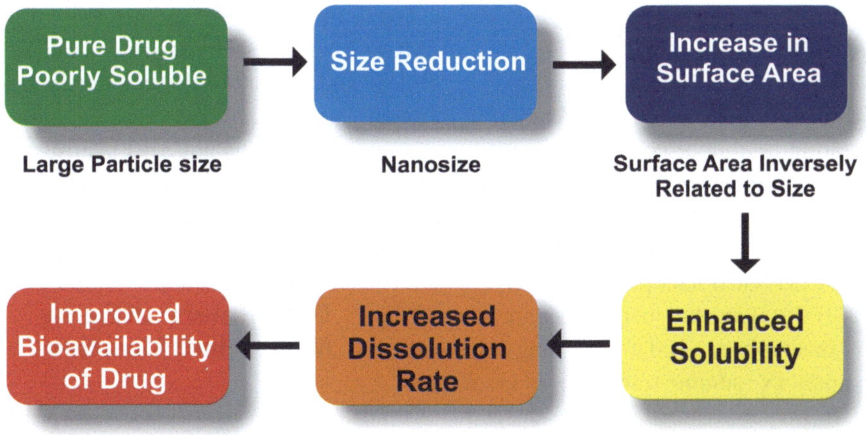

Fig. 2.6 Mechanism of bioavailability enhancement by nanosuspension

technique for delivering poorly soluble drugs owing to their nanosize subsequently solving the bioavailability issues (Fig. 2.6) (Goel et al. 2019).

Studies have shown that nanotechnology can be used for drugs which are insoluble in both water and organic solvents. Hydrophobic drugs such as naproxen, omeprazole, nimesulide, amphotericin B, omeprazole, nifedipine and baicalin (Jin et al. 2019) are formulated as nanosuspensions.

2.4.2 Nanosuspensions in Pulmonary Administration

The pulmonary route is a non-invasive way of administering the drug for both local and systemic action. This route has benefit of high permeability and vascularity as compared to oral route. The pulmonary route presents direct delivery of the drug to the site of action that minimizes the drug dose and the side effects. Conventional pulmonary delivery systems provide only rapid drug release, have poor residence time and lack selectivity. Nanosuspensions can solve problems of poor drug solubility in pulmonary secretions and lack of selectivity through direct delivery to target pulmonary cells.

Nanosuspensions increase the adhesiveness and hence the staying time of drug at the site. They also avoid the undesirable presence of drug in the oral cavity. Thus, nanosuspensions preclude the issues of bioavailability and optimize drug delivery (Patil and Sarasija 2012).

Nanosuspensions can be easily nebulized for lung delivery. Muller and team studied the administration of budesonide nanoparticles for asthmatic conditions through ultrasonic nebulizer that resulted in improved bioavailability parameters (Muller et al. 2000). Qelliny and co-workers also exploited budesonide potential in colon targeting by formulating it into Eudragit S 100-tailored nanoparticles in colitis-induced rat model. Disease activity score, macroscopic examination, blood glucose level and histopathological assessment showed marked improvements over free drug suspension. Obtained results demonstrate that the budesonide-loaded Eudragit S 100 nanocapsules are an effective colon-targeting nanosystem for the treatment of inflammatory bowel disease (Qelliny et al. 2019).

The failure of conventional TB therapy had been a serious concern for ages. A novel antitubercular drug delivery system aims at the direct delivery of drugs to the lungs. Antitubercular drugs have been successfully entrapped and delivered in biodegradable and biocompatible polymers. Zahoor and team have reported inhalable alginate nanoparticles as antitubercular drug carriers against experimentally induced tuberculosis in guinea pigs. The outcomes revealed significantly improved bioavailability of the drug as compared to oral route (Zahoor et al. 2005).

2.4.3 Nanosuspensions in Drug Targeting

Nanosuspensions have the potential of targeting and accumulating in tumour cells. This is attributed to their size and other surficial properties. The nanosuspensions can be designed for active and passive targeting by employing various coating materials. PEGylated nanoparticles with size range of 10–100 nm in the suspension prevent engulfing by macrophages and enable long-term circulation upon IV administration (Rai et al. 2019). Kayser prepared mucoadhesive suspension of buparvaquone for targeting *Cryptosporidium parvum* through oral route (Kayser 2001).

Similarly, pulmonary aspergillosis was targeted by amphotericin B, in the form of pulmonary nanosuspensions (Kohno et al. 1997). Gao and team also reported about the IV injection of curcumin nanosuspension for the effective treatment of cancer (Gao et al. 2011).

2.4.4 Applications of Nanosuspension in the Management of Diabetes

Diabetes mellitus is one of the most prevalent disorders globally. It is classified as type I and type II diabetes. The former occurs when the pancreas fails to prepare insulin leading to hyperglycaemia. This condition requires daily administration of insulin. About 90% of diabetics are type II patients who need administration of glibenclamide-like drugs that suffer from bioavailability issues. Panda and team reported the metformin-loaded PLGA nanosuspensions for the treatment of type II diabetes. Poloxamer 188 was used as a versatile excipient in the preparation of nanocrystals for enhancing the bioavailability of metformin (Panda et al. 2018). Wang and co-workers have studied the efficiency of berberine in nanosuspension in streptozocin-induced diabetes in mice; results depicted that berberine NS produced better hypoglycaemic effect (Wang et al. 2015). Curcumin-NS presented much higher cytotoxicity to Hela and MCF-7 cell lines in vitro and showed less irritability and lower erythrocytic haemolysis compared to the reported curcumin solution, suggesting that the aqueous nanosuspension is a good choice for intravenous administration of poorly soluble curcumin (Gao et al. 2011).

2.5 Dendrimers: Utilizing Multivalent Moieties

Dendrimers are nanosized, outwardly uniform particles with properly distinct standardized and monostrewed assembly consisting of branched structures (Bosman et al. 1999). These subdivided branched structures were discovered by Fritz Vogtle in 1978 for the very first time, followed by modification through Donald Tomalia and team during the 1980s. The structure of dendrimers consists of monodispersed molecules fabricated around an atom, which gives them a thematic look, and they are not a compound (Fig. 2.7). Additionally, their tailoring needs careful construction, so that they can be functionalized for further modification in physicochemical or natural properties (Abbasi et al. 2014). As per reports from Janaszewska and team, dendrimers require chemical modifications so that their intrinsic cytotoxicity can be dazed. Their complexation with various bioactive molecules can be perfectly optimized while being delivery-specific and safe for both the cell and the cargo (Janaszewska et al. 2019).

2.5.1 Dendrimer-Based Antivirals

Over the past few years, linking of dendrimers with various biomolecules has been tested on antiviral grounds, out of which linking of dendrimers with carbohydrates usually called "glycodendrimers" was most common (Reuter et al. 1999). Glycodendrimers were comprehensively assessed on influenza virus. Reuter et al. were the first to investigate the utilization of sialic acid derivatized dendrimers explicitly as a novel "restorative methodology" for influenza. Their

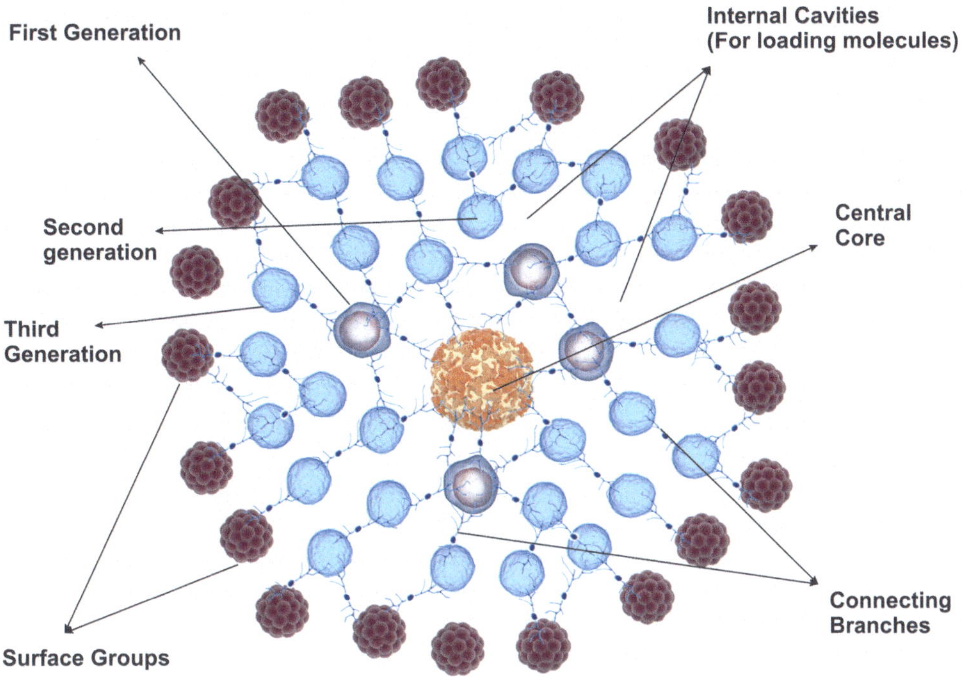

Fig. 2.7 Basic structure of dendrimer

outcomes showed that sialic corrosive connected by means of a musky spacer to various sorts of dendrimers was up to 5x104-overlay better at restraining hemagglutination than monomeric sialic corrosive. Straight polymers were less viable than dendritic types of sialic corrosive yet more successful than free sialic corrosive. In another study by landers et al, authors reported about development of "Polyvalent, generation 4 (G4) SA-conjugated polyamidoamine (PAMAM) dendrimer (G4-SA)", which was evaluated for prevention of adhesion of 3 influenza A subtypes (H1N1, H2N2, and H3N2). Results of in vivo studies depicted that, developed G4-SA totally prohibited infection by a H3N2 subtype in a murine influenza pneumonitis model (Landers et al. 2002).

Studies have also revealed that complex viruses like herpes simplex and HIV has binding efficiency with polyanionic compounds (Luganini et al. 2011). The rationale behind this tendency is supported by the fact that sulphated polysaccharides are potential inhibitors of viral infection (Gong et al. 2002). In a study by Bernstein and team, dendrimers loaded with sulphonated and carboxylated polylysine have achieved immense success in blocking herpes simplex virus. Results also depicted that viral infection-induced animals (mice and guinea pigs), when administered with dendrimers, showed maximal intravaginal protection against viruses (Bernstein et al. 2003). Further, it was also found that sulphonated dendrimers obstructed late-stage multiplication of virus by inhibiting synthesis of virus DNA in the infected cells (Schinazi et al. 2003). The study proved that anionically tailored dendrimers have potential to prevent the infection but also their further inhibition.

Peptide conjugation with dendrimers is also another interesting class of dendrimer series that have achieved success in delivery of drugs and bioactive compounds especially in antineoplastic segment (Knauer et al. 2019). The fundamental rationale of peptide delivery relies upon the fact that bioactive molecules can be easily associated or entangled inside peptide structure. Delivery of anticancer agent is based on penetration inside target cells, and this is difficult in case of peptide dendrimers because of their large structure. Yan et al. researched with a motive to explore chemical artefacts of peptide dendrimers and conjugated linear peptides which have the ability to penetrate cells with PAMAM dendrimers. Further these conjugates were tagged with fluorescent dye and companioned with Tat-peptide (GRKKRRQRRRPQ), which is a human immunodeficiency transcription derivative. It was found that cell internalization was subsequently proportional to the conjugation frequency between Tat-peptide and PAMAM. Cytotoxicity reports showed that PAMAM conjugate was less toxic than free dendrimer (Yan et al. 2015).

2.5.2 Dendrimers in Cancer

As mentioned earlier in this chapter, dendrimers are monodispersed macromolecules having huge number of peripheral groups attached in a tree-like fashion. This feature makes them an ideal candidate for delivery of numerous therapeutic agents, and also with these, further assessments can also be explored like polymer sizing, configuration and construction of bioactive-associated characteristics like lipid bilayer interaction, toxicity profiling, internalization, blood plasma retain time profile, biologic distributions and tumour studies. Over the past few years, dendrimers have gained significant attention in therapeutic and diagnostic applications towards treatment of cancer, which includes progressive delivery of antineoplastic agents and neutron and photon capture therapy.

2.5.2.1 Dendrimer as Potential Tool in RNA-/DNA-Based Cancer Therapy

Dendrimers have acquired substantial popularity over the last 10 years in therapeutic management, diagnostic imaging and investigation of cancer, which is evidenced by the market success of Doxil® (Barenholz 2012). Following this, many explorations have emerged in using dendrimer for cancer therapy, like double-stranded RNA consisting of tiny inquisitive RNA which specifically interferes with expression of genes that restricts their conversion into proteins. These proteins are principally involved in cancer; if synthesis of these is prohibited by targeting specific protein, then prospective of conquering the medical condition increases (Xu et al. 2019).

siRNA consists of exonucleases, due to which they cannot be delivered directly, and requires an appropriate transporter, which could successfully contribute to its cellular uptake. siRNA and DNA both contain phosphate groups in their structure which can be easily coupled with charged dendrimers (positive); this coupled group is also called dendriplexes. In an umbrella-like structure, dendriplexes are situated in endosomes, which emancipates siRNA and DNA; this release is accelerated by addition of proton to dendriplexes which eventually enhances its hydrodynamic ration, and finally siRNA/DNA shreds off from dendriplexes (Fig. 2.8) (Liu et al. 2014).

Monteagudom et al. in their study utilized amino-terminated G1 PAMAM dendrimer as a carrier for targeting p42 MAPK in prostate cancer. Results depicted better stability and potential effects when from dendrimer in contrast to marketed products Lipofectamine and HiPerFect (Monteagudom et al. 2012). In another study, Huang and the team developed and explored G5 PAMAM-dendrimer (EDAcore), in which its surface was transformed into 3,5-diamino-triazines. This system was successfully complexed with siRNA complexes which furnished outstanding performance both in vitro and in vivo of the expression of MDM2 gene, which is a chief player in non-small cell lung cancer (Huang et al. 2016). Marcinkowska and team developed and synthesised two PAMAM dendrimer-trastuzumab conjugates that carried docetaxel or paclitaxel, specifically targeted to cells which overexpressed HER-2. Results depicted that AMAM-drug-trastuzumab conjugates in particular showed extremely high toxicity toward the HER-2-positive SKBR-3 cells and very low toxicity towards to HER-2-negative MCF-7 cells. This confirmed the high selectivity of PAMAM-doc-trastuzumab and PAMAM-ptx-trastuzumab conjugates for HER-2-positive cells, and demonstrated the utility of trastuzumab as a targeting agent (Marcinkowska et al. 2019).

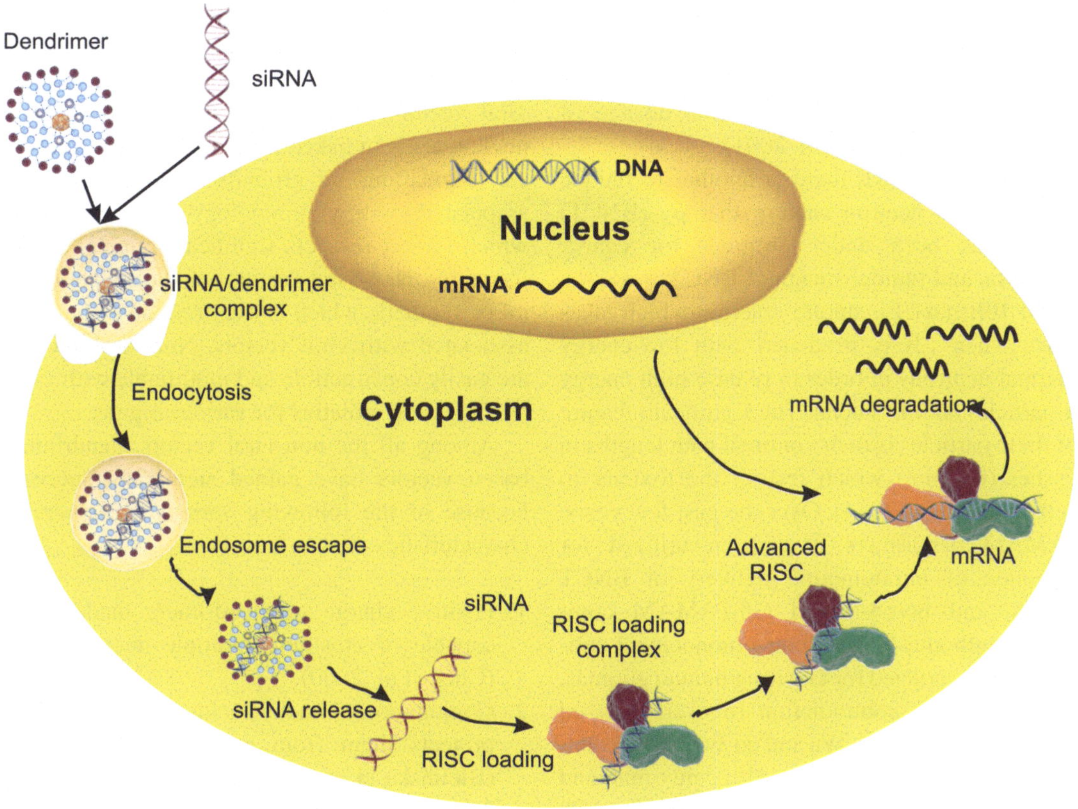

Fig. 2.8 Schematic representation of siRNA loading and unloading by dendrimer

2.5.2.2 Dendrimer Nanoarchitectures for Cancer Diagnosis

The precise identification of cancer is the very first and fundamental step towards effectual therapeutic management and further preventive measures for patients. The therapeutic management of cancer is classified according to various types of cancer; hence, its precise diagnosis becomes highly imperative. Several dendrimer-based therapeutic strategies have been explored so far which utilize cell type-reliant tumour-targeting prospective, which not only identifies explicitly cancer in its early stage but also remains fruitful from an economic and sentiment point of view. Magnetic resonance imaging (MRI) has already proven its utility in the field of cancer diagnosis (Caravan 2006), but the discovery of "dendrimer-based nanodevices" in MRI applications has significantly boosted this application.

The very first application of dendrimer in MRI-based cancer diagnosis was executed by Wiener et al. in the early 1990s. In their research, they tailored novel contrasting agent gadolinium chelates with PAMAM dendrimer. They found out that in contrast to plain gadolinium, dendrimer complexed with gadolinium triggered longitudinal relaxation more promptly and precisely. While the dendrimer without complexation has almost no effect on rates of relaxation, the rationale behind this is attributed to the fact that it is the high molecular weight of dendrimer that is responsible for significant alternations in the properties of gadolinium (Wiener et al. 1994).

In another study, a dendrimer-based contrasting agent has been utilized to explore micro-MRI. In this, DAB-AM64-(1B4M-Gd)64 contrast agent was administered at 0.03 mmol dose, to detect colon carcinoma tumour cells in mouse. Results depicted that DAB-AM64-

(1B4M-Gd)64 showed better images with enhanced intensity (without any background noise) of tumour in contrast to another agent utilizing dimeglumine-DTPA-Gd at a dosage of 0.1 mmol (Kobayashi et al. 2001).

Along with MRI, there is another technique named boron neutron capture therapy (BNCT) which has been under progress for cancer diagnosis and tumour imaging. BNCT works on lethal 10B(n,α)7Li capture reaction which takes place when $_{10}B$ is irradiated with low-energy thermal neutrons in order to release high energy α-particles and $_7Li$ nuclei. The significant feature of these particles is their confined path lengths in tissues (b_{10} mm) which restrict the toxicity to cells only (Moss 2014). Over the past few years, PAMAM dendrimers have been utilized for detection of intratumoural delivery of BNCT agents, and boron-loaded G5-PAMAM complexed with anti-EGF receptor monoclonal antibodies were utilized for targeting human gliomas, which acted in contradiction to overexpressed tumour cell receptors. Wu and co-workers in their study conjugated dendrimer with cetuximab and assessed its effect in vitro and in vivo on F98 cells in contrast to free cetuximab. Results showed that after intratumoural injections in rats, there was 13.8 times increment in tumour boron content for the targeted dendrimer in comparison with unchanged boron-mediated G5-PAMAM (Wu et al. 2004).

2.5.2.3 Dendrimers as Nanocarriers for Nucleic Acid and Drug Delivery in Cancer Therapy

Therapeutic management based on nucleic acid has already gained significant interest among researchers because of their biological compatibility and preciseness in contrast to generic chemotherapies. However, nucleic acids suffer from one drawback: because of their hydrophilic structure, it is very difficult for them to pass through cell membranes due to which they become susceptible to deprivation by enzymes in the blood vessels. Hence, there is a high demand for a potential delivery system that could not only prevent nucleic acids from such degradation but also transport and deliver them safely at specified locations. In order to resolve this issue, two major carriers have evolved for delivery of nucleic acid: viral- and non-viral-based vectors. Nonetheless, viral vectors bear higher efficiency to deliver nucleic acids in naked form which leads to critical trepidations on grounds of adverse effects associated with immunology and oncology, which further restricts significant clinical manifestations. Non-viral vectors are made up of natural or synthetic which is free from all difficulties associated with viral vectors. Non-viral vectors are easily constructible and modifiable with various targeting moieties for various organs.

Among all the non-viral vectors, dendrimer-based vectors have gained significant success, because of the following various idiosyncratic characteristics:

1. Positive charge on dendrimers made them capable of attaching multiple nucleic acids (Chen et al. 2000).
2. Conjugation of nucleic acids with dendrimers protects them from enzymatic degradation (Bielinska et al. 1996; Bielinska et al. 1997; Tang and Szoka 1997).
3. The presence of tertiary amines in the structure of dendrimers simplifies the release of nucleic acid molecules with the help of "proton sponge" effect (Behr 1997).
4. Dendrimers bear talented surface which is capable enough to modify various functional groups as well as other targeting moieties.
5. Specific delivery of nucleic acids at a targeted location makes dendrimers superior over conventional polymers on the grounds of biological and chemical properties.

2.6 Quantum Dots (QDs): Potentials in Biomedical and Pharmaceutical Research

QD also is known as semiconductor nanocrystal, which consists of two basic parts, i.e. "core" and "shell", in which electrons in semiconductors invigorate to an excited state after receiving energy and emit radiations on returning to

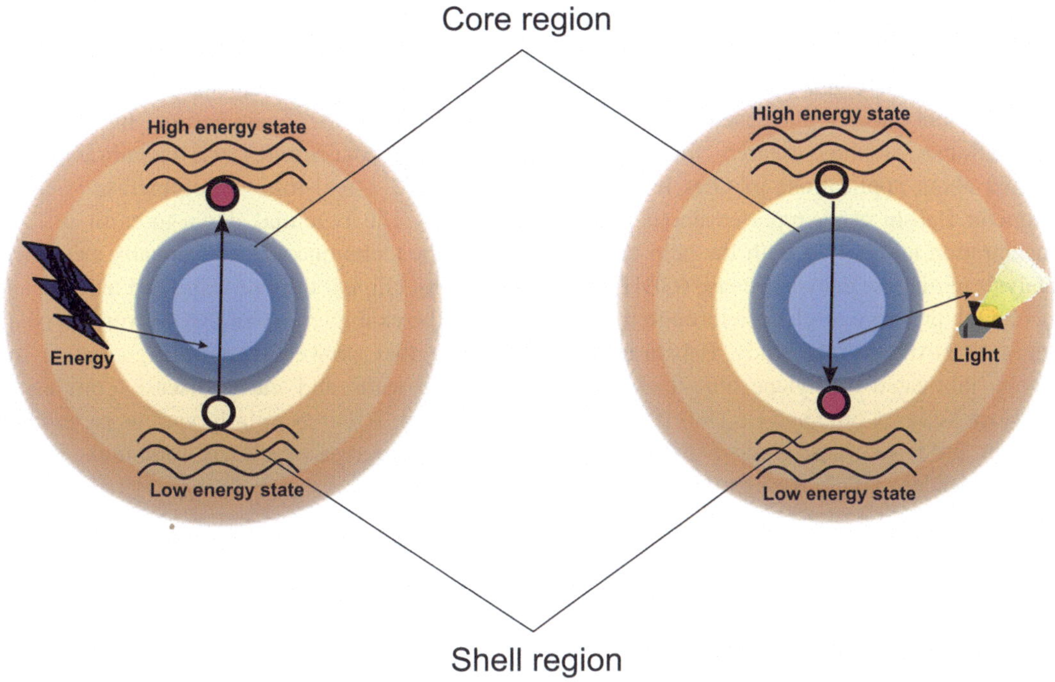

Fig. 2.9 Structure of QDs

the ground state (Fig. 2.9) (Valizadeh et al. 2012). Over the past few years, ODs have emerged as an impactful tool in biomedical research in the form of fluorescence imaging. The rationale behind QD's popularity is attributed to their enormous utility as luminous probing tool and as carrier for biomedical solicitation (Bera et al. 2010). QDs bear a wide range of applicability, but their size range especially between 1 and 10 nm allows them to glow remarkably upon excitation by various light sources especially lasers. Along with success of QDs in biomedical imaging (Wagner et al. 2019), QDs have also been utilized in clinical and translational research. Among which, one of the most significant applications of QDs is in drug delivery since they have the capability of explicating the pharmacokinetic and pharmacodynamics characteristics of therapeutic agents, which proffers the opportunities of fabricating principles for further drug and carrier engineering. In the subsequent sections, we will try to explore various potentials of QDs in pharmaceuticals.

2.6.1 Quantum Dots in Drug Delivery

The ability of QDs to specifically target debilitated cells and preclude healthy cells made QDs a potential option in drug delivery. Along with this, QDs can be easily loaded as fluorescent labels into complicated architecture or we can say complex drug delivery systems which proves them as impactful candidates in theranostic applications (Matea et al. 2017). Zhao et al. exploited hybrid silica nanocapsules in theranostic approach by loading them with ZnSe:Mn/ZnS core shell and anticancer drug paclitaxel; they utilized the set in chemotherapy and fluorescent imaging. The results of the study depicted solubility enhancement of paclitaxel up to 600 times (Zhao et al. 2017). Tailoring of QDs with various elements and allotropes has also come up as a good option in drug delivery; in one of the recent studies, graphene QDs were conjugated with neuroprotective peptide glycine-proline-glutamate and tested in APP/PS1 transgenic mice to combat against Alzheimer's disease. Results furnished exciting outcomes, the set-up promoted inhibitory effect on the accumulation of amyloid-β fibrils and the population of newly generated neuronal precursor cells substantially increased (Xiao et al. 2016). Some of the research findings also reported about applications of QDs in diabetes treatment; Bahshi et al. reported about glucose concentration monitoring with the help of QDs. Catalysis of glucose dehydrogenase (GDH) takes place in the presence of glucose through the production of NADH; in the study, Bahshi and co-workers fabricated methylene blue-loaded QDs with Hops Yellow Core Shell EviDots (CdSe/ZnS QDs) in order to track glucose oxidation by NAD^+-dependent GDH. Results depicted detection limit of glucose of up to 1×10^{-5} $_M$ (Bahshi et al. 2009).

2.6.2 Quantum Dots as Biosensors

QDs have also made their strong position in the field of biodetection analysis since they have the capability of accelerating the sensitivity and its reliability. Li et al. conducted fruitful research on exploring the potential of QDs in detection of levels of ceruloplasmin in human plasma. Ceruloplasmin is a very important enzymatic molecule of human blood since it consists more than 95% of total copper in individual's plasma, and low levels of this component indicate serious health concerns like Wilson disease and Menkes disease. Li and co-workers fabricated QDs with lateral flow test strip which was utilized to smidgen the quantity of ceruloplasmin. Results depicted that the developed system was proficient enough to measure 1 ng mL_{-1} nitrated ceruloplasmin just within 10 min (Li et al. 2010). In another study by Deng et al., QDs were utilized as biosensor in miRNA conjecture. In this exploration, QDs were utilized as splendid photostable names that preferred great discovery effectiveness for the biosensor. A target-recycled enhancement system dependent on sequence-specific barrette strand relocation process without the help of chemicals was furthermore acquainted with the framework to expand affectability. The detecting stage could distinguish miRNAs in the focus scope of 2–200 fmol with a point of confinement of 200 amol. In addition, miRNA examination in different tumour cell concentrates was tantamount with quantitative real-time polymerase chain response. The potential down-to-earth utilization of the technique was additionally examined by testing clinical tumour tests, and a dominant part of the examples (16 of 20) delivered a positive flag that showed incredible guarantee for straightforward and early disease conclusion (Deng et al. 2017). Similarly various researches are under progress which will soon make QDs a market success.

2.6.3 Quantum Dots in Cell Labelling

QDs possess a widespread absorption profile, due to which they can be excited at any wavelength which makes them an ideal candidate for long-term multicolour cell labelling. QD bears the advantage of being resistant towards photobleaching in contrast to traditional organic dyes. One of the studies from the past depicted potential utilization of QDs in which actin filaments were targeted by utilizing phalloidin by exposing to streptavidin and biotinylated QDs in a double-packed layered system; charged QDs successfully labelled the nucleus (Bruchez et al. 1998). In another study, QDs were labelled with transferrin and delivered into HeLa cells and compared with plain QDs; result depicted successful delivery of transferrin-labelled QDs. This study proved QDs as potential performer as fluorophores inside the cells, which can be utilized as successful strategy for intracellular delivery (Chan and Nie 1998). From there on several exploratory findings reported about cellular labelling by QDs. Jaiswal and co-workers utilized luminescent QDs to label live cells and determine their utility in long-term multicolour imaging. They developed two process systems, one for endocytic uptake of QDs and another for selective labelling of cell surface protein on the conjugation of QDs with antibodies. Results furnished positive outcomes in the form of consistently labelled cells which retained for more than a week (Jaiswal et al. 2003).

2.6.4 Quantum Dots in Diagnostics

QDs are also known for their high photoluminescence (PL), extinction coefficients and photostability characteristics which parade interesting photosensitive and electrical behaviours. These properties have accelerated immense interest among research persons working on relationship between quantum computing and high sensitivity in vivo diagnostics, which give birth to numerous productive outcomes that revolutionized the world of medical and pharmaceutical science.

2.6.4.1 Immunolabelling

QDs are miniscule light-transmitting particles on the nanometre scale and signify another class of fluorescent marks for medical and pharmaceutical science. In contrast to traditional fluorophores, organic colours and fluorescent proteins, QDs have exceptional optical properties, presenting focal points for biomedical application. These are size-adjustable symmetric, limited discharge range, expansive assimilation range and high protection from photobleaching. In malignant growth diagnostics, fluorescent nanoparticles, for example, QDs combined with malignancy explicit focusing on bearers are exceedingly encouraging operators for fluorescent labelling and assurance of resistant status of tumours, just as for picturing of fringe metastases (Gao et al. 2004).

2.6.4.2 Nucleic Acid Detection

Two-shading natural colours are typically utilized for happenstance recognitions and single-pair fluorescence reverberation vitality transfer detection (spFRET) (Wabuyele et al. 2003); conversely their utilitarian restrictions, for example, the spectral crosstalk and non-uniform fluorophore photograph fading rates, make resulting evaluation examination obfuscated. In alternate to this, QDs have expansive excitation and size-tunable photograph glow spectra with limited emanation data transfer capacity (fullwidth at half-limit of ~25–40 nm), remarkable photochemical steadiness and relative high quantum yield (Bruchez et al. 1998; Chan et al. 1998; Patolsky et al. 2003; Alivisatos 2004; Medintz et al. 2005). QDs have been utilized as fluorescent markers in the genomic examination, immunoassay, fluorescence imaging and medication delivery. Over the past recent few years, they have been utilized as a FRET benefactor in biosensors to recognize DNA and protein (Zhang et al. 2005).

2.6.4.3 Toxicity Quantification

Every individual sort of QD has its own kind of physicochemical properties, which thusly decides its potential poisonous quality or scarcity in that department. When all is said and done, there are errors in the present literature with respect to the poisonous quality of QDs that can be credited to a few factors: the absence of toxicology-based examinations, the assortment of QD dose/introduction fixations as mentioned in various literature and the generally shifting physicochemical properties of individual QDs (Akerman et al. 2002). Concentrates explicitly intended for toxicologic evaluation (e.g. portion, term, recurrence of introduction, instruments of activity) are not many. Huge numbers of the examinations from which QD toxicity data is determined and that have been referred to in reference to QD poisonous quality were performed by nanotechnology specialists as opposed to toxicologists or wellbeing researchers (Aldana et al. 2001).

Significantly, and a potential cradle of disarray in evaluating QD toxicity, QD toxicity relies upon various variables from both individual QD physicochemical properties and natural conditions: QD estimate, charge, focus, external covering bioactivity (topping material, utilitarian gatherings) and oxidative, photolytic and mechanical solidness have each been demonstrated to decide factors in QD toxicity (Beaurepaire et al. 2004). For instance, some QDs have been observed to be cytotoxic simply after oxidative or potentially photolytic debasement of their centre coatings. Lastly, in light of the fact that QD dose/introduction focuses revealed in the literature differ in their units of estimation (e.g. milligrams per millilitre, molarity, milligrams per kilogram body weight, number of QDs per cell), relating measurement crosswise over current investigations is testing.

2.7 Liposomes: Leading to Nanopharmaceuticals

Nanoliposomes (NPs) are modified artefacts of liposomes, having lipid vesicles of nanosized range (Abreu et al. 2011). NPs bear similar physical, structural and thermodynamic characteristics similar to liposomes except one factor, that is, stability. The bilayer lipid vesicle system in NPs imparts them long-term stability which conserves their nano-metric size range during storage and application (Mozafari 2010). Over the past few years, NPs have gained immense popularity in targeted therapy, which can be achieved via both mechanisms, i.e. active and passive. NPs provide freedom of fabricating or conjugating them with various bioactive/carrier systems to one or more targeting ligands like tissue or cell-explicit molecules in order to acquire active targeting (Sun et al. 2019). On the other hand, passive targeting is executed by complexation of NPs with bioactive carriers and release of bioactive agents from complex in vivo sites explicitly (Riaz et al. 2018). NPs have shown significant success in various medical conditions, especially in diabetes.

Prevalence of diabetes especially type II needs no more introduction now. Its increasing incidences worldwide are demanding novel and potential approaches for its better and stable therapeutic management. In contrast to conventional therapy, several novel approaches have been introduced so far in order to combat type II diabetes, among which NP formulation systems have satisfied formulation scientists up to a considerable limit. In one of the famous and recent studies, Yücel and co-workers established the forte of NPs in enhancing the potential of popular anti-diabetic molecule resveratrol (RSV). In the study, researchers had developed two different RSV-loaded NP systems and assessed them for anti-diabetic performance and oxidative stress. Results showed that novel NP system has significantly reduced blood glucose level in diabetic cell groups along with extended antioxidant activity against oxidative stress in contrast to pure RSV solution (Yücel et al. 2018).

2.8 Challenges for Nanoformulations

Augmentation in the efficacy of active therapeutic moieties and their ameliorated uptake is the chief factor behind evolution of nanoformulation system of drugs. In addition, try-outs on nanoformulations of drugs are consistently under progress with a motive to overcome concerns associated with conventional formulation system like stability of the developed formulation; improvisation in drug delivery; prevention of drugs from pre-expected degradation; and satisfactorily meeting FDA quality, standards and regulations. But the fulfilment of these criteria is not so easy for pharmaceutical research and industries formulating nanoformulations. The significant rationale behind this difficulty is the high propensity of nanoformulations towards self-aggregation especially at lower concentrations, eventually leading to deprived stability of final formulation (Barenholz et al. 1993; Barenholz 2012) and crucial variations in entrapment efficiency of drugs which are probably due to high polydispersity indexing (Tiyaboonchai 2003; Kharia et al. 2012). This speculation is supported by some research findings conducted in the past. For example, Berenholz and team fabricated doxorubicin in nanoformulation to improvise its efficacy, but unfortunately outcomes weren't fruitful. Doxorubicin underwent self-aggregation because of elevated ionic efficiency which enlarged its size and ultimately affected its stability (Barenholz 2007; Gabizon and Barenholz

2010) and solubility in biological solutions (Liu et al. 2008).

Similarly one of the remarkable formulation "nanocapsules" works on mechanism of "swelling" in order to deliver drug at targeted site, but this mechanism turned upside down for formulators since the intended swelling increases the size of formulation, which understandably affects the bioavailability and solubility (Choi et al. 2006) of the drug. However, trials are still being carried out to resolve this issue, e.g. in one of the recent researches, fruitful outcomes have come up, in which a pH-sensitive coating agent is utilized to control the swelling mechanism up to an optimum limit (Iyisan and Landfester 2019). With these obstacles, it is very difficult for pharmaceutical research and industries to successfully meet FDA standards and GMP criteria, and eventually this aspect makes nanoformulations ineligible for large-scale production.

2.9 Conclusion and Future Prospects

Undoubtedly, NNI initiation has done and will continue to put significant influence in the progress of novel therapeutic, diagnostic and/or theranostic methodologies. The amazing amalgamation between nanoscience, nanotechnology and pharmaceuticals unlocked several new horizons, which set new platforms for discovery and development of novel formulation systems. Upcoming researchers will get new opportunities for effective utilization of distinctive characteristics of nanosized materials in pharmaceuticals, which can combat critical and prevailing medical conditions with more impact. In addition, the focus must also be given on exploring new ways for manufacturing of nanopharmaceuticals at large scale along with satisfactory compliance with FDA standards and regulations, so that applicability of engineered nanopharmaceuticals can be taken to the next level and their fruitful applications can be made to produce nanomedicines with extraordinary benefits for clinical outcomes.

References

Abbasi E, Aval SF, Akbarzadeh A, Milani M, Nasrabadi HT, Joo SW, Hanifehpour Y, Koshki KN, Asl RP (2014) Dendrimers: synthesis, applications, and properties. Nanoscale Res Lett 9(1):247

Abreu AS, Castanheira EMS, Queiroz M, Ferreira P, Silva L, Pinto E (2011) Nanoliposomes for encapsulation and delivery of the potential antitumoral methyl 6-methoxy-3-(4-methoxyphenyl)-1H-indole-2-carboxylate. Nanoscale Res Lett 6(1):482

Akerman ME, Chan WCW, Laakkonen P, Bhatia SN, Ruoslahti E (2002) Nanocrystal targeting *in vivo*. Proc Natl Acad Sci U S A 99(20):12617–12621

Akhtar J, Siddiqui HH, Fareed S, Aqil M (2016) Nanoemulsion: for improved oral delivery of repaglinide. Drug Deliv 23(6):2026–2034

Aldana J, Wang YA, Peng X (2001) Photochemical instability of CdSe nanocrystals coated by hydrophilic thiols. J Am Chem Soc 123:8844–8850

Alivisatos AP (2004) The use of nanocrystals in biological detection. Nat Biotechnol 22:47–52

Aslan B, Ozpolat B, Sood AK, Berestein GL (2013) Nanotechnology in cancer therapy. J Drug Target 21(10):904–913

Babu A, Templeton AK, Munshi A, Ramesh R (2014) Nanodrug delivery systems: a promising technology for detection, diagnosis, and treatment of cancer. AAPS Pharm Sci Tech 15(3):709–721

Bahshi L, Freeman R, Gill R, Willner I (2009) Optical detection of glucose by means of metal nanoparticles or semiconductor quantum dots. Small 5:676–680

Baloch J, Sohail MF, Sarwar HS, Kiani MH, Khan GM, Jahan S, Rafay M, Chaudhry MT, Yasinzai M, Shahnaz G (2019) Self-Nanoemulsifying Drug Delivery System (SNEDDS) for improved oral bioavailability of chlorpromazine: in vitro and in vivo evaluation. Medicina (Kaunas) 55(5):210

Bangham AD, Standish MM, Watkins JC (1965) Diffusion of univalent ions across the lamellae of swollen phospholipids. J Mol Biol 13:238–252

Barenholz Y (2007) Amphipathic weak base loading into preformed liposomes having a transmembrane ammonium ion gradient: from the bench to approved DOXIL. In: Liposome technology: entrapment of drugs and other materials into liposomes, New York: Informa Healthcare. (3rd edn) vol 2, pp 1–25

Barenholz Y (2012) Doxil® – the first FDA-approved nano-drug: lessons learned. J Control Release 160(2):117–134

Barenholz Y, Amselem S, Goren D, Cohen R, Gelvan D, Samuni A, Golden EB, Gabizon A (1993) Stability of liposomal doxorubicin formulations: problems and prospects. Med Res Rev 13(4):449–491

Beaurepaire E, Buissette V, Sauviat MP, Giaume D, Lahlil K, Mercuri A (2004) Functionalized fluorescent oxide nanoparticles: artificial toxins for sodium channel targeting and imaging at the single-molecule level. Nano Lett 4(11):2079–2083

Behr JP (1997) The proton sponge: a trick to enter cells the viruses did not exploit. Chimia 51:34–36

Bera D, Qian L, Tseng T, Holloway P (2010) Quantum dots and their multimodal applications: a review. Materials (Basel) 3(4):2260–2345

Bernstein DI, Stanberry LR, Sacks S, Ayisi NK, Gong YH, Ireland J, Mumper RJ, Holan G, Matthews B, McCarthy T, Bourne N (2003) Evaluations of unformulated and formulated dendrimer-based microbicide candidates in mouse and guinea pig models of genital herpes. Antimicrob Agents Chemother 47(12):3784–3788

Bielinska AU, Kukowska-Latallo JF, Baker JR Jr (1996) Regulation of in vitro gene expression using antisense oligonucleotides or antisense expression plasmids transfected using starburst PAMAM dendrimers. Nucleic Acids Res 24:2176–2182

Bielinska AU, Kukowska-Latallo JF, Baker JR Jr (1997) The interaction of plasmid DNA with polyamidoamine dendrimers: mechanism of complex formation and analysis of alterations induced in nuclease sensitivity and transcriptional activity of the complexed DNA. Biochim Biophys Acta 1353:180–190

Binnewies M, Edward W, Kersten RK, Chan V, Fearon DF, Merad M, Coussens LM, Gabrilovich DI, Rosenberg SO, Hedrick CC, Vonderheide RH, Pittet MJ, Jain RK, Zou W, Howcroft TK, Woodhouse EC, Weinberg RA, Krummel MF (2018) Understanding the tumor immune microenvironment (TIME) for effective therapy. Nat Med 24(5):541–550

Bosman AW, Janssen HM, Meijer EW (1999) About dendrimers: structure, physical properties, and applications. Chem Rev 99(7):1665–1688

Bruchez M, Moronne M, Gin P, Weiss S, Alivisatos AP (1998) Semiconductor nanocrystals as fluorescent biological labels. Science 281:2013–2016

Caravan P (2006) Strategies for increasing the sensitivity of gadolinium based MRI contrast agents. Chem Soc Rev 35:512–523

Chan WC and Nie S (1998) Quantum dot bioconjugates for ultrasensitive nonisotopic detection. Science 281(5385): 2016–2018

Chen W, Turro NJ, Tomalia DA (2000) Using ethidium bromide to probe the interactions between DNA and dendrimers. Langmuir 16:15–19

Chingunpituk J (2007) Nanopsuspention technology for drug delivery. Walailak J Sci Technol 4(2):139–153

Choi SH, Lee JH, Choi SM, Park TG (2006) Thermally reversible pluronic/heparin nanocapsules exhibiting 1000-fold volume transition. Langmuir 22(4):1758–1762

Choi SR, Britigan BE, Narayanasamy P (2019) Treatment of Virulent Mycobacterium tuberculosis and HIV coinfected macrophages with gallium nanoparticles inhibits pathogen growth and modulates macrophage cytokine production. mSphere 24(4). pii: e00443–19

Deng H, Liu Q, Wang X, Huang R, Liu H, Lin Q, Zhou X, Xing D (2017) Quantum dots-labeled strip biosensor for rapid and sensitive detection of microRNA based on target-recycled nonenzymatic amplification strategy. Biosens Bioelectron 87:931–940

Din F, Aman W, Ullah I, Qureshi OS, Mustapha O, Shafique S, Zeb A (2017) Effective use of nanocarriers as drug delivery systems for the treatment of selected tumors. Int J Nanomedicine 12:7291–7309

Deoli M (2012) Nanosuspension technology for solubilizing poorly soluble drugs. International J. Drug Dev. and Research 4(4):40–49

Espinoza LC, Silva-Abreu M, Calpena AC, Rodríguez-Lagunas MJ, Fábrega MJ, Garduño-Ramírez ML, Clares B (2019) Nanoemulsion strategy of pioglitazone for the treatment of skin inflammatory diseases. Nanomedicine 19:115–125

Fofaria NM, Qhattal HS, Liu X, Srivastava SK (2016) Nanoemulsion formulations for anti-cancer agent piplartine – characterization, toxicological, pharmacokinetics and efficacy studies. Int J Pharm 498(1–2):12–22

Forssen EA, Tökès ZA (1981) Use of anionic liposomes for the reduction of chronic doxorubicin-induced cardiotoxicity. Proc Natl Acad Sci U S A 78(3):1873–1877

Gabizon AA, Barenholz Y (2010) Method for drug loading in liposomes. Google Patents

Ganta S, Singh A, Kulkarni P, Keeler AW, Piroyan A, Sawant RR, Patel NR, Davis B, Ferris C, O'Neal S, Zamboni W, Amiji MM, Coleman TP (2015) EGFR targeted theranostic nanoemulsion for image-guided ovarian cancer therapy. Pharm Res 32(8):2753–2763

Gao X, Cui Y, Levenson RM, Chung WK, Nie S (2004) In vivo cancer targeting and imaging with semiconductor quantum dots. Nat Biotechnol 22(8):969–976

Gao Y, Sun M, Guo C, Yu A, Xi Y, Cui J, Lou H, Zhai G (2011) Preparation and characterization of intravenously injectable curcumin nanosuspension. Drug Deliv 18(2):131–142

Ge W, Hu P, Huang Y, Wang XM, Zhang XM, Sun YJ, Li ZS, Si SY, Sui YF (2009) The antitumor immune responses induced by nanoemulsion-encapsulated MAGE1-HSP70/SEA complex protein vaccine following different administration routes. Oncol Rep 22(4):915–920

Gladwin MT, Plorde JT, Martin TR (1998) Clinical application of the Mycobacterium Tuberculosis direct test: case report, literature review and proposed clinical alogrothim. Chest 114(1):317–323

Goel S, Sachdeva M, Agarwal V (2019) Nanosuspension technology: recent patents on drug delivery and their characterizations. Recent Pat Drug Deliv Formul 13:91. https://doi.org/10.2174/187221131366619061 4151615

Gong Y, Matthews B, Cheung D, Tam T, Gadawski I, Leung D, Holan G, Raff J, Sacks S (2002) Evidence of dual sites of action of dendrimers: SPL-2999 inhibits both virus entry and late stages of herpes simplex virus replication. Antivir Res 55(2):319–329

Gonzales J, Kossatz S, Roberts S, Pirovano G, Brand C, Medina CP, Donabedian P, de la Cruz MJ, Mulder WM, Reiner T (2018) Nanoemulsion-based delivery of fluorescent PARP inhibitors in mouse models of small cell lung cancer. Bioconjug Chem 29(11):3776–3782

Gradishar WJ, Jjulandin S, Davidson N, Shaw H, Desai N, Bhar P, Hawkins M, Shaughnessy JO (2005) Phase III trial of NP albumin bound paclitaxel compared with polyethylated castor oil based paclitaxel in women with breast cancer. J Clin Oncol 23(31):7794–7803

Gupta D, Nguyen PYM (2014) Nanoparticles for superior pharmacokinestics and enhanced efficacy. J Dev Drug 3:2

Gupta A, Eral HB, Hatton TA, Doyle PS (2016) Nanoemulsions: formation, properties and applications. Soft Matter 12(11):2826–2841

Huang Q, Li L, Li L, Chen H, Dang YY, Zhang JS, Shao NM, Chang H, Zhou ZJ, Liu CY, He BW, Wei HF, Xiao JR (2016) MDM2 knockdown mediated by a triazine-modified dendrimer in the treatment of non-small cell lung cancer. Oncotarget 7(28):44013–44022

Iyisan B, Landfester K (2019) Modular approach for the design of smart polymeric nanocapsules. Macromol Rapid Commun 40(1):e1800577. https://doi.org/10.1002/marc.201800577

Jaiswal JK, Mattoussi H, Mauro JM, Simon SM (2003) Long-term multiple color imaging of live cells using quantum dot bioconjugates. Nat Biotechnol 21(1):47–51

Jaiswal M, Dudhe R, Sharma PK (2015) Nanoemulsion: an advanced mode of drug delivery system. Biotech 5(2):123–127

Janaszewska A, Lazniewska L, Trzepiński P, Marcinkowska M, Maculewicz K (2019) Cytotoxicity of dendrimers. Biomolecules 9(8):330

Jin X, Yijing L, Yang L, Yueqin M, Pengfei Y, Ming Y (2019) Novel redispersible nanosuspensions stabilized by co-processed nanocrystalline cellulose–sodium carboxymethyl starch for enhancing dissolution and oral bioavailability of baicalin. Int J Nanomedicine 14:353–369

Kaul G, Amiji MJ (2002) Long- circulating poly(ethyleneglycol)-modified gelatin nanoparticles for intracellular delivery. Pharm Res 19:1062–1068

Kayser O (2001) A new approach for targeting to cryptosporidium parvum using mucoadhesive nanosuspension: research and application. Int J Pharm 214:83–85

Kharia A, Singhai A, Verma R (2012) Formulation and evaluation of polymeric nanoparticles of an antiviral drug for gastroretention. Int J Pharm Sci Nanotechnol 4:1557–1562

Kim JE, Park YJ (2017a) Improved antitumor efficacy of hyaluronic acid-complexed paclitaxel nanoemulsions in treating non-small cell lung cancer. Biomol Ther (Seoul) 25(4):411–416

Kim JE, Park YJ (2017b) Paclitaxel-loaded hyaluronan solid nanoemulsions for enhanced treatment efficacy in ovarian cancer. Int J Nanomedicine 12:645–658

Knauer N, Pashkina E, Apartsin E (2019) Topological aspects of the design of nanocarriers for therapeutic peptides and proteins. Pharmaceutics 11(2):91

Kobayashi H, Saga T, Kawamoto S, Sato N, Hiraga A, Ishimori T, Konishi J, Togashi K, Brechbiel MW (2001) Dynamic micro – magnetic resonance iimaging of liver micrometastasis in mice with a novel liver macromolecular magnetic resonance contrast agent DAB-Am64-(1B4M-Gd)64. Cancer Res 61:4966–4970

Kohno S, Otuubo T, Tanaka E, Maruyaana K, Hara K (1997) Amphotericin B encapsulated in polyethylene glycol immunoliposomes for infectious disease. Adv Drug Del Rev 24:325–329

Kotta S, Khan AW, Pramod K, Ansari SH, Sharma RK, Ali J (2012) Exploring oral nanoemulsions for bioavailability enhancement of poorly water-soluble drugs. Expert Opin Drug Deliv 9(5):585–598

Krittika S, Indhumathi P, VedhaHari BN, Devi DR, Yadav P (2019) Evidence of nanoemulsion as an effective control measure for fruit flies Drosophila melanogaster. Sci Rep 9:10578

Kruk ME, Gage AD, Joseph NT, Danaei G, Saisó SG, Salomon JA (2018) Mortality due to low-quality health systems in the universal health coverage era: a systematic analysis of amenable deaths in 137 countries. Lancet 392(10160):2203–2212

Kuplennik N, Lang K, Steinfeld R, Sosnik A (2019) Folate receptor alpha-modified nanoparticles for the targeting of the central nervous system. ACS Appl Mater Interfaces 11:39633. https://doi.org/10.1021/acsami.9b14659

Landers JJ, Cao Z, Lee I, Piehler LT, Myc PP, Myc A, Hamouda T, Galecki AT, Baker JR (2002) Prevention of influenza pneumonitis by sialic acid-conjugated dendritic polymers. Infect Dis 186:1222

Langer R, Folkman J (1976) Polymers for the sustained release of proteins and other macromolecules. Nature 263:797–800

Leone F, Cavalli R (2015) Drug nanosuspensions: a ZIP tool between traditional and innovative pharmaceutical formulations. Expert Opin Drug Deliv 12(10):1607–1625

Leong KW, Mao HQ, Truong LVL (1998) DNA- polycation nanospheres as non viral gene delivery vehicles. J Control Release 53:183–193

Li Z, Wang Y, Wang J, Tang Z, Pounds JG, Lin Y (2010) Rapid and sensitive detection of protein biomarker using a portable fluorescence biosensor based on quantum dots and a lateral flow test strip. Anal Chem 82(16):7008–7014

Liu Z, Jiao Y, Wang Y, Zhou C, Zhang Z (2008) Polysaccharides-based nanoparticles as drug delivery systems. Adv Drug Deliv Rev 60(15):1650–1662

Liu XX, Liu C, Catapano CV, Peng L, Zhou JH, Rocchi P (2014) Structurally flexible triethanolamine-core poly(amidoamine) dendrimers as effective nanovectors to deliver RNAibased therapeutics. Biotechnol Adv 32(4):844–852

Luganini A, Nicoletto SF, Pizzuto L, Pirri G, Giuliani A, Landolfo S, Gribaudo G (2011) Inhibition of herpes simplex virus type 1 and type 2 infections by peptide-derivatized dendrimers. Antimicrob Agents Chemother 55(7):3231–3239

Mahto R (2017) Nanoemulsion as targeted drug delivery system for cancer therapeutics. J Pharm Sci Pharmacol 3:83–97
Marcinkowska M, Stanczyk M, Janaszewska A, Sobierajska E, Chworos A, Klajnert-Maculewicz B (2019) Multicomponent conjugates of anticancer drugs and monoclonal antibody with PAMAM dendrimers to increase efficacy of HER-2 positive breast cancer therapy. Pharm Res 36(11):154
Marty JJ, Oppenheim RC, Speiser P (1978) Nanoparticles – a new colloidal drug delivery system. Pharm Acta Helv 53(1):17–23
Matea CT, Mocan T, Tabaran F, Pop T, Mosteanu O, Puia C, Iancu C, Mocan L (2017) Quantum dots in imaging, drug delivery and sensor applications. Int J Nanomedicine 12:5421–5431
Medintz IL, Uyeda HT, Goldman E, Mattoussi H (2005) Quantum dot bioconjugates for imaging, labelling and sensing. Nat Mater 4:437–446
Migotto A, Carvalho VFM, Salata GC, da Silva FWM, Yan CYI, Ishida K, Costa-Lotufo LV, Steiner AA, Lopes LB (2018) Multifunctional nanoemulsions for intraductal delivery as a new platform for local treatment of breast cancer. Drug Deliv 25(1):654–667
Mittal N, Kaur G (2019) Investigations on polymeric nanoparticles for ocular delivery. Adv Polym Technol 2019:1–14
Monteagudom S, Perez-Martinez FC, Perez-Carrion MD, Guerra J, Merino S, Sanchez-Verdu MP, Cena V (2012) Inhibition of p42 MAPK using a nonviral vector-delivered siRNA potentiates the anti-tumor effect of metformin in prostate cancer cells. Nanomedicine 7(4):493–506
Moss RL (2014) Critical review, with an optimistic outlook, on boron neutron capture therapy (BNCT). Appl Radiat Isot 88:2–11
Mozafari MR (2010) Nanoliposomes: preparation and analysis. Methods Mol Biol 605:29–50
Muhamad N, Plengsuriyakarn T, Bangchang KN (2018) Application of active targeting nanoparticle delivery system for chemotherapeutic drugs and traditional/herbal medicines in cancer therapy: a systematic review. Int J Nanomedicine 13:3921–3935
Muller RH, Gohla S, Dingler A, Schneppe T, Wise D (2000) Handbook of pharmaceutical controlled release technology. Marcel Dekker. Large-scale production of solid-lipid nanoparticles (SLN) and nanosuspension (Dissocubes), New York, pp 359–375
Mustapha O, Kim KS, Shafique S, Kim DS, Jin SG, Seo YG, Youn YS, Oh KT, Lee BJ, Park YJ, Yong CS, Kim JO, Choi HG (2016) Development of novel cilostazol-loaded solid SNEDDS using a SPG membrane emulsification technique: physicochemical characterization and in vivo evaluation. Colloids Surf B Biointerfaces 150:216–222
Muzammil AS, Naidu VG, Harishankar N, Kishan V (2016) Albumin anchored docetaxel lipid nanoemulsion for improved targeting efficiency – preparation, characterization, cytotoxic, antitumor and in vivo imaging studies. Drug Deliv 23(4):1355–1363
Nakhlband A, Eskandani M, Omidi Y, Saeedi N, Ghaffari S, Barar J, Garjani A (2018) Combating atherosclerosis with targeted nanomedicines: recent advances and future prospective. Bioimpacts 8(1):59–75
Nasimi P, Haidari M (2013) Medical use of nanoparticles: drug delivery and diagnosis diseases. Int J Green Nanotechnol 1:194308921350697. https://doi.org/10.1177/1943089213506978
Nasiruddin M, Neyaz MK, Das S (2017) Nanotechnology based approaches in tuberculosis treatment. Tuberc Res Treat 4920209:12
Nasr A, Gardouh A, Ghorab M (2016) Novel Solid Self-Nanoemulsifying Drug Delivery System (S-SNEDDS) for oral delivery of olmesartan medoxomil: design, formulation, pharmacokinetic and bioavailability evaluation. Pharmaceutics 8(3):20–29
Panda BP, Kirshnamoorthy R, Hawala NK, Gowda S, Patnaik S (2018) Influence of poloxamer 188 on design and development of second generation PLGA nanocrystals of metformin HCL. Nano Biomed Eng 10(4):334–343
Pandey R, Sharma S, Khuller GK (2004) Nebulisation of liposomes encapsulated antitubercular drugsin guinea pigs. Int J Antimicrob Drugs 24(1):93–94
Pandey R, Sharma S, Khuller GK (2005) Oral solid lipid nanoparticlesbased antitubercular chemotherapy. Tuberculosis 85(5–6):415–420
Pangeni R, Choi SW, Jeon OC, Byun Y, Park JW (2016) Multiple nanoemulsion system for an oral combinational delivery of oxaliplatin and 5-fluorouracil: preparation and in vivo evaluation. Int J Nanomedicine 11:6379–6399
Pardridge WM (2012) Drug transport across the blood–brain barrier. J Cereb Blood Flow Metab 32(11):1959–1972
Pastar I, Stojadinovic O, Yin NC, Raminez H, Nusbaum AG, Sawaya A, Patel SB, Khalid L, Isseroff RR, Canic MT (2014) Epithilisation in wound healing: a comprehensive review. Adv Wound Care 3(7):445–464
Patel VR, Agrawal YK (2011) Nanosuspension: an approach to enhance solubility of drugs. J Adv Pharm Technol Res 2(2):81–87
Patil JS, Sarasija S (2012) Pulmonary drug delivery strategies: a concise, systematic review. Lung India 29(1):44–49
Patolsky F, Gill R, Weizmann Y, Mokari T, Banin U, Willner I (2003) Electron-transfer quenching of nucleic acid-functionalized CdSe/ZnS quantum dots by doxorubicin: a versatile system for the optical detection of DNA, aptamer–substrate complexes and telomerase activity. J Am Chem Soc 125:13918–13919
Prabhakaran D et al (2018) The changing patterns of cardiovascular diseases and their risk factors in the states of India: the global burden of disease study 1990–2016. Lancet Glob Health 6(12):e1339–e1351
Qelliny MR, Aly UF, Elgarhy OH, Khaled KA (2019) Budesonide-loaded Eudragit S 100 nanocapsules for the treatment of acetic acid-induced colitis in animal model. AAPS PharmSciTech 20(6):237

Rahman MA, Mujahid M (2018) Development of self-nanoemulsifying tablet (SNET) for bioavailability enhancement of sertraline. Braz J Pharm Sci 54. https://doi.org/10.1590/s2175-97902018000117232

Rai R, Alwani S, Badea I (2019) Polymeric nanoparticles in gene therapy: new avenues of design and optimization for delivery applications. Polymers (Basel) 11(4):745

Rajendran NK, Sundar S, Kumar D, Houreld NN, Abrahamse H (2018) A review on nanoparticle based treatment for wound healing. J Drug Deliv Sci Technol 44:421–430

Reuter JD, Myc A, Hayes MM, Gan Z, Roy R, Qin D, Yin R, Piehler LT, Esfand R, Tomalia DA, Baker JR Jr (1999) Inhibition of viral adhesion and infection by sialic-acid-conjugated dendritic polymers. Bioconjug Chem 10:271

Riaz MK, Riaz MA, Zhang X, Lin C, Wong KH, Chen X, Zhang G, Lu A, Yang Z (2018) Surface functionalization and targeting strategies of liposomes in solid tumor therapy: a review. Int J Mol Sci 19(1):195

Roberts S, Andreou C, Choi C, Donabedian P, Jayaraman M, Edwinn C, Tang PB, Medina C, Cruz J, Mulder W, Grimm J, Kircher M, Reiner T (2018) Sonophore-enhanced nanoemulsions for optoacoustic imaging of cancer. Chem Sci 9(25):5646–5657

Sahu P, Das D, Mishra VK, Kashaw V, Kashaw SK (2017) Nanoemulsion: a novel eon in cancer chemotherapy. Mini Rev Med Chem 17(18):1778–1792

Schinazi RF, Brettreich M, Hirsch A (2003) In United States patent and trademark office; number 20030036562; www.uspto.gov

Shahba AW, Mohsin K, Alanazi FK (2012) Novel Self-Nanoemulsifying Drug Delivery Systems (SNEDDS) for oral delivery of cinnarizine: design, optimization, and in-vitro assessment. AAPS PharmSciTech 13(3):967–977

Shahba AA, Ahmed AR, Mohsin K, Abdel-Rahman SI, Alanazi FK (2017) Solidification of cinnarizine self-nanoemulsifying drug delivery systems by fluid bed coating: optimization of the process and formulation variables. Pharmazie 72(3):143–151

Shanmugapriya K, Kim H, Kang HW (2019) In vitro antitumor potential of astaxanthin nanoemulsion against cancer cells via mitochondrial mediated apoptosis. Int J Pharm 5(560):334–346

Shi R, Hong L, Wu D, Ning X, Chen Y, Lin T, Fan D, Wu K (2005) Enhanced immune response to gastric cancer specific antigen peptide by coencapsulation with CpG oligodeoxynucleotides in nanoemulsion. Cancer Biol Ther 4(2):218–224

Shinde UA, Joshi PN, Jain DD, Singh K (2019) Preparation and evaluation of N-trimethyl chitosan nanoparticles of flurbiprofen for ocular delivery. Curr Eye Res 44(5):575–582

Silva GA (2008) Nanotechnology approaches to crossing the blood brain barrier and delivery to the CNS. BMC Neurosci 9:54

Sultana S, Khan R, Kumar M, Kumar S (2012) Nanoparticle mediated drug delivery approaches for cancer targeting: a review. J Drug Target 21(2):712130

Sun Y, Wang H, Wang P, Zhang K, Geng X, Liu Q, Wang X (2019) Tumor targeting DVDMS-nanoliposomes for an enhanced sonodynamic therapy of gliomas. Biomater Sci 7(3):985–994

Tang MX, Szoka FC (1997) The influence of polymer structure on the interactions of cationic polymers with DNA and morphology of the resulting complexes. Gene Ther 4:823–832

Tiyaboonchai W (2003) Chitosan nanoparticles: a promising system for drug delivery. Naresuan Univ J 11(3):51–66

Tong Y, Wang Y, Yang M, Yang J, Chen L, Chu X, Gao C, Jin Q, Gong W, Gao C (2018) Systematic development of self-nanoemulsifying liquisolid tablets to improve the dissolution and oral bioavailability of an oily drug, vitamin K1. Pharmaceutics 10(3). https://doi.org/10.3390/pharmaceutics10030096

Valizadeh A, Mikaeili H, Samiei M, Farkhani SS, Zarghami N, Kouhi M, Akbarzadeh A, Davaran S (2012) Quantum dots: synthesis, bioapplications, and toxicity. Nanoscale Res Lett 7(1):480

Wabuyele MB, Farquar H, Stryjewski W, Hammer RP, Soper SA, Cheng Y, Barany F (2003) Approaching real-time molecular diagnostics: single-pair fluorescence resonance energy transfer (spFRET) detection for the analysis of low abundant point mutations in K-ras oncogenes. J Am Chem 125:6937–6945

Wagner AM, Knipe JM, Orive G, Peppas NA (2019) Quantum dots in biomedical applications. Acta Biomater 94:44–63

Wang Z, Wn J, Zhou O, Wang Y, Chen T (2015) Berberine nanosuspension enhances hypoglycemic efficacy on streptozatocinn induced diabetic C57BL/6 mice. Evid Based Complement Altern Med 239479:5

Wiener EC, Brechbiel MW, Brothers H, Magin RL, Gansow OA, Tomalia DA, Lauterbur PC (1994) Dendrimer – based metal chelates: a new class of magnetic resonance imaging contrast agents. Magn Reson Med 31:1–8

Wu G, Barth RF, Yang W, Chatterjee M, Tjarks W, Ciesielski MJ, Fenstermaker RA (2004) Site-specific conjugation of boron-containing dendrimers to anti-EGF receptor monoclonal antibody cetuximab (IMCC225) and its evaluation as a potential delivery agent for neutron capture therapy. Bioconjug Chem 15:185–194

World Health Organization (2018). Newsroom factsheet on cancer. Retrieved from who.int/news-room/fact-sheets/detail/cancer.

Xiao S, Zhou D, Luan P, Gu B, Feng L, Fan S, Liao W, Fang W, Yang L, Tao E, Guo R, Liu J (2016) Graphene quantum dots conjugated neuroprotective peptide improve learning and memory capability. Biomaterials 106:98–110

Xu J, Wang H, Xu L, Chao Y, Wang C, Han X, Dong Z, Chang H, Peng R, Cheng Y, Liu Z (2019) Nanovaccine based on a protein-delivering dendrimer for effective antigen cross-presentation and cancer immunotherapy. Biomaterials 207:1–9

Yan C, Gu J, Hou D, Jing H, Wang J, Guo Y, Katsumi H, Sakane T, Yamamoto A (2015) Improved tumor targetability of Tat-conjugated PAMAM dendrimers as a novel nanosized anti-tumor drug carrier. Drug Dev Ind Pharm 41(4):617–622

Yan S, Zeng X, Tang Y, Liu BF, Wang Y, Liu X (2019) Activating antitumor immunity and antimetastatic effect through polydopamine-encapsulated core-shell upconversion nanoparticles. Adv Mater 31(46):e1905825

Yücel Ç, Karatoprak GŞ, Aktaş Y (2018) Nanoliposomal resveratrol as a novel approach to treatment of diabetes mellitus. J Nanosci Nanotechnol 18(6):3856–3864

Zahoor A, Sharma S, Khuller GK (2005) Inhalable alginate nanoparticles as antitubercular drug carriers against experimental tuberculosis. Int J Antimicrobial Agents 26:298–303

Zhang CY, Yeh HC, Kuroki MT, Wang TH (2005) Single-quantum-dot-based DNA nanosensor. Nat Mater 4:826–831

Zhao T, Liu X, Li Y, Zhang M, He J, Zhang X, Liu H, Wang X, Gu H (2017) Fluorescence and drug loading properties of ZnSe:Mn/ZnS-Paclitaxel/SiO2 nanocapsules templated by F127 micelles. J Colloid Interface Sci 490:436–443

Zhao CY, Cheng R, Yang Z, Tian ZM (2018) Nanotechnology for cancer therapy based on chemotherapy. Molecules 23(4):826

Zhou HY, Hao JL, Wang S, Zeng Y, Zhang WS (2013) Nanoparticles in ocular drug delivery. Int J Opthalmol 6(3):390–396

3 Preformulation Challenges: The Concept Behind the Selection, Design and Preparation of Nanoformulations

Krishna Kumar Patel, Ashish Kumar Agrawal, and Sanjay Singh

Abstract

Nano-drug delivery carriers have fascinated researchers worldwide for the last two to three decades. The nanoformulations are preferred over conventional dosage forms as they provide improved drug solubility, bioavailability, drug stability under adverse external or physiological conditions, controlled drug release for prolonged action and target specificity using ligand binding and many more. Multiple essential aspects must be carefully studied and implemented for the development of efficient drug delivery vehicles. These aspects include rationale of nanoparticle preparation; use of polymeric or lipid nanoparticle; selection of polymer, lipid and excipients; method of preparation; screening of critical formulation or process parameters that affect the critical quality attributes; optimization of process to obtain the desired formulation characteristics; characterization of nanoparticles; strategy to improve the low entrapment efficiency and stability, etc. This chapter comprehensively summarizes all these aspects of nanoformulation development and proposes solutions for these challenges. Although a variety of nanoformulations have been described in literature, this chapter is restricted to discuss in detail the liposomes and polymeric and lipid nanoparticles.

Keywords

Nanoformulation · Polymeric nanoparticles · Liposomes · Lipid nanoparticles · Characterization of nanoparticles · Micelles · Design of experiments

K. K. Patel · A. K. Agrawal (✉)
Department of Pharmaceutical Engineering & Technology, Indian Institute of Technology (Banaras Hindu University), IIT (BHU), Varanasi, Uttar Pradesh, India
e-mail: ashish.phe@iitbhu.ac.in

S. Singh
Department of Pharmaceutical Engineering & Technology, Indian Institute of Technology (Banaras Hindu University), IIT (BHU), Varanasi, Uttar Pradesh, India

Babasaheb Bhimrao Ambedkar University, Lucknow, Uttar Pradesh, India

3.1 Introduction

Nanotechnology, a multifaceted development in science, has emerged as a breakthrough providing superiority over conventional technology due to robustness, accuracy and higher efficiency over the conventional approaches. Specifically, in medical science, researchers have explored several applications of nanotechnology including diagnostics, medical devices, imaging systems,

S. Talegaonkar, M. Rai (eds.), *Nanoformulations in Human Health*,
https://doi.org/10.1007/978-3-030-41858-8_3

drug delivery, etc. For the past few decades, extensive research conducted worldwide has directed us to learn the broader and multiple applications of nanotechnology in drug delivery. The delivery system, with improved pharmaceutical aspects, encapsulating the drug within the nanostructured matrix ranging from 50 to 500 nm, is generally considered as a nano-drug delivery carrier. Nano-drug delivery system commendably overcomes the limitation of conventional dosage forms (tablets, capsules, powders, gels, etc.) such as low solubility, low bioavailability, frequent dosing, high dose, low stability, toxicity, low permeation across the skin and many more (Jain et al. 2014a, b, c; Kaler et al. 2014; Uchechi et al. 2014; Agrawal et al. 2017a, b).

Mostly, the nanoparticle matrix is either polymeric or lipid-based (solid lipid nanoparticle, nanostructured lipid carrier), and the optimization process of nanoparticles involves the consideration of several critical issues. Interestingly, the rationale of nanoformulation; the selection of polymer, lipid and excipients; solvent system; and method of preparation further depend upon the drug's physicochemical properties, application purpose and route of administration. Moreover, the optimization of nanoformulations with desired characteristics, improvement of drug encapsulation within the matrix and production of stable formulation are the most challenging tasks while preparing the nano-drug delivery system. This chapter covers all such aspects precisely and elaborates on the importance of each step during the preparation of nanoformulations.

3.2 Rationale of Nanoformulations

Nanoformulations possess several advantages over the conventional delivery systems and thus were found to have several applications depending upon the need. Examples of various nanoparticles developed in contemporary research with various objectives/rationales are listed in Table 3.1. A list of marketed nanoformulation has also been provided in Table 3.2.

The rational of developing nanoformulations has been illustrated in Fig. 3.1 and described in the following sections.

3.2.1 Increase the Solubility of Poorly Soluble Drugs

Several studies based on nanotechnology approaches to improve the solubility and thus the absorption and bioavailability of drugs, which ultimately reduces the required dose, have been reported (Jain et al. 2013a, b; Rai et al. 2016). Approximately, 40% of the available drugs in the market are either weak acid or weak base and mostly suffer from low solubility in water or physiological fluids (Lipinski 2002). Even though the lipophilic drugs show higher diffusion coefficient and absorbance from the gut, the drug with low water solubility (lipophilic) possesses low bioavailability (dissolution is an essential criterion for absorption, and only solubilized or molecularly dispersed drug can diffuse across the biological membranes; thus, insoluble drugs impede the diffusion of drug across the biological membrane). The nanoparticles have proven to improve the water solubility of the entrapped drug by enhancing the surface area-to-volume ratio and thereby offer the higher surface area for dissolution in vitro or in vivo. Thus, improving the dissolution rate ultimately improves diffusion and bioavailability (Chen et al. 2011). Apart from that, a drug with low water solubility requires a higher dose to meet the therapeutic need and concentration in blood. The nanoparticle efficiently reduces the dose by improving solubility, permeation and bioavailability (Hu et al. 2004).

The dissolution phenomenon can be easily understood by Noyes-Whitney equation:

$$\frac{dC}{dt} = \frac{\text{Diffusion coefficient of the drug in solution} \times \text{Surface area}}{\text{thickness of diffusion layer}} \times \left(C_s - C\right) \tag{3.1}$$

Table 3.1 A summary of different applications of nanoparticles to overcome the challenges of drug delivery

Drug	Nanoformulation and objective	References
Nanoparticle for improving the solubility and bioavailability		
Cyclosporine	Solid lipid nanoparticles of cyclosporine developed successfully and demonstrated improved water solubility and oral bioavailability	El-Shabouri (2002), Potta et al. (2010)
Raloxifene	Raloxifene loaded HPMC nanoparticles was optimized to improve the water solubility	Suthar et al. (2011)
Risperidone	Spray-dried polymeric nanoparticles of risperidone is fabricated which claimed to improve the solubility of drug and its bioavailability	Nair et al. (2019)
Vinpocetine	Solid lipid nanoparticles of vinpocetine is developed and exhibited improved oral bioavailability	Luo et al. (2006)
Insulin	Dextran sulphate/chitosan nanoparticle enriched with insulin shown to improve oral bioavailability due to improved stability	Sarmento et al. (2007)
Curcumin	Oral bioavailability of curcumin was improved multiple-fold when encapsulated in the biodegradable polymeric nanoparticles	Shaikh et al. (2009)
Doxorubicin	The doxorubicin was efficiently encapsulated in the dendrimers to increase its oral bioavailability	Ke et al. (2008)
Nanoparticle reduces the toxicity of drugs		
Temozolomide	The cardiac toxicity and nephrotoxicity of temozolomide is significantly minimized when loaded in the solid lipid nanoparticles. Moreover, the dose was also reduced	Huang et al. (2008)
Doxorubicin	The polyalkylcyanoacrylate nanoparticles of doxorubicin considerably reduced the systemic toxicity induced by doxorubicin	Couvreur et al. (1982)
Amphotericin B	Gelatin nanoparticles of amphotericin B with the objective to reduce the dosing frequency and severe nephrotoxicity side effects and toxicity	Nahar et al. (2008)
Imaging and diagnosis		
Temozolomide	Temozolomide-entrapped PLGA superparamagnetic nanoparticles were developed successfully for MRI and malignant glioma therapy	Ling et al. (2012)
Docetaxel	The polymeric nanoparticles simultaneously encapsulating the docetaxel and superparamagnetic iron oxide were developed to improve cancer targeting and tracking of nanoparticle distribution and aggregation simultaneously	Ling et al. (2011)
Brain targeting		
Doxorubicin	This study efficiently improved the brain fluid concentration up to 60 times when administered in the form of polysorbate 80-coated biodegradable poly(butyl cyanoacrylate) nanoparticles. Polysorbate 80-coated nanoparticles proved to achieve the higher brain targeting due to endocytosis by the brain blood vessel endothelial cells	Gulyaev et al. (1999)
Estradiol	The nanoparticle proposed to have higher nose to brain absorption. This study proved the nasal-to-brain targeting of the estradiol-loaded chitosan nanoparticles as a safe and effective delivery of drug for achieving sufficient concentration in the brain	Wang et al. (2008)
Rivastigmine	Rivastigmine loaded in chitosan nanoparticles was developed to improve the brain targeting of the drug for the prevention and treatment of Alzheimer's disease	Fazil et al. (2012)
	Lactoferrin proved to improve brain targeting across the blood-brain barrier. This study proved that lactoferrin-attached PEG-PLA nanoparticles improved the brain delivery in vivo	Hu et al. (2009)
	PEG-polylactic acid nanoparticle conjugated with TGN and QSH to target the amyloid plaques to effectively treat Alzheimer's disease. TGN bind to specific receptor present at the blood-brain barrier, while QSH target $A\beta_{1-42}$, a key component of amyloid plaque, and to improve the contration in brain	Zhang et al. (2014)

(continued)

Table 3.1 (continued)

Drug	Nanoformulation and objective	References
Cancer targeted drug delivery		
Cisplatin	The Pt(IV)-loaded PLGA-PEG nanoparticles decorated with aptamer targeting the prostate-specific membrane antigen on prostate cancer demonstrated higher anticancer activity than cisplatin	Dhar et al. (2008)
Doxorubicin	Integrin $\alpha_v\beta_3$ receptor was targeted with cyclic pentapeptide cRGD-conjugated polymeric micelles of doxorubicin which exhibited enhanced concentration of nanoparticles in the tumour due to increased endocytosis by tumour endothelium	Nasongkla et al. (2004)
Doxorubicin	The tumour was actively targeted with anti-MT1-MMP antibody-conjugated PEG liposomes of doxorubicin to improve anticancer potential and reduce side effect	Hatakeyama et al. (2007)
Irinotecan	The thermosensitive liposome of irinotecan demonstrating promising anticancer results on colon cancer cells due to higher uptake of the liposomes	Casadó et al. (2014)
Transdermal delivery		
Minoxidil	Transdermal delivery of minoxidil-loaded poly(ε-caprolactone)-block-poly(ethyleneglycol) potentiated the transdermal flux of minoxidil across the skin due to lower particle size and improved partitioning in the skin	Shim et al. (2004)
Flurbiprofen	Lipid nanoparticles of flurbiprofen successfully delivered the drug across the skin by transdermal route. The aim of the study was to improve the short half-life and circumvent the high first-pass metabolism	Bhaskar et al. (2009)
Triamcinolone acetonide acetate	Evaluated the permeation efficiency of solid lipid nanoparticles of triamcinolone acetonide acetate across the stratum corneum when administered with iontophoresis	Liu et al. (2008)
Aceclofenac	Chitosan-egg albumin nanoparticles for transdermal aceclofenac delivery were prepared to enhance permeation across the skin	Jana et al. (2014)
Indomethacin	PLGA nanoparticles of indomethacin significantly improved the transdermal permeation by iontophoresis	Tomoda et al. (2011)
Melatonin	Lecithin/chitosan nanoparticles for transdermal delivery of melatonin proved to have high permeation flux compared to pure melatonin	Hafner et al. (2011)
Ophthalmic drug delivery		
Indomethacin	The solid lipid nanoparticle and nanostructured lipid carrier enhanced the availability or concentration of indomethacin in posterior chamber of eye when administered by ocular route. The enhanced bioavailability is perhaps due to higher permeability of lipid nanoparticle across the cornea and higher and retention	Balguri et al. (2016)
Levofloxacin	Polymeric nanoparticles of levofloxacin effectively improve the permeation of drug across the cornea in controlled way	Gupta et al. (2011)
Carprofen	The PLGA nanoparticles of carprofen were developed successfully for improving transcorneal permeation to achieve higher anti-inflammatory effect	Parra et al. (2015)
Dorzolamide	*Chitosan nanoparticle of dorzolamide was fabricated to improve the treatment of glaucoma*	Katiyar et al. (2014)
Carteolol	Carteolol was successfully incorporated in the dendrimer to treat ocular hypertension and glaucoma	Spataro et al. (2010)
Regenerative medicine and wound healing		
	Stem cell aligned growth induced by CeO_2 nanoparticles in PLGA scaffolds with improved bioactivity for regenerative medicine	Mandoli et al. (2010)
VEGF and bFGF growth factor	Diabetic wounds are chronic condition that displays difficulty in wound healing. This study proved that VEGF and bFGF nanoparticle accelerated the wound healing process when incorporated in fibrin scaffold	Losi et al. (2013)

(continued)

Table 3.1 (continued)

Drug	Nanoformulation and objective	References
Curcumin	The study demonstrated the accelerated wound healing property of Curcumin-loaded nanoparticles	Krausz et al. (2015)
Improved stability		
Camptothecin	Camptothecin has low water solubility and lactone ring highly unstable. Camptothecin formulation as chitosan nanoparticle improves stability and tumour targeting	Min et al. (2008)
Insulin	Multilayered nanoparticle enhances stability of entrapped insulin in the presence of gastric pH and enzyme and improves the absorption of insulin across the gut after oral administration	Woitiski et al. (2010)
Antimicrobial resistance		
Ciprofloxacin	Ciprofloxacin loaded in alginate lyase-functionalized chitosan nanoparticles significantly eliminated biofilm-mediated *P. aeruginosa* infection. Moreover it also improved the minimum inhibitory concentration performance in terms of duration	Patel et al. (2019a, b, c, d)
Moxifloxacin	Moxifloxacin polybutyl cyanoacrylate nanoparticles demonstrated higher internalization in cell and improve the therapeutic efficacy against mycobacterium tuberculosis	Kisich et al. (2007)
Azithromycin and rifampin	Azithromycin and rifampin PLGA nanoparticle significantly reduced intracellular chlamydial count, indicating higher therapeutic value of nanoparticle due to higher penetration	Toti et al. (2011)
Levofloxacin	The inhalable polymeric nanoparticle of levofloxacin was fabricated to effectively reduce *E. coli* count in the biofilm established in the airway track	Cheow et al. (2010)

Here, C is a drug concentration in solution, C_s is equilibrium solubility of the drug (the concentration of drug in diffusion medium is equivalent to the C_s), and $(C_s - C)$ represents the concentration gradient. So according to Eq. 3.1, the higher the surface area of the formulation, the more is the dissolution.

3.2.2 Improve the Half-Life and Reduce the Dosing Frequency

Nanoformulations provide controlled release over time which improves the half-life of the drug in the systemic circulation which ultimately reduces the dosing frequency (Agrawal et al. 2015a, b, 2017a, b; Aqil et al. 2017a, b, 2019). The drug release is a critical parameter that meaningfully affects the performance in vivo. The modification in release profile may bring alteration in the onset of action, duration of action, drug's half-life in the systemic circulation and consequently therapeutic potential. The drug encapsulated within the polymeric or lipid matrix of nanoparticles releases in a controlled manner for an extended period. The nanoformulations improve the systemic half-life of the drugs by encapsulating and releasing the drug at a controlled rate for longer duration and, therefore, maintain the minimum therapeutic drug level in the systemic circulation for longer duration and thereby reduce the need of multiple dosing (Zhang et al. 2008; Wen and Park 2010; Aqil et al. 2017a, b; Gade et al. 2019).

3.2.3 Reduce the Toxicity

Typically, the immediate-release dosage form may elicit drug toxicity by reaching the systemic drug concentration above the maximum tolerable dose or if the drugs have inherent fatal toxicity on the vital body organ or tissues. Nanoparticle modifies the release of drug from the matrix and maintains the drug concentration below the maximum tolerable concentration or within the therapeutic window and, therefore, has the potential to reduce drug toxicity. Moreover, the cytotoxic drugs (anticancer) are highly toxic and elicit the

Table 3.2 List of FDA-approved drug nanoformulation for various indications

Drug name	Brand name and formulation	Mechanism	Indication	Approval year
Amphotericin B	AmBisome® (liposome)	Monocyte phagocytic system (MPS) targeting. Negative charge and small size (70–90 nm) promote the accumulation in MPS	Systemic fungal infection (intravenous)	1997
Daunorubicin citrate	DaunoXome® (Liposome)	Enhanced permeability and retention (EPR) effect contribute to elevated concentration in the tumour	Intravenous administration in HIV-associated Kaposi's sarcoma	1996
Doxorubicin hydrochloride	Doxil® (Stealth Liposome; 100 nm)	Improve the targeting of drug at diseased site by enhanced permeability and retention	IDS-related KS, multiple myeloma, ovarian cancer	1995
Vincristine sulphate	Marqibo® (liposome; 100 nm)	Passive targeting by EPR effect	Acute lymphoid leukaemia, Philadelphia chromosome-negative	2012
Verteporfin	Visudyne® (Liposome)	Higher drug solubility imparting the easy intravenous administration	Ocular histoplasmosis syndrome	2000
Amphotericin B	Abelcet® (lipid based non liposomal)	MPS targeting	Systemic fungal infections	1995
Aprepitant's nanocrystal	Emend®	Improved the bioavailability duet to enhanced solubility	Emesis, antiemetic	2003
Rapamycin nanocrystal	Rapamune®	Improved the bioavailability due to accelerated dissolution and drug absorption across the gut	Immunosuppressant (oral)	2002
Paclitaxal (albumin nanoparticle)	Abraxane®	Passive targeting via EPR effect	Metastatic breast cancer	2005
Leuprolide acetate (polymeric nanoparticles)	Eligard®	Sustained release	Advanced prostate cancer (subcutaneous)	2002

fatal adverse events on normal human body cells also due to systemic exposure and accumulation in the organs. Targeted nanoparticles show selective accumulation at the diseased site and thus protect the normal body cell from unnecessary higher drug exposure by releasing the drug at the diseased site and reducing the occurrence of potential side effects (Jain et al. 2013a, b, 2015a, b; Kushwah et al. 2018a, b, c, d). Doxorubicin-loaded polyalkylcyanoacrylate nanoparticles have been reported to show reduced systemic toxicity due to encapsulation and less accumulation at myocardial muscle toxicity (Couvreur et al. 1982). Exosomes (biological nanoparticles), having lipid and protein as major structural components, have been reported to reduce the general toxicity (Aqil et al. 2016; Munagala et al. 2017).

3.2.4 Improve the Permeability and Retention

The skin has been used as a drug delivery route for several therapeutic moieties in the form of gels, ointments and lotions. But the low permeability of drugs across the skin due to stratum corneum limits the application of this route only for potent drugs (maximum dose of 20 mg per day) or for local treatments (skin disease). The advantages of the transdermal route such as avoidance of the first-pass metabolism and slow and steady

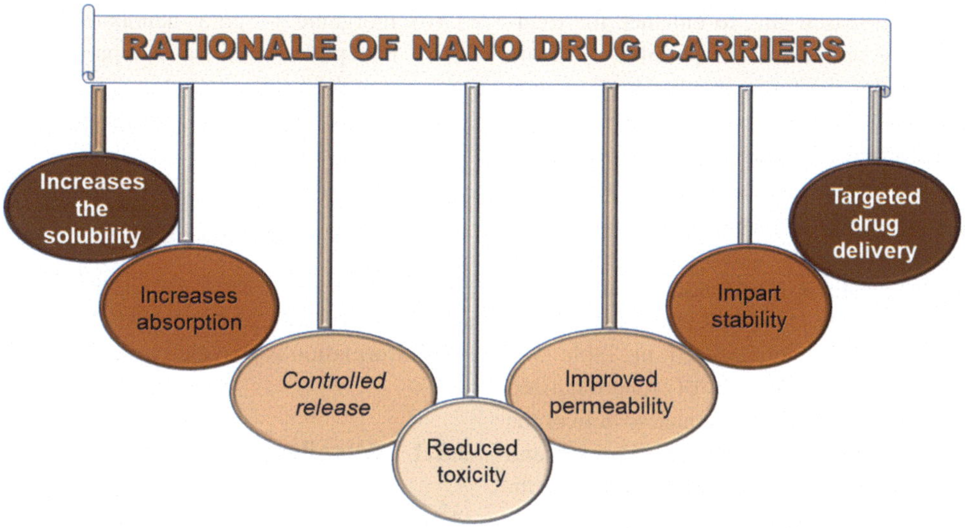

Fig. 3.1 Rationales for the design of nanoformulations

release of drugs for a longer period always fascinated the researchers. A variety of inorganic and organic nanoparticles, specifically solid lipid nanoparticles and nanostructured lipid carriers, have been reported to show higher retention within the skin and permeation across the skin as compared to the conventional dosage form (gels, ointment, etc.) (Agrawal et al. 2010; Tomoda et al. 2011; Kaler et al. 2014). Similarly, the nanoparticles had a profound effect on the ocular permeability of the drugs. Nanoparticles significantly improve the corneal permeation and enhance the ocular bioavailability of drugs (Agrawal et al. 2012).

3.2.5 Regenerative Medicine

Nanotechnology has extended its application in the area of regenerative medicine including bone and neural tissue fabrication. The nanomaterial can be easily engineered to produce the crystal mineral human structure analogous to the bone tissue having the same strength and characteristics. Moreover, several successful attempts have been made to regenerate the human organ by growing the complex tissue within a day. Apart from that, the researchers are also working on quick healing of spinal cord injury using graphene nanoribbons, and preliminary studies performed have shown outstanding results with the growth of neurons (Engel et al. 2008; Mandoli et al. 2010).

3.2.6 Impart Stability at Different Environmental and Physiological Conditions

Several drugs, specifically protein-based drugs, degrade and lose their activity at various temperatures, humidity, sunlight and varying physiological conditions such as pH and presence of enzyme before it reaches the site of action (Harde et al. 2015a, b, c, d, e, f). Nanoparticles can overcome such limitations by protecting the drug within the polymeric or lipid matrix. Several studies have proved the protection from degradation following the encapsulation within the nanoparticles. Nanoparticles have demonstrated excellent insulin stability in gastric conditions and resulted in good oral bioavailability (Agrawal et al. 2013; Urimi et al. 2019).

3.2.7 Targeted Drug Delivery

The administered drug reaches every organ or tissue of the body by systemic circulation. So achieving the desired drug concentration selectively at the diseased site, to enhance the treatment efficacy or reduce the possible systemic toxicity, remains the foremost challenge for formulation scientists. Nanoparticles offer a larger surface area and easy surface modification for targeting the specific site using the ligands. These ligands are either adsorbed on the surface or covalently bind to specific groups present on the surface of the nanoparticles for active targeting to the pathogenic site. Some of the examples of ligands and targets are enlisted in Table 3.1. Recently, the potential use of functionalized nanoparticles is widely investigated to deliver the drug at a specific site for efficient therapy and reduced toxicity. These unconventional techniques utilize small molecules, peptides, antibodies, engineered proteins or nucleic acid aptamers as ligands (Byrne et al. 2008, Friedman et al. 2013, Agrawal et al. 2015a, b).

3.2.8 Diagnostic Imaging

The imaging techniques, viz. CT scan and MRI, depend on the contrast agent administered intravenously to evaluate the physiological condition and diagnosis of the disease. Apart from rapid diagnosis, the contrast agent currently in use has some limitation including the lack of specificity and potential systemic toxicity. Several investigations to explore the application of nanoparticles in the diagnosis purpose have revealed that nanoparticles are more sensitive and provide specific information without eliciting the significant systemic toxic effect (Xie et al. 2010; Rosen et al. 2011) by providing higher selectivity and accumulation to the targeted site along with the drug having therapeutic efficacy.

3.3 Classification of Nanoparticles

Nanoparticles can be classified in many ways:

1. Classification based on origin
   (a) Organic – dendrimer, polymeric nanoparticles, lipid nanoparticles, etc.
   (b) Inorganic – gold nanoparticles, silver nanoparticles, silica nanoparticles, quantum dots, fullerene, etc.
2. Classification based on application
   (a) Diagnostic
   (b) Imaging
   (c) Therapy

As this chapter is restricted to discuss liposomes and polymeric and lipid nanoparticles, a piece of brief information is provided here.

3.3.1 Micelles

Micelles are the colloidal spherical arrangement of the amphiphilic (have both hydrophilic and lipophilic end) lipids or polymers in the aqueous system (Fig. 3.2a). Micelles have a hydrophobic core and hydrophilic surface. Similarly, the reverse micelles with hydrophilic core and hydrophobic outer surface can be formed in the organic solvent. Micelles can easily accommodate the water-soluble drugs in the core and amphiphilic moiety within the structure. These are the stable arrangement with extended systemic circulation due to hydrophilic surface (Letchford and Burt 2007). Micelles have shown their potential to efficiently entrap the lipophilic drug, enhance the stability of the drug, penetrate the biological membrane and improve the therapeutic potential and targeted drug delivery.

3.3.2 Liposomes

Liposomes are bilayer spherical vesicles (Fig. 3.2b) made up of amphiphilic phospholipids and cholesterol. Liposomes are biocompatible and proven to be promising carriers for hydrophilic as well as hydrophobic drug moieties. The properties including surface charge and size may vary with lipid composition and the method of preparation. Moreover, the lipid constituents may also alter the rigidity and fluidity of the membrane. The phospholipids (unsaturated) with natural origin (egg and soybean phosphatidylcholine) tend to produce unstable, permeable

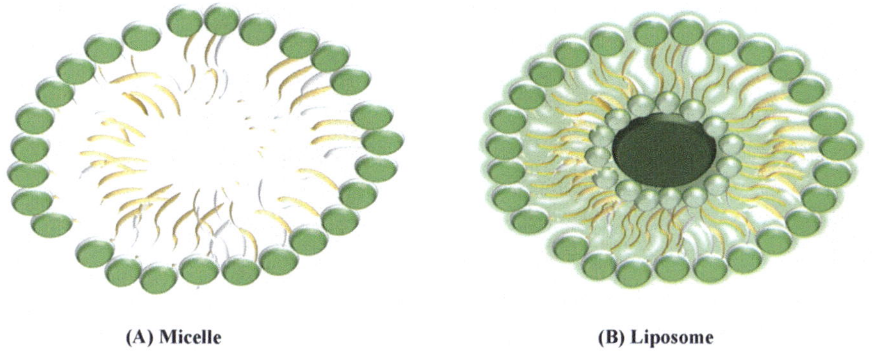

Fig. 3.2 Schematic diagram of micelles (**a**) and liposomal bilayer (**b**)

and more fluidized bilayer; however, the saturated phospholipids, having long acyl chains like dipalmitoylphosphatidylcholine, produce comparatively more rigid and impermeable bilayer. Liposomes have fascinated researchers worldwide due to the use of physiological phospholipids which have been proven to be biocompatible, biodegradable and non-toxic for clinical applications (Jain et al. 2012). Most importantly, the liposomes can reduce the drug toxicity and target the drugs to the diseased site. The liposomes can be classified based on their application as a diagnostic and therapeutic purpose having entrapped various disease markers and bioactive molecules (Akbarzadeh et al. 2013).

3.3.3 Lipid Nanoparticles

Solid lipid nanoparticles (SLNs) are the most widely used nanoparticles, among the different lipid nanoparticles, which are prepared by using various physiological solid lipids. Another name under this category is nanostructured lipid carriers (NLCs) which are made up of solid as well as the liquid lipids and have shown improved encapsulation efficiency and stability. Generally, SLNs possess similar kind of molecules or crystals and on storage, temperature or relative humidity conditions trigger crystalline change from unstable state (irregular arrangement of crystal lattice) to more stable one (regular crystal) leading to the expulsion of encapsulated drug and instability of the system. However, NLCs possess two different kinds of lipids and thus are unable to rearrange in regular shape and provide the regular void for drug accommodation and thereby improve drug entrapment and stability. Lipid nanoparticles have been reported to deliver the drugs through various routes to even have liver and brain targeting (Müller et al. 2002; Schäfer-Korting et al. 2007). An in vivo study on lipid nanoparticles of flurbiprofen reported having improved transdermal permeation flux across the skin (Bhaskar et al. 2009). Similarly, the solid lipid nanoparticles of indomethacin have been reported to improve the transcorneal distribution of indomethacin in anterior and posterior lobe (Balguri et al. 2016). Several other studies have also been summarized to effectively deliver the drugs by using lipid nanoparticles (Harde et al. 2015a, b, c, d, e, f). A new class of nanoparticles, liquid crystalline nanoparticles, has also been reported to impart stability and improve the oral bioavailability of proteins (Singh et al. 2018).

3.3.4 Polymeric Nanoparticles

Polymeric nanoparticles, developed by using various polymers of either natural or synthetic origin, have been widely reported as drug delivery vehicles (Jain et al. 2015a, b; Kushwah et al. 2017). The polymeric nanoparticles may further be differentiated as nanospheres (Fig. 3.3a) and nanocapsules (Fig. 3.3b). In nanospheres, the drug is usually distributed uniformly in the polymeric matrix, while in nanocapsules, the drug is

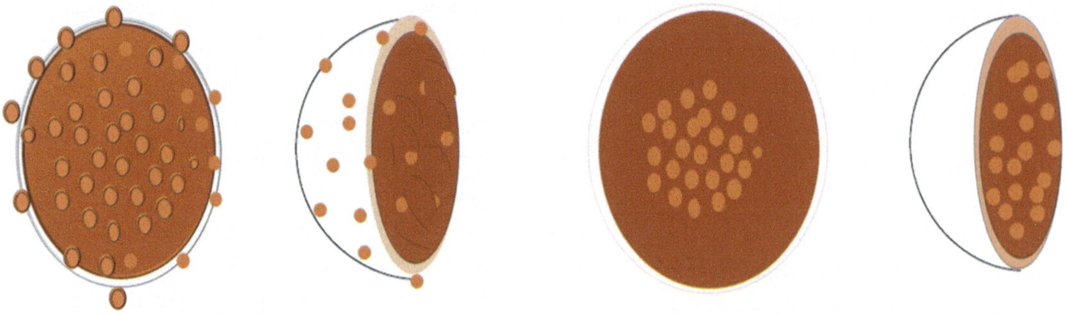

Fig. 3.3 Diagrammatic representation of polymeric nanoparticles: (**a**) nanosphere and (**b**) nanocapsule

dispersed or dissolved within the liquid reservoir (either aqueous or oil) in the core covered by solid polymeric coating.

3.4 Formulation Development of Nanoformulation

3.4.1 Selection of Drug

The rationale of nanoparticle development as a drug delivery vehicle is dependent upon certain limitations associated with the physicochemical properties of the drug and the biological barriers and the disease's pathophysiology.

3.4.1.1 Low Water Solubility

Most of the drugs are either weak acid or weak base and possess low solubility in water which results in poor dissolution rate, leading to poor absorption and thus poor bioavailability. Ultimately, it affects the pharmacokinetics and pharmacodynamics of the drug leading to low efficacy, slow onset of action and higher dose to achieve effective blood concentration. By entrapping the drug in the molecularly dispersed form inside the polymeric matrix, nanoparticles have been reported to improve dissolution, bioavailability, onset of action and therapeutic efficacy which is further helpful in reducing the dose size.

3.4.1.2 Short Half-Life

The systemic half-life of a drug is the time at which half of the total drug reaching the blood eliminates from the body. The basic reason for fast elimination or short half-life can be high polarity (easy renal excretion) or fast metabolism. The drugs with shorter half-life require frequent dosing to keep the effective blood concentration within the therapeutic window. Nanoparticles entrap the drug in the matrix and can overcome the fast metabolism and elimination. Simultaneously, the nanoparticles release the drug in a controlled and sustained way for longer duration which helps in maintaining the constant blood concentration and thus reducing the dosing frequency (Madan et al. 2013).

3.4.1.3 High Toxicity

Some drugs with high therapeutic efficacy induce severe systemic toxicity to other vital organs. Specifically, anticancer drugs along with their cytotoxic effect on cancerous cell induce lethal toxicity such as hepatotoxicity, nephrotoxicity, bone marrow depression, etc. Developing a nanoformulation for the delivery may overcome the toxicity by the restricted distribution of the nanoparticles to the diseased site (Sengupta et al. 2012).

3.4.1.4 High First-Pass Metabolism

The orally administered drug first undergoes the first-pass metabolism in the liver which is a presystemic metabolic in which fraction of absorbed drug is metabolized in the liver by microsomal enzymes after absorption from intestine before reaching to the systemic circulation. Consequently, the required concentration of drugs in blood is not attained and thus the higher dose is needed. Nanoparticles can evade the first-pass metabolism by enhancing the absorption of the drug from the lymphatic system which does not pass through the liver. Moreover, the systemically absorbed nanoparticles efficiently avoid the direct exposure of the drug to the enzyme and circumvent the metabolism. The drugs with the highest first metabolism are propranolol, raloxifene, morphine, pethidine, diazepam, lidocaine, midazolam, etc. There are several reports which indicated the bypass of the first-pass metabolism following the entrapment of drug into the nanoparticles (Yao et al. 2015).

3.4.1.5 Drug with Low Skin/Ophthalmic Permeation/Retention

Drugs intended to treat skin diseases or ocular ailments or drugs administered by transdermal route generally have low retention locally in the skin and low ocular and transdermal bioavailability perhaps due to low permeation across the skin, cornea and other ocular barriers. Several studies conducted on the efficiency on nanoparticles prepared for topical, transdermal and ophthalmic application proved to improve skin retention for local skin therapy, skin permeation and corneal permeation, and hence the drugs having the above-mentioned problems are good candidates to develop nanoformulations (Naik et al. 2004; Shim et al. 2004; Sahoo et al. 2008).

3.4.1.6 Chronic Pathophysiological Conditions

Chronic pathophysiological disease conditions such as diabetes, AIDS, tuberculosis and many others require long-term treatment regimen. Therefore, a strategy that can efficiently reduce rapid drug administration is desired for the patient's compliance. Nanoparticles can maintain the required drug concentration in blood by extending the drug release from hours to several days, and hence developing nanoformulations for such drugs might be a good approach to improve the efficacy (El-Shabouri 2002; Sarmento et al. 2007).

3.4.2 Selection of Polymers and Lipids

It is mandatory to evaluate some of the parameters before starting the optimization of nanoformulation to achieve the nanoparticles with desired particle characteristics (particle size, zeta potential, polydispersity index, entrapment efficiency and in vitro release) and the desired therapeutic effect. At the same time, toxicity profiling is a regulatory mandate to assure the safety of the formulation on the human subject. Polymer or lipid (Table 3.3) used to form the nano-reservoir for the drug is selected based on numerous factors. The selection of polymers and/or lipids is again dependent upon multiple factors.

3.4.2.1 Physicochemical Compatibility with the Selected Drug Moiety

The polymer or lipid should not show any chemical interaction with the drug to ensure the inherent therapeutic activity and avoid the unwanted effects. Therefore, various techniques such as Fourier transform infrared spectroscopy (FTIR), differential scanning calorimetry (DSC) and X-ray diffraction are conducted to assess the possible interaction among the drug, polymer/lipid and other excipients (Patel et al. 2019a, b, c, d).

3.4.2.2 Biocompatibility and Toxicity

Neither polymer/lipid nor the metabolites should elicit harmful effect on human vital organs or tissues on short-term or long-term exposure. Therefore, toxicity profiling is very important before the selection of any polymer/lipid for nanoformulation development.

3.4.2.3 Biodegradability

The nanoformulations intended to be administered orally or systemically should be degraded in the human physiological environment to confirm its easy elimination from the body. The polymers with higher molecular weight may have slower elimination and thus may accumulate within different body tissues and induce severe toxicity (Seymour et al. 1987).

Table 3.3 Classification of different polymers and lipids generally used for the development of nanoformulation for the drug delivery purpose

Polymers	
Based on origin	
Natural	Chitosan, alginate, albumin, cellulose
Semisynthetic	Methyl cellulose (MC), carboxymethyl cellulose (CMC), hydroxypropyl methylcellulose (HPMC), dextrin
Synthetic	Polyacrylamate, Poly epsilon caprolactum (PCL), Poly lactic acid (PLA), Poly glycolic acid (PGA), Poly-lactic acid co glycolic acid (PLGA)
Based on structure	
Linear	Poly glycolic acid (PGA), Poly-lactic acid co glycolic acid (PLGA)
Branched chain	Poly (amidoamine) (PAMAM), Poly(propylene imine) (PPI), Polyether-copolyester (PEPE)
Stimuli-responsive polymers	
Thermoresponsive	Xyloglucan, N-Isopropylacrylamide (NIPAAm), Poloxamers
pH sensitive	Carbopols, Chitosan
Ion sensitive	Gellan gum, Sodium alginate
Lipids	
Based on physical state	
Liquid	Hydrogenated oils, Compritol
Solid	Triglycerides (e.g. tristearin), Diglycerides (e.g. glycerolbahenate), monoglycerides (e.g. glycerol monostearate), fatty acids (e.g. stearic acid, Behenic acid), steroids (e.g. cholesterol)
Based on source	
Natural	Cholesterol, Phosphocholine
Semisynthetic	1,2-Dipalmitoyl-sn-glycero-3-phosphocholine, 1,2-Dipalmitoyl-sn-glycero-3-phosphoethanolamine
Synthetic	Dioleoylphosphatidylcholine, Dioleoylphosphatidylethanolamine, Distearoylphosphatidylethanolamine
Based on structure	
Phospholipids	Phosphatidylcholine, Phosphatidylinositol, Phosphatidylserine
Sphingolipids	Sphingomyelins
Glycerolipids	Digalactosyldiacylglycerols

3.4.2.4 Desirable Particle Size

Polymeric and lipid nanoparticle size increases with an increased molecular weight of the polymer and lipid, respectively. Moreover, the lipid nanoparticles have been used to have a higher particle size range as compared to the polymeric nanoparticles. Hence, based on the desired application and route of administration, the polymer/lipid is selected.

3.4.2.5 Anticipated Release Profile

Nanoparticles have shown to have a controlled or sustained release profile (Yoo et al. 1999). The molecular weight of polymer/lipid is deciding property for the desired release profile. The polymer/lipid with higher molecular weight increases the release time for a longer period. Therefore, depending on the therapeutic need, the matrix component can be selected.

3.4.2.6 Inherent Properties of the Drug

This is a very common practice to select either the polymeric matrix or lipid matrix based on the drug solubility characteristic and its logP value. At the same time, the drug solubility in the lipids is determined to achieve the maximum possible encapsulation while optimizing the SLNs and NLCs.

3.4.2.7 Surface Charge and Permeability

The nature of the surface charge on the nanoparticles determines the interaction of particles with body cells and tissues.

3.4.2.8 Nonirritant

The formulation intended for the topical or ophthalmic purpose should be evaluated for the irritancy potential on the skin before the use. Therefore, the irritancy is one of the criteria to be considered while selecting the polymer or lipids for delivering a drug through these routes.

3.4.3 Selection of Solvents

The solvent system is a liquid vehicle used to prepare the solution or suspension of a particular compound for carrying out the experimentation. The solvent may be aqueous or organic. USFDA has classified the solvents into four different classes (Dixit et al. 2015) based on permissible residual limit in the formulation or drug products.

Class 1 The use of class I solvent is prohibited owing to its fatal toxicity on human or harmful effects on the environment until their use is necessary to complete the process for obtaining the product of significant therapeutic value. In that case, the residual limit should be validated according to the ICH Q3C guidelines, and the residual limits with their harmful effects are listed in Table 3.4.

Class 2 These solvents are again toxic and not allowed to use in drug unless mandatory. The permissible limit of residual solvents, of class 2, is shown in Table 3.5.

Class 3 The solvents belonging to this category are least toxic and have a lower risk to human health. None of the solvents in this class produce toxicity at its accepted limit level. The permissible quantity that can be allowed for human uptake is 5000 ppm or 50 mg/day or less without any prior clarification. The available data of toxicity is for short-term exposure and has never elicited genotoxicity. However, long-term toxicity and carcinogenic assessment on chronic exposure is needed to be performed for many of these solvents. The solvent of this class is depicted in Table 3.6.

While preparing the nanoparticles, selection of organic solvents or the combination of solvents, volume and their ratio affect the critical quality parameter of the final product and hence the selection of solvent should be done carefully to optimize the product. Moreover, solvent selection for any pharmaceutical manufacturing mainly depends on the following criteria:

3.4.3.1 Toxicity

As described above the solvent system used for any process or manufacturing should be less toxic, or the use of solvents with high toxicity should be justified and should be limited. Moreover, the residual limit should be maintained according to the guidelines.

3.4.3.2 The Solubility of Drugs/ Excipients

Most of the experiments and manufacturing processes are performed in the solubilize state or by preparing the suspension, and there comes the

Table 3.4 Different solvent in class 1 category

Class 1		
Solvent	Residual limit	Toxicity/concern
Benzene	2	Carcinogenic
Carbon tetrachloride	4	Toxic and environmental hazard
1,2-Dichloroethane	5	Toxic
1,1-Dichloroethene	8	Toxic
1,1,1-Trichloroethane	1500	Environmental hazard

Table 3.5 FDA-approved class 2 solvent with their permitted daily exposure and residual limit

Class 2		
Solvent	Permitted daily exposure (mg/day)	Residual limit (ppm)
Acetonitrile	4.1	410
Chlorobenzene	3.6	360
Chloroform	0.6	60
Cyclohexane	38.8	3880
Cumene	0.7	70
1,2-Dichloroethene	18.7 18.7	1870
Dichloromethane	6.0	600
1,2-Dimethoxyethane	1.0	100
N,N-Dimethylacetamide	10.9	1090
N,N-Dimethylformamide	8.8	880
1,4-Dioxane	3.8	380
2-Ethoxyethanol	1.6	160
Ethyleneglycol	3.1	310
Formamide	2.2	220
Hexane	2.9	290
Methanol	30.0	3000
2-Methoxyethanol	0.5	50
Methylbutyl ketone	0.5	50
Methylcyclohexane	11.8	1180
Methylisobutylketone2	45	4500
N-Methylpyrrolidone	5.3	530
Nitromethane	0.5	50
Pyridine	2.0	200
Sulfolane	1.6	160
Tetrahydrofuran	7.2	720
Tetralin	1.0	100

Table 3.6 FDA-approved least toxic class 3 solvents permitted to be used in drug products

Class 3 solvents	
Acetic acid	Heptane
Acetone	Isobutyl acetate
Anisole	Isopropyl acetate
1-Butanol	Methyl acetate
2-Butanol	3-Methyl-1-butanol
Butyl acetate	Methylethyl ketone
tert-Butylmethyl ether	2-Methyl-1-propanol
Dimethyl sulfoxide	Pentane
Ethanol	1-Pentanol
Ethyl acetate	1-Propanol
Ethyl ether	2-Propanol
Ethyl formate	Propyl acetate
Formic acid	Triethylamine3

role of solvents. Therefore, solubility is one of the critical parameters while selecting the solvent to get the product with the desired quality and high yield.

3.4.3.3 Volatility

Most of the drugs and excipients are solubilized in the organic solvents, and hence the use of an organic solvent is necessary for manufacturing purposes. However, organic solvent provokes human toxicity at a certain level. The solvent used should be volatile for easy removal after completion of the process.

3.4.4 Selection of the Excipients/Surfactants

According to the USFDA guideline, any substances intended to human use should be "generally recognized as safe (GRAS)". Excipients are the chemicals or substances commonly used as drug carriers, bulking agents, disintegrators, binders or surfactants. Each class has a specific and important role in optimizing the product with the desired characteristic while preparing the drug product. Specifically, surfactants play a critical role in attaining stable nanoparticles with higher drug encapsulation and are reported to increase the oral bioavailability of a variety of nanoformulations (Jain et al. 2017; Shilpi et al. 2017). The surfactant may be anionic, cationic or non-ionic, and depending upon the intended use, the appropriate surfactant is selected. The regulatory authority needs assurance in terms of safety and efficacy data for approval of particular excipients. Besides several other factors, the following are the important factors that are considered before the final selection of the surfactant for formulation development.

3.4.4.1 Toxicity

On selecting the particular excipients, safety in clinic remains a major concern. The excipient should not be toxic. Therefore, long-term toxicity and short-term profiling need to be checked, if available, or evaluated, if not available.

3.4.4.2 Inertness

The compound/surfactant should be inert, i.e. should not interact chemically or physically, which may affect the efficacy of the drug product in terms of lost or diminished therapeutic activity or may exhibit toxicity.

3.4.4.3 Required Surface Charge

Depending upon the use and application, the surfactant can be utilized during the preparation of nanoparticles to impart specific charges (positive or negative). Charged particle stability depends on the zeta potential; however, non-ionic surfactants are long-chain polymers that provide stability by steric hindrance. Surfactant molecules adsorb on the newly formed nanoparticle surface while processing and provide stability and also prevent drug expulsion from the matrix. Therefore, the surfactant is the key factor for optimizing the formulation with the highest stability and encapsulation efficiency (Khdair et al. 2008).

3.4.4.4 Application

Excipients/surfactants are chosen based on the area or route of administration because the excipients used topically may have toxicity on systemic consumption. Therefore, the surfactant and excipients can also be grouped based on topical and systemic use.

3.4.5 Selection of Method of Preparation

There are several methods enlisted in the literature for the preparation of the drug nanoparticles. The selection of the method depends on the type of nanoparticles and physicochemical properties of polymer and drug. Factors which influence the choice of the apposite technique are enlisted below:

- The solubility of drug and polymer
- Thermal sensitivity of the drug
- Type of nanoformulations

Several methodologies, commonly practised to fabricate the different kinds of nanoparticles in contemporary research, are elaborated below.

3.5 Method of Preparation for Polymeric/Lipid Nanoparticles

3.5.1 Solvent Evaporation Method

Solvent evaporation technique is the most extensively used process for nanoparticle preparation of hydrophobic drug and polymer. Briefly, there are two phases, one organic containing the dissolved drug and polymer and second aqueous phase supplemented with the desired surfactant to form the o/w emulsion (appropriate concentration). The organic phase is gradually mixed to the aqueous phase to produce the o/w type emulsion followed by high-speed homogenization or sonication to produce the desired nanoparticle size. Finally, the solvent is allowed to evaporate to initiate the polymer precipitation by reducing the pressure or by continuous stirring. The commonly used solvents are dichloromethane, chloroform or ethyl acetate. In this method, the particle size can be controlled by adjusting the polymer concentration, stabilizer, sonication time, viscosity of organic phase, homogenization speed and temperature (Lee et al. 2006).

3.5.2 Double-Emulsion and Evaporation Method

This is the modification of the solvent evaporation method to overcome the limitation to successfully incorporate the hydrophilic drug in the nanoparticles up to a maximum extent. Precisely, the drug-containing aqueous phase is added to an organic system containing w/o type emulsifier to form the primary w/o emulsion. Subsequently, the primary w/o emulsion is steadily mixed with a surfactant solution to produce the w/o/w emulsion at high homogenization speed. Eventually, the system is kept for the solvent removed to obtain the nanoparticles. The polymer concentration, drug quantity, organic to aqueous ratio and homogenization speed are the crucial factors that majorly affect the particle size and entrapment efficiency of the nanoparticles (Zambaux et al. 1998).

3.5.3 Solvent Displacement/Precipitation Method

This is one of the frequently used methods for preparing the nanoformulations of hydrophobic drugs. Moreover, this technique can be efficiently utilized to obtain the nanoparticles of thermosensitive drugs. Concisely, a water-miscible organic solvent is selected to dissolve the drug and polymer and form the organic phase. The most frequently used organic solvent is acetone; however, ethanol can also be used. Secondly, the preformed polymeric organic phase is injected slowly at a particular rate in the surfactant-rich aqueous phase. The surfactant system is kept at a magnetic stirrer at an optimized speed sufficient enough to break the drops and produce the nano-droplets. Once the organic phase comes into contact with water, it starts diffusing in water gradually due to hydrophilic affinity. The diffusion of organic solvent leads to supersaturation and nucleation of drug-polymer and induces the formation of nanoparticles. Formulation parameters such as drug/polymer ratio, polymer quantity and organic-to-aqueous phase ratio can be optimized to achieve the desired nanoparticle characteristics. Likewise, process parameters, viz. stirring rate and injection rate, also affect the quality of the particle (Lince et al. 2011).

3.5.4 Coacervation or Ionic Gelation Method

Nanoparticle formulation by ionic gelation method depends upon the alteration of pH of polymeric solution and formation of electrostatic bonding between the charged group of the polymer and the crosslinking agents (sodium TPP). This method is commonly employed to prepare the nanoparticles of hydrophilic polymers such as gelatin, sodium alginates and chitosan. For making the chitosan nanoparticles, the aqueous solution of chitosan in acetic acid is mixed with polyanion sodium tripolyphosphate (TPP) with continuous stirring. The anionic phosphate group of TPP is crosslinked electrostatically with an amino group of chitosan and forms the coacervates of nanosize range. The existence of strong electrostatic interaction between two aqueous phases results in the conversion of liquid into a gel-like matrix (Fan et al. 2012; Harde et al. 2014).

3.5.5 Supercritical Fluid Technology

Unlike all the above conventional techniques, supercritical fluid techniques do not require the use of organic solvents. Apart from that, supercritical fluid technology produces particles with a minimum size and uniform size distribution. It may be considered as the second-generation method for the preparation of nanoparticles which is not harmful to the environment and health but requires specialized equipment and supercritical fluids. These are the fluids that remain in the liquid phase and unaffected by pressure above its critical temperature. The most commonly used cheap, non-toxic supercritical fluid is CO_2. This technique of nanoparticle preparation involves two major methods:

- *Supercritical fluid anti-solvent technique (SAS)*

In this method drug solution in an organic solvent (anti-solvent) is mixed with supercritical CO_2. The quick dissolution of supercritical CO_2 into organic solvent results in the precipitation of drug molecules in the form of nanoparticles (Reverchon 1999). The nanoparticles of a hydrophilic drug such as dexamethasone phosphate have been successfully prepared using this technology.

- *The rapid expansion of supercritical solution (RESS)*

In this method, drug and polymer are directly solubilized in the supercritical fluid and sprayed through the nozzles for expansion. Rapid expansion results in an abrupt decrease in pressure leading to precipitation in the form of nanoparticles (Sun et al. 2005). The nozzle size, type of supercritical fluid, spraying rate and polymer concentration affect particle size and particle size distribution significantly.

3.5.6 Polymerization Method

This method was firstly reported for the grafting of nanoparticles using the polymerization of butyl cyanoacrylate into polybutyl cyanoacrylate. This method involves the preparation of nanoparticles using the monomer and can be easily controlled to attain the required particle size and uniform particle distribution. Interestingly, the drug can be either incorporated in the polymerization medium before polymerization or adsorbed on the nanoparticle surface after polymerization. Particle size and other particle characteristics can be controlled by optimizing the concentration of the monomer in the reaction mixture, surfactant concentration and reaction time (Gnanakan et al. 2009).

3.5.7 High-Pressure Homogenization

High-pressure homogenization is an extensively employed technique to produce solid lipid nanoparticles and nanostructured lipid carriers on a laboratory scale. It can be further classified as cold homogenization and hot homogenization.

- *Hot homogenization*

In this technique, the drug is dissolved or dispersed evenly in the lipid melt and homogenized at high speed in the melt state only. Finally, the preformed dispersion is homogenized at high pressure to form the nanoparticles. Unfortunately, this method cannot be applied to thermossensitive drugs (Jenning et al. 2002).

- *Cold homogenization*

The SLNs and NLCs of highly temperature-sensitive drugs can be obtained by using cold homogenization. At the same time, hydrophilic active moiety, which might show phase separation in water, can be entrapped into the lipid nanoparticles using this technique. The drug is dissolved in the lipid matrix on short time exposure cooled down to produce solid mass and micronized. Finally, the micronized particles are dispersed in an aqueous solution containing stabilizer and homogenized at high pressure to achieve the nanoparticles.

3.6 Preparation of Liposomes

Liposomes can be fabricated by several methods reported in the literature (Akbarzadeh et al. 2013). The following section briefly describes such methods to prepare liposomes.

3.6.1 Membrane Hydration Method

The membrane hydration technique is the most commonly used method to produce large unilamellar vesicles (LUV). The organic solution (usually chloroform and ethanol combination) of lipid is placed in the round bottom flask and allowed to rotate with the simultaneous application of vacuum to form the thin lipid layer in the round bottom flask. Further addition of aqueous phase and rotation without vacuum result in the formation of LUVs. Both hydrophobic and hydrophilic drugs can be incorporated by adding in the lipid solution at the time of film formation or aqueous solution at the time of hydration, respectively. These LUVs can be converted to small unilamellar vesicles (SUVs) by using sonication or extrusion.

3.6.2 Mechanical Dispersion Methods

There are various methods categorized under mechanical dispersion for liposome preparation:

- *Sonication*

Sonication is the most preferred method to prepare liposomal formulation. The multilamellar vesicles (MLVs) are sonicated to produce SUVs by using sonic energy. Even being most preferred method, the sonication process is associated with some limitations in terms of polydispersity, low entrapment, low vesicular internal volume, metal contamination, phospholipid's degradation, high energy wave generates the high temperature in the formulation that may degrade temperature-sensitive active compounds (proteins, peptides).

- *French pressure cell*

This method is preferred for the temperature-sensitive (proteins and peptides) compounds that cannot be entrapped into the liposomes by sonication. It does not affect the internal structure of proteins and peptides and is therefore preferred for sensitive molecules. Precisely, preformed MLVs are passed through the fine orifices of the French press at high pressure to generate the small vesicles. Moreover, the stability of SUVs is higher concerning the expulsion of the drug from the liposome compared to those formed by sonication. Unlike the sonication, it can process only very low volume at a time.

3.6.2.1 Solvent Dispersion Methods

- *Ether injection (solvent vaporization)*

In this method, the lipid solution prepared in the diethyl ether or in a combination of methanol is slowly injected to the buffer at a temperature above the melting point of lipid or under reduced pressure. Subsequently, the solution is kept under reduced pressure to eliminate the ether and initiate the formation of liposomal vesicles. The major drawbacks of this method are (1) formation of an azeotropic mixture of ether with water which is difficult to remove from the final formulation and (2) production of a heterogeneous population of liposomes.

- *Ethanol injection*

Lipid is dissolved in the ethanol instead of ether in this process and gradually injected into the excess aqueous buffer to create the MLVs. Finally, the formulation is allowed to remove the ethanol under reduced pressure. Moreover, heterogeneous vesicle formation and the presence of residual ethanol in the final formulation are the major drawbacks associated with this method.

- *Reverse phase evaporation method*

Reverse phase evaporation technique is an advanced method for achieving the liposomes with high entrapment efficiency (maximum up to 65%) for hydrophilic moiety and high aqueous space to lipid ratio. Interestingly, this method forms the inverted micelles. Concisely, the lipid dissolved in an organic solvent is dispersed in the aqueous buffer supplemented with drug and subsequently sonicated to arrange the phospholipid molecule into liposomal vesicles. Finally, the inverted micelles are generated while removing the organic phase gradually from the mixture under vacuum. The isopropyl ether, diethyl ether, chloroform and their mixture are the most commonly used organic solvents for dissolving phospholipid. Moreover, the method has already been investigated for encapsulation of several compounds including small, medium and large molecules. Major drawbacks include the residual solvent and denaturing of sensitive molecules like proteins and peptides.

3.6.2.2 Microencapsulation Vesicles (MCV)

The MCV is a highly reproducible preparation technique for liposome that competently creates the liposome with uniform particle size and higher entrapment efficiency. This method can encapsulate the water-soluble, lipophilic as well as amphiphilic drugs. The drugs can be dissolved either in the aqueous phase or organic phase before the preparation of liposome. The method is a two-step process; initially, w/o emulsion is prepared by dispersing the lipid dissolved in the organic phase in the aqueous phase with continuous stirring. Finally, the primary w/o emulsion is gradually added to the water to produce the w/o/w emulsion and kept at stirring to remove the organic phase using the vacuum and produce the liposome (Nii and Ishii 2005).

3.7 Identification of Variables

There are mainly two kinds of variables:

1. Dependent variable/critical quality attributes
2. Independent variables/formulation/process variables

3.7.1 Critical Quality Parameters or Dependent Variables

Critical quality attributes are the characteristics of the final formulation that will have a direct impact on the therapeutic performance of the developed formulation. These are also known as dependent variables because their values depend on the independent variables. So before starting the optimization of the process for fabricating the quality product, quality parameters are needed to be identified, and the desired limit should be set. Particle size, polydispersity index (PDI), zeta potential and entrapment efficiency are generally considered as major dependent variables for any kind of nanoformulation. Particle size is an important parameter as it directly affects the nanoparticle uptake, while PDI is responsible for the homogeneity of the formulation. Zeta potential plays a crucial role in nanoformulation's stability as well as cellular uptake, while entrapment efficiency is a direct measure of the efficiency of the delivery vehicle in carrying the maximum amount of drug to the target site.

3.7.2 Formulation and Process Factors or Independent Variables

After setting the limits of desired quality attributes, critical formulation or process parameters, which significantly affect the critical quality attributes of the formulation, need to be identified to further optimize the process. Depending on the method, type and formulation, there are several factors (Sharma et al. 2016) that play a crucial role in achieving the quality product. The identified parameters that affect the quality of nanoparticles are as follows:

(i) Organic-to-aqueous phase ratio
(ii) Drug-to-polymer/lipid ratio
(iii) Amount of polymer/lipid
(iv) Surfactant concentration
(v) Homogenization speed
(vi) Working temperature
(vii) Sonication time
(viii) Vacuum pressure
(ix) Rotation speed
(x) Homogenization time
(xi) Injection rate
(xii) pH of the working solutions

Depending on the extent of their influence on the quality, the factors are selected for further optimization while keeping the remaining factors constant. The factors and their required levels can be designated based on the knowledge, previous studies reported in the literature and experimental approach. In an experimental approach, keeping all other factors constant, a single factor is varied to measure its influence on particle size, PDI, zeta potential and entrapment efficiency. At last, depending on the comparative analysis of data for each factor, significantly affecting factors are selected for the final process to be optimized.

3.8 Optimization of Process and Product

Process optimization is a step where all the critical steps are controlled to produce the product with desired quality. Similarly, in nanoformulations, the process and formulation parameters affecting the process and formulation quality are identified and controlled to obtain the product with predefined quality.

Once the critical quality attributes and the factors affecting those attributes are identified, experiments are designed with the varying combination of independent levels to obtain the nanoparticles with desired particle size, PDI, zeta potential and entrapment efficiency. The formulation with the best set of nanoparticle responses is selected as optimized and further evaluated for the respective studies. Design of experiments, a statistical tool, is now available to get the formulation with desired quality attributes (Turk et al. 2014).

During optimization, various models can be used from preliminary screening of factors to select their level and for the final study of their effect. It will again depend on the formulator to choose a suitable model for study and help in minimizing the experimentation time.

3.9 Design of Experiments

It is a statistical method to optimize the formulation systematically. It involves the well-organized experimental approach to design the experiments and attains the optimized product by finding the optimized levels of variables from the statistical analysis of responses (for dependent variables) obtained in the experiments. Simultaneously, with optimized levels, it also explains the effect of variables on the response and their interaction. The design of experiments is an emerging tool for pharmaceutical product development that ensures the quality, safety and efficacy of the drug products. Moreover, it reduces the time consumption and resource wastage and improves process performance.

The design of experiment is completed in four basic steps:

1. Based on the requirements, a number of factors and their selected levels, experiments are generated using the various DOE models.
2. Experiments are performed and the responses are recorded for each experiment set.
3. Statistical analysis of data to predict the optimized level of each independent variable along with the predicted response. Moreover, it also generates the polynomial equation elaborating on the effect of the variables on the responses.
4. The optimized batch with predicted levels is prepared, and the responses are compared with predicted responses to determine the standard deviation (should not be more than 10% to assure the authenticity of the process).

3.10 Factorial Design

Though the factorial design is ideally chosen for the screening of primary factors affecting the formulation to further design the experiments, it can be used to optimize the process also (Vandervoort and Ludwig 2002). There are several numbers of factorial designs available and selected according to suitability:

- Two-level factorial designs

2–21 factors with two-level (−1–1) can be studied at a time by full and fractional designs each factor to only two levels. Fractional factorials are an effective method to screen out the factors having a significant effect on the process and product. At the same time, it can predict the effect of factor interaction.

- General factorial designs

This is a special experimental design in which factors (1–12 maximum) have a different level (2 to 299) used to determine the critical factor. The method generates all possible combinations of factors with different levels.

- Plackett-Burman designs

This is a useful technique to evaluate up to 31 factors by assuming that the factors do not possess a significant effect.

- Taguchi designs

Not more than 63 factors can be studied simultaneously. There are number of designs available based on the number of factors to reduces the number of experiments.

3.11 Response Surface Design Selection

Response surface method (RSM) designs quantitatively determine the effect of various factors on the responses in terms of a polynomial equation and plot them as a surface plot to elaborate the effect. Moreover, it predicts the optimized level in the space with predicted responses from the statistical analysis of the responses generated in the experiment for a designed set of experiments. The levels are predicted by the desirability method; the desired responses selected (maximum or minimum or may be quantitatively selected) over the range of stable responses consequently predict the optimized level point. For this method, the level of the factor should be defined numerically or quantitatively. All the responses can be predicted with a combined set of factors.

3.12 Box-Behnken Design

When the process has three to ten factors to optimize and had three levels, the Box-Behnken is preferred. This design requires only three levels, coded as −1, 0 and + 1. The advantage of this design over the other is that very few experiments are needed to attain the designs with anticipated statistical properties. The quadratic model is the best model to explain the obtained findings and effect of a single factor or interaction of factor on the response, as the factors only have three levels and have been reported to optimize a variety of nanoformulations for oral immunization (Harde et al. 2015a, b, c, d, e, f).

3.13 Central Composite Design (CCD)

The CCD is a widely preferred response surface method to design the experiments and optimize the process (Hao et al. 2012). It can be divided into three groups of design points:

(a) Two-level factorial or fractional factorial design points
(b) Axial points
(c) Centre points

3.14 Mixture Design Selection

This method is generally preferred over another method if:

1. The components add to a fixed total. For instance, A is 10% of the mixture, B is 30% and C is the remaining 60%. If the percentage of one component is increased, then the percentage of one or more of the other components must be decreased. If the component amounts do not depend on each other, then response surface designs should be preferred over mixture designs (Choisnard et al. 2005).
2. The response must be a function of the proportions of the components. For example, the flavour of ice cream depends on the relative proportions of the ingredients, not on the total amount of ice cream. If the response is not related to the ingredient proportions, then response surface designs should be used.

3.15 Characterization of Nanoparticles

There are various characterization methods performed to evaluate the quality of the nanoparticles. The characterization techniques are depicted in Fig. 3.4 and briefly described below.

3.15.1 Particle Size and Polydispersity Index

Particle size and polydispersity index are very important parameters for any nanoformulation as they may directly affect the therapeutic performance (Harde et al. 2015a, b, c, d, e, f). Particle size analysis is conducted by photon correlation spectroscopy also called dynamic light scattering. The particle size is obtained as a function of correlation of scattered intensity to the particle's

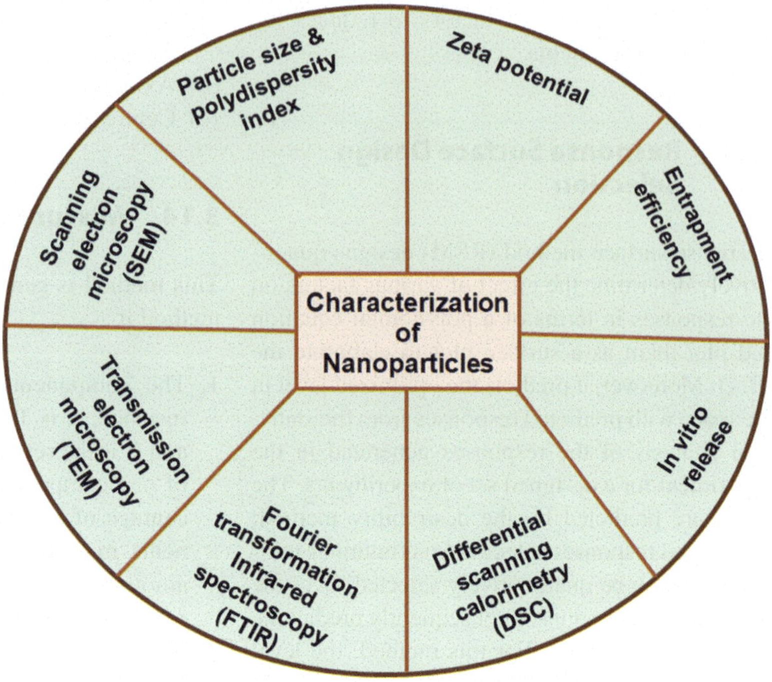

Fig. 3.4 Various characterization techniques employed to evaluate the nanoformulations

diffusion coefficient. It measures the change in the intensity of scattered light during the analysis concerning the volume of particles. The polydispersity index is a measure of particle distribution over the size range. The higher polydispersity index is the indication of heterogeneity in the particle size range.

3.15.2 Zeta Potential

The zeta potential has been considered as one of the very important parameters for the nanoformulation optimization as this is considered as stability of nanoformulations in suspension form (Harde et al. 2015a, b, c, d, e, f). The zeta potential measurement is based on the movement of charged nanoparticles dispersed in liquid in the direction of cathode or anode (depending on the charge on NPs) on applying the electric field in the sample. Briefly, the electric field is applied across the sample to induce mobility. Further, the electrophoretic mobility is determined in terms of the ratio of nanoparticle velocity and the electric field. Finally, the zeta potential is calculated using the Henry equation.

3.15.3 Entrapment Efficiency

Entrapment efficiency is calculated to find out the total drug encapsulated within the nanoparticles. The entrapment efficiency can be measured by either direct method or indirect method. The direct method measures the drug entrapped within the nanoparticles while in the indirect method the unentrapped drug is determined to calculate the drug entrapped within the nanoparticles (Harde et al. 2015a, b, c, d, e, f).

3.15.4 In Vitro Release

Determining the in vitro release is a very important parameter to predict the in vivo response in different physiological pH conditions (Das et al. 2014; Jain et al. 2014a, b, c). The nanoparticles or the formulation to be tested is suspended in the simulated physiological fluid or buffer of particular pH maintained at 37 °C and constant stirring. The conditions vary according to the route of administration to mimic the corresponding physiological conditions. The samples of dissolution medium are collected at various time intervals and analysed using the UV spectroscopy or HPLC depending on the suitability and sensitivity, to determine the drug concentration. Finally, the amount of drug released is calculated for each sampling period.

3.15.5 Scanning Electron Microscopy (SEM)

SEM has been widely reported to study the shape and surface morphology of a variety of novel formulations (Choudhary et al. 2010). This is direct visualization of prepared nanoparticles. Along with shape and morphology, actual particle size can also be measured by SEM. Before SEM analysis, properly diluted nanosuspension is dried over the copper strip and coated with gold to make it electrically conducting using the coater equipment. Then the coated nanoparticles are scanned by an electron beam over the focused area, and the secondary electron emitted from the surface is collected to attain the evidence about the surface morphology and shape of the particles.

3.15.6 Transmission Electron Microscopy (TEM)

In addition to the SEM, transmission electron microscopy is an excellent and widely reported tool for determining the exact shape and particle size of the nanoparticles (Jain et al. 2014a, b, c). A high potential electron beam is bombarded on the thin sample prepared in the metallic mesh (TEM grid), and once the electron beam interacts with the surface of the particles, it transmits the electrons which are captured by the detector to generate the crystal structure and shape and calculate the particle size. High-resolution TEM is an accurate technique generally applied to evaluate the quality, shape, size and density of nanoparticles. The TEM utilizes the high-potential electron for analysis rather than using the light rays. The magnification of TEM is much higher than other imaging techniques as the technique uses a low-wavelength electron beam.

3.15.7 Fourier Transform Infrared Spectroscopy (FTIR)

Fourier transform infrared spectroscopy is an analysis technique that determines the presence of specific functional groups in the compound in the form of transmittance peak in FTIR spectra corresponding to specific wavenumbers. During the processing, the drug may interact physically or chemically with the formulation component and can lose the activity or may elicit unwanted toxicity. FTIR is one of the widely conducted studies to assess the possible interaction (Patel et al. 2019a, b, c, d). Loss of peak corresponding to a specific functional group in the drug or appearance of some unknown peak in the spectra indicates the interaction. Moreover, the technique also qualitatively evaluates the drug entrapment in polymeric or lipid matrix.

3.15.8 Differential Scanning Calorimetry (DSC)

DSC is a thermal analysis usually conducted to define the melting point, glass transition temperature and melting enthalpy. This information can give us an idea about the crystalline nature qualitatively or quantitatively. Moreover, the interaction can also be evaluated with a significant shift in the melting point of the drug (Patel et al. 2019a, b, c, d). The sample equivalent to 10–20 mg is placed in the metallic pan and scanned over a certain temperature range. The endothermic peak gives the value of the melting point, while the disappearance of endothermic peak or intensity reduction signifies the loss of crystalline structure or conversion of the drug into an amorphous form. The % crystallinity can be calculated from the melting enthalpy. Melting enthalpy is directly proportional to crystallinity, and by keeping the pure drug 100% crystalline, the crystallinity of another sample can be obtained.

3.15.9 X-Ray Diffraction (XRD)

XRD is performed to determine the crystalline or amorphous structure of a compound and can be considered a universally accepted technique for the determination of drugs following the entrapment within the nanoformulation (Patel et al. 2019a, b, c, d). For taking the XRD spectra, the powdered sample is placed on the goniometer and thrown with the X-ray beam at a varying angle of diffraction (2θ; 10–80°). The diffracted beam of X-ray is collected by the detector to generate the X-ray diffraction pattern. The X-ray diffraction pattern of crystalline material exhibits high-intensity diffraction peaks at certain diffraction angles and has a specific arrangement for a particular compound. However, the amorphous compound does not possess a highly intense diffraction pattern. Interestingly, the nanoparticles convert the crystalline material into amorphous; thus, XRD is employed to determine the change in the crystalline structure of the drug.

3.16 Major Challenges

Though research in the field of nanomedicine has attained considerable success, very few nanoformulations got FDA approval in the last two to three decades of nanomedicine research. The safety, efficacy, scalability and regulatory compliance for nanoformulations are the major challenges.

3.17 Safety or Toxicity

Manufacturers have the responsibility to submit the appropriate and sufficient human toxicity data to regulatory agencies for approval of the drug product to assure the safety of drugs intended to be used in the clinic. The companies have to perform preclinical and clinical trials to generate sufficient toxicity data to fill the new drug application (NDA) or investigational new drug application (INDA) for FDA approval. Therefore, pharmacokinetics should be studied for any new product proposed for therapeutic use. Intensive study of the absorption, distribution, metabolism and excretion to establish complete pharmacokinetic profile to ensure safety is needed.

3.18 Scalability

Scalability, a process of manufacturing at an industrial level for clinical use, is a major challenge faced by the manufacturers. The optimization of the process for the efficient production of nanoformulations on a large scale is a difficult task. The unavailability of capable equipment, process controls and trained personnel and non-compliance with current good manufacturing practices pose impediments to manufacturing the nanoformulations at commercial level. Moreover, the unavailability of clear-cut regulatory guidelines is another challenge in maintaining quality standards.

3.19 Conclusion

Nanoformulations have been presented as a solution to overcome many of the challenges with conventional drug delivery; however, critical evaluation of different process and formulation variables, viz. selection of the right delivery system, polymer/lipid and solvent, method of preparation and exhaustive characterization, is needed to develop nanoformulations with the desired quality attributes for better therapeutic performance. Although extensive research in this field has resulted in the development of a handful of clinically approved products, finding a biocompatible material with minimal possible toxicity and scalability is the major issue that needs attention.

References

Agrawal A, Gupta P, Khanna A, Sharma R, Chandrabanshi H, Gupta N, Patil U, Yadav S (2010) Development and characterization of in situ gel system for nasal insulin delivery. Pharmazie 65(3):188–193

Agrawal AK, Das M, Jain S (2012) In situ gel systems as 'smart'carriers for sustained ocular drug delivery. Expert Opin Drug Deliv 9(4):383–402

Agrawal AK, Harde H, Thanki K, Jain S (2013) Improved stability and antidiabetic potential of insulin containing folic acid functionalized polymer stabilized multilayered liposomes following oral administration. Biomacromolecules 15(1):350–360

Agrawal AK, Urimi D, Harde H, Kushwah V, Jain S (2015a) Folate appended chitosan nanoparticles augment the stability, bioavailability and efficacy of insulin in diabetic rats following oral administration. RSC Adv 5(127):105179–105193

Agrawal AK, Urimi D, Jain S (2015b) Multifunctional polymeric nano-carriers in targeted drug delivery. In: Targeted drug delivery: concepts and design. Springer, Cham, pp 461–500

Agrawal AK, Aqil F, Jeyabalan J, Spencer WA, Beck J, Gachuki BW, Alhakeem SS, Oben K, Munagala R, Bondada S (2017a) Milk-derived exosomes for oral delivery of paclitaxel. Nanomedicine 13(5):1627–1636

Agrawal AK, Kumar K, Swarnakar NK, Kushwah V, Jain S (2017b) "Liquid crystalline nanoparticles": rationally designed vehicle to improve stability and therapeutic efficacy of insulin following oral administration. Mol Pharm 14(6):1874–1882

Akbarzadeh A, Rezaei-Sadabady R, Davaran S, Joo SW, Zarghami N, Hanifehpour Y, Samiei M, Kouhi M, Nejati-Koshki K (2013) Liposome: classification, preparation, and applications. Nanoscale Res Lett 8(1):102

Aqil F, Kausar H, Agrawal AK, Jeyabalan J, Kyakulaga A-H, Munagala R, Gupta R (2016) Exosomal formulation enhances therapeutic response of celastrol against lung cancer. Exp Mol Pathol 101(1):12–21

Aqil F, Jeyabalan J, Agrawal AK, Kyakulaga A-H, Munagala R, Parker L, Gupta RC (2017a) Exosomal delivery of berry anthocyanidins for the management of ovarian cancer. Food Funct 8(11):4100–4107

Aqil F, Munagala R, Jeyabalan J, Agrawal AK, Gupta R (2017b) Exosomes for the enhanced tissue bioavailability and efficacy of curcumin. AAPS J 19(6):1691–1702

Aqil F, Munagala R, Jeyabalan J, Agrawal AK, Kyakulaga A-H, Wilcher SA, Gupta RC (2019) Milk exosomes-natural nanoparticles for siRNA delivery. Cancer Lett 449:186–195

Balguri SP, Adelli GR, Majumdar S (2016) Topical ophthalmic lipid nanoparticle formulations (SLN, NLC) of indomethacin for delivery to the posterior segment ocular tissues. Eur J Pharm Biopharm 109:224–235

Bhaskar K, Anbu J, Ravichandiran V, Venkateswarlu V, Rao YM (2009) Lipid nanoparticles for transdermal delivery of flurbiprofen: formulation, in vitro, ex vivo and in vivo studies. Lipids Health Dis 8(1):6

Byrne JD, Betancourt T, Brannon-Peppas L (2008) Active targeting schemes for nanoparticle systems in cancer therapeutics. Adv Drug Deliv Rev 60(15):1615–1626

Casadó A, Sagristá ML, Mora M (2014) Formulation and in vitro characterization of thermosensitive liposomes for the delivery of irinotecan. J Pharm Sci 103(10):3127–3138

Chen H, Khemtong C, Yang X, Chang X, Gao J (2011) Nanonization strategies for poorly water-soluble drugs. Drug Discov Today 16(7–8):354–360

Cheow WS, Chang MW, Hadinoto K (2010) Antibacterial efficacy of inhalable levofloxacin-loaded polymeric nanoparticles against E. coli biofilm cells: the effect of antibiotic release profile. Pharm Res 27(8):1597–1609

Choisnard L, Géze A, Bigan M, Putaux J-L, Wouessidjewe D (2005) Efficient size control of amphiphilic cyclodextrin nanoparticles through a statistical mixture design methodology. J Pharm Sci 8(3):593–600

Choudhary H, Agrawal A, Malviya R, Yadav S, Jaliwala Y, Patil U (2010) Evaluation and optimization of preparative variables for controlled-release floating microspheres of levodopa/carbidopa. Pharmazie 65(3):194–198

Couvreur P, Kante B, Grislain L, Roland M, Speiser P (1982) Toxicity of polyalkylcyanoacrylate nanoparticles II: doxorubicin-loaded nanoparticles. J Pharm Sci 71(7):790–792

Das M, Jain R, Agrawal AK, Thanki K, Jain S (2014) Macromolecular bipill of gemcitabine and methotrexate facilitates tumor-specific dual drug therapy with higher benefit-to-risk ratio. Bioconjug Chem 25(3):501–509

Dhar S, Gu FX, Langer R, Farokhzad OC, Lippard SJ (2008) Targeted delivery of cisplatin to prostate cancer cells by aptamer functionalized Pt (IV) prodrug-PLGA–PEG nanoparticles. Proc Natl Acad Sci 105(45):17356–17361

Dixit K, Athawale RB, Singh S (2015) Quality control of residual solvent content in polymeric microparticles. J Microencapsul 32(2):107–122

El-Shabouri M (2002) Positively charged nanoparticles for improving the oral bioavailability of cyclosporin-A. Int J Pharm 249(1–2):101–108

Engel E, Michiardi A, Navarro M, Lacroix D, Planell JA (2008) Nanotechnology in regenerative medicine: the materials side. Trends Biotechnol 26(1):39–47

Fan W, Yan W, Xu Z, Ni H (2012) Formation mechanism of monodisperse, low molecular weight chitosan nanoparticles by ionic gelation technique. Colloids Surf B: Biointerfaces 90:21–27

Fazil M, Md S, Haque S, Kumar M, Baboota S, Sahni JK, Ali J (2012) Development and evaluation of rivastigmine loaded chitosan nanoparticles for brain targeting. Eur J Pharm Sci 47(1):6–15

Friedman AD, Claypool SE, Liu R (2013) The smart targeting of nanoparticles. Curr Pharm Des 19(35):6315–6329

Gade S, Patel KK, Gupta C, Anjum MM, Deepika D, Agrawal AK, Singh S (2019) An ex vivo evaluation of moxifloxacin nanostructured lipid carrier enriched in situ gel for transcorneal permeation on goat cornea. J Pharm Sci 108(9):2905–2916

Gnanakan SRP, Rajasekhar M, Subramania A (2009) Synthesis of polythiophene nanoparticles by surfactant-assisted dilute polymerization method for high performance redox supercapacitors. Int J Electrochem Sci 4(9):1289–1301

Gulyaev AE, Gelperina SE, Skidan IN, Antropov AS, Kivman GY, Kreuter J (1999) Significant transport of doxorubicin into the brain with polysorbate 80-coated nanoparticles. Pharm Res 16(10):1564–1569

Gupta H, Aqil M, Khar R, Ali A, Bhatnagar A, Mittal G (2011) Biodegradable levofloxacin nanoparticles for sustained ocular drug delivery. J Drug Target 19(6):409–417

Hafner A, Lovrić J, Pepić I, Filipović-Grčić J (2011) Lecithin/chitosan nanoparticles for transdermal delivery of melatonin. J Microencapsul 28(8):807–815

Hao J, Wang F, Wang X, Zhang D, Bi Y, Gao Y, Zhao X, Zhang Q (2012) Development and optimization of baicalin-loaded solid lipid nanoparticles prepared by coacervation method using central composite design. Eur J Pharm Sci 47(2):497–505

Harde H, Agrawal AK, Jain S (2014) Development of stabilized glucomannosylated chitosan nanoparticles using tandem crosslinking method for oral vaccine delivery. Nanomedicine 9(16):2511–2529

Harde H, Agrawal AK, Jain S (2015a) Tetanus toxoid-loaded layer-by-layer nanoassemblies for efficient systemic, mucosal, and cellular immunostimulatory response following oral administration. Drug Deliv Transl Res 5(5):498–510

Harde H, Agrawal AK, Jain S (2015b) Tetanus toxoids loaded glucomannosylated chitosan based nanohoming vaccine adjuvant with improved oral stability and immunostimulatory response. Pharm Res 32(1):122–134

Harde H, Agrawal AK, Jain S (2015c) Trilateral '3P' mechanics of stabilized layersomes technology for efficient oral immunization. J Biomed Nanotechnol 11(3):363–381

Harde H, Agrawal AK, Katariya M, Kale D, Jain S (2015d) Development of a topical adapalene-solid lipid nanoparticle loaded gel with enhanced efficacy and improved skin tolerability. RSC Adv 5(55):43917–43929

Harde H, Siddhapura K, Agrawal AK, Jain S (2015e) Development of dual toxoid-loaded layersomes for complete immunostimulatory response following peroral administration. Nanomedicine 10(7):1077–1091

Harde H, Siddhapura K, Agrawal AK, Jain S (2015f) Divalent toxoids loaded stable chitosan–glucomannan nanoassemblies for efficient systemic, mucosal and cellular immunostimulatory response following oral administration. Int J Pharm 487(1–2):292–304

Hatakeyama H, Akita H, Ishida E, Hashimoto K, Kobayashi H, Aoki T, Yasuda J, Obata K, Kikuchi H, Ishida T (2007) Tumor targeting of doxorubicin by anti-MT1-MMP antibody-modified PEG liposomes. Int J Pharm 342(1–2):194–200

Hu J, Johnston KP, Williams RO III (2004) Nanoparticle engineering processes for enhancing the dissolution rates of poorly water soluble drugs. Drug Dev Ind Pharm 30(3):233–245

Hu K, Li J, Shen Y, Lu W, Gao X, Zhang Q, Jiang X (2009) Lactoferrin-conjugated PEG–PLA nanoparticles with improved brain delivery: in vitro and in vivo evaluations. J Control Release 134(1):55–61

Huang G, Zhang N, Bi X, Dou M (2008) Solid lipid nanoparticles of temozolomide: potential reduction of cardial and nephric toxicity. Int J Pharm 355(1–2):314–320

Jain S, Patil SR, Swarnakar NK, Agrawal AK (2012) Oral delivery of doxorubicin using novel polyelectrolyte-stabilized liposomes (layersomes). Mol Pharm 9(9):2626–2635

Jain S, Kumar S, Agrawal AK, Thanki K, Banerjee UC (2013a) Enhanced transfection efficiency and reduced cytotoxicity of novel lipid–polymer hybrid nanoplexes. Mol Pharm 10(6):2416–2425

Jain S, Sharma JM, Agrawal AK, Mahajan RR (2013b) Surface stabilized efavirenz nanoparticles for oral bioavailability enhancement. J Biomed Nanotechnol 9(11):1862–1874

Jain S, Harde H, Indulkar A, Agrawal AK (2014a) Improved stability and immunological potential of tetanus toxoid containing surface engineered bilosomes following oral administration. Nanomedicine 10(2):431–440

Jain S, Indulkar A, Harde H, Agrawal AK (2014b) Oral mucosal immunization using glucomannosylated bilosomes. J Biomed Nanotechnol 10(6):932–947

Jain S, Jain R, Das M, Agrawal AK, Thanki K, Kushwah V (2014c) Combinatorial bio-conjugation of gemcitabine and curcumin enables dual drug delivery with synergistic anticancer efficacy and reduced toxicity. RSC Adv 4(55):29193–29201

Jain S, Kumar S, Agrawal A, Thanki K, Banerjee U (2015a) Hyaluronic acid–PEI–cyclodextrin polyplexes: implications for in vitro and in vivo transfection efficiency and toxicity. RSC Adv 5(51):41144–41154

Jain S, Spandana G, Agrawal AK, Kushwah V, Thanki K (2015b) Enhanced antitumor efficacy and reduced toxicity of docetaxel loaded estradiol functionalized stealth polymeric nanoparticles. Mol Pharm 12(11):3871–3884

Jain S, Garg T, Kushwah V, Thanki K, Agrawal AK, Dora CP (2017) α-Tocopherol as functional excipient for resveratrol and coenzyme Q10-loaded SNEDDS for improved bioavailability and prophylaxis of breast cancer. J Drug Target 25(6):554–565

Jana S, Manna S, Nayak AK, Sen KK, Basu SK (2014) Carbopol gel containing chitosan-egg albumin nanoparticles for transdermal aceclofenac delivery. Colloids Surf B: Biointerfaces 114:36–44

Jenning V, Lippacher A, Gohla S (2002) Medium scale production of solid lipid nanoparticles (SLN) by high pressure homogenization. J Microencapsul 19(1):1–10

Kaler A, Mittal AK, Katariya M, Harde H, Agrawal AK, Jain S, Banerjee UC (2014) An investigation of in vivo wound healing activity of biologically synthesized silver nanoparticles. J Nanopart Res 16(9):2605

Katiyar S, Pandit J, Mondal RS, Mishra AK, Chuttani K, Aqil M, Ali A, Sultana Y (2014) In situ gelling dorzolamide loaded chitosan nanoparticles for the treatment of glaucoma. Carbohydr Polym 102:117–124

Ke W, Zhao Y, Huang R, Jiang C, Pei Y (2008) Enhanced oral bioavailability of doxorubicin in a dendrimer drug delivery system. J Pharm Sci 97(6):2208–2216

Khdair A, Gerard B, Handa H, Mao G, Shekhar MP, Panyam J (2008) Surfactant– polymer nanoparticles enhance the effectiveness of anticancer photodynamic therapy. Mol Pharm 5(5):795–807

Kisich K, Gelperina S, Higgins M, Wilson S, Shipulo E, Oganesyan E, Heifets L (2007) Encapsulation of moxifloxacin within poly (butyl cyanoacrylate) nanoparticles enhances efficacy against intracellular Mycobacterium tuberculosis. Int J Pharm 345(1–2):154–162

Krausz AE, Adler BL, Cabral V, Navati M, Doerner J, Charafeddine RA, Chandra D, Liang H, Gunther L, Clendaniel A (2015) Curcumin-encapsulated nanoparticles as innovative antimicrobial and wound healing agent. Nanomedicine 11(1):195–206

Kushwah V, Agrawal AK, Dora CP, Mallinson D, Lamprou DA, Gupta RC, Jain S (2017) Novel gemcitabine conjugated albumin nanoparticles: a potential strategy to enhance drug efficacy in pancreatic cancer treatment. Pharm Res 34(11):2295–2311

Kushwah V, Jain DK, Agrawal AK, Jain S (2018a) Improved antitumor efficacy and reduced toxicity of docetaxel using anacardic acid functionalized stealth liposomes. Colloids Surf B: Biointerfaces 172:213–223

Kushwah V, Katiyar SS, Agrawal AK, Gupta RC, Jain S (2018b) Co-delivery of docetaxel and gemcitabine using PEGylated self-assembled stealth nanoparticles for improved breast cancer therapy. Nanomedicine 14(5):1629–1641

Kushwah V, Katiyar SS, Agrawal AK, Saraf I, Singh IP, Lamprou DA, Gupta RC, Jain S (2018c) Implication of linker length on cell cytotoxicity, pharmacokinetic and toxicity profile of gemcitabine-docetaxel combinatorial dual drug conjugate. Int J Pharm 548(1):357–374

Kushwah V, Katiyar SS, Dora CP, Agrawal AK, Lamprou DA, Gupta RC, Jain S (2018d) Co-delivery of docetaxel and gemcitabine by anacardic acid modified self-assembled albumin nanoparticles for effective breast cancer management. Acta Biomater 73:424–436

Lee M, Cho YW, Park JH, Chung H, Jeong SY, Choi K, Moon DH, Kim SY, Kim I-S, Kwon IC (2006) Size control of self-assembled nanoparticles by an emulsion/solvent evaporation method. Colloid Polym Sci 284(5):506–512

Letchford K, Burt H (2007) A review of the formation and classification of amphiphilic block copolymer nanoparticulate structures: micelles, nanospheres, nanocapsules and polymersomes. Eur J Pharm Biopharm 65(3):259–269

Lince F, Marchisio DL, Barresi AA (2011) A comparative study for nanoparticle production with passive mixers via solvent-displacement: use of CFD models for optimization and design. Chem Eng Process Process Intensif 50(4):356–368

Ling Y, Wei K, Luo Y, Gao X, Zhong S (2011) Dual docetaxel/superparamagnetic iron oxide loaded nanoparticles for both targeting magnetic resonance imaging and cancer therapy. Biomaterials 32(29):7139–7150

Ling Y, Wei K, Zou F, Zhong S (2012) Temozolomide loaded PLGA-based superparamagnetic nanoparticles for magnetic resonance imaging and treatment of malignant glioma. Int J Pharm 430(1–2):266–275

Lipinski C (2002) Poor aqueous solubility—an industry wide problem in drug discovery. Am Pharm Rev 5(3):82–85

Liu W, Hu M, Liu W, Xue C, Xu H, Yang X (2008) Investigation of the carbopol gel of solid lipid nanoparticles for the transdermal iontophoretic delivery of triamcinolone acetonide acetate. Int J Pharm 364(1):135–141

Losi P, Briganti E, Errico C, Lisella A, Sanguinetti E, Chiellini F, Soldani G (2013) Fibrin-based scaffold incorporating VEGF-and bFGF-loaded nanoparticles stimulates wound healing in diabetic mice. Acta Biomater 9(8):7814–7821

Luo Y, Chen D, Ren L, Zhao X, Qin J (2006) Solid lipid nanoparticles for enhancing vinpocetine's oral bioavailability. J Control Release 114(1):53–59

Madan J, Pandey RS, Jain V, Katare OP, Chandra R, Katyal A (2013) Poly (ethylene)-glycol conjugated solid lipid nanoparticles of noscapine improve biological half-life, brain delivery and efficacy in glioblastoma cells. Nanomedicine 9(4):492–503

Mandoli C, Pagliari F, Pagliari S, Forte G, Di Nardo P, Licoccia S, Traversa E (2010) Stem cell aligned growth induced by CeO2 nanoparticles in PLGA scaffolds with improved bioactivity for regenerative medicine. Adv Funct Mater 20(10):1617–1624

Min KH, Park K, Kim Y-S, Bae SM, Lee S, Jo HG, Park R-W, Kim I-S, Jeong SY, Kim K (2008) Hydrophobically modified glycol chitosan nanoparticles-encapsulated camptothecin enhance the drug stability and tumor targeting in cancer therapy. J Control Release 127(3):208–218

Müller RH, Radtke M, Wissing SA (2002) Solid lipid nanoparticles (SLN) and nanostructured lipid carriers (NLC) in cosmetic and dermatological preparations. Adv Drug Deliv Rev 54:S131–S155

Munagala R, Aqil F, Jeyabalan J, Agrawal AK, Mudd AM, Kyakulaga AH, Singh IP, Vadhanam MV, Gupta RC (2017) Exosomal formulation of anthocyanidins against multiple cancer types. Cancer Lett 393:94–102

Nahar M, Mishra D, Dubey V, Jain NK (2008) Development, characterization, and toxicity evaluation of amphotericin B–loaded gelatin nanoparticles. Nanomedicine 4(3):252–261

Naik A, Kalia YN, Guy RH, Fessi H (2004) Enhancement of topical delivery from biodegradable nanoparticles. Pharm Res 21(10):1818–1825

Nair A, Khunt D, Misra M (2019) Application of quality by design for optimization of spray drying process used in drying of risperidone nanosuspension. Powder Technol 342:156–165

Nasongkla N, Shuai X, Ai H, Weinberg BD, Pink J, Boothman DA, Gao J (2004) cRGD-functionalized polymer micelles for targeted doxorubicin delivery. Angew Chem Int Ed 43(46):6323–6327

Nii T, Ishii F (2005) Encapsulation efficiency of water-soluble and insoluble drugs in liposomes prepared by the microencapsulation vesicle method. Int J Pharm 298(1):198–205

Parra A, Mallandrich M, Clares B, Egea MA, Espina M, García ML, Calpena AC (2015) Design and elaboration of freeze-dried PLGA nanoparticles for the transcorneal permeation of carprofen: ocular anti-inflammatory applications. Colloids Surf B: Biointerfaces 136:935–943

Patel KK, Agrawal AK, Anjum MM, Tripathi M, Pandey N, Bhattacharya S, Tilak R, Singh S (2019a) DNase-I functionalization of ciprofloxacin-loaded chitosan nanoparticles overcomes the biofilm-mediated resistance of Pseudomonas aeruginosa. Appl Nanosci 10:563. https://doi.org/10.1007/s13204-019-01129-8

Patel KK, Gade S, Anjum MM, Singh SK, Maiti P, Agrawal AK, Singh S (2019b) Effect of penetration enhancers and amorphization on transdermal permeation flux of raloxifene-encapsulated solid lipid nanoparticles: an ex vivo study on human skin. Appl Nanosci 9(6):1383–1394

Patel KK, Surekha DB, Tripathi M, Anjum MM, Muthu M, Tilak R, Agrawal AK, Singh S (2019c) Antibiofilm potential of silver sulfadiazine-loaded nanoparticle formulations: a study on the effect of DNase-I on microbial biofilm and wound healing activity. Mol Pharm 16(9):3916–3925

Patel KK, Tripathi M, Pandey N, Agrawal AK, Gade S, Anjum MM, Tilak R, Singh S (2019d) Alginate lyase immobilized chitosan nanoparticles of ciprofloxacin for the improved antimicrobial activity against the biofilm associated mucoid P. aeruginosa infection in cystic fibrosis. Int J Pharm 563:30–42

Potta SG, Minemi S, Nukala RK, Peinado C, Lamprou DA, Urquhart A, Douroumis D (2010) Development of solid lipid nanoparticles for enhanced solubility of poorly soluble drugs. J Biomed Nanotechnol 6(6):634–640

Rai VK, Mishra N, Agrawal AK, Jain S, Yadav NP (2016) Novel drug delivery system: an immense hope for diabetics. Drug Deliv 23(7):2371–2390

Reverchon E (1999) Supercritical antisolvent precipitation of micro-and nano-particles. J Supercrit Fluids 15(1):1–21

Rosen J, Yoffe S, Meerasa A, Verma M, Gu F (2011) Nanotechnology and diagnostic imaging: new advances in contrast agent technology. J Nanomed Nanotechnol 2:115

Sahoo SK, Dilnawaz F, Krishnakumar S (2008) Nanotechnology in ocular drug delivery. Drug Discov Today 13(3–4):144–151

Sarmento B, Ribeiro A, Veiga F, Ferreira D, Neufeld R (2007) Oral bioavailability of insulin contained in polysaccharide nanoparticles. Biomacromolecules 8(10):3054–3060

Schäfer-Korting M, Mehnert W, Korting H-C (2007) Lipid nanoparticles for improved topical application of drugs for skin diseases. Adv Drug Deliv Rev 59(6):427–443

Sengupta P, Basu S, Soni S, Pandey A, Roy B, Oh MS, Chin KT, Paraskar AS, Sarangi S, Connor Y (2012) Cholesterol-tethered platinum II-based supramolecular nanoparticle increases antitumor efficacy and reduces nephrotoxicity. Proc Natl Acad Sci 109(28):11294–11299

Seymour L, Duncan R, Strohalm J, Kopeček J (1987) Effect of molecular weight (M w) of N-(2-hydroxypropyl) methacrylamide copolymers on body distribution and rate of excretion after subcutaneous, intraperitoneal, and intravenous administration to rats. J Biomed Mater Res 21(11):1341–1358

Shaikh J, Ankola D, Beniwal V, Singh D, Kumar MR (2009) Nanoparticle encapsulation improves oral bioavailability of curcumin by at least 9-fold when compared to curcumin administered with piperine as absorption enhancer. Eur J Pharm Sci 37(3–4):223–230

Sharma N, Madan P, Lin S (2016) Effect of process and formulation variables on the preparation of parenteral paclitaxel-loaded biodegradable polymeric nanoparticles: a co-surfactant study. Asian J Pharm Sci 11(3):404–416

Shilpi D, Kushwah V, Agrawal AK, Jain S (2017) Improved stability and enhanced oral bioavailability of atorvastatin loaded stearic acid modified gelatin nanoparticles. Pharm Res 34(7):1505–1516

Shim J, Kang HS, Park W-S, Han S-H, Kim J, Chang I-S (2004) Transdermal delivery of mixnoxidil with block copolymer nanoparticles. J Control Release 97(3):477–484

Singh S, Kushwah V, Agrawal AK, Jain S (2018) Insulin- and quercetin-loaded liquid crystalline nanoparticles: implications on oral bioavailability, antidiabetic and antioxidant efficacy. Nanomedicine 13(5):521–537

Spataro G, Malecaze F, Turrin C-O, Soler V, Duhayon C, Elena P-P, Majoral J-P, Caminade A-M (2010) Designing dendrimers for ocular drug delivery. Eur J Med Chem 45(1):326–334

Sun YP, Meziani MJ, Pathak P, Qu L (2005) Polymeric nanoparticles from rapid expansion of supercritical fluid solution. Chem Eur J 11(5):1366–1373

Suthar AK, Solanki SS, Dhanwani RK (2011) Enhancement of dissolution of poorly water soluble raloxifene hydrochloride by preparing nanoparticles. J Adv Pharm Educ Res 2:189–194

Tomoda K, Terashima H, Suzuki K, Inagi T, Terada H, Makino K (2011) Enhanced transdermal delivery of indomethacin-loaded PLGA nanoparticles

by iontophoresis. Colloids Surf B: Biointerfaces 88(2):706–710
Toti US, Guru BR, Hali M, McPharlin CM, Wykes SM, Panyam J, Whittum-Hudson JA (2011) Targeted delivery of antibiotics to intracellular chlamydial infections using PLGA nanoparticles. Biomaterials 32(27):6606–6613
Turk CTS, Oz UC, Serim TM, Hascicek C (2014) Formulation and optimization of nonionic surfactants emulsified nimesulide-loaded PLGA-based nanoparticles by design of experiments. AAPS PharmSciTech 15(1):161–176
Uchechi O, Ogbonna JD, Attama AA (2014) Nanoparticles for dermal and transdermal drug delivery. In: Application of nanotechnology in drug delivery. IntechOpen, London, UK
Urimi D, Agrawal AK, Kushwah V, Jain S (2019) Polyglutamic acid functionalization of chitosan nanoparticles enhances the therapeutic efficacy of insulin following oral administration. AAPS PharmSciTech 20(3):131
Vandervoort J, Ludwig A (2002) Biocompatible stabilizers in the preparation of PLGA nanoparticles: a factorial design study. Int J Pharm 238(1–2):77–92
Wang X, Chi N, Tang X (2008) Preparation of estradiol chitosan nanoparticles for improving nasal absorption and brain targeting. Eur J Pharm Biopharm 70(3):735–740
Wen H, Park K (2010) Oral controlled release formulation design and drug delivery. Theory to practice, pp 169–183, Wiley, USA
Woitiski CB, Neufeld RJ, Veiga F, Carvalho RA, Figueiredo IV (2010) Pharmacological effect of orally delivered insulin facilitated by multilayered stable nanoparticles. Eur J Pharm Sci 41(3–4):556–563
Xie J, Lee S, Chen X (2010) Nanoparticle-based theranostic agents. Adv Drug Deliv Rev 62(11):1064–1079
Yao M, McClements DJ, Xiao H (2015) Improving oral bioavailability of nutraceuticals by engineered nanoparticle-based delivery systems. Curr Opin Food Sci 2:14–19
Yoo HS, Oh JE, Lee KH, Park TG (1999) Biodegradable nanoparticles containing doxorubicin-PLGA conjugate for sustained release. Pharm Res 16(7):1114–1118
Zambaux M, Bonneaux F, Gref R, Maincent P, Dellacherie E, Alonso M, Labrude P, Vigneron C (1998) Influence of experimental parameters on the characteristics of poly (lactic acid) nanoparticles prepared by a double emulsion method. J Control Release 50(1–3):31–40
Zhang L, Gu F, Chan J, Wang A, Langer R, Farokhzad O (2008) Nanoparticles in medicine: therapeutic applications and developments. Clin Pharm Ther 83(5):761–769
Zhang C, Wan X, Zheng X, Shao X, Liu Q, Zhang Q, Qian Y (2014) Dual-functional nanoparticles targeting amyloid plaques in the brains of Alzheimer's disease mice. Biomaterials 35(1):456–465

Theranostics Nanoformulations: Merging Diagnostics and Nanotherapeutics

4

Shubham Khot, Shruti U. Rawal, and Mayur M. Patel

Abstract

Since the emergence of the concept of theranostics in 1998, the field has constantly evolved. With a unique amalgamation of diagnostic and therapeutic applications, theranostics has gained profound attention from researchers worldwide. More recently, researchers have attempted to augment the paradigm with the concept of "nanotheranostics," which offers multimodal medical and biomedical applications. "Nanotheranostics" are specially devised drug delivery systems/nanoformulations that comprise nanocarriers/nanoparticles for theranostics applications. "Nanotheranostics" confers special attributes to theranostics, thereby potentiating their efficacy. Spurred on by advances in material chemistry and nanoformulations, scientists have exploited distinctive electrical, magnetic and optical properties of several types of nanocarriers for theranostics applications. The present chapter discusses the nanocarriers of several types for diverse applications in disease state monitoring, treatment monitoring, personalized medicine, image-guided drug delivery, molecular imaging and pharmacogenomics. Besides offering the above-stated advantages, nanotheranostics can offer a safer and more efficient therapy to the patients, obviating redundant treatment and saving overall cost of therapy. Other aspects such as biological processes governing theranostics fundamentals, their applications in several diseases and medical conditions, regulatory aspects, commercial aspects and future perspectives have been discussed in the chapter.

Keywords

Theranostics · Nanomaterials · Diagnostics · Upconversion nanoparticles · Dendrimers

Nomenclature

CEO	Chief executive officer
Cy5	Cyanine 5
E. coli	*Escherichia coli*
MUC1	Mucin1
PDT	Photodynamic therapy
PEG	Polyethylene glycol
RBCs	Red blood cells
ROS	Reactive oxygen species
US	United States of America
USD	United states dollar
UV	Ultraviolet

S. Khot · S. U. Rawal · M. M. Patel (✉)
Department of Pharmaceutics, Institute of Pharmacy, Nirma University, Ahmedabad, Gujarat, India

S. Talegaonkar, M. Rai (eds.), *Nanoformulations in Human Health*, https://doi.org/10.1007/978-3-030-41858-8_4

4.1 Introduction

The term "theranostics" was coined in 1998 by John Funkhouser to address the integrated science of therapy and diagnosis (Idée et al. 2013). Hence, theranostics can be ascribed as a multidisciplinary therapeutic paradigm, utilizing innumerable imaging, therapeutic and targeting agents, enabling real-time diagnosis and therapeutic drug monitoring in the future of personalized medicine.

Although the term theranostics was coined in late twentieth century, the use of theranostic formulations dates back to 1940s. Thus, the concept of theranostics is not entirely new to the field of medicine. It started with the use of radionuclides in diagnosis as well as in therapy. The use of radioactive iodine (I-131)-based formulation was first reported in 1941 by Saul Hertz for diagnosis and treatment of hyperthyroidism. In 1946, radioactive iodine was first ever to be reported for metastatic thyroid cancer therapy. Moreover, the biochemical moiety "Haem" was utilized in diagnostic imaging for cancer in the 1920s. Another biochemical moiety "phthalocyanine" was also used in positron emission-based diagnosis around the 1950s, whereas "porphyrin" was used as a contrast agent in magnetic resonance imaging around the 1980s. Since its inception till date, theranostics has been fostering remarkable tailored and targeted therapy.

Theranostics is most widely employed in the treatment of the majority of inflammatory diseases such as cardiovascular disease, neurodegenerative disease and cancer. Neurodegenerative diseases such as Alzheimer's, Parkinson's, epilepsy and Huntington's have been investigated for treatment with theranostics. The majority of cardiovascular diseases such as atherosclerosis, ischemia, hypertension, myocardial infarction and thromboembolism are potentially fatal and require precise treatment measures offered by theranostics nanomedicine. Further, life-threatening diseases such as cancer (breast, lung, brain, pancreatic and colon), multiple sclerosis and some of the autoimmune diseases are also reported to have been investigated for the employment of theranostics. The global theranostics market size was estimated at USD 6.22 billion in 2017 and is anticipated to gain significant traction over the coming years. Theranostic nanomedicine has offered promising and potential medical intervention by taking advantage of the high-payload nanoconstructs for both imaging and therapeutic function biomedicine (Bulte and Modo 2008). The advantages and disadvantages of theranostic delivery systems have been schematized in Fig. 4.1.

4.2 Fundamentals Governing Nanotheranostics

The use of nanotechnology in the field of medicine is emerging and expanding, since advances in scientific research spurred in the late twentieth century. Numerous examples of nanomedicines exist that have undergone thorough and extensive research from preclinical stage to clinical stage. Moreover, various nanocarrier-based systems have been extensively investigated such as liposomes, micelles, dendrimers and inorganic nanoparticles. These systems can be modified into less toxic, multifunctional and biocompatible nanoscaled vectors that have an enhanced biodistribution. In contrast to small molecules, theranostics nanomaterials render paramount potential in enhancing site-specific delivery of pharmacological agents. Moreover, multifunctionality of these theranostics agents depicts superior therapeutic efficiency and reduced adverse effects. Such diversified theranostics nanoplatforms are fabricated by combination of drugs and contrast agents for simultaneous imaging and therapy intended for active as well as passive targeted and controlled drug delivery. Engineering multifunctional theranostic nanoparticles present numerous challenges as mentioned below:

1. Limited choice of materials with inherent imaging and therapeutic properties which can be employed for designing such systems.
2. Inherent toxicity of individual components.
3. Lack of adequate storage and loading capacity as well as insufficient or inconsistent in vivo stability.

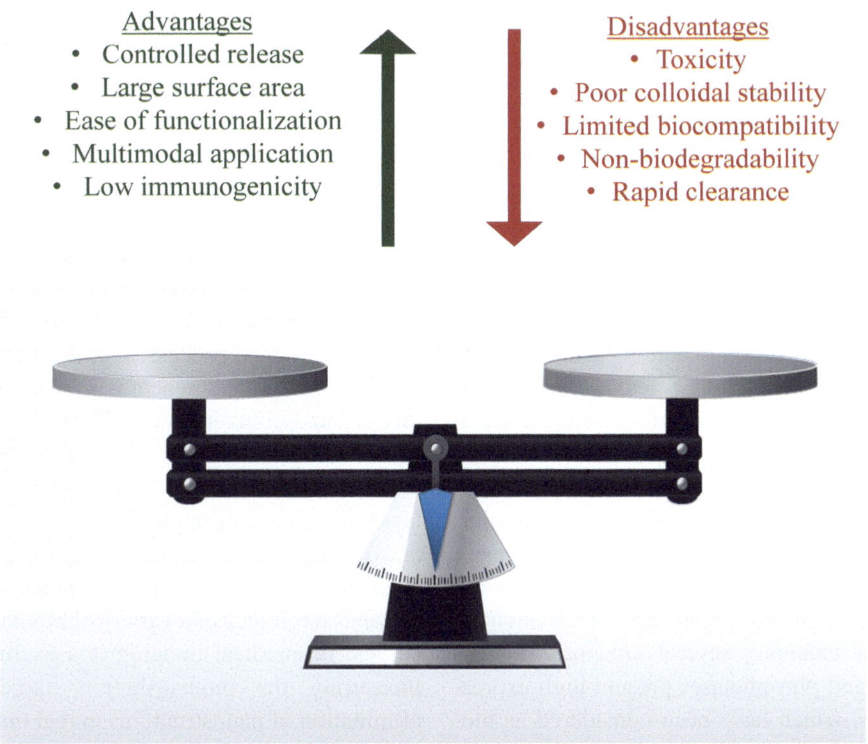

Fig. 4.1 Advantages and disadvantages offered by theranostic delivery systems

4. Complex fabrication process posing practical difficulties for industrial scalability and a high degree of variation in batch production.
5. Manufacturing cost incurred is often high.
6. Regulatory obstacles which impede clinical translation, development and progress.

Designing an ideal theranostics formulation requires a thorough screening and careful evaluation of drug and excipients. For example, a contrast agent for imaging in ideal conditions functions via faster binding to the target tissue and rapid systemic clearance, whereas drug delivery approach requires prolonged systemic circulation to achieve maximum uptake by target tissue. Similarly, physical characteristics and parameters of drug-loaded cargos (e.g. lipophilic drugs, lipophobic image contrast agent and polyionic nucleic acids) are subjected to considerable variation in order to achieve effective and optimum loading capacities by using different materials and strategies. Thus, it becomes difficult for any approach to provide a generalized theranostics platform for diverse applications. In order to integrate theranostics with nanotechnology, one must have a clear understanding of nanoscaled materials and their inherent physicochemical properties.

Nanoparticles can be defined as nanostructured constructs with particle size range of 10 nm to few hundred nanometres. In comparison with atoms or molecules, the nanoparticulate system possesses a significantly high surface area-to-volume ratio. Nanoparticulate systems are designed in particular fashion to enhance its magnetic, optical, electrical and immunological properties. Moreover, the technological advancements have enabled us to harness and alter their potential for utilization and widespread applications. These systems can be modulated into different sizes and shapes, surfaces, porosity and polarity. Theranostics nanoplatforms have been integrated with several stimuli-responsive agents, thereby enhancing their theranostics potential and providing a more accurate diagnosis as well as higher therapeutic efficiency and precision.

The stimulus can be classified as endogenous (e.g. pH, enzymes, hypoxia and redox) and exogenous (e.g. temperature, light, ultrasound, magnetic field). Furthermore, enzymes possessing inherent characteristics such as a high degree of relevance in several diseases in presence of precise and specific substrate selectivity and high catalytic activity are more likely and widely employed candidates for designing stimuli-responsive theranostics. Mechanism of catalysis mainly involves redox reaction with substrate leading to bond formation or cleavage. Numerous research studies have depicted widespread use of proteases, kinases, oxidoreductases and phosphatases in fabrication of stimuli-responsive systems. As a representative endogenous stimulus, enzymes are involved in a variety of key physiological processes and exhibit altered expression levels in many disease-associated microenvironments. For example, several enzymes such as proteases and phosphatases present high expression levels, which have been considered as biomarkers for the diagnosis and treatment of cancer, inflammation and neurodegeneration. A few examples of popularized commercial theranostics are listed in Table 4.1.

The following sections focus on various nanovectors, their applications in theranostics as well as their toxicity, pharmacokinetics, characteristics and compositions.

4.3 "Nanotheranostics": Nanomaterials for Theranostics Applications

4.3.1 Biomedical Imaging and Therapeutic Payloads

Imaging can provide valuable information about tissue composition, morphology and function, as well as quantitative descriptions of many fundamental biological processes. In recent years, biomedical imaging science has matured into a distinct and coherent set of ideas and concepts, and it has attained a position of central importance in medical research. In particular, numerous studies have been published on how imaging is evolving from qualitative visual depictions of anatomy into a science that contributes quantitative measurements of a variety of biomedical processes. Biomedical imaging is a useful tool for measuring the biodistribution, targeting and elimination of nanostructures in real time. This is especially needed at the whole organism level. In order to provide sufficient imaging contrast, biomedical nanodevices can be designed with reporting functions or moieties that provide a signal in conventional medical imaging modalities. These include gamma scintigraphy, magnetic resonance imaging (MRI), computed tomography (CT), positron emission tomography (PET)

Table 4.1 Commercial theranostic products

Brand name	Agent/system employed	Intent	Reference
Resovist®	Superparamagnetic iron oxide nanoparticles	MRI contrast agent in patients with liver diseases such as cirrhosis and hepatocellular carcinoma	Reimer and Balzer (2003)
Supravist®	Ultrasmall superparamagnetic iron oxide nanoparticles	MRI contrast agent in patients with multiple sclerosis and nephrogenic systemic fibrosis	Neuwelt et al. (2009), Engberink et al. (2010)
Neotect®	Technitium 99 m Depreotide	Used in oncotherapy for diagnosis and treatment.	Weiner and Thakur (2005)
Zevalin®	Yttrium-90 labelled ibritumomab and rituximab	Radioimmunotherapy for non-Hodgkin's lymphoma	Goldsmith (2010)
Bexxar®	Iodine-131 labelled tositumomab		
Folatescan™	Technetium-99 m etarfolatide or Technetium-99 m EC20	Treatment of rheumatoid arthritis, metastatic renal cell carcinoma and ovarian carcinoma	Naveed et al. (2004), Matteson et al. (2009), Marchetti et al. (2014)
Lipiodol®	I-131 poppy seed oil	Radiocontrast agent in hepatocellular carcinoma	Dumortier et al. (2014), Gallicchio et al. (2016)

and ultrasound (US) imaging. Additionally, digital radiography such as X-ray imaging has produced a spectrum of methods for interrogating intact 3D structure of the body non-invasively. A variety of new microscopies have also flourished, making use of novel phenomena such as non-linear photon interactions and the sensing of atomic forces at surfaces. Of these, the functional imaging modalities are particularly useful given that nanomedicine targets processes at the cellular and molecular level.

Biomedical imaging involves the complex chain of acquiring, processing and visualizing structural or functional images of living objects or systems, including extraction and processing of image-related information. Several techniques are utilized for optical imaging such as near-infrared (NIR) fluorescence imaging (Hong et al. 2017; Hu et al. 2017), photodynamic therapy (Näkki et al. 2017) and photoacoustic and photothermal imaging therapy (Rong et al. 2015). Ultrasound-assisted imaging and therapy is another effective non-invasive method that can be utilized in designing potential theranostics (Emi et al. 2019). Moreover, nuclear chemistry is an effective and useful tool for imaging and therapy by utilizing radiolabeled nanoparticles. With the help of radio imaging techniques, these radiolabeled nanoparticles can be successfully employed for theranostics in cancer and other therapeutic applications (Liu et al. 2015; Dai et al. 2018). Theranostics nanomaterials are designed based on their physical and chemical properties such as optical, magnetic, thermal and radioactive properties.

In contrast to the conventional approach of using a single imaging tool, recently researchers are adopting multiple imaging approaches. The multi-imaging approach or multimodal approach has been extensively investigated in preclinical and clinical research. Few examples of multimodal approach are the use of a combination of imaging techniques such as MRI/PET, MRI/CT, MRI/PET/US, etc. Recently discovered photoacoustic imaging is yet another multimodal approach which serves as theranostics platform. This technique especially offers high-level precision and accuracy in imaging of endophytic tumours in contrast with other single modal imaging. Photoacoustic imaging possesses an ability to convert light signals into ultrasound, to yield a high contrast optical image and ultrasonic spatial resolution with deep tissue penetration in a single modality. Photoacoustic imaging has a wide range of applications in multiscale and multi-contrast visualization from cells to organs and anatomy to physiology. Moreover, innovations in photoacoustic techniques have rendered even better and advanced imaging, such as photoacoustic microscopy, photoactivated localization microscopy, stochastic optical reconstruction microscopy, confocal microscopy, photoacoustic endoscopy and CT (Liu et al. 2016).

The therapeutic payload includes a wide array of bioactives like the small molecules, peptides and proteins which are loaded with a carrier system for enhancing their efficiency through targeted delivery. Several such carrier systems are employed in preclinical and clinical research for enhancement in drug delivery. Inorganic nanostructures offer unique and desirable physicochemical properties and have been employed as molecular payloads for peptide delivery (Bertucci et al. 2018). Magnetic nanoconstructs have been employed as multifunctional therapeutic payloads for all in one cancer therapy (immune, thermal, chemo and radiotherapy). Such magnificent multifunctional payloads could address and overcome the challenges offered by conventional cancer therapy leading towards a new paradigm in modern cancer theranostics (Datta et al. 2016). Similarly, porous silicon nanoconstructs depict excellent materialistic properties and advanced theranostics applications for incorporation of therapeutic payloads (Kumeria et al. 2017). Furthermore, Janus-like nanoparticles have been synthesized and investigated in cancer treatment. These nanoparticles comprised of magnetite and gold nanohybrids exhibiting dual nature and were found superior as compared to pre-existing commercial MRI contrast agents (Efremova et al. 2018). Other than inorganic nanomaterials, several other bio-inspired materials are also under investigation as potential theranostics agents. Antibody-drug conjugates have been employed as potential tumour cell-specific targeted payloads in cancer theranostics (Miller et al. 2018). Newer therapeutic payloads have been designed using non-pathogenic *E. coli*. The novel designs have shown high efficiency and excellent biocompatibility as drug delivery systems (González-Prieto and Lesser 2018). Moreover, RBCs have also been utilized as multifunctional bio-inspired cargos as potential cancer theranostics agent. The multifunctionality and high payload capability of RBC can render multimodal cancer therapy. Additionally, these cargos have low off-target toxicity and excellent biocompatibility and safety in simultaneous monitoring and treatment (Wu et al. 2015). Bio-inspired nanomaterials will continue to gain popularity and significance because of their advantages in circumventing the biological barriers, which are huge hurdles for use of conventional nanovectors in drug delivery (Evangelopoulos et al. 2018). The role of theranostics in cancer therapy has been exemplified in Fig. 4.2.

4.3.2 Nanotheranostics Carriers

Various nanocarriers that have been employed for diagnostic and therapeutic application are discussed in the present section.

4.3.2.1 Polymeric Nanocarriers

Polymeric Micelles

Polymeric micelles are composed of units of natural or synthetic polymers which condense and precipitate under suitable process conditions to give nanospheres or nanoparticles. Upponi et al. (2018) described a polymeric nanoformulation comprising of PEG and phosphatidylethanolamine for diagnosis and treatment of cancer. The prepared micellar formulation was utilized for the loading of hydrophobic and water-insoluble paclitaxel and superparamagnetic iron oxide nanoparticles. The former is a functional chemotherapeutic agent, and the latter one is used as an MRI contrast agent. These polymeric micelles were found to be stable with minimum interaction between the loaded therapeutic and diagnostic agents. Moreover, the developed formulation depicted significant retention in magnetic properties as well as enhanced tumour cell apoptosis in murine breast cancer and melanoma as compared to single-agent-loaded micelles. Furthermore, the development of such nanotheranostics displays a high degree of synergism, enabling it to be more efficient in treatment as well as real-time analysis in contrast to conventional ex vivo diagnosis. Such nanosystems can be further integrated with targeted therapies such as multimodal photodynamic therapy, magnetic hyperthermia and radiotherapy.

Polymer-Drug Conjugates

Nagel et al. (2018) have described stimuli-responsive cleavable motif-based nanoscaled polymer-drug conjugates for cancer therapy. The authors have developed a novel theranostics system triggered by cell-mediated stimuli. The

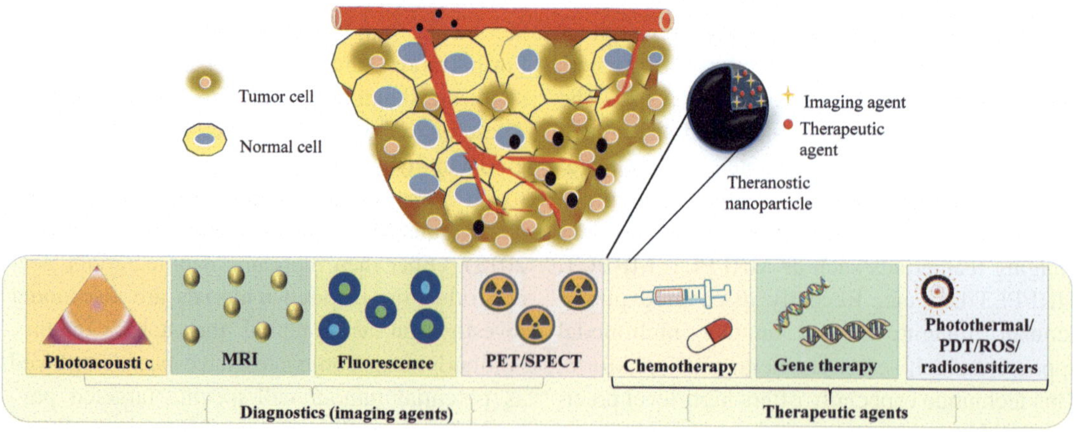

Fig. 4.2 Role of theranostics in cancer therapy

system was integrated by embedding two different linker molecules in dendritic polyglycerol matrix, i.e. a pH-responsive and enzyme-responsive linker for aldoxorubicin and doxorubicin, respectively. Moreover, the prodrug was conjugated with the thiol functional group intended for interaction with the cysteine residue of albumin to prolong its circulation and controlled drug release in the tumour microenvironment. The developed system was activated optically at the excitation wavelength of 490 nm, resulting in emissions at 590 nm (for doxorubicin) and 670 nm (for indidocarbocyanine). Both drug and dye conjugated to polymer depict inherent fluorophoric properties. In order to enhance the efficiency of the system, the donor fluorophore (doxorubicin) and acceptor fluorophore (indidocarbocyanine) were spaced 10 nm apart. Subsequently, the stimuli-responsive linker was selected in a particular manner to render drug conjugation and attachment for quencher fluorophore in close proximity to the drug. Furthermore, in vitro release studies of doxorubicin carried out using fluorescence microscopy and flow cytometry depicted enhanced and targeted drug release as compared to free drug. The authors reported superior performance of the pH-responsive system vs. enzyme-responsive one, due to the occurrence of premature drug release when acted upon by extracellular proteases. This had a pronounced effect on the treatment of a multidrug-resistant cell line where an intracellular drug release is crucial to overcome the resistance mechanisms. Therefore, the developed system was successful in the treatment of cancer and provided targeted and controlled drug release in response to tumour microenvironment making it a potential theranostics candidate for future cancer therapy.

Polymeric Nanogel

Polymeric nanogel is a broader term to describe the novel delivery system which incorporates polymers via cross-linking into a nanogel system. Gyawali et al. (2018) described a novel biodegradable polymeric nanogel-loaded doxorubicin for anticancer treatment. The novel synthesized polymer possessed inherent photostability and fluorescent properties. The theranostics potential of the prepared polymer was enhanced by surface functionalization with cyclic arginine-glycine-aspartic acid (cRGD) peptide for targeted and pH-dependent release in the tumour microenvironment. The authors synthesized photocross-linkable photoluminescent polymer by using biodegradable monomers such as citric acid, PEG, L-cysteine and maleic acid. Moreover, the prepared nanogels displayed excellent biological stability, biocompatibility along with strong fluorescent properties and enhanced uptake by the tumour cell. Fluorescence-guided imaging depicted cytoplasmic accumulation of doxorubicin in prostate cancer cells which resulted in augmented cell death. In conclusion, this novel synthesized polymer can be used as a potential theranostics platform for simultaneous tumour diagnosis and real-time pH-responsive drug monitoring. Chambre et al. (2018) described the synthesis of a novel polymeric nanogel obtained via cross-linking of reactive copolymers. Furthermore, drug conjugation was achieved via carbamate linkage and embedded in thiol-maleimide-functionalized PEG. The cRGD peptide was employed for surface functionalization of developed nanogel intended for targeted delivery of doxorubicin. The developed polymeric nanogel, which is comprised of a self-assembled cross-linked copolymer, was thus intended for thermo-responsive anticancer therapy. The functionalized maleimide-thiol PEG was responsible for the cross-linking ability of the nanogel. Succinimidyl-dicarbonate was employed to render carbonate functionalized doxorubicin-conjugated polymer, responsible for forming an acid labile carbamate linkage in response to drug release in the tumour microenvironment. Furthermore, the Cy5 dye was added to the nanogel system to render fluorescence imaging properties. In conclusion, the developed system depicted enhanced drug release and superior uptake as well as cytotoxicity in L929 fibroblast and MDA-MB-231 breast cancer cells in vitro. It can be envisioned that facile fabrication and multifunctionalization of these reactive nanogels offer a modular platform that can be configured as a theranostics agent for addressing challenges in conventional therapy of various diseases.

4.3.2.2 Lipid Nanocarriers

Liposomes

Liposomes are bilayered phospholipid vesicles that are formed spontaneously in the presence of aqueous solutions. Zhang et al. (2018) described a liposomal system loaded with hypoxia-activated chemotherapeutic prodrug combined with photodynamic therapy for anticancer treatment. The authors demonstrated the fabrication of 2-nitroimidazole-conjugated PEG-based theranostic liposome. Tirapazamine prodrug, lipophilic chlorine 6 and miRNA 155 as gene probe were encapsulated in the developed liposomal system. The gene probe was labelled with a fluorescent dye and quencher, which in the absence of target shows quenching of fluorescence by the dye in close proximity and upon target hybridization resulted into the separation of dye producing fluorescence imaging. Chlorine 6 renders photosensitizer functionality which was activated upon laser irradiation at 670 nm producing photodynamic therapy and severe hypoxia. This triggered the liposome disassembly, thereby activating tirapazamine prodrug to produce a cytotoxic anticancer effect. Encapsulated gene probe yielded enhanced fluorescent imaging along with differentiating cancer cell uptake vs. normal cells. The developed liposomes depicted enhanced in vitro and in vivo performance by significantly improved antitumor activity compared to conventional PDT. Thus, fabrication of nano-liposomal theranostics platform may contribute to the design of a hypoxia-responsive multifunctional system for tumour diagnosis and hypoxia-activated chemotherapy combined with PDT for synergetic therapy, holding great potential for future cancer therapy.

Solid Lipid Nanoparticle (SLN)

Shen et al. (2019) described a combination of magnetic hyperthermia and chemotherapy-based theranostics nanocarriers for oral anticancer treatment. The authors demonstrated the fabrication of doxorubicin and superparamagnetic iron oxide nanoparticle-loaded SLN theranostic for colon targeted delivery. These SLNs were further functionalized using folic acid/TPGS and octadecanol-modified dextran via layer-by-layer encapsulation. This developed system provided hyperthermic action of superparamagnetic iron oxide nanoparticles and chemotherapeutic effect of doxorubicin upon activation by the high-frequency magnetic field in orthotopic colon cancer. Folic acid-decorated doxorubicin and superparamagnetic iron oxide nanoparticle-loaded SLN encapsulated in dextran shell demonstrated successful evasion from systemic uptake, thereby enhancing local delivery in the colon. Employing folic acid/TPGS on to SLN allowed selective uptake by folic acid overexpressed cancer cells. The literature review revealed the presence of folate receptors in the small intestine as well, thereby limiting the colon targeting action. Hence, modified dextran was employed to overcome the challenge of preventing intestinal uptake. Furthermore, selective degradation of dextran shell was found upon the action of dextranase secreted in the colon. This functionalization yields highly effective and targeted delivery in colon cancer. Therefore, the developed system was highly efficient in providing a synergistic anticancer effect and a significant reduction in off-target toxicity. The system also depicted enhanced cell uptake and tumour growth inhibition in vitro and in vivo via magnetothermal and chemotherapeutic combination therapy.

Nanostructured Lipid Carriers (NLC)

Fernandes et al. (2018) described doxorubicin and docosahexaenoic acid-loaded NLCs for targeted cancer delivery. The in vitro and in vivo performance depicted superior activity as compared to free drug. Moreover, technetium-99 m labelling was employed for enhanced theranostics application of developed NLCs. Scintigraphy and biodistribution studies of NLC were performed in 4 T1 breast cancer cell-bearing mice depicting the enhanced anticancer activity of encapsulated doxorubicin compared to its free form. Radiolabelling enabled precise imaging potential of preferential nanoparticle uptake by tumour cells. Furthermore, the developed system depicted prolonged circulation, high therapeutic payload and superior anticancer effect.

Docosahexanoic acid and Doxorubicin co-loaded NLCs displayed synergistic and augmented antitumor effects. Additionally the system was found to produce reduced off-target toxicity. Therefore, the developed system may serve as a potential theranostics candidate for real-time drug monitoring and diagnostic imaging in breast cancer.

Lipid-Polymer Hybrids

Lipid-polymer can be defined as a combination system involving the use of polymer with predetermined function in lipid nanosystems. Huang et al. (2019) described Pt(IV) prodrug-loaded lipid-polymer nanohybrids for treatment of ovarian cancer. The nanohybrid system is comprised of the liquid core of perfluorohexane, a lipopolymer shell of PLGA-PEG and DSPE-PEG-Pt(IV) as well as cRGD peptide as targeting ligand. The perfluorohexane core was employed as an ultrasound contrast agent for enhanced and real-time imaging. The developed nanohybrids displayed multifunctionality and reduction in sensitive tumour targeting. The cRGD peptide was conjugated to the nanohybrid system for enhanced targeted delivery. The developed system displayed enhanced US imaging, drug release, cell uptake, cytotoxicity and cell apoptosis in vitro and in vivo. Thus, the developed hybrid can serve as a highly efficient theranostics platform for the treatment of ovarian cancer. You et al. (2018) described a pH-responsive system based on reactive oxygen species (ROS) triggered under NIR irradiation for cancer therapy. The authors demonstrated the fabrication of succinic peroxide-conjugated PLGA with Fenton-activated Pt/Fe_3O_4 lipo-polymersome. The presence of Fenton reactive species triggers the production of OH radicals as a source of ROS in cancer therapy. The developed system was rapidly internalized with further depolymerization leading to the formation of loose structures disintegrated with an increase in temperature as a consequence of NIR irradiation. Consequently, the release of ferrous ions and dissociate succinic peroxide triggered the formation of OH radicals in response to NIR irradiation when exposed to the tumour microenvironment. Cisplatin-loaded system depicted enhanced antitumor efficacy in vitro and in vivo. Furthermore, the developed system displayed multifunctionality, excellent biocompatibility, reduced off-target toxicity, high yield of ROS and enhanced uptake and accumulation in tumour cells. Moreover, the developed system also demonstrated excellent in vitro and in vivo performance in suppressing MCF-7 tumour cells. Thus, fabrication of lipo-polymersome nanohybrids can serve as a potential theranostics platform towards clinical translation for cancer therapy (Huang et al. 2019).

4.3.2.3 Dendrimers

Dendrimers are highly branched, star-shaped macromolecules with nanometer-scale dimensions. Dendrimers are defined by three components: a central core, an interior dendritic structure (the branches) and an exterior surface with functional surface groups. Alibolandi et al. 2018 described poly(amidoamine) dendrimer-based multifunctional nanotheranostics platform. Gold nanoparticles and curcumin were loaded onto the poly(amidoamine) dendrimer and conjugated with MUC1 aptamer for selective and enhanced tumour targeting. The developed system was intended for CT imaging and drug delivery to C26 tumour cells in vitro and in vivo. Moreover, MUC1 aptamer was conjugated via thiol functionalization to heterofunctional PEG. This developed nanosystem displayed marked targeting to MUC1 in HT29 and C26 cancer cell. Furthermore, the system also depicted high cell uptake, cytotoxicity and enhanced anticancer efficacy. In conclusion, the developed nanotheranostics system depicts good X-ray attenuation and is a desirable probe for CT imaging while demonstrating high therapeutic index against colorectal cancer. Jędrzak et al. 2019 described the synthesis of poly(amidoamine) functionalized magnetic nanoparticles encapsulated with polydopamine for advanced cancer therapy. Fifth-generation nanohybrids were employed for combination photothermal and chemotherapy in liver cancer treatment. The developed nanoparticles displayed no toxicity in healthy cells and exhibited strong photothermal properties. The developed system demonstrated a high degree of drug loading and the synergistic additive effect of photothermal therapy as well as chemotherapy. In vitro and in vivo studies depicted apoptosis-induced cell death instead of necrosis, thereby confirming highly efficient and versatile nature of the developed system. Moreover, the developed system displayed excellent MRI contrast properties. Overall, the functionality of dendrimers has been extended by merging them with magnetic nanoparticles resulting in multifunctional hybrid nanostructures making them a promising smart drug delivery system for cancer therapy.

4.3.2.4 Inorganic Nanocarriers

SPIONs and Magnetic Nanocarriers

Superparamagnetic iron oxide nanoparticles are iron oxide nanoparticles which have different electromagnetic properties due to their nanosize, a phenomenon called superparamagnetism. Gholami et al. (2019) described the fabrication of doxorubicin and superparamagnetic iron oxide nanoparticle-loaded polyarginine/chitosan nanoparticles. The developed system was fabricated using ionic gelation loaded with biodegradable chitosan for dual application, i.e. diagnosis and therapy. In vitro release studies depicted burst release from the developed system in an acidic environment, hence exhibiting pH-dependent release behaviour suitable for release in the tumour microenvironment. Moreover, flow cytometric analysis and fluorescence microscopy demonstrated rapid internalization of the developed system into the tumour cells. Consecutively, the in vitro uptake was corroborated by drug accumulation in intracellular space of C6 glioma cells using MRI. Additionally, the developed system depicted excellent biocompatibility, long-term stability and safety along with cytotoxicity against cancer cells. In conclusion, the developed system may serve as a promising theranostics platform for glioblastoma intervention in futurized clinical applications. Abedin et al. (2018) described essentiality of functionalized inorganic nanoparticles in nanomedicine to address the issue of dispersibility in physiological environments. The authors demonstrated modulation of colloidal stability of gold-iron oxide nanoparticles by employing a polymer coating of poly-L-lysine. The polymer-coated inorganic nanoparticles were found to remain as a stable dispersion in aqueous and physiological media, thus causing rapid internalization of nanoparticles in cells. The multifunctional NIR-responsive gold-iron oxide nanoparticles were intended for simultaneous imaging and photoactivated hyperthermic treatment of breast cancer cells. Surface-coated inorganic nanoparticles demonstrated the formation of a physical barrier around inorganic nanoparticles as a function of the polymer coating, thereby imparting stability and preventing its aggregation. The physicochemical properties of inorganic materials can render a multimodal nanoplatform, e.g. gold nanoparticles possess surface plasmon resonance and superparamagnetic properties which can be successfully employed for photothermal ablation as well as enhanced MRI contrast, respectively. The developed nanoparticles, which were investigated in BT-474 and MDA-MB-231 breast cancer, depicted enhanced cell uptake in NIR-assisted photothermal therapy. Moreover, the developed nanoparticles were able to promote and enhance tumour growth inhibition more significantly as compared to nanoparticles without NIR activation. In conclusion, the developed nanoparticles displayed excellent optical, magnetic and therapeutic properties by integrating diagnostic and therapeutic functions into a single multimodal nanotheranostics platform for translational cancer therapy.

Quantum Dots

Quantum dots are tiny particles or nanocrystals of a semiconducting material with diameters in the range of 2–10 nanometres. Quantum dots display unique electronic properties, intermediate between those of bulk semiconductors and discrete molecules, which are partly the result of the unusually high surface-to-volume ratios for these particles. The most apparent result of this is fluorescence, wherein the nanocrystals can produce distinctive colours determined by the size of the particles. Chang et al. (2019) described multifunctional quantum dot-based theranostics nanoformulation rendering diverse platform to address heterogeneity in cancer therapy. The authors demonstrated the development of a hybrid peptide for simultaneous diagnosis and cancer therapy. The research study involved isolation of two functional peptides A and B from *E. coli* and their conjugation with streptavidin-loaded quantum dots and magnetic nanoparticles, respectively. Furthermore, these functional peptides were coupled by promoting interaction between appropriate domains of both peptides. The developed hybrid system is comprised of streptavidin-loaded quantum dots, magnetic nanoparticles and targeting ligand designed for the treatment of HER2-positive breast cancer. The developed multifunctional hybrid system was efficient in the detection and inhibition of tumour growth of HER2-positive breast cancer. The developed hybrid system was equipped with ZH2 affibody which enabled specific targeting of HER2 receptor. To achieve optimum therapeutic efficacy, the developed hybrid system was employed for simultaneous quantum dot-assisted fluorescence imaging and magnetic hyperthermia for breast cancer treatment. The developed hybrid system is simple and flexible equipped with tunable modules rendering protein-protein interaction domains for lowering the immunogenicity. In conclusion, the developed hybrid system is highly useful in numerous biological applications serving as a potential theranostics platform in the development of an advanced bioassay for early cancer detection.

Metallic Nanoparticles

Nanoparticles are prepared from metals like iron, silver, gold, cobalt, zinc, etc. by various physical and chemical techniques to get nanoparticles in size range of 5–20 nm. Sakr et al. (2018) have described the development of a potential nanotheranostics system comprising of I-131-doped silver nanoparticles functionalized using PEG. The authors have integrated cancer therapy silver nanoparticles and radiolabelling. The nanoparticles were fabricated using a one-step synthesis of PEG-encapsulated silver nanoparticles doped with I-131. The developed system depicted excellent radiolabelling yield (~98%) along with significant stability in aqueous and physiological media in vitro. The developed system depicted temperature-sensitive behaviour and hence was administered in cold condition. Moreover, the developed system was safe and biocompatible and showed reduced off-target toxicity. The developed system depicted a high amount of radioactivity in tumour-bearing mice with enhanced tumour uptake upon post-intravenous as well as intratumoural injection. Thus, the developed system may serve as great potential in cancer theranostics. Liu et al. (2018) described a novel theranostics nanoconstruct comprising of hyaluronate-based cationic bovine serum albumin-encapsulated gold nanocluster for targeted drug delivery in cancer therapy. The authors demonstrated modulation of particle size by altering the hyaluronate to cationic bovine serum albumin-encapsulated gold nanocluster which was investigated for its targeting and pharmacokinetic potential. This preliminary screening then led to the selection of the developed system with size of 200 nm based on optimal EPR effect. Moreover, the developed system possessed red fluorescence providing real-time imaging and inherent drug binding sites. Therefore, the developed system was further utilized for loading of indocyanine green dye and lipophilic paclitaxel providing photothermal and chemotherapy, respectively, and nitric oxide for modulating the tumour microenvironment and enhancing drug delivery. Hyaluronate incorporation into the developed system imparted protection to charged nanoparticles, in turn, prolonging its systemic circulation and reduced off-target toxicity. Furthermore, the developed system depicted active targeting ability and facilitated penetration due to size reduction triggered by a degradation of hyaluronate shell in the tumour microenvironment. The developed system depicted high accumulation in breast cancer cells. Consequently, the developed system demonstrated in situ suppression of tumour growth (~95%) as well as lung metastatic growth inhibition (~88%). In conclusion, the developed system was safe and biocompatible intended targeted delivery and sufficient suppression of breast cancer.

Upconversion Nanoparticles

Jin et al. (2019) described a facile fabrication of NIR-assisted theranostics nanoconstructs via encapsulation of upconversion nanoparticles and a luminogen {2-(2,6-bis((E)-4-(phenyl(40-(1,2,2-triphenylvinyl)-[1,10-biphenyl]-4-yl)amino)styryl)-4H-pyran-4-ylidene)malononitrile} (TTD) within an amphiphilic polymer-based nanohybrid system. To obtain cancer cell targeting, the developed system was further conjugated with cRGD peptide to yield hybrid nanoparticles. A class of fluorogens has emerged to serve as an efficient and potential fluorescent material useful in theranostics applications. These fluorogens exhibit aggregation-induced emission properties, which can be described as non-emissive materials in appropriate solutions but can render high emission properties upon aggregation. Mechanism of aggregation can be explained via restricted intramolecular rotations that prevent dissipation of energy through non-radiative channels. Therefore, aggregation-induced emission-based photosensitizer has been employed widely as key materials for single-unit multimodal imaging and photodynamic therapy. Upconversion nanoparticles possess the ability to harness NIR frequency and upconvert into higher frequency such as visible or UV light. Therefore, selection of appropriate upconversion nanoparticles having similar emission spectra to that of aggregation-induced emission photosensitizer can render a potential platform for NIR-assisted nanotheranostics in the treatment of deeply situated tumours. The authors have discussed the encapsulation of hydrophobic luminogen (TTD) and upconversion nanoparticles into a biocompatible lipid-PEG polymer hybrid surface decorated with cRGD peptide for targeted action. This developed system depicted NIR-assisted multifunctional probes intended for photodynamic therapy in cancer cells. Furthermore, the developed system depicted efficient generation of ROS upon NIR excitation in the presence of thick tissue. Additionally, the developed system depicted highly efficient targeting and significant in vitro anticancer activity against MDA-MB-231 breast cancer cells. Moreover, in vivo studies depicted enhanced accumulation of developed system and significant tumour growth inhibition. Also intravenous injection of the developed system could illuminate the tumours and induced significant apoptosis in tumour cells. The developed system showed excellent photostability and was able to maintain its fluorescent properties for a longer duration (1 month). Theranostic probes composed of a combination of upconversion nanoparticles and photosensitizers may serve as a platform for NIR-assisted imaging and phototherapy of deeply situated tumors. Wang et al. (2019) described precision-based theranostics nanoplatforms for image-guided tumour-targeted delivery of chemotherapeutic drugs. Lanthanide-doped upconversion nanoparticles are attractive systems for the design of theranostic platforms which serve as a potential candidate in laser components, NIR probes, low-background bioimaging and solar energy conversion. The intrinsic NMR properties of gadolinium (Gd) ions can be employed for multimodal imaging. Furthermore, rare-earth co-doped elements ytterbium (Yb^{3+}) and erbium (Er^{3+}) can offer absorption of NIR excitation photon and emission upconversion luminescence, respectively, which can be applied to fluorescence labelling and luminescence resonance energy transfer. The developed nanoplatform comprised of Gd/Yb^{3+}/Er^{3+} upconversion nanoparticles and gold nanodots encapsulated bovine serum albumin in a layer-by-layer manner which was further conjugated to folic acid. This developed nanohybrid system was then successively employed for loading of doxorubicin. The upconversion nanoparticles provided photothermal effect along with NIR conversion and depicted excellent luminescent properties, X-ray attenuation and photothermal ablations. Moreover, bovine serum albumin was rendered as a template for doxorubicin binding, thereby enhancing its anticancer efficacy via photothermal therapy. The developed system was efficient in the delivery of doxorubicin within the tumour microenvironment, thereby reducing the off-target toxicity during treatment regime. Meanwhile, in vivo anticancer efficacy was improved by the pH-responsive release of doxorubicin in association with NIR excitation-induced heat. The developed system was highly effective in rendering multimodal imaging and potent anticancer response as well as tumour growth inhibition via deep penetration ability of photothermal therapy. The bovine serum albumin and folic acid coating provided prolonged circulation and a replacement for conventional surfactants to further render non-toxic, biocompatible and safe theranostics nanoplatform for in vivo cancer therapy. In conclusion, the development of such nanohybrids may serve as potential novel theranostics strategies which can be employed in simultaneous multifunctional diagnosis and therapy.

Silica and Other Nanoparticles

Su et al. (2019) described the fabrication of functional theranostics mesoporous silica-coated gold nanostars as combination photothermal therapy and chemotherapy in the treatment of cancer. The authors demonstrated the synthesis of mesoporous silica-coated gold nanostars using sodium hydroxide etching. The silica-coated nanoparticles were functionalized by grafting PEG and further loaded with doxorubicin. The developed system displayed good dispersibility in aqueous and physiological media. Moreover, the developed system depicted good drug-loading capacity and pH as well as light-responsive drug release. Upon NIR excitation, the developed system depicted excellent photothermal effects. Also the combination therapy in HeLa and cervical cancer cell lines consequently displayed superior anticancer efficacy than chemotherapy or photothermal therapy alone. The developed nanocomposites depicted excellent biocompatibility with low toxicity. In conclusion, the developed nanocomposite system serves as a multimodal theranostics platform for treating cancer. Victor et al. (2018) described the fabrication of calcium phosphate-based ceramic nanoparticles present as a unique drug delivery system. The developed system renders functional, biocompatible and biodegradable properties in vivo. The in vitro studies depicted rapid internalization of nanoparticles. Furthermore, the developed system depicted prolonged systemic circulation at physiological pH with low systemic toxicity. Moreover, the developed system was doped with neodymium encapsulated with alginic acid for pH-responsive drug release. Acetylsalicylic acid was loaded onto the developed functionalized nanocarrier for orally administered colon targeted delivery. The drug-loaded nanoparticles of 20–40 nm in size displayed negative surface charge, thereby facilitating simultaneous imaging and pH-responsive drug delivery. In conclusion, the lanthanide-doped calcium phosphate-based nanotheranostics may serve a potential for simultaneous imaging and therapy in the treatment of solid tumours. Cipreste et al. (2018) described the fabrication of hydroxyapatite nanoparticles doped with an array of radionuclides intended for theranostics applications in the treatment of various types of cancer. The authors demonstrated the synthesis of functionalized nanocomposite comprised of hydroxyapatite and CuO (known as tenorite) for PET imaging and simultaneous diagnosis and treatment of osteosarcoma. Copper serves as a potential candidate for modulation of hydroxyapatite nanoparticles to yield certain desirable theranostics properties. Activation of this metal by a neutron flux can produce 64Cu, a positron and beta radiation. The emitted beta radiation can be employed to kill cancer cells, and the positron radiation could be used to generate diagnostic images in PET systems. ^{64}Cu and ^{32}P were the two radionuclides, which were doped to the prepared nanocomposites, and upon activation inside the hydroxyapatite matrix can produce desirable theranostics material. Moreover, the developed system was found to stable and biocompatible in physiological conditions and serve as an excellent theranostics agent against osteosarcoma. The developed system was conjugated with folic acid to render active targeting to folate-overexpressed osteosarcoma cells. Wyszogrodzka et al. (2018) described a facile fabrication of novel metal-organic framework Fe-MIL-101-NH2 as a theranostics platform for antituberculous drug therapy. Several nanosized iron-based metal-organic frameworks (MIL-88A, MIL-89 and MIL-101-NH2) have been synthesized as drug cargos rendering good MRI contrast properties. The developed system was able to depict multifunctionality, significant drug loading, excellent

MRI contrast agent and low level of toxicity. The developed hybrid metal-organic frameworks, which were loaded with isoniazid and were investigated for its cytotoxicity against fibroblasts L929, depicted enhanced accumulation inside the cells. The proposed drug delivery system can also serve as the MRI contrast agent. Dissolution studies of the developed nanohybrids depicted an extended-release pattern. In conclusion, the developed system was found suitable for the extended-release inhalable system in drug delivery of isoniazid along with monitoring of drug-loaded hybrid system distribution within the lung tissue. Theranostics is widely employed for cancer treatment, but numerous other examples do exist for effective treatment and local drug delivery. The developed system demonstrates that Fe-MIL-101-NH2-based metal-organic framework can serve as an effective theranostics carrier for first-line antitubercular treatment with isoniazid. Additionally, MRI imaging of the developed system suspended in HPMC demonstrated the contrast ability of the novel theranostics platform. The proposed features such as efficient drug delivery and excellent imaging properties, in combination, describe a single all-in-one carrier system allowing it to be classified as a potential theranostics agent for tuberculosis treatment.

4.3.2.5 Carbon-Based Nanomaterials

Fullerenes Nanoparticles

Fullerenes were first discovered back in 1985 by Harold Kroto and his group at the University of Sussex, England. Kroto described fullerene as large and hollow spheroidal molecule composed of 60 or more carbon atoms. Fullerenes are produced chiefly by the action of arc discharge between carbon electrodes in an inert atmosphere. Misra et al. (2018) described functionalized C60 fullerenes as a potential theranostics platform in drug delivery of antiviral drugs employed for HIV treatment. The derivatives of fullerene C60 exhibited inhibition of HIV proteases via complex formation, among which dendrofullerene was found to have the highest inhibitory activity. Interestingly, amino acid-modified fullerene C60 was found to inhibit HIV replication in humans. Moreover, C60 fullerene has been utilized for potential medical application based on its photo-excitable properties. N-vinylpyrrolidone-functionalized C60 can form highly hydrophilic copolymer complex for photodynamic therapy. Fullerene C60 is also an inherent antioxidant as a consequence of its unique chemistry. Functionalization of fullerenes has been investigated in numerous activities such as radioprotective drug delivery, MRI contrast and photodynamic and gene therapy. Furthermore, researchers have discovered that under specific conditions, these fullerenes possess the ability to stimulate the generation of ROS and killer cells. He et al. (2019) developed a multifunctional contrast agent intended for simultaneous imaging and synergistic high-intensity focused ultrasound-assisted therapy. The authors described fabrication of perfluorohexane-encapsulated fullerene nanosphere, which was subsequently employed in US/CT dual-modality and high-intensity focused ultrasound ablation therapy. The developed system significantly enhanced integrated US/CT imaging along with enhanced high-intensity focused ultrasound ablation in dissected livers. In conclusion, the developed composite nanospheres demonstrate potential theranostics application as a multifunctional contrast agent for dual-modal biological imaging and highly efficient synergistic imaging-guided high-intensity focused ultrasound ablation.

Carbon Nanotubes

Carbon nanotubes can be classified as a subcategory of fullerene derivatives with similar and widespread application in the medical, biomedical and pharmaceutical field. Structurally carbon nanotubes are cylindrical nanoconstructs having a high length to diameter ratio. Two functional carbon nanotubes have been described for its use in biomedical field, viz. single- and multi-walled carbon nanotubes. Like fullerenes, carbon nanotubes also possess numerous optical fluorescence properties making them a potential material in photothermal cancer therapy. Fiegel et al. (2018) described the fabrication of carbon-based nanotubes for designing potential theranostics nanoconstructs. The developed nanoconstructs based on carbon nanotubes depicted high drug loading capacity with combination of photothermal therapy and imaging property. To overcome the poor hydrophilicity of carbon nanotubes, mesoporous silica shell was grafted which was further encapsulated with human serum albumin to form nanofilms via isobutyramide cross-linking. Curcumin and camptothecin were loaded onto the developed system. The porous silica rendered sites for drug loading. Thus, the developed nanocomposite system was found to be biocompatible and safe with reduced side toxicity. Hence, such systems can be utilized in the future for phototherapy and NIR-assisted drug delivery. Such novel nanocomposites are expected to be very promising new theranostics systems ensuring drug delivery, imaging and photothermal properties.

Carbon Nanodots

Carbon nanodots belong to a novel class of small theranostics nanoplatforms with size range below 10 nm, capable of exhibiting excellent optical and non-toxic properties. These unique properties of carbon nanodots are utilized in designing of ideal platforms for multifunctional cancer targeting. Numerous applications of carbon dots in cancer theranostics have been reported during the past decade. Ortega-Liebana et al. (2019) described the fabrication of nitrogen-doped carbon nanodots, which were employed as dual-modal theranostics, rendering NIR-assisted imaging and photodynamic therapy. The developed nanodots were rapidly internalized inside tumour cells via selective uptake and did not show cytotoxicity prior to NIR irradiation. The developed nanodots depict excellent photodynamic properties, along with highly efficient simultaneous imaging as well as cancer therapy. Cancer therapy was found to be efficient and displayed good luminescent properties upon NIR excitation which triggered in situ ROS generation. This ROS generation induced cell apoptosis in U251 cells in vitro visualized by flow cytometry.

Graphene Nanoparticles

Usman et al. (2018) described the fabrication of graphene oxide-based theranostic nanoconstructs for cancer imaging and therapy. The graphene oxide was employed for loading of anticancer protocatechuic acid and gadolinium nitrate hexahydrate as an MRI contrast agent. Gold nanoparticles were also employed as a contrast material for diagnosis. The graphene oxide nanosheets were conjugated with protocatechuic acid which was further conjugated to gadolinium nitrate. A similar process was followed to obtain gold-coated graphene oxide nanosheets. The developed system depicted significant cytotoxicity and excellent MRI contrast properties. The cytotoxicity studies depicted significant cytotoxicity in human liver hepatocellular cancer cell lines, but apparently, no significant cytotoxicity was observed in fibroblast cell lines. Moreover, the gold-coated nanosheets depicted superior contrast activity as compared to gadolinium-coated nanosheets. Therefore, the developed system has good prospects of serving as a future theranostics platform for cancer chemotherapy and diagnosis. Shervedani et al. (2018) described fabrication of novel graphene-based theranostics nanoplatform for cancer therapy. The authors demonstrated the synthesis of a multifunctional hybrid system comprising of partially reduced graphene oxide functionalized by polydopamine. This reduced graphene-polydopamine system was further grafted onto bovine serum albumin which was decorated with diethylenetriaminepentaacetic acid-Mn (II) employed as a diagnostic agent and loaded with chemotherapeutic agent methotrexate. In vitro studies depicted enhanced drug release and cell uptake which can be accounted to bovine serum albumin facilitating internalization and uptake.

4.4 Conclusion and Future Perspectives

To summarize briefly, the design of current and future theranostics deals with three important components, viz. imaging/diagnostic agent, therapeutic moiety and a targeting agent. All three components mentioned above have been extensively investigated in the design, development and evaluation of tailored theranostics applications. Great achievements have been made in the past decade to fabricate very small nanostructures, with smart stimuli-responsive architectures. It has also demonstrated methods to well decorate surface for enhanced colloidal stability with capabilities to carry both therapy and diagnostic agents. Even satisfactory in vitro and in vivo results have been achieved for most of the research works. Moreover, theranostics depicts great potential to revolutionize modern therapeutics and imaging. Further developments in using such nano-architectures for gene delivery would make the theranostics more personalized and customizable based on individual medical history and genomics. We still have to overcome a lot of obstacles, such as the reproducibility of such complex formulations, which is very difficult with current capabilities. The next hurdle would be to develop such facilities and instruments which would scale up these nanoformulations to higher volumes.

With application of nanomaterials, theranostics approaches depict a more promising medical intervention over conventional treatment strategies. However, the full potential of these materials is yet to be explored. Recently developed green synthesis of nanoparticles is a novel and emerging approach with low capital and operating expenses, in addition to being environmentally benign and enhanced biostability and compatibility. Hence, green synthesis is highly advantageous over traditional chemical and physical methods of nanoparticle synthesis. Theranostics nanovectors face a major challenge of lab-to-industrial-scale translation in terms of manufacture and technology development. This difficulty leads to compromise of stability, structural integrity and shelf life of nanotheranostics formulations. A key factor for maintenance of shelf life of the theranostics formulation is concerned with fragility and reduced activity of the employed targeting agents (i.e. antibodies) during manufacture and use. Nanotheranostics has afforded a novel class of personalized medicine for efficient delivery of therapeutics with reduced off-target toxicity via novel and advanced treatment strategies for individual patients. Moreover, recent advances in designing of multifunctional and modal nanoparticles as delivery technologies serve and promote next-generation molecular and nuclear imaging in clinics for rapid diagnosis and therapy. The blood-brain barrier offers structural and functional complexity, thereby limiting the use of theranostics platforms in clinical translation and personalized treatment of several neurological disorders.

Based on an extensive survey by Grand View Research statistics, the market for nanomedicine is expected to rise up to $ 350 billion worldwide by 2025. A majority of deaths occurring worldwide are associated with cancer metastasis, which is diagnosed late and only revealed upon surgical biopsy. Moreover, some other types of cancer such as lung cancer are more difficult to access for biopsy or require a liquid biopsy-based diagnosis. The liquid biopsy renders information regarding presence of circulating tumour cells (often referred as CTCs). Hence, early detection of cancer with help of nanoscaled diagnostic agents may serve as beneficial breakthrough in medical intervention. Diagnostics play a crucial role in paving road for precise and accurate treatment along with advanced medical interventions for various diseases. Recent reports and published data represent rapid advancement in search of novel biomarkers for disease subtypes, which is further developed by academic researchers and pharmaceutical industries to enhance well-defined and well-designed biomaterials with more individualized treatment strategy, depicting its potential into clinical translation. Modern research displays a paradigm shift in the field of medicine by utilizing integrated, multifunctional, multimodal nanotheranostics. This is rather a steady and slowly progressing field, advancing towards highly efficient personalized medicine along with the companion diagnostic agents at intermediate step. However, more detailed investigation and exploration for use and design of such nanotheranostics are essential.

The question continues to arise over the past few years regarding what will be the future of theranostics. Integrating nanotechnology and next-generation materials won't be enough for treating severe and deadly diseases. Recently researchers have developed approaches beyond multimodal techniques for next-generation imaging and therapy. An example of such a technique is the 4D-XCAT (four-dimensional extended cardiac-torso) imaging tool. 4D-XCAT is in silico or computer-assisted simulation tool for multiscale and multifunctional modelling of physiological and anatomical features. Techniques such as 4D-XCAT display highly advanced imaging with marked precision and accuracy in imaging therapy (Segars et al. 2018). Furthermore, in assistance to computer simulation for imaging and therapy, in silico designed microscaled multifunctional robots have been fabricated, transcending from conventional to next-generation theranostics. These microbots are specifically designed synthetic or biohybrid constructs for safe, biocompatible therapeutic interventions, aiming towards controlled delivery of bioactives. These miniaturized microbots are highly advanced programmable complex systems, intended for deep cellular access and performing multifunctional molecular diagnostics and therapeutics. Additionally, these micro- and nanomachines possess similar function and physicochemical properties as those of conventional theranostics materials. Moreover, these are highly efficient in performing predefined tasks as well as remote-controlled modulation in preprogrammed function. Depicted as emergent future theranostics, microbots upheld the potential in merging pre-existing drug delivery systems with the next-generation in silico tools. Therefore, it can significantly enhance the drug loading capacity, highly specified targeting and protection against opsonization and more importantly can reduce off-target accumulation as future-generation nanotheranostic systems (Erkoc et al. 2019).

In conclusion, the field of nanotheranostics is rapidly growing and enabling the transition from traditional "trial and error"-based medicine towards a more personalized approach serving as potential and superior clinical outcomes. Nanotheranostics offers a unique and useful tool in classifying, stratifying and selection of patients via prediction of molecular phenotype affirmative response of drug in particular. Nanotheranostics depicts the ability to improve the potency of therapeutic agent, thereby assisting physicians to better understand the highest benefits of particular drugs in individual patients. Moreover, the specific targeting virtues of nanotheranostics will render enhancement in monitoring and maintaining drug safety profile, also reducing off-target toxicity which commonly occurred during traditional chemotherapy. Furthermore, from an economic view, nanotheranostics can lead to cost-effective therapeutic regimes guiding preclinical development or clinical investigation to aid in amplifying the possible research outcomes.

Acknowledgements The authors are grateful for the financial support (Major Research Project) from Nirma University (NU/Ph.D./Major Res Pro/IP/16-17/669). Mr. Shubham Khot and Ms. Shruti Rawal are also thankful to Nirma University for providing the Junior Research Fellowship.

References

Abedin MR, Umapathi S, Mahendrakar H, Laemthong T, Coleman H, Muchangi D, Santra S, Nath M, Barua S (2018) Polymer coated gold-ferric oxide superparamagnetic nanoparticles for theranostic applications. J Nanobiotechnol 16(1):80

Alibolandi M, Hoseini F, Mohammadi M, Ramezani P, Einafshar E, Taghdisi SM, Ramezani M, Abnous K (2018) Curcumin-entrapped MUC-1 aptamer targeted dendrimer-gold hybrid nanostructure as a theranostic system for colon adenocarcinoma. Int J Pharm 549(1–2):67–75

Bertucci A, Silvestrini S, Corradini R, De Cola L (2018) Loading of PNA and other molecular payloads on inorganic nanostructures for theranostics. In DNA nanotechnology 1811:65–77

Bulte JW, Modo MM (2008) Introduction: the emergence of nanoparticles as imaging platform in biomedicine. In Nanoparticles in biomedical imaging, Springer, New York, NY 102:1–5

Chambre L, Degirmenci A, Sanyal R, Sanyal A (2018) Multi-functional nanogels as theranostic platforms: exploiting reversible and nonreversible linkages for targeting, imaging, and drug delivery. Bioconjug Chem 29(6):1885–1896

Chang CH, Tsai IC, Chiang CJ, Chao YP (2019) A theranostic approach to breast cancer by a quantum dots- and magnetic nanoparticles-conjugated peptide. J Taiwan Inst Chem Eng 97:88–95

Cipreste MF, de Rezende MR, Hneda ML, Peres AM, Cotta AAC, de Carvalho Teixeira V, de Almeida Macedo WA, de Sousa EMB (2018) Functionalized-

radiolabeled hydroxyapatite/tenorite nanoparticles as theranostic agents for osteosarcoma. Ceram Int 44(15):17800–17811
Dai L, Jones CM, Chan WTK, Pham TA, Ling X, Gale EM, Rotile NJ, Tai WCS, Anderson CJ, Caravan P, Law GL (2018) Chiral DOTA chelators as an improved platform for biomedical imaging and therapy applications. Nat Commun 9(1):857
Datta NR, Krishnan S, Speiser DE, Neufeld E, Kuster N, Bodis S, Hofmann H (2016) Magnetic nanoparticle-induced hyperthermia with appropriate payloads: Paul Ehrlich's "magic (nano) bullet" for cancer theranostics? Cancer Treat Rev 50:217–227
Dumortier J, Decullier E, Hilleret MN, Bin-Dorel S, Valette PJ, Boillot O, Partensky C, Letoublon C, Ducerf C, Leroy V, Vuillez JP (2014) Adjuvant intraarterial lipiodol or 131I-lipiodol after curative treatment of hepatocellular carcinoma: a prospective randomized trial. J Nucl Med 55(6):877–883
Efremova MV, Naumenko VA, Spasova M, Garanina AS, Abakumov MA, Blokhina AD, Melnikov PA, Prelovskaya AO, Heidelmann M, Li ZA, Ma Z (2018) Magnetite-gold nanohybrids as ideal all-in-one platforms for theranostics. Sci Rep 8(1):11295
Emi T, Michaud K, Orton E, Santilli G, Linh C, O'Connell M, Issa F, Kennedy S (2019) Ultrasonic generation of pulsatile and sequential therapeutic delivery profiles from calcium-crosslinked alginate hydrogels. Molecules 24(6):1048
Engberink RDO, Van Der Pol SM, Walczak P, Van Der Toorn A, Viergever MA, Dijkstra CD, Bulte JW, De Vries HE, Blezer EL (2010) Magnetic resonance imaging of monocytes labeled with ultrasmall superparamagnetic particles of iron oxide using magnetoelectroporation in an animal model of multiple sclerosis. Mol Imaging 9(5):7290–2010
Erkoc P, Yasa I, Ceylan H, Yasa O, Alapan Y, Metin Sitti M (2019) Mobile microrobots for active therapeutic delivery. Adv Ther 2(1):1800064
Evangelopoulos M, Parodi A, Martinez J, Tasciotti E (2018) Trends towards biomimicry in theranostics. Nanomaterials 8(9):637
Fernandes RS, Silva JO, Mussi SV, Lopes SC, Leite EA, Cassali GD, Cardoso VN, Townsend DM, Colletti PM, Ferreira LA, Rubello D (2018) Nanostructured lipid carrier co-loaded with doxorubicin and docosahexaenoic acid as a theranostic agent: evaluation of biodistribution and antitumor activity in experimental model. Mol Imaging Biol 20(3): 437–447
Fiegel V, Harlepp S, Begin-Colin S, Begin D, Mertz D (2018) Design of protein-coated carbon nanotubes loaded with hydrophobic drugs through sacrificial templating of mesoporous silica shells. Chem Eur J 24(18):4662–4670
Gallicchio R, Nardelli A, Mainenti P, Nappi A, Capacchione D, Simeon V, Sirignano C, Abbruzzi F, Barbato F, Landriscina M, Storto G (2016) Therapeutic strategies in HCC: radiation modalities. Biomed Res Int 2016:1295329
Gholami L, Tafaghodi M, Abbasi B, Daroudi M, Kazemi Oskuee R (2019) Preparation of superparamagnetic iron oxide/doxorubicin loaded chitosan nanoparticles as a promising glioblastoma theranostic tool. J Cell Physiol 234(2):1547–1559
Goldsmith SJ (2010) Radioimmunotherapy of lymphoma: Bexxar and Zevalin. In Seminars in nuclear medicine, WB Saunders 40(2):122–135
González-Prieto C, Lesser CF (2018) Rationale redesign of type III secretion systems: toward the development of non-pathogenic E. coli for in vivo delivery of therapeutic payloads. Curr Opin Microbiol 41:1–7
Gyawali D, Kim JP, Yang J (2018) Highly photostable nanogels for fluorescence-based theranostics. Bioactive Mater 3(1):39–47
He K, Ran H, Su Z, Wang Z, Li M, Hao L (2019) Perfluorohexane-encapsulated fullerene nanospheres for dual-modality US/CT imaging and synergistic high-intensity focused ultrasound ablation. Int J Nanomedicine 14:519
Hong G, Antaris AL, Dai H (2017) Near-infrared fluorophores for biomedical imaging. Nature Biomed Eng 1(1):0010
Hu P, Wu T, Fan W, Chen L, Liu Y, Ni D, Bu W, Shi J (2017) Near infrared-assisted Fenton reaction for tumor-specific and mitochondrial DNA-targeted photochemotherapy. Biomaterials 141:86–95
Huang H, Dong Y, Zhang Y, Ru D, Wu Z, Zhang J, Shen M, Duan Y, Sun Y (2019) GSH-sensitive Pt (IV) prodrug-loaded phase-transitional nanoparticles with a hybrid lipid-polymer shell for precise theranostics against ovarian cancer. Theranostics 9(4):1047
Idée JM, Louguet S, Ballet S, Corot C (2013) Theranostics and contrast-agents for medical imaging: a pharmaceutical company viewpoint. Quant Imaging Med Surg 3(6):292
Jędrzak A, Grześkowiak BF, Coy E, Wojnarowicz J, Szutkowski K, Jurga S, Jesionowski T, Mrówczyński R (2019) Dendrimer based theranostic nanostructures for combined chemo-and photothermal therapy of liver cancer cells in vitro. Colloids Surf B: Biointerfaces 173:698–708
Jin G, He R, Liu Q, Lin M, Dong Y, Li K, Tang BZ, Liu B, Xu F (2019) Near-infrared light-regulated cancer theranostic nanoplatform based on aggregation-induced emission luminogen encapsulated upconversion nanoparticles. Theranostics 9(1):246
Kumeria T, McInnes SJ, Maher S, Santos A (2017) Porous silicon for drug delivery applications and theranostics: recent advances, critical review and perspectives. Expert Opin Drug Deliv 14(12):1407–1422
Liu Y, Liu Y, Bu W, Xiao Q, Sun Y, Zhao K, Fan W, Liu J, Shi J (2015) Radiation–/hypoxia-induced solid tumor metastasis and regrowth inhibited by hypoxia-specific upconversion nanoradiosensitizer. Biomaterials 49:1–8
Liu Y, Nie L, Chen X (2016) Photoacoustic molecular imaging: from multiscale biomedical applications towards early-stage theranostics. Trends Biotechnol 34(5):420–433
Liu R, Xiao W, Hu C, Xie R, Gao H (2018) Theranostic size-reducible and no donor conjugated gold nano-

cluster fabricated hyaluronic acid nanoparticle with optimal size for combinational treatment of breast cancer and lung metastasis. J Control Release 278:127–139

Marchetti C, Palaia I, Giorgini M, De Medici C, Iadarola R, Vertechy L, Domenici L, Di Donato V, Tomao F, Muzii L, Panici PB (2014) Targeted drug delivery via folate receptors in recurrent ovarian cancer: a review. Onco Targets Ther 7:1223

Matteson EL, Lowe VJ, Prendergast FG, Crowson CS, Moder KG, Morgenstern DE, Messmann RA, Low PS (2009) Assessment of disease activity in rheumatoid arthritis using a novel folate targeted radiopharmaceutical Folatescan™. Clin Exp Rheumatol 27(2):253

Miller ML, Shizuka M, Wilhelm A, Salomon P, Reid EE, Lanieri L, Sikka S, Maloney EK, Harvey L, Qiu Q, Archer KE (2018) A DNA-interacting payload designed to eliminate cross-linking improves the therapeutic index of antibody–drug conjugates (ADCs). Mol Cancer Ther 17(3):650–660

Misra C, Yadav AB, Verma RK (2018) Carbon-based nanofibers: fullerenes, diamond, and carbon nanostructures. In: Barhoum A, Bechelany M, Makhlouf A (eds) Handbook of nanofibers. Springer, Cham, pp 1–14

Nagel G, Tschiche HR, Wedepohl S, Calderón M (2018) Modular approach for theranostic polymer conjugates with activatable fluorescence: impact of linker design on the stimuli-induced release of doxorubicin. J Control Release 285:200–211

Näkki S, Martinez JO, Evangelopoulos M, Xu W, Lehto VP, Tasciotti E (2017) Chlorin e6 functionalized theranostic multistage nanovectors transported by stem cells for effective photodynamic therapy. ACS Appl Mater Interfaces 9(28):23441–23449

Naveed F, Fisher R, Engel JS, Lu J, Low P, Amato RJ (2004) Folate-scan in subjects with suspected metastatic renal cell carcinoma. J Clin Oncol 22(14):4751–4751

Neuwelt EA, Hamilton BE, Varallyay CG, Rooney WR, Edelman RD, Jacobs PM, Watnick SG (2009) Ultrasmall superparamagnetic iron oxides (USPIOs): a future alternative magnetic resonance (MR) contrast agent for patients at risk for nephrogenic systemic fibrosis (NSF)? Kidney Int 75(5):465–474

Ortega-Liebana MC, Encabo-Berzosa MM, Casanova A, Pereboom MD, Alda O, Hueso JL, Santamaria J (2019) Upconverting carbon nanodots from EDTA as near-infrared activated phototheranostic agents. Chem Eur J 25(21):5539–5546

Reimer P, Balzer T (2003) Ferucarbotran (Resovist): a new clinically approved RES-specific contrast agent for contrast-enhanced MRI of the liver: properties, clinical development, and applications. Eur Radiol 13(6):1266–1276

Rong P, Huang P, Liu Z, Lin J, Jin A, Ma Y, Niu G, Yu L, Zeng W, Wang W, Chen X (2015) Protein-based photothermal theranostics for imaging-guided cancer therapy. Nanoscale 7(39):16330–16336

Sakr TM, Khowessah OM, Motaleb MA, El-Bary AA, El-Kolaly MT, Swidan MM (2018) I-131 doping of silver nanoparticles platform for tumor theranosis guided drug delivery. Eur J Pharm Sci 122:239–245

Segars W Paul et al (2018) Application of the 4-D XCAT Phantoms in Biomedical Imaging and Beyond. IEEE Transactions on Medical Imaging 37(3): 680–92

Shen MY, Liu TI, Yu TW, Kv R, Chiang WH, Tsai YC, Chen HH, Lin SC, Chiu HC (2019) Hierarchically targetable polysaccharide-coated solid lipid nanoparticles as an oral chemo/thermotherapy delivery system for local treatment of colon cancer. Biomaterials 197:86–100

Shervedani RK, Foroushani MS, Kefayat A, Torabi M, Rahsepar FR (2018) Construction and characterization of a theranostic system based on graphene/manganese chelate. Biosens Bioelectron 117:794–801

Su G, Miao D, Yu Y, Zhou M, Jiao P, Cao X, Yan B, Zhu H (2019) Mesoporous silica-coated gold nanostars with drug payload for combined chemo-photothermal cancer therapy. J Drug Target 27(2):201–210

Upponi JR, Jerajani K, Nagesha DK, Kulkarni P, Sridhar S, Ferris C, Torchilin VP (2018) Polymeric micelles: Theranostic co-delivery system for poorly water-soluble drugs and contrast agents. Biomaterials 170:26–36

Usman M, Hussein M, Kura A, Fakurazi S, Masarudin M, Ahmad Saad F (2018) Graphene oxide as a nanocarrier for a theranostics delivery system of protocatechuic acid and gadolinium/gold nanoparticles. Molecules 23(2):500

Victor SP, Paul W, Sharma CP (2018) Calcium phosphate nanoplatforms for drug delivery and theranostic applications. In: Drug delivery nanosystems for biomedical applications. Sharma CP, Elsevier, pp 163–179

Wang C, Xue R, Gulzar A, Kuang Y, Shao H, Gai S, Yang D, He F, Yang P (2019) Targeted and imaging-guided chemo-photothermal ablation achieved by combining upconversion nanoparticles and protein-capped gold nanodots. Chem Eng J 370:1239–1250

Weiner RE, Thakur ML (2005) Radiolabeled peptides in oncology. BioDrugs 19(3):145–163

Wu Z, de Ávila BEF, Martín A, Christianson C, Gao W, Thamphiwatana SK, Escarpa A, He Q, Zhang L, Wang J (2015) RBC micromotors carrying multiple cargos towards potential theranostic applications. Nanoscale 7(32):13680–13686

Wyszogrodzka G, Dorożyński P, Gil B, Roth WJ, Strzempek M, Marszałek B, Węglarz WP, Menaszek E, Strzempek W, Kulinowski P (2018) Iron-based metal-organic frameworks as a Theranostic carrier for local tuberculosis therapy. Pharm Res 35(7):144

You, Chaoqun, et al. (2018) Near Infrared Radiated Stimulus-Responsive Liposomes Based on Photothermal Conversion as Drug Carriers for Co-Delivery of CJM126 and Cisplatin. Materials Science and Engineering C 80: 362–70

Zhang K, Zhang Y, Meng X, Lu H, Chang H, Dong H, Zhang X (2018) Light-triggered theranostic liposomes for tumor diagnosis and combined photodynamic and hypoxia-activated prodrug therapy. Biomaterials 185:301–309

Nanoparticles: Importance and Need for Regulations

5

Meenakshi Bajpai, Huma Shafi, and Shalini Kumari

Abstract

Nanoparticles are a boon to mankind. They exist in nature as volcanic ashes, proteins, chitins, etc. and can also be engineered. All nanoparticles have an impact on human health and environment, and recent research has focused on these aspects. Ayurveda and Siddha systems also have various examples of nanomedicines. However, use of nanomaterials raises safety concerns as the physical, chemical, and biological properties undergo changes at nanolevel. Thus, the importance and need of regulations are self-evident. Various agencies around the world regulate nanotechnology-based products as per norms and regulations framed for this purpose. The need for regulations, specifically for nanoparticle-based products, is felt, and regulations on relevant aspects should be drafted and implemented.

Keywords

Nanoparticles · Engineered nanoparticles · Nanomedicines · Regulations

Abbreviations

ADME	Absorption, distribution, metabolism and excretion
Al	Aluminium
API	Active pharmaceutical ingredient
ASTM	American Society for Testing and Materials
Ca	Calcium
CAS	Chemical Abstracts Service
CEN	European Committee for Standardization
DBT	Department of Biotechnology
DDS	Drug delivery system
DSIR	Department of Scientific and Industrial Research
DST	Department of Science and Technology
EU	European Union
FDA	Food and Drug Administration
Fe	Iron
ISO	International Organization for Standardization
JRC	Joint Research Centre
NIOSH	National Institute for Occupational Safety and Health
OECD	Organisation for Economic Co-operation and Development
OSHA	Occupational Safety and Health Administration
PAMAM	Poly(amidoamine)
PLA	Poly(lactic acid)

M. Bajpai (✉) · H. Shafi · S. Kumari
Institute of Pharmaceutical Research, GLA University, Mathura, India
e-mail: meenakshi.bajpai@gla.ac.in

S. Talegaonkar, M. Rai (eds.), *Nanoformulations in Human Health*,
https://doi.org/10.1007/978-3-030-41858-8_5

PLGA	Poly(lactic-co-glycolic acid)
PPE	Personal protective equipment
R&D	Research and Development
REACH	Registration, Evaluation, Authorisation and Restriction of Chemicals
Si	Silicon
STM	Scanning tunnelling microscope

5.1 Introduction

The prefix "nano" is derived from the Greek word νᾶνος which means "dwarf" (Latin – *nanus*) (Nikalje 2015). The general conference on weights and measures endorsed the usage of nano as a prefix in 1960. Nano means one billionth (10^{-9}) and is used for prefixing units of time and length. The term nanometre was first proposed by Richard Zsigmondy in 1925 for characterising particle size.

Properties of substances at the nanoscale are different from the properties of a single atom and molecules. The concept of nanotechnology in the modern times is started by physicist Richard Feynman in a lecture entitled "There's Plenty of Room at the Bottom" delivered at the meeting of the American Physical Society on December 29, 1959, at the California Institute of Technology. He discussed that scientists would manipulate atoms and molecules to build small things.

The term nanotechnology was given by Norio Taniguchi in 1974. As per the literature available, nanomaterials have been in use since the fourth century AD (Krukemeyer et al. 2015):

- Romans used nanosized metals to decorate cups, for example, Lycurgus cup (gold and silver nanoparticles embedded in a glass) (Fig. 5.1).
- Medieval stained glass windows used in churches (Fig. 5.2).
- Italians also used nanosized metals to produce iridescent or metallic glazes, for example, Deruta ceramics (particles of copper and silver metal).

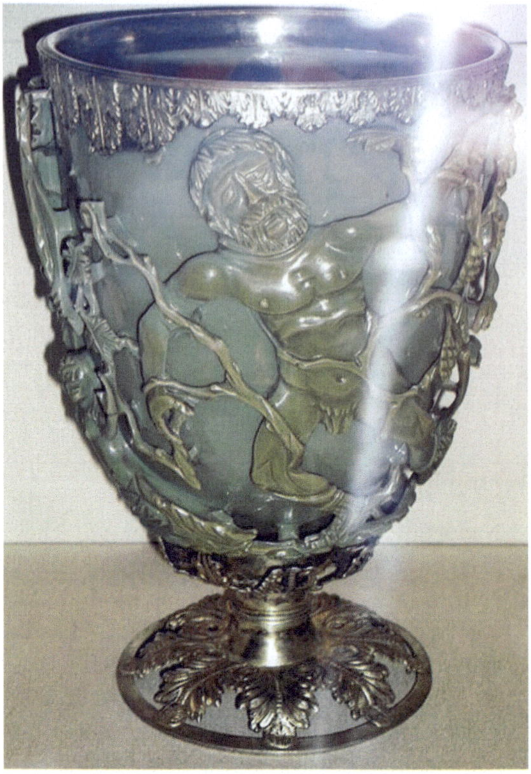

Fig. 5.1 Lycurgus cup. (From Wikimedia Commons, the free media repository. https://commons.wikimedia.org/wiki/File:Brit_Mus_13sept10_brooches_etc_044.jpg)

In 1981 Gerd Binnig and Heinrich Rohrer working at IBM, Zurich, invented the scanning tunnelling microscope (STM). In 1985 atomic force microscope was invented and fullerenes were discovered. These instruments gave a major impetus to the study of nanomaterials.

The beginning of this century saw an increased use of nanotechnology, and all walks of human life have felt its impact. Today, nanoparticles find applications in almost all areas of human requirement. For example, nanotechnology is used in production, processing, packaging and safety of foods (McClements and Xiao 2017). Some examples of use of nanotechnology in commercial products are manufacturing scratch-proof eyeglasses, crack-resistant paints, sunscreens, self-cleaning windows, stain-repellent fabrics and coating for solar cells. Nanoparticles can be used as fillers in tyres; to improve the

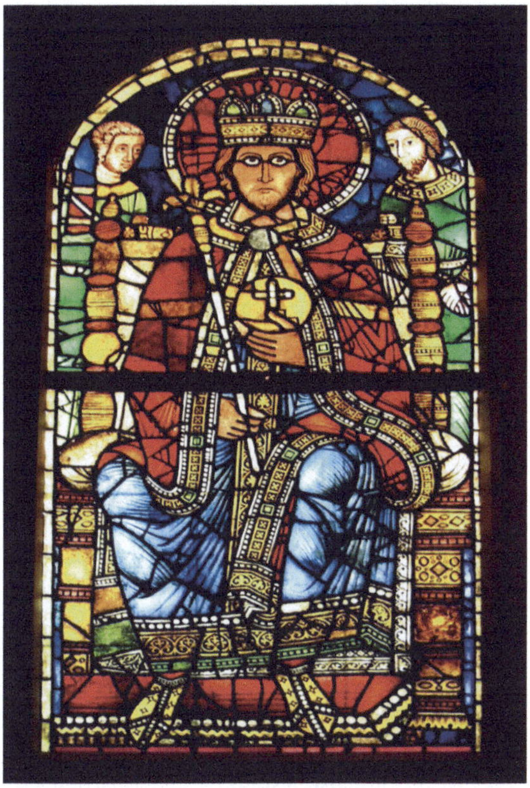

Fig. 5.2 Stained glass window. (From Wikimedia Commons, the free media repository. Romanesque stained glass from Strasbourg Cathedral, located in the Cathedral Museum. Subject: the Emperor Charlemagne. By photo Rama - Wikimedia Commons, CC BY-SA 2.0 fr, https://commons.wikimedia.org/w/index.php?curid=20737795)

stiffness of the car body, nanoparticle-strengthened steels are used (https://ec.europa.eu/health/scientific_committees/opinions_layman/en/nanotechnologies/l-3/5-nanoparticles-consumer-products.htm). Nanoparticles find extensive use in biology and medicine-drug delivery, gene therapy, tissue engineering, nanoscale biochips, DNA probes, microsurgical technology, separation and purification of biological molecules, etc.

5.2 Diversity of Nanoparticles

As per ISO and ASTM standards, nanoparticles, either engineered or naturally occurring, are broadly defined as particles of sizes ranging from 1 to 100ηm with one or more dimensions. The properties of nanoparticles are different from that of their bulk material, which include spatial confinement, high surface energy, large fraction of surface atoms and reduced imperfections. Classification of nanoparticles can be done according to their nature of origin, physical and chemical properties, size, morphology, etc. Classification of nanoparticles according to the nature of their origin (Fig. 5.3), i.e. natural nanoparticles and engineered nanoparticles, is discussed below (Ealias and Saravanakumar 2017; Ray 2018).

5.2.1 Natural Nanoparticles

Nature is an excellent nanotechnologist, and therefore the word "nano" should not always be associated with "synthetic".

There are countless types of nanoparticles found in nature which include inorganic materials such as volcanic ash, clays and soot; naturally occurring silver nanoparticles as a result of weathering, etc.; interstellar natural nanoparticles which originated from the influence of comets and asteroids on earth; natural inorganic thin films; and a variety of organic nanostructures from living organisms such as proteins, chitins (insect and crustacean shells), wing ribs, epidermal projections, etc. Examples of some naturally occurring nanoparticles along with their sizes (ηm) are given in Table 5.1. There is an increasing interest in the development of natural nanoproducts in the areas of phyto- and phyconanotechnology (Buzea et al. 2007; Pachapur et al. 2015; Griffin et al. 2018; Cuffari et al. 2018).

Nanoparticles, whether natural or engineered, should be studied for their impact on the environment and health; therefore recently numerous researches have been dedicated to investigating the structural and chemical varieties of naturally occurring nanoparticles (Cuffari et al. 2018).

Classification of natural nanoparticles:

1. Inorganic nanoparticles: These are nanoparticles which occur naturally but are not biological; they are the result of a natural phenomenon such as volcanic eruptions, fire, ocean splash, etc.

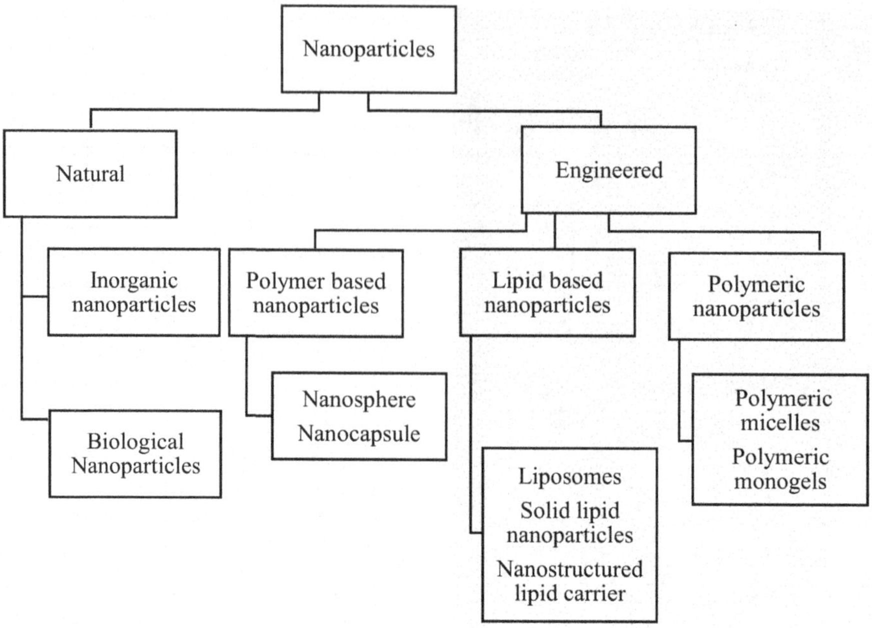

Fig. 5.3 Classification of nanoparticles

Table 5.1 List of some naturally occurring nanoparticles and their sizes

Sr. No.	Name of the naturally occurring nanoparticles	Size (nm)
1	Haemoglobin	5.5
2	1 strand of DNA	2
3	Proteins	1–20
4	Insulin	5
5	Glucose	1
6	Virus	100–300
7	Tryptophan (longest amino acid)	1.2
8	Volcanic ashes	100–200
9	Casein micelles	50–250

- Volcanic ash: Volcanic eruption and erosion are sources of natural nanoparticles. During volcanic eruptions the ash is released which reaches the atmosphere and water sources; chemical interaction with the environment leads to deposition of nanoparticles which may have an adverse impact on health.
- These particles are in the size range of 100–200 nm in diameter and therefore are easily suspended in the air. This suspension within the atmosphere is easily inhaled and deposited in the respiratory tract leading to serious respiratory disorders.
- Deserts as source of nanoparticles: Dust storms are also a source of nanoparticles in the atmosphere; 50% of total aerosols in the troposphere are minerals which originated from the deserts as the result of dust storms. The chemical composition of nanoparticles originating from deserts consists of high concentration of silicon and traces of aluminium, iron and calcium.
- A study carried out in China (in Xian) revealed that the dust transported from the Gobi desert contained high carbon and nitrogen concentrations, nitrates, sulphates and ammonium ions (Wang et al. 2013).

2. Biological nanoparticles

Microorganisms such as *Shewanella* and *Lactobacillus* (species of bacteria) which cause the fermentation of milk proteins also reduce selenite to elemental selenium nanoparticles. The biological origin of nanoparticles plays an important role in removing environmental contaminants like heavy metals and inorganic and organic pollutants. Nanoparticles from bacteria, plants, fungi, etc. are environment friendly and are important alternatives to traditional methods of removal of environmental contaminants.

Microorganisms like *Saccharomyces cerevisiae* and *Staphylococcus carnosus* have been investigated by scientists to produce homogenous selenium nanoparticles for use in food supplements and antimicrobial agents. This holds promise for the agriculture industry, for enriching soil with selenium and thus providing plants with a natural defence system is a future technology against harmful pathogens that damage crops.

The semi-living organisms such as viruses also come under the category of natural biological nanoparticles. Proteins, lipids, carbohydrates, haemoglobins and other inorganic biomolecules are also of nanosized levels.

Natural nanomaterials possess the unique property of molecular recognition; thus they can self-assemble. They also remain in a colloidal state without coagulating for many hours after which they tend to aggregate at an increasing rate. This indicates that they possess good stability. These particles have a large surface area to volume ratio due to their minute sizes making them much more reactive and efficient. Most of the active ingredients of plant extract or animal serum occur in nanoscale (Rochishnu et al. 2009). A list of some naturally occurring nanoparticles and their sizes is summarised in Table 5.1.

5.2.2 Engineered Nanoparticles

Engineered nanoparticles are a heterogeneous group of substances, which differ in size, shape, surface area, chemical composition and biopersistence, thus strongly affecting their potential impact on health. Nanoparticles possess unique characteristics at molecular, atomic and cellular levels. Their geometrical shape influences behaviour and uses. Synthetic or engineered nanomaterials are those which are synthesised either by physical, chemical, biological or hybrid methods (Patra et al. 2018; Jeevanandam et al. 2018; Urbanska et al. 2019).

Types of engineered nanoparticles (U.S. Environmental Protection Agency 2017; Patra et al. 2018) are as follows

Carbon-based nanoparticles (spherical nanoparticles, fullerenes; cylindrical nanoparticles, nanotubes).

Metallic nanoparticles (gold, silver, iron, copper, platinum, selenium, metal oxides like cerium dioxide, titanium dioxide nanoparticles, etc.)

Quantum dots (semiconductor nanocrystals, with a diameter of 2–10 ηm; optical properties of quantum dots change by changing their size)

Dendrimers (monodisperse, highly bifurcated, well-defined and three-dimensional structures, for example, poly(amidoamine) (PAMAM), core-shell, chiral, peptide, glycodendrimers, etc.)

Composites (engineered nanosized clays)

Polymeric nanoparticles (nanospheres, nanocapsules)

Phospholipids (liposomes, micelles)

Biopolymeric nanoparticles (nanoparticles synthesised from chitosan, alginates, etc.)

Inorganic nanoparticles (silver, gold, iron oxide, silica nanoparticles, etc.)

Nanocrystals

Protein and polysaccharide nanoparticles (natural biopolymers extracted from plants, animals, microorganisms, etc.)

Superparamagnetic iron oxide nanoparticles

Nanoparticles synthesised from natural products (metals, metal oxides and sulphide nanoparticles synthesised using various microorganisms like bacteria, fungi, yeasts, etc.) or from plant extracts

5.3 Nanoparticles in Medicines

Nanomedicine is the application of nanotechnology in the field of biomedical sciences and healthcare (Farokhzad and Langer 2006; Sayes et al. 2017). The US federal authorities have provided more than $1.4 billion funding for the National Nanotechnology Initiative, which confirms the importance of nanotechnology. Nanotechnology has attracted huge attention around the world. According to a recent report by Forbes, nanotechnology is one of the fifth biggest growth technologies to watch over the coming decade (Iyer et al. 2015; Desai and Rustomjee 2016).

Nanotechnology has an enormous role in today's biomedical sciences (https://www.understandingnano.com/medicine.html). Nanotechnology in medicine application includes cancer therapy, drug delivery, early detection and prevention,

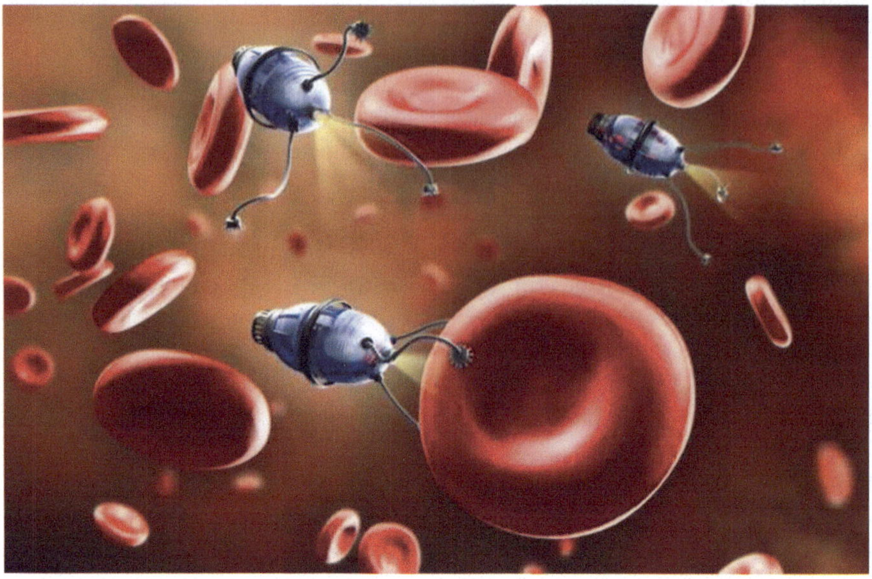

Fig. 5.4 A nanorobot treating blood cell. https://ashutoshviramgama.com/molecular-nanotechnology-nano-robotics/

diagnostic technique, antibacterial treatment, wound treatment, cell repair and nanorobot-based nanomedicine. Nanorobots (Fig. 5.4) are the future of nanomedicine. They are programmed to repair specific diseased cells, eliminate bacterial infections, perform surgery at the cellular level and act in a similar way to antibodies in our natural healing processes. They can even be programmed to increase the human lifespan by repairing cellular level conditions that cause the body to age. Ethnomedicines are also part of nanomedicines.

However, in Ayurveda nanotechnology has been used in the form of nanomedicine as Ayurvedic Bhasmas. These are herbo-mineral-metallic compounds in the range of 5–50 ηm and products of Ayurveda Rasa Shastra. Bhasmas of metals and minerals are in use since the seventh century.

Few examples of Bhasmas:

Swarna Bhasma (gold nanoparticles: 27 ± 3 ηm) is used in the treatment of arthritis.

Mukta Shukti Bhasma (pearl-oyster nanoparticles: 22.52 ± 0.45 ηm) is used in the treatment of cough, asthma, etc. and is also used to increase bone mineral density.

Tamra Bhasma (copper nanoparticles) is used as antioxidant and hepatoprotective.

Bhasmikarana converts the metals from their zerovalent state to a higher oxidation state. This eliminates the toxic nature of metals and their oxides and produces metal oxide into medicinal value.

However, safety concerns should be addressed, and guidelines taking care of safety, ecology and environment should be framed (Sarkar and Chaudhary 2010; Kapoor 2010; Pal et al. 2014; Palkhiwala and Bakshi 2014; Rohit and Prajapati 2018).

The Siddha medicine system which uses raw materials from plant, animal, metal and mineral origins also uses the concept of nanotechnology in most of its medicines. There are nearly 212 varieties of chemico-metallurgical medicines in Siddha medicine system for example, minerals, metals, salts, gold, silver, mercury, sulphur, etc. Most medicines of Siddha medicine system from the category of Parpam, Chenduram, Chunnam, Kattu and Padhangam were found to contain nanoparticles.

Few examples of nano-based medicine in Siddha medicine system are as follows:

Siddha system uses nano-mercury (sulphide of mercury is commonly used) in the treatment of cancer, rheumatoid arthritis, systemic lupus erythematosus, chronic ulcers, etc.

Nano-gold in its oxide or sulphide form is used in Siddha medicine system as Thanga Parpam (globular particles of gold with size of 56–57 ηm) or Chenduram for the treatment of reproductive disorders, autoimmune diseases, skin diseases, respiratory diseases and other chronic diseases.

In Siddha medicine system nanosilver (velli) is used in the treatment of respiratory diseases, venereal diseases, haemorrhoids, etc. The Siddha system of medicine uses herbo-mineral drugs. The herbs are selected depending on the metal or mineral used. These herbo-mineral drugs are soaked in herbal juice/decoction and then triturated with the same.

The triturated drug is then subjected to incineration or else sublimation for certain hours in an earthen pot, cooled and triturated again. These tedious processes result in physico-chemical transformation of drug, which leads to particle size reduction and change in chemical composition and thus enhances the efficacy and reduces the toxicity (Kandasamy 1998; Shailaja and Sugunthan 2016).

In the modern system of medicine, these nanopharmaceuticals are either nanocrystalline-based or lipid-based formulations (liposomes, solid lipid nanoparticles, nanostructured lipid carriers) or polymeric or metallic nanoformulations (Agarwal et al. 2018; Farjadian et al. 2018). Presently there are a variety of FDA-approved nano-based pharmaceuticals in the market. These are the products from various companies across the world. Some of the nanopharmaceuticals are given in Table 5.2.

Table 5.2 List of some FDA-approved nanopharmaceuticals currently available in the market

Sr. No.	Trade name/company	Drug/type of formulation	FDA approval
1	Emend® Merck & Co., Inc., NJ, USA	Nanocrystalline form of aprepitant	2003
2	Megace ES® Elan Pharma International Limited, a subsidiary of Elan Corporation, plc Par Pharmaceutical Companies, Woodcliff Lake, New Jersey, USA	Megestrol acetate Nanocrystalline form of megestrol acetate	2005
3	Triglide® SkyePharma/Sciele Pharma, Inc. (formerly known as First Horizon Pharmaceutical Corp.), Atlanta, Georgia, USA	Fenofibrate Nanocrystalline form of fenofibrate	2005
4	Tricor® Abbott Laboratories	Fenofibrate Nanocrystalline form of fenofibrate	2004
5	DaunoXome® Galen, Craigavon, UK	Liposomal daunorubicin citrate	1996
6	DepoCyt® Pacira Pharmaceuticals, NJ, USA	Liposomal formulation of cytarabine	1999/2007
7	Feraheme® AMAG Pharmaceuticals, MA, USA	Ferumoxytol Carbohydrate-coated, superparamagnetic iron oxide nanoparticles	2009
8	Macugen® Eyetech Pharmaceuticals	Pegaptanib sodium, anti-VEGF (vascular endothelial growth factor) aptamer PEGylated anti-VEGF aptamer	2004
9	Cimzia® UCB, Brussels, Belgium	Certolizumab pegol (Fab fragment of a humanised anti-TNF-alpha antibody) PEGylated antibody	2008

(continued)

Table 5.2 (continued)

Sr. No.	Trade name/company	Drug/type of formulation	FDA approval
10	Adagen® Enzon, Inc., NJ, USA	Pegademase bovine (adenosine deaminase) PEGylated adenosine deaminase	1990
11	Neulasta® Amgen, Inc., CA, USA	Recombinant methionyl human G-CSF (granulocyte colony-stimulating factor) PEGylated form of filgrastim (granulocyte colony-stimulating factor)	2002
12	Oncaspar® Enzon Pharmaceuticals Inc., NJ, USA	Asparaginase PEGylated L-asparaginase	1994
13	Pegasys® Previously the Hoffmann-La Roche Inc. and currently the Genentech USA, Inc., CA, USA	Interferon alfa-2a Interferon alfa-2a PEGylated	2002
14	Somavert® Pfizer Pharmaceuticals, CT, USA	hGH (human growth hormone) Pegvisomant (B2036-PEG) is the PEGylated analogue of human growth hormone	2003

5.4 Regulatory Framework

Nanotechnology has potential applications in almost all areas pertaining to human existence. However, use of nanomaterials also raises safety concerns as the physical, chemical and biological properties of substance undergo changes at the nanolevel. Thus the role of regulatory bodies around the world becomes very important to address these safety concerns.

There are various agencies which regulate nanotechnology-based products as per the norms, regulations and legislations framed for this purpose.

In this chapter, we have focused on the following:

1. Regulations in the USA (cosmetic and drug products)
2. Regulations in Europe
3. Regulations in India

5.4.1 Regulations in the USA

5.4.1.1 Guidelines for Cosmetics

Regulations in the USA fall under the purview of the Food and Drug Administration (FDA). The FDA has issued a guidance document (https://www.fda.gov/regulatory-information/search-fda-guidance-documents/guidance-industry-safety-nanomaterials-cosmetic-products) for the industry for the safety of nanomaterials in cosmetic products which include the following considerations:

(i) Nanomaterial characterisation

Nanomaterials vary in compositions, morphologies, characteristics, etc. and therefore are not a uniform group of substance. They may have physical, chemical, or biological properties that are different from those of large-scale materials with the same chemical composition.

A. Physico-chemical properties

Nanomaterials in cosmetics require the following information:

- Name of nanoparticles.
- CAS number.
- Structural formula.
- Elemental and molecular composition (degree of purity, any known impurities or additives).
- Proper evaluation of nanomaterials should be done to determine whether the product formulated is safe for future use; the characterisation must include measurement of particle size and distribution, aggregation and agglomeration characteristics, surface

chemistry (zeta potential/surface charge, surface coating, fictionalising, catalytic activity), morphology (shape, surface, surface topology, crystallinity), solubility, density, stability and porosity.

B. Impurities: Change in starting material of cosmetic results in altered composition and thus different impurities. Use of additional agents and impurities should be taken into account in safety aspects of nanomaterials in cosmetic products.

(ii) Toxicology consideration

The suitability of toxicological testing is based on the intended use, exposure level and potential toxicity of ingredients or formulations.

(a) Routes of exposure

The safety of ingredients depends on the potential for exposure and relevant routes of exposure that are determined by its intended use.

(b) Uptake and absorption

The physico-chemical properties of the nanoparticles are different, so there must be safety assessment through which regulation of dose of the nanoparticles could be increased or decreased so that it could cross the blood-brain barrier.

(c) Toxicity testing

The earliest step for the determination of the safety estimation of cosmetic formulation is to perform toxicity testing which is generally based on the toxicological profile of the ingredients as well as routes of exposure.

5.4.1.2 Guidelines for Drug Products

The FDA has issued a guidance document for industry *drug products, including biological products, that contain nanomaterials* (https://www.fda.gov/media/109910/download). The main features are:

- Scope
- Potential risk factors for products with nanomaterials
- Quality: Chemistry, manufacturing and controls
  - Description of nanomaterials
  - Nanomaterial quality attribute, structural characterisation
  - Nanomaterial physico-chemical characterisation methods
  - Dissolution/in vitro drug release methods for quality testing
  - Manufacturing process and process control
  - Excipients
  - Stability
  - Postmarket CMC changes
- Nonclinical studies for drug products
  - General applicability of existing guidance
  - Absorption, distribution, metabolism, and excretion (ADME) considerations
  - Risk consideration for specific routes of administration

    Topical/subcutaneous/inhalation/intravenous/oral
  - Testing of the representative nanomaterial
  - Bridging toxicology – a drug product not containing nanomaterials to a drug product containing nanomaterials
- Clinical developments

5.4.1.3 Fact Sheet on Working Safely with Nanomaterials

The *Occupational Safety and Health Administration (OSHA)* has come forward with the fact sheet entitled "Working Safely with Nanomaterials" (https://www.osha.gov/Publications/OSHA_FS-3634.html) (OSHA is part of the United States Department of Labor; it was created in 1971. The OSHA mission is to protect workers' health and safety. It ensures safety of work and healthy working environment for workers in the USA).

This fact sheet delivers researchers, employers and workers with the essential information on the understanding of possible hazards related to nanotechnology and various methods to avoid exposure to nanomaterials in the workplace as the workers and researchers using nanotechnology for research and production may absorb nanomaterials through ingestion, skin contact or inhalation.

Workplaces that use nanomaterials include pharmaceutical labs or industries, chemical laboratories and plants, medical hospitals, construction sites, etc. In these workshops nanoparticles possess greater hazards if they are easily dispersed in the form of powders, droplets or sprays or if they are not contained or isolated.

Such workplaces should provide information about the nanoparticles being in use, and the workers should be trained at least about the following:

- Nanomaterial identification and the processes in which it is used
- What are the results associated with exposure to nanomaterials at the workplace
- Identification and working of personal protective equipment (PPE)
- Uses and limitations of personal protective equipment
- Emergency measures in case of exposures or spills of nanomaterials

The fact sheet covers some important topics such as:

- Health hazards resulting from exposure to nanomaterials
- Current occupational exposure limits for nanomaterials
- Assessing worker exposures to nanomaterials
- Methods employers can use to reduce worker exposure to nanomaterials, which include:
  - Engineering controls
  - Administrative controls
  - Personal protective equipment (PPE)
  - Medical screening and surveillance
- OSHA Standards that may apply to nanomaterial hazards
- How OSHA can help employers/workers (https://www.osha.gov/consultation)

5.4.2 European Union

In September 2017 the European Commission's research centre had considered the legislation on nanomaterials and realised that better implementation and safety evaluation were needed. The existing regulatory guidelines cover legislations on particular products containing nanomaterials, which include labelling and safety assessments, and therefore they have come forth with a suggested definition of nanotechnology so that regulators are able to recognise and describe nanoparticles. This is essential because then only nano-specific rules can apply. Many policies mandate a hazard evaluation of nanomaterials before their use. Regulators need to confirm that existing test procedures and guidance are compatible with nanomaterials; otherwise, nano-specific tests need to be developed.

The *JRC (Joint Research Centre)* is the science and knowledge service of the European Commission. It is spread across five different countries Belgium, Germany, Italy, the Netherlands and Spain (EU Science Hub; https://ec.europa.eu/jrc/en). The JRC forms the backbone of EU efforts to study nanomaterials and is part of collaborative research with European and international partners.

Methods for assessing the safety of nanomaterials are related to OECD test guidelines. It collaborates with the European Committee for Standardization (CEN) and International Organization for Standardization (ISO).

The Joint Research Centre (JRC) does the following:

- It supports the development and implementation of EU policy for nanomaterial safety assessment.
- It provides scientific and technical advice concerning nanomaterials to other commission services.
- It contributes to standardisation and harmonisation of methods for nanomaterials.
- Scientists participate in about ten FP7 (seventh Framework Programme for Research and Technological Development. It lasted for 7 years from 2007 till 2013).
- It hosts the web platform on nanomaterials.

EU regulations on consumer products – biocides, cosmetics and foods – have specific provisions for nanomaterials. Ingredient labelling is based on the definition of "nanomaterial". Nanomaterials are covered by the EU chemical legislation (REACH Regulation).

JRC scientists have contributed to reducing uncertainties related to the potential impact of nanomaterials on environment and health and are helping in the development of regulatory guidelines by providing advice with scientific credentials.

5.4.3 Regulations in India

In India, "Nano mission" was unveiled in 2007 to streamline investment into R&D. The Ministry of Science and Technology is responsible for the promotion of R&D in this area through three agencies: Department of Science and Technology (DST), Department of Biotechnology (DBT) and Department of Scientific and Industrial Research (DSIR). Nano mission is implemented by the DST (Srivastava and Chowdhury 2006). Some of the nanotechnology-based pharmaceutical drugs and substances are listed in Table 5.3.

5.4.3.1 Guidelines and Best Practices for Safe Handling of Nanomaterials in Research Laboratories and Industries

The Centre for Knowledge Management of Nanoscience and Technology has published guidelines and best practices for safe handling of nanomaterials in research laboratories and industries (https://dst.gov.in/sites/default/files/Draft-Guidelines%20.pdf):

- Document based on regulatory reports published by the ISO, OECD, NIOSH, OSHA and others.
- The report covers "identifying hazards, pathways and common tasks that could result in exposure, exposure control strategies, Best practices to be followed while handling nanoparticles, Best practices and adequate approaches regarding making and handling of nanopowders and use of products relating to food and healthcare, Safety practices".
- Engineered nanomaterials like nanospheres, nanotubes, nanowires and nanosheets possess a unique combination of properties – biological, physical, chemical, mechanical, electrical and thermal – making them capable for a variety of applications. Due to high reactivity, large surface area and small dimensions, nanoparticles are able to penetrate living cells. The unique nano-features make them hazardous for the environment and health. Extensive research activity is being undertaken in various R&D institutions, universities and industries across the world to evaluate the toxicity and critical exposure levels of nano material,

Table 5.3 Nanotechnology applications developed in India

Sr. No.	Technology/process	Description	Owner/developer
1	Abraxane	A formulation of paclitaxel for targeted drug delivery	Biocon Bengaluru
2	Antimicrobial spray	Through use of silver nanoparticles	Bhaskar Center for Innovation and Scientific Research Chennai
3	Drug scanner	Nanotechnology-based spurious drug detection scanner machine	Bilcare Research Pune
4	Estrasorb	DDS for oestrogen therapy (drug loaded within the nanoparticle formulation)	Bharat Biotech (with Novavax) Hyderabad
5	Nanoxel	Paclitaxel-based drug delivery systems (DDS) for cancer drugs	Dabur (Fresenius Kabi Oncology Ltd.) Haryana
6	Water-soluble carbon nanotube-based cancer drug delivery system	Water-soluble carbon nanotubes that have functional groups on the walls for conjugation with cancer drugs	Cromoz Inc./IIT Kanpur

5.4.3.2 Guidelines for Evaluation of Nanopharmaceuticals

Guidelines for evaluation of nanopharmaceuticals in India have been published by the Government of India in October 2019 (http://164.100.117.97/WriteReadData/userfiles/Guidelines%20For%20Evaluation%20of%20Nanopharmaceuticals%20in%20India_24.10.19.pdf).

The aim of these guidelines is to ensure the quality, safety and efficacy of nanopharmaceuticals and to encourage commercialisation of nanotechnology-based inventions by increasing benefit-to-risk ratio.

The scope applies to the nanopharmaceuticals in the form of finished formulation as well as API of a new molecule or an already-approved molecule with altered nanoscale dimensions, properties or phenomena associated with the application of nanotechnology intended to be used for treatment, in vivo diagnosis, mitigation and cure or prevention of diseases and disorders in humans.

These do not apply to conventional drugs with incidental presence of nanoparticles or drug products containing microorganisms or proteins, which are naturally present in the nanoscale range. These are not applicable to medical devices, in vitro diagnostics, tissue-engineered products using nanotechnology and nanoparticle-modified cell-based therapies.

These guidelines have defined and categorised nanopharmaceuticals as described below:

Nanopharmaceutical is a "pharmaceutical preparation containing nanomaterials intended for internal use or external application on human for the purpose of therapeutics, diagnostics and health benefits. The nanomaterial is generally defined as material having particle size in the range of 1–100 nm in at least one dimension. However, if a material exhibits physical, chemical or biological phenomenon or activity which are attributable to its dimension beyond nanoscale range up to 1000 nm, the material should also be considered as nanomaterial. Therefore, any pharmaceutical containing such material should also be considered as nanopharmaceutical".

In particle-size distribution of the nanopharmaceutical, the nanosized range should be declared in the product specification. Further, the particles should be within the claimed nanosized range in all given testing conditions during the claimed stability period and final product.

The guideline has categorised the nanopharmaceuticals according to various categories as follows:

1. According to degradability of nanomaterial
    (a) Biodegradable (PLA, PLGA, etc.)
    (b) Non-biodegradable (gold, silver, platinum, etc.)
2. According to nature of nanomaterial
    (a) Organic nanomaterials
        (i) Biodegradable (carbohydrates, lipids, liposomes, polymers, proteins or their conjugates or composites)
        (ii) Non-biodegradable (carbon nanotube, fullerene, graphene, etc.)
    (b) Inorganic nanomaterials
        (i) Biodegradable (biominerals)
        (ii) Non-biodegradable (metallic nanoparticles, semiconductor quantum dots, iron oxides, etc.)
    (c) Multicomponent nanomaterials (magnetic liposomes)
3. According to nanoform of the ingredient
    (a) Nanocarriers loaded with active pharmaceutical ingredient (dendrimers, liposomes, gold nanoparticles, etc.)
    (b) API converted to nanoform (nanocrystals of tacrolimus, cyclosporin, griseofulvin, etc.)

The key features are:

- Scientific rationality for development of nanopharmaceuticals
- Stability testing of nanopharmaceuticals
- Animal pharmacology data
- Animal toxicology data
- Clinical trial data
- Evaluation of nanopharmaceuticals
- Pharmacovigilance of nanopharmaceuticals

5.5 Conclusion and Future Perspectives

It has been reported that there are large data gaps which indicate the need to augment over conventional toxicity methods (Hulla et al. 2015; Walker and Bucher 2009; https://www.greenfacts.org/en/risks-nanotechnologies-nanomaterials/index.html).

The four main areas which need to be focused on are:

1. Insufficient data: there is no specific data regarding nanoparticles and nanomaterials and even no information or data about the use of the same in products and release from products.
2. Scientific understanding of nanotoxicological behaviour needs to be improved to facilitate the next step of generalisation and abstraction.
3. Nanotoxicological data needs to address existing and future areas of development in nanomaterials.
4. There are limited risk assessment and regulatory guidelines available.

The government, society, scientists and business houses need to cooperate to develop an action plan to deal with developments in materials and the associated risks. This would provide the foundation for increased data availability and mutual understanding.

Various agencies around the world regulate nanotechnology products as per existing norms and regulations. Regulations specifically for nanoparticle-based products are essential and regulations regarding the same need to be drafted and implemented.

References

Agarwal V, Bajpai M, Sharma A (2018) Patented and approval scenario of nanopharmaceuticals with relevancy to biomedical application, manufacturing procedure and safety aspects. Recent Pat Drug Deliv Formul 12:40–52

Buzea C, Blandino IIP, Robbie K (2007) Nanomaterials and nanoparticles: sources and toxicity. Biointerphases 2(4):MR17

Cuffari B (2018) What nanomaterials exist in nature? AZoNano. https://www.azonano.com/article.aspx?ArticleID=4837

Desai PP, Rustomjee MT (2016) Business Potential of Advanced Drug Delivery Systems. CRS Indian Local Chapter Newsletter 8:29–34. Retrieved from https://www.google.com/url?sa=t&source=web&rct=j&url=http://www.crsic.org/pdf/newsletter- 2016.pdf&ved=2ahUKEwiI1IeN6fXoAhVY83MBHda6CdoQFjAAegQIARAB&usg=AOvVaw2a_GUGoJsDYEfOnnWCn7TV

Ealias AM, Saravanakumar MP (2017) A review on the classification, characterisation, synthesis of nanoparticles and their application. IOP Conf Ser Mater Sci Eng 263:1–15

EU Science Hub, The European Commission's science and knowledge service (https://ec.europa.eu/jrc/en/research-topic/nanotechnology, https://ec.europa.eu/research/fp7/understanding/fp7inbrief/what-is_en.html, https://ec.europa.eu/jrc/en)

Farjadian F, Ghasemi A, Gohari O, Roointan A, Karimi M, Hamblin MR (2018) Nanopharmaceuticals and nanomedicines currently on the market: challenges and opportunities. Nanomedicine (Lond). https://doi.org/10.2217/nnm-2018-0120

Farokhzad OC, Langer R (2006) Nanomedicine: developing smarter therapeutic and diagnostic modalities. Adv Drug Deliv Rev 58(14):1456–1459

Griffin S, Masood MI, Nasim MJ, Muhammad Sarfraz, Ebokaiwe AP, Schäfer KH, Cornelia M. Keck, Jacob C (2018) Natural Nanoparticles: A Particular Matter Inspired by Nature. Antioxidants 7(3):1–21. https://doi.org/10.3390/antiox7010003; www.mdpi.com/journal/antioxidants

Guidelines and Best Practices for Safe Handling of Nanomaterials in Research Laboratories and Industries. Compiled for Nano Mission, DST, Govt. of India (with inputs from Nanoregulatory Task Force) By Centre for Knowledge Management of Nanoscience & Technology (A Project of ARCI, Department of Science & Technology, Govt. of India)

Hulla JE, Sahu SC, Hayes AW (2015) Nanotechnology: history and future. Hum Exp Toxicol 34(12):1318–1321

Iyer R, Hsia CC, Nguyen KT (2015) Nano-therapeutics for the lung: state-of-the-art and future perspectives. Curr Pharm Des 21(36):5233–5244

Jeevanandam J, Barhoum A, Chan YS, Dufresne A, Danquah MK (2018) Review on nanoparticles and nanostructured materials: history, sources, toxicity and regulations. Beilstein J Nanotechnol 9:1050–1074

Kandasamy NP (1998) History of Siddha medicine, 2nd edn. Dept. of Indian Medicine and Homoeopathy, Chennai

Kapoor RC (2010) Some observations on the metal based preparations in the Indian system of medicine. Indian J Tradit Knowl 9:562–575

Krukemeyer MG, Krenn V, Huebner F, Wagner W, Resch R (2015) History and possible uses of nanomedicine based on nanoparticles nanotechnological progress. J Nanomed Nanotechnol 6(6):1–7

McClements DJ, Xiao H (2017) Is nano safe in foods? Establishing the factors impacting the gastrointestinal fate and toxicity of organic and inorganic food-grade nanoparticles. npj Sci Food 1:6. https://doi.org/10.1038/s41538-017-0005-1

Nikalje PA (2015) Nanotechnology and its application in medicine. Med Chem 5(2):081–089

Pachapur V, Brar SK, Verma M, Surampalli RY (2015) Nano-ecotoxicology of natural and engineered nanomaterials for animals and humans. Chapter 16. In: Nanomaterials in the environment, pp 421–437. https://doi.org/10.1061/9780784414088.ch16

Pal D, Sahu CK, Haldar A (2014) Bhasma: the ancient Indian nanomedicine. J Adv Pharm Technol Res 5(1):4–12

Palkhiwala S, Bakshi SR (2014) Engineered nanoparticles: revisiting safety concerns in light of ethno medicine. Ayu 35(3):237–242

Patra JK, Das G, Fraceto LF, Campos EVR, Rodriguez-Torres Maria del Pilar, Acosta-Torres LS, Diaz-Torres LA, Grillo R, Swamy MK, Sharma S, Habtemariam S, Shin H (2018) Nano based drug delivery systems: recent developments and future prospects. J Nanobiotechnol 16:71

Ray U (2018) What are the different types of nanoparticles? AZoNano. https://www.azonano.com/article.aspx?ArticleID=4938

Rochishnu D, Brahmachary RL (2009) Natural nanoparticles: an overview. LAP Lambert Academic Publishing. ISBN: 3838335074

Rohit S, Prajapati PK (2018) Nanotechnology in medicine: leads from Ayurveda. J Pharm Bio Allied Sci 8(1):80–81

Sarkar PK, Chaudhary AK (2010) Ayurvedic bhasma: the most ancient application of nanomedicine. J Sci Ind Res 69:901–905

Sayes CM, Aquino GV, Hickey AJ (2017) Nanomaterial drug products: manufacturing and analytical perspectives. AAPS J 19(1):18–25

Shailaja R, Sugunthan S (2016) Concept of nano technology in Siddha medical literatures. World J Pharma Res 5(10):276–284

Srivastava N and Chowdhury N (2006) Nanotechnology regulation in India: a framework for exploring the risks and opportunities. Chapter 11 nanotechnology and state regulation (India), 241–260

U.S. Environmental Protection Agency (2017, July 31) Classification of nanomaterials, the four main types of intentionally produced nanomaterials. AZoNano

Urbanska AM, Sefat F, Yousaf S, Kargozar S, Milan PB, and Mozafari M (2019) Nanoengineered biomaterials for intestine regeneration. Nanoengineered Biomaterials for Regenerative Medicine. Micro and Nano Technologies Chapter 16: 363–378 (Elsevier, ScienceDirect journals and books) https://www.sciencedirect.com/topics/engineering/engineered-nanoparticles

Walker NJ, Bucher JR (2009) A 21st century paradigm for evaluating the health hazards of nanoscale materials. Toxicol Sci 110:251–254

Wang GH, Zhou BH, Cheng CL, Cao JJ, Li JJ, Meng JJ, Tao J, Zhang RJ, Fu PQ (2013) Impact of Gobi desert dust on aerosol chemistry of Xi'an, inland China during spring 2009: differences in composition and size distribution between the urban ground surface and the mountain atmosphere. Atmos Chem Phys 13:819–835

Websites

https://www.nano.gov/nanotech-101/what/definition

https://www.sciencedirect.com/topics/engineering/taniguchi

http://nano%2D%2Dtech.blogspot.com/p/history.html

https://www.understandingnano.com/medicine.html

https://www.fda.gov/regulatory-information/search-fda-guidance-documents/guidance-industry-safety-nanomaterials-cosmetic-products

https://www.osha.gov/Publications/OSHA_FS-3634.html

https://www.osha.gov/consultation

https://dst.gov.in/sites/default/files/Draft-Guidelines%20.pdf

https://www.greenfacts.org/en/risks-nanotechnologies-nanomaterials/index.htm

https://www.greenfacts.org/en/risks-nanotechnologies-nanomaterials/index.html

https://ec.europa.eu/jrc/en/research-topic/nanotechnology

https://ec.europa.eu/research/fp7/understanding/fp7in-brief/what-is_en.html, https://ec.europa.eu/jrc/en

https://www.sciencedirect.com/topics/engineering/engineered-nanoparticles

https://www.fda.gov/media/109910/download

https://www.fda.gov/media/82686/download

http://164.100.117.97/WriteReadData/userfiles/Guidelines%20For%20Evaluation%20of%20Nanopharmaceuticals%20in%20India_24.10.19.pdf

http://dbtindia.gov.in/sites/default/files/DBT_Draft1-Nano-Agri_Input_nd_Nano-Agri_Products.pdf

http://ris.org.in/images/RIS_images/pdf/DP%20193%20Amit%20Kumar.pdf

https://timesofindia.indiatimes.com/city/varanasi/Bhasmas-are-nano-medicine-of-ancient-times/articleshow/7438242.cms

https://www.fda.gov/science-research/nanotechnology-programs-fda/nanotechnology-fact-sheet

https://www.nature.com/scitable/knowledge/library/the-environmental-significance-of-natural-nanoparticles-105737311

https://www.fda.gov/science-research/nanotechnology-programs-fda/fdas-approach-regulation-nanotechnology-products

https://www.nano.gov/nanotech-101/special

https://copublications.greenfacts.org/en/nanotechnologies/l-2/4-nanoparticle-formation.htm

https://www.fda.gov/science-research/nanotechnology-programs-fda/nanotechnology-fact-sheet
http://www.ipc.org/4.0_Knowledge/4.1_Standards/test/2.3.2.pdf
https://www.nature.com/scitable/knowledge/library/the-environmental-significance-of-natural-nanoparticles-105737311
https://repository.law.umich.edu/mjeal/vol7/iss2/7/
https://www.osha.gov/Publications/OSHA_FS-3634.pdf
www.nanowerk.com/news2/newsid=26583.php
https://cdsco.gov.in/opencms/resources/UploadCDSCOWeb/2018/UploadPublic_NoticesFiles/newdrunoti7march.pdf
https://www.researchgate.net/publication/289522360_NanoEcotoxicology_of_Natural_and_Engineered_Nanomaterials_for_Animals_and_Humans
http://nanomission.gov.in/What_new/Draft_Guidelines_and_Best_Practices.pdf
https://www.researchgate.net/publication/265533479_Drug_Regulation_History_Present_and_Future_1
https://www.azonano.com/article.aspx?ArticleID=4837

Part II

Nanoformulations in Drug Targeting

6 Conventional and Nonconventional Approaches to Site-Specific Targeting of Nanotherapeutics in Some Infectious Diseases and Metabolic Disorders

Biswajit Mukherjee, Samrat Chakraborty, Iman Ehsan, Apala Chakraborty, Leena Kumari, Alankar Mukherjee, and Shounak Sarkhel

Abstract

Systemic fungal infection in pulmonary tissue and viral infections affecting peripheral nerve claim millions of lives every year. The inability of therapeutics to reach the diseased sites at an optimum concentration, lack of patient-friendly delivery strategies, and inability of delivery strategies to penetrate and/or release the therapeutic payload at the diseased sites, keeping the normal cells unaffected, are some of the reasons which demand alternative or other methods to successfully deliver drug to affected sites. Since the end of the last century, a novel drug delivery system (drug-nanocarrier system) has reached a new benchmark with the application of nanomedicine in the treatment of fatal metabolic disorders and infectious diseases. Despite its ability to increase permeability and penetrability to cells/tissues/organs, its uncontrolled biodistribution may cause cytotoxicity to nontargeted cells, resulting in improper therapeutic management. Therefore, ligand-based active targeting strategies are most popularly exploited by researchers around the world to develop site-specific targeting of diseased sites. A plethora of site-specific nanomedicines has been developed on the laboratory scale based on conventional active targeting strategies with ligands. Even after a lot of sincere efforts, the translation of laboratory to clinic is very limited due to toxicity, stability, and the nonspecific nature of ligands. Therefore, certain nonconventional approaches of targeting therapeutics, such as gene-silencing technology, management of glioma by incorporation of brain-mimicking lipid in nanoliposomal formulations, chemical-mediated nanoliposomal formulations specifically targeted to peripheral nervous systems (PNS), and innovation of novel delivery devices, offer significant promise for effective therapeutic management. This chapter focuses on the pros and cons and future prospects of various conventional and nonconventional approaches of drug targeting with an insight to develop powerful therapeutic weapons for effective therapeutic management of deadly diseases.

B. Mukherjee (✉) · S. Chakraborty · I. Ehsan · A. Chakraborty · L. Kumari · A. Mukherjee · S. Sarkhel
Department of Pharmaceutical Technology, Jadavpur University, Kolkata, West Bengal, India
e-mail: biswajit.mukherjee@jadavpuruniversity.in; biswajit55@yahoo.com

S. Talegaonkar, M. Rai (eds.), *Nanoformulations in Human Health*,
https://doi.org/10.1007/978-3-030-41858-8_6

Keywords

Conventional drug-targeting · Nonconventional drug targeting · Ligand-conjugated drug targeting · Antisense RNA-mediated targeting · siRNA-mediated targeting · drug targeting at PNS

6.1 Introduction

Combating the mortality associated with various systemic diseases, such as fungal infection in pulmonary tissues, viral infections in peripheral nerves, metabolic disorders including malignant tumors, diabetes, etc., faces lots of challenges due to multiple factors, namely, (i) lack of specificity of therapeutics at the diseased sites, resulting in severe toxicity in normal tissues; (ii) poor penetration and retention of therapeutics in the diseased sites; (iii) feeble therapeutic outcome due to frequent dosing, resulting in poor patient compliance, etc. (Li et al. 2016). Nanomedicine (application of nanotechnology in medicine) offers a considerable promise to provide significant improvement in therapeutic response to combat those challenges of metabolic disorders or fungal/viral infections in humans/animals (Sinha et al. 2013). However, issues such as nonspecific biodistribution of nanoformulations upon systemic administration are an obstacle that need to be addressed for better therapeutic management of diseases. These drawbacks have shifted the attention of researchers around the globe toward the development of ligand-based site-specific delivery of nanocarriers to the diseased sites for radical improvement in therapeutic response and outcome. Furthermore, ongoing understandings of these diseases at the molecular level help to design ligands with superior affinity for the diseased sites. Although many so far explored ligands have shown superiority in delivering therapeutics to the diseased sites, their nonspecific biodistribution, especially in healthy normal cells/tissues, cannot be fully tackled. Most of the ligands target specific overexpressed proteins of the diseased cells and the normal cells are often found to express those proteins (may be at a low amount). The treatment of diseases of the central nervous systems (CNS), such as glioblastoma and neurodegenerative disorders, imposes another hurdle to biomedical scientists due to the strategic location of the blood-brain barrier (BBB), which allows very selective transport of molecules between the systemic circulation and the interstitial fluid to maintain homeostasis.

A plethora of ligands such as peptides, antibodies, aptamers, and small molecules such as vitamins and sugars are heavily exploited globally for the development of powerful therapeutics (as illustrated in Table 6.1). Despite several approaches by scientists to develop ligand-based active therapeutics, their limited success is due to many reasons, a few of them are: (i) nonspecificity due to their inability to target proteins solely expressed by diseased cells/tissues, (ii) in vivo instability, (iii) toxicity, (iv) high cost, and (v) saturation of target proteins by targeting ligands, etc. These drawbacks have instigated researchers to explore certain nonconventional site-specific drug delivery approaches that show significant opportunity for the development of powerful therapeutic weapons in order to strengthen the armory of humankind. These concepts of targeting include use of certain indigenous components of tissues, use of chemicals which have a natural affinity for the target sites, and direct gene-silencing technology to prevent the expressions of the corresponding proteins responsible for metabolic disorders. Therefore, the fundamental focus of the present chapter is to highlight various pros and cons of the conventional and nonconventional methods of drug targeting in order to accelerate translation of research from laboratory scales to clinics to utilize those technologies to prevent humankind from the fatality of these diseases.

At the outset, we should explain our thoughts related to defining conventional and nonconventional approaches to site-specific nanosize drug delivery. Various ligand-mediated drug delivery systems for transporting the drug cargo to the specific cells or tissues are conventional approaches of drug targeting. Several such widely targeted ligands are monoclonal antibodies,

Table 6.1 Conventional approaches for site specific targeting of therapeutics

Disease	Targeting moieties		Specific targeted site	References
Cancer	*Monoclonal antibodies*	IgG1	CD20 (in low-grade B-cell non-Hodgkin lymphoma)	Cardarelli et al. (2002)
			HER2/neu (in metastatic breast cancer)	Holgado et al. (2018)
			CD52 (in chronic lymphocytic leukemia)	Mone et al. (2006)
			VEGF and EGFR (in metastatic colorectal cancer)	Ohhara et al. (2016)
		IgG4/calicheamicin	CD33 (in acute myeloid leukemia)	van der Velden et al. (2001)
		IgG1/90Y	CD20 (in relapsed or refractory non-Hodgkin lymphoma)	Sharkey et al. (2010)
		IgG2a/ 131I	CD20 (non-Hodgkin' lymphoma refractory to Rituximab and relapsed following chemotherapy)	Kaminski et al. (2000)
	Peptide-mediated targeting	Bombesin (QQRLGNQWAVGHLM)	GRP receptors (in small cell lung, glioblastomas, gastric, pancreatic, prostate, breast, cervical, and colon cancers)	Accardo et al. (2019)
		Somatostatin (AGCKNFFWKTFTSC)	Somatostatin receptors (in small cell and non-small cell lung cancers)	Kiaris et al. (2001)
		FSH β chain carrying peptide FSH-33 (YTRDLVYKDPARPKIQKTCTF)	FSH receptors (in ovarian cancer)	Hong et al. (2013)
		LyP-1 peptide (CGNKRTRGC)	p32 protein (in MDA-MB-435 melanoma cancer cells)	Song et al. (2019)
		Fibroblast growth factor analogs (KRLYCKNGGF FLRIHPDGRV DGVREKSDPH IKLQLQAEER GVVSIKGVCA NRYLAMKEDG RLLASKCVTD ECFFFERLES NNYNTY)	Fibroblast growth factor receptors (FGFRs) (on both tumor cells and neovasculature)	Schmidt et al. (2015)
		Liver cancer targeting peptide (FQHPSFI)	HepG2 (in hepatocarcinoma cells)	Zhang et al. (2007)
		Peptide GFE (CGFECVRQCP ERC) and peptide F3 (KDEPQRRSAR LSAKPAPPKP EPKPKKAPAK K)	Endothelial cells of lung blood vessels and tumor vasculature	Åkerman et al. (2002)
		Tripeptide RGD	αvβ6 integrin (in head and neck cancers)	Ahmedah et al. (2017)
		Alpha melanocyte stimulating hormone (α-MSH peptide)	α-MSH receptors (on metastatic melanoma cells)	Quinn et al. (2010)
	Aptamer-mediated targeting	Enterotoxin (STh) from Escherichia coli (NSSNYCCELC CNPACTGCY)	guanylate cyclase C receptor (on the surface of human colon cancer cells)	Pitari et al. (2001)

(continued)

Table 6.1 (continued)

Disease	Targeting moieties		Specific targeted site	References
Cancer	*Aptamer-mediated targeting*	A9 and A10	PSMA (in prostate cancer cells)	Fan et al. (2016)
		TTA-1	Tenascin-C (in glioblastoma cells)	Hicke et al. (2001)
		5TR1	MUC1 (in mammary gland, esophagus, stomach, duodenum, colon, pancreas, uterus, prostate, lungs, and hematopoietic cells)	Moosavian et al. (2018)
		J18	EGFR (in breast, lung, esophageal, and head and neck cancer)	Li et al. (2010)
		D4	RET (in pheochromocytoma and multiple endocrine neoplasis)	Cerchia et al. (2005)
		Sgc8	Protein tyrosine kinase 7 (in T cell acute lymphoblastic leukemia cells)	Taghdisi et al. (2010)
		TD05	Membrane-bound immunoglobulin heavy μ-chain (in Burkitt's lymphoma cells)	Mallikaratchy et al. (2007)
	Folate-mediated targeting	Folic acid	FR-α (in adenocarcinomas of the ovary, uterus and cervix, testicular choriocarcinoma, ependymal brain tumors, malignant pleural mesothelioma, and nonfunctioning pituitary adenocarcinoma)	Cheung et al. (2016)
			FR-β (in chronic (CML) and acute (AML) myelogenous leukemia)	Lynn et al. (2015)
			FR-γ (in ovarian, cervical and uterine carcinoma)	Shen et al. (1995)
	Transferrin-mediated targeting	Transferrin	TFR1 (in brain, breast, colon, liver, lung, ovarian and prostate cancer)	Shen et al. (2018)
			TFR2 (in ovarian cancer, colon cancer and glioblastoma cell lines)	Calzolari et al. (2007)

(continued)

Table 6.1 (continued)

Disease	Targeting moieties		Specific targeted site	References
Diabetics	Protein-mediated targeting	Lectin	Intestinal epithelial cells absorption enhancement	Woitiski et al. (2008)
	Polysaccharides	Double coating with chitosan and alginate	Enhancing of the NPs' electrostatic interactions with the intestinal cells	Li et al. (2017)
		Tri-methyl chitosan chloride[1], Chitosan–6 mercaptonicotinic acid (chitosan–6-MNA)[2]	mucoadhesion	Lui et al. (2015), Millotti et al. (2014)
	Boric acid derivative	Phenyl boronic acid-containing block copolymer	Glucose responsive micelles with faster response in physiological pH	Yang et al. (2013)
	Protease inhibitor	Diethylene triaminepenta acetic acid (DTPA) as chelating agent	Inhibits intestinal protease activity	Su Fy et al. (2012)
		Trypsin or achymotrypsin inhibitors, such as soybean trypsin inhibitor[1] FK-448[2] Ca3ostatmesylate[2], aprotinin[3]		Kinesh et al. (2010), Pandit and Joshi (2015), Cliek et al. (2005)
	PEG conjugated	PEGylation of insulin	nonimmunogenic, nontoxic, nonallergic variants of insulin	Zhang et al. (2008)
	Peptides	CPP (molecular weight protamine[1], arginine[2], lysine[2], penetratin[3], R9[4])	Enhance penetration of negatively charged cell surface	Sheng et al. (2016), Wearly (1991), Kamei et al. (2015), Araújo et al. (2016)
	Biotinylation	Lys34-,Lys26,34–biotin–GLP-1 derivatization	Actively traverses the intestine membrane via sodium-dependent multivitamin transport	Youns et al. (2008)
Peripheral targeting	peptidomimetics	Claudin-1	Barrier opener to transport hydrophilic analgesic	Zwanziger et al. (2012), Sauer et al. (2014), Staat et al. (2015)
	Bacterial neurotoxins	Tetanus toxins[1] Tet-1[2]	Ganglioside GT1b receptor	Surana et al. (2018), Liu et al. (2005)
		Botulinum neurotoxin A (BoNT/A)	Motor neurons	Marinelli et al. (2012)
		Cholera toxin subunit B, or CTB	Ganglioside GM1.	Porras et al. (2016)
	Monoclonal antibody	–	To target intercellular adhesion molecule (ICAM)-1	Lengert et al. (2013)
	Others	dioleoyl-phosphatidylcholine (DOPC)	Preferentially targeted peripheral neurons and Schwann cells	Lee et al. (2013)
Pulmonary fungal infection	Surface functionalization	Chitosan	Increases mucoadhesion in pulmonary fungal infection	Paul et al. (2018)
	Delivery devices	Nebulizer	Direct deposition of drugs to pulmonary site	Monforte et al. (2010)

peptides, aptamers, carbohydrate compounds, vitamins, and many more. However, nonconventional site-specific drug delivery approaches highlight the approaches to deliver drug to the target cells/organs/tissues without using any ligands. They may include charge-dependent drug carrier, drug delivery to a systemic tissue directly for prolonged action of drug in the tissue as drug depot, using indigenous components of tissues in the carrier systems, use of chemical compounds in the drug carrier, which has natural affinity to the target site, or even approaches to directly silencing genes or protein expression to stop development of malfunctioning proteins responsible for causing the disease.

Due to the chapter's limited scope, we describe here only a few selective conventional and nonconventional nanosize site-specific drug delivery systems.

6.2 Conventional Approaches for Targeting

Some selective ligand-mediated approaches have been described below in a nutshell.

6.2.1 Monoclonal Antibodies

The unique characteristics of antibodies such as molecular homogeneity, high specificity, and binding affinity of monoclonal antibodies (mAbs) make them attractive ligands for cancer cell targeting. Monoclonal antibodies are widely explored on various cell-surface proteins, such as epidermal growth factor receptor (EGFR), vascular endothelial growth factor receptor (VGFR), human epidermal receptor (HER2), etc. Antibodies can be used either to recognize the target proteins on the surface of the cells or to function as therapeutics. Therapeutic mAbs are engineered to make them fully humanized or chimeric antibodies in order to avoid untoward toxicity. Despite their potential as targeting ligands and as therapeutics, their toxicity, stability, and size are the serious drawbacks limiting the translation of their potential from preclinical stage to clinical trial to the clinic. Some examples depicting antibody-mediated active targeting of nanoparticles are given below:

(a) The monoclonal antibody PDL1 – functionalized polyethylene glycol-poly(ε-caprolactone) nanoparticles were developed by Xu et al. (2019) for the effective management of gastric cancer, as the expression of PDL1 is upregulated in gastric cancer following the infection with *Helicobacter pylori*. They reported that mAb PDL1 binds with the extracellular domain of protein PDL1, thus preventing its interaction with receptor PD-1, which plays very crucial role in the downregulation of the immune system as well as promotes self-tolerance by the suppression T-Cell inflammatory activity.
(b) Nagesh et al. (2016) developed docetaxel-loaded superparamagnetic iron oxide nanoparticles which were functionalized with antibody J591 to target prostate-cancer-specific membrane antigen (PSMA) for the effective management of prostate cancer.
(c) Overexpression of the epidermal growth factor is seen in various cases of small lung cancer. This overexpressed epidermal growth factor was exploited by Karra et al. (2013) for site-specific targeting by developing cetuximab-conjugated paclitaxel-loaded polylactide-co-glycolide (PLGA) nanoparticles. Results of their investigation revealed that EFGR-targeted nanoparticles might have the potential for effective management of lung cancers.

6.2.2 Peptides

Peptides are widely explored as targeting ligands due to their small size, resulting in superior penetration into the target sites as compared to antibodies and proteins, and their ability to interact with the surface protein of the target sites through protein-protein interaction, resulting in higher binding affinity and specificity compared to other targeting ligands. Comparatively low immunogenicity, large-scale synthesis by relatively inexpensive phase-display technology, and biocompatible chemical properties are the additional advantages of paptides. A plethora of peptide molecules has been explored as anticancer peptides, as targeting ligands for site-specific delivery of chemotherapeutics, and in the development of cancer vaccine against various types of malignancies. However, susceptibility towards proteolysis, especially after in vivo delivery is the serious drawback encountered by peptide ligands, and thus it probably hinders their translation from laboratory scale to clinic, and very few peptides have entered into clinical trials in order to serve humankind by developing efficient therapeutic weapons to combat fatal diseases. Lo et al. (2008) developed nanoliposomal doxorubicin conjugated with peptide SP94 for the development of site-specific targeting in hepatocellular carcinoma. In vitro study in malignant hepatocytes cells and in vivo investigations in tumor-bearing xenograft mice revealed that the peptide SP94 enhanced penetration of liposomal doxorubicin in malignant liver cells and tissues. Wang et al. (2016) developed arginyl-glycinyl-aspartic acid (RGD)-peptide-modified, lipid-coated nanoparticles for the dual delivery of sorafenib and quercetin. The prepared nanoformulations had been characterized on the basis of physicochemical investigations of different parameters such as particle size, zeta potential, etc. In vitro study in malignant hepatocytes has been performed, which showed excellent efficacy of the nanoformulation. Further in vivo study was performed in tumor-bearing xenograft mice. Results of a series of in vitro and in vivo investigations revealed that RGD-peptide-functionalized modified lipid-coated nanoparticles had significant potential in controlling hepatocellular carcinoma (HCC).

6.2.3 Aptamers

Single-stranded DNA or RNA oligonucleotides are known as aptamers, which are popularly used as targeting ligands due to their numerous positive features such as low molecular weight, ease of manufacturing, nonimmunogenicity, and high binding affinities for a wide range of target molecules, which include peptides, enzymes, antibodies, and various cell-surface receptors. Systemic evolution of ligands through exponential enrichment (SELEX) techniques enables to generate aptamers with high selectivity and sensitivity (Li et al. 2016; Ladju et al. 2018; Zhuo et al. 2017). Furthermore, durability of aptamers in biological fluids has been enhanced by chemical modifications (such as phosphorothioate, methylphosphonate backbone modifications, etc.) which make them resistant against nucleases and peptidase enzymes (Toprkiewicz et al. 2015). Despite enormous potential of aptamers as targeting ligand, the development of aptamer-functionalized nanocarriers is still at its infancy as most of the aptamer-binding proteins that are overexpressed by cancer cells, also express in normal healthy cells (may be low in amount) resulting in toxicity in the noraml healthy cells.

Azhdarzadeh et al. (2016) developed gold-coated superparamagnetic iron oxide nanoparticles (SPIONs) as theranostics for magnetic resonance imaging and photodermal therapy. They prepared the SPIONs by microemulsion technique and modified by gold coating. Thiol-modified mucin-1 aptamer was attached on the surface of the gold modified SPIONs for the development of site-specific targeting therapy against colon cancer. Results of magnetic resonance imaging (MR) revealed that they had the significant potential to enhance the contrast enhancement agent. They concluded that the prepared gold-coated SPIONs could serve as potential theranostic agents in the management of colon cancer.

Zhang et al. (2010) developed a dot-labeled aptamer bioprobe (QD-Apt) by conjugating streptavidin-modified quantum dots (SA-QDs) with biotin-modified mouse liver hepatoma cell line, known as MEAR (BNL1MEA.7R.1)-specific single-stranded DNA aptamer (TLS9a). The developed QD-Apt specifically recognized the MEAR cells but could not recognize BNL cells (normal liver cells). Furthermore, results of this investigation showed that the developed probe was biocompatible and had the potential for live-cell imaging.

Glypican-3 (GPC-3) is recognized as a cellular membrane proteoglycan and is one of the potential and selective biomarkers for HCC diagnosis. Dong et al. (2018) screened 19 GPC-3 bound aptamers by capillary electrophoresis (CE)-SELEX technology. Among them, aptamer AP613-1 was found to be useful for specifically targeting GPC-3 with a dissociation constant (k_d) of 55.85 nM. Upon modification by phosphorothioate linkage, the k_d value dropped down to 15.48 nm and designated phosphorothioate modified AP613-1 as APS613-1. Results of in vitro investigations in malignant hepatocytes cells such as Huh-7 and in vivo study of xenograft nude mice revealed that APS613-1 had significant potential in imaging and diagnosis GPC-3-positive HCC.

6.2.4 Saccharide and Polysaccharide Ligands

Various glycoproteins and proteoglycans present in the outer surface of cells get upregulated due to transformation of normal cells into malignant cells. These upregulated expressions lead researchers to explore saccharides and polysaccharides as targeting ligands for the development of site-specific delivery strategies against different types of malignancies, especially HCC (Zhong et al. 2014; Jain et al. 2012). The expressions of asialoglycoprotein (ASGPR) receptors are upregulated in HCC. Therefore, the development of various targeted delivery vehicles against HCC has been designed by targeting the asialoglycoprotein receptors. D-galactose (Gal) and N-acetyl galactosamine residues bind with the asialoglycoprotein receptors with high affinity and specificity. Asialoglycoprotein receptors are also present in normal hepatocytes resulting in penetration of chemotherapeutics, and also leading to drug-related adverse effects, in normal hepatocytes. Apart from galactose and N-acetyl galactosamine, lactobionic acid, lactose, and polysaccharides, such as hyaluronic acid (HA), pectin, and pullulan, are some examples of saccharides as ligands (Li et al. 2016; Chitttasupho et al. 2013). Nonimmunogenic lectins are the multidomain proteins that are widely explored to target various glycans overexpressed in various malignant tumors (Lepenies et al. 2013).

6.2.5 Vitamins as Targeting Ligand

Vitamins represent a series of organic compounds which are essential micronutrients for myriad metabolic processes responsible for survival. The requirement of vitamins by cancer cells is upregulated due to their rapid proliferation. Among the various types of vitamins, cancer cells especially require excess quantities of folate, biotin, retinoic acid, vitamin B_{12}, and dehydroascorbic acid (DHAA) for their growth and survival (Li et al. 2016; Chen et al. 2010). Higher expression of receptors for these vitamins in cancer cells has been evidenced compared to normal cells (Li et al. 2016). Nanocarriers functionalized with vitamins have been attempted by the researchers for the development of site-specific delivery strategy in different types of malignant tumors as described below.

(i) Overexpression of transcobalamin-II receptors is one of the characteristic features of different types of malignancies in the ovaries, kidney, uterus, testis, brain, colon, lung, and myelocytic blood cells. Therefore, B_{12}-decorated nanocarriers offer significant promise for site-specific delivery of therapeutics and as imaging agents (Toprkiewicz et al. 2015).

(ii) Folic acid or folate, one of the key members in the vitamin B complex family, plays a pivotal role in the transfer of one-carbon unit into various biosynthetic pathways especially in de novo biosynthesis of purine and pyrimidine nucleotides. Cellular internalization of folate takes place through reduced folate carrier (RFC) and folate receptors (FR). The affinity of folate for FR is much higher compared to its affinity for RFC and upregulated expression of FR has been observed in various malignant tumors such as ovarian, brain, head and neck, renal, and breast cancers (Ai et al. 2012; Chen et al. 2013; Lemon and Low 2001; Lucock 2000). That is why folate-decorated nanocarriers have been developed to target the overexpressed folate receptors for the site-specific delivery of theranostics (personalized and precision-based medicine).

(iii) Like FR, overexpression of biotin receptors (even more than FR) is seen in various cancer cells, namely, breast, colon, lungs, and renal cancer and leukemia. The overexpression of biotin receptors encourages researchers to develop delivery strategies with biotin to achieve site-specific targeting of malignant cells (Russel-Jones et al. 2004).

(iv) Retinoic acid, the metabolite of vitamin A, has established its potential against HCC as it exerts its cytotoxic potential by different mechanisms, such as (i) regulation of apoptosis and differentiation, (ii) modulating the sensitivity of tumor cells to the innate immune response, etc. It has been reported in the literature that among the different subtypes of RA receptors (α, β, and γ), the subtype γ is upregulated in HCC (Sano et al. 2003). Investigations reveal that RA-functionalized chitosan-albumin nanoparticles showed much better apoptotic potential than nonfunctionalized chitosan-albumin nanoparticles in HCC (Varshosaz et al. 2013).

(v) Cancer cells upregulate the glycolysis pathway which enables them to meet their high energy demand in hypoxic environment (Kim et al. 2006). Subsequently, the expression of GLUT 1 (glucose transporter isoform 1), the representative member of GLUT family, is enhanced due to its regulatory role in transporting D-glucose inside neoplastic cells. The structural similarity between dehydroascorbic acid (DHAA) and D-glucose drives the researchers to develop DHAA-decorated nanocarriers for site-specific targeting of neoplastic hepatocytes due to the overexpression of GLUT 1 isoforms in HCC (Guo et al. 2015).

Despite the exploration of the ability of different vitamin-derivative analogs for the development of site-specific delivery strategies to combat cancer, the normal expression of the receptors (where they also bind) is a real concern and it may decrease the interest in their site-specific targeting potential.

6.2.6 Transferrin

Transferrin, the 80 kDa iron-transporting glycoprotein secreted by the liver and cancer cells, has a high demand for iron due to its rapid proliferation. Therefore, the expression of transferrin receptor (Tfr) is upregulated in different types of malignant tumors, such as HCC, glioma, etc., compared to its expression in normal cells. Site-specific targeting of therapeutic entity towards malignant cells has been attempted by surface decoration of carriers with transferrin. However, expression of Tfr in normal cells results in significant accumulation of therapeutic payloads in normal cells leading to drug-related toxicity.

Apart from holo-transferrin and apo-transferrin (iron-removed transferrin), lactoferrin (mammalian iron-binding glycoproteins) has also been exploited especially in glioma for its ability to efficiently cross the BBB as the present expression of lactoferrin receptor is found in the endothelial cells constituting the BBB. Glioma stem cells are the subpopulation of tumor cells and they are responsible for developing resistance to radiotherapy and chemotherapy after surgery. Sun et al. (2017) developed holo-transferrin (holoTf)-conjugated nanoparticulate carriers encapsulating temozolamide. Results showed that developed nanoformulation was highly effective in crossing the BBB and delivered temozolomide in therapeutically effective concentrations to the glioma stem cells.

Kumar et al. (2017) developed temozolomide-loaded lactoferrin nanoparticles with an objective to accelerate transcytosis across the BBB through the lactoferrin present in the matrix of nanoparticles. Results of in vitro and in vivo investigations revealed sustained accumulation of temozolamide in the brain with improved pharmacokinetic profiles. Furthermore, temozolomide induced powerful apoptosis, leading to significant reduction of tumor volume and improved median survival of tumor-bearing mice. Therefore, they concluded that lactoferrin nanoparticles provided an efficient delivery platform for the successful delivery of temozolamide to tackle glioma in a much effective manner.

In the above discussion, we have explored the potentials of conventional targeting (i.e., ligand-mediated) approaches of drug carriers, along with their advantages and disadvantages. Now we will focus on a few selective nonconventional drug targeting approaches of nanoformulations.

6.3 Nonconventional Methods of Drug Targeting

6.3.1 Nonconventional Gene Silencing Method of Drug Targeting

Radical advancements in the field of molecular biology and computer-aided drug design help in the development of a plethora of ligands, resulting in the development of potential site-specific therapeutic weapons against different types of cancers and other diseases. However, active targeting of therapeutics always precedes passive targeting as passive targeting causes more accumulation of chemotherapeutics in normal cells leading to severe side-effects. This may probably be a prime reason because of which the severe mortality associated with cancer could not be tackled in an efficient manner (Yao et al. 2016; Li et al. 2016). To overcome these drawbacks, genomics-based approaches such as antisense technology and RNA inference (RNAi) are recognized as much more vibrant technologies compared to ligand-based active targeting to achieve radical improvement in therapeutic outcomes. The revolution in the field of molecular biology in the recent decade has resulted in specific and effective identification of gene(s) responsible for malignant transformation, and thus triggers the efficient designing of genomic-based therapeutics capable of selectively blocking the expression of mutated gene(s) or its downstream products such as mRNA. A general active targeting mechanism of antisense oligonucleotides to block gene expression in cancer cells is depicted in Fig. 6.1.

The concept of their designing and their potentials as anticancer therapeutics are discussed below.

6.3.2 Antisense Oligonucleotide-Mediated Gene Silencing

Antisense oligonucleotides (ASOs), short oligonucleotide fragments (<50 nucleotides long) discovered by Paul Zamecnik and Mary Stephenson in 1978 is an example of direct targeting of gene/mRNA and it is a nonconventional approach of drug targeting. Upon their entry into the cells, they bind with mRNA of a gene or with a gene against which it is designed, resulting in selective cellular depletion of mRNA molecules and subsequent depletion of corresponding proteins (Fig. 6.1). Thus, gene silencing by ASOs has been explored to block the expressions of malfunctioning proteins or genes such as oncogenes to achieve much better therapeutic outcome, especially in metabolic disorders or human genetic diseases (Watts and Corey 2012; Ghosh et al. 2014). Different mechanisms have been proposed regarding the action of antisense oligonucleotides and the mechanisms are described below.

6.3.3 Modulation of Splicing Mechanism

The formation of functionally active mature mRNA requires a splicing mechanism to remove introns. ASOs prevent the splicing of mRNA in different ways, such as interaction with different components responsible for splicing and binding with sequences required for splicing, resulting in blockage in the expressions of mRNA and subsequent production of oncogenic proteins.

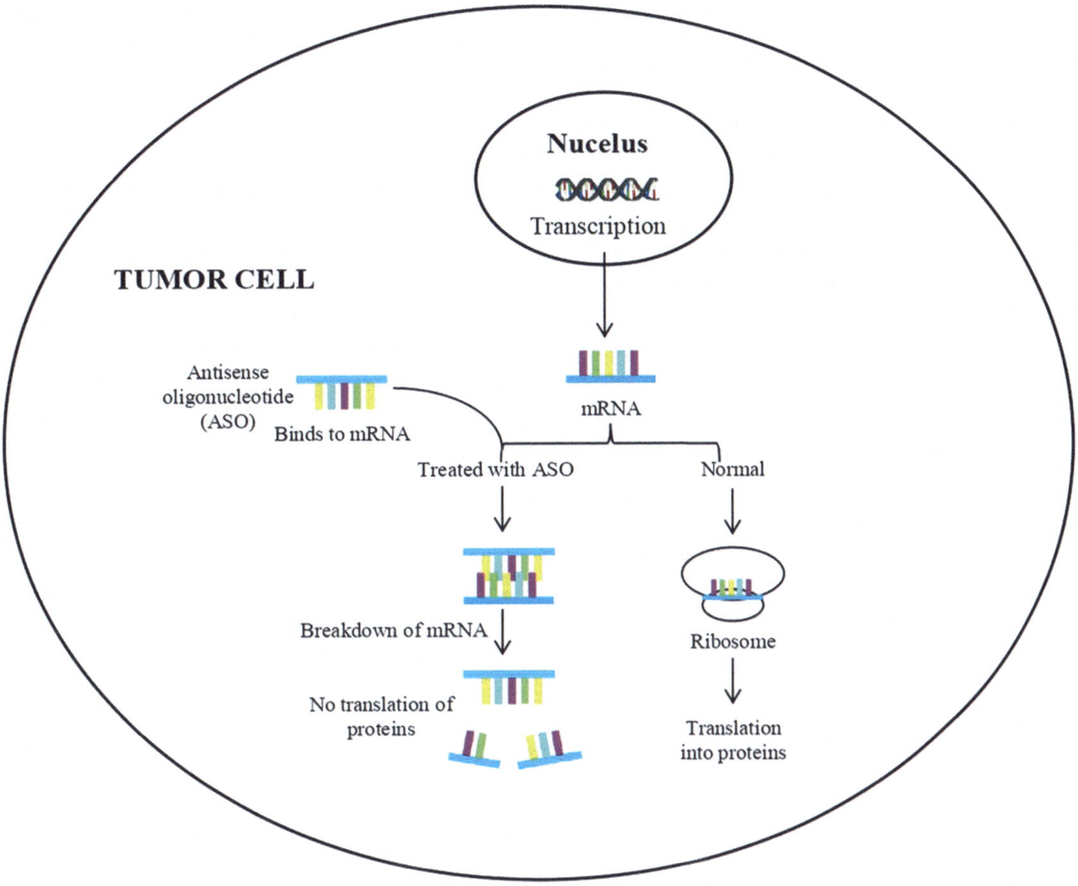

Fig. 6.1 Antisense oligonucleotide (ASO)-mediated mRNA dysfunction for inhibiting undesired protein production

6.3.4 Translational Arrest

ASOs can promote translational arrest by binding with the initiation codon of translation. Furthermore, ASOs lacking the contiguous stretch of DNA (or DNA-like oligonucleotides) can suppress translation by acting as steric blockers to block the function of the ribosome in protein synthesis.

6.3.5 Activation of RNase H

ASOs have the ability to bind with a complementary region of target mRNA by following the rules of Watson-Crick base pairing leading to activation of RNase H activity. Activated Rnase H results in the degradation of RNA from the DNA-RNA duplex leading to suppression of gene expression and subsequent production of oncogenic proteins (Minshull and Hunt 1986; Devi 2006).

6.3.6 Targeting microRNA (miRNA)

An endogenous small RNA known as microRNA plays a crucial role in physiological processes and affects metabolic disorders. ASOs have the ability to block miRNA. Researchers have designed ASO against miRNA, (miR-122), which is abundantly present in the liver of patients with HCC and hepatitis C virus infection. ASOs provided therapeutic benefit by inhibiting the replication of the hepatitis C virus and improved the function of the liver (Oliveira et al. 2006).

Apart from exerting their roles as mentioned above, ASOs can interrupt stability, and transport of mRNA from the nucleus to cytoplasm by blocking 5′-capping and polyadenylation (Shen et al. 2018).

6.3.7 Cellular Delivery of ASOs

Unmodified ASOs are very much unstable as they are prone to degradation by nucleases. Therefore, several chemical modifications have been developed to impart the stability to ASOs. Majority of modifications have been done either at 2′ position of sugar moiety, such as 2′-O-methyl (2′-O-Me), 2′-fluro (2′-F), and 2′-O-methoxyethyl (2′-MOE), or at the phosphodiester linkage, such as modification by the phosphorothioate linkage. Furthermore, the affinity of ASOs can be increased by modifying them with locked nucleic acids (LAA) which contain a methylene bridge between the 2′ and 4′ positions of ribose. This methylene bridge is responsible for locking of ribose in a conformation ideal for binding with the complementary sequence with high affinity (Devi 2006; Watts and Corey 2012).

Cationic lipids have been explored widely for intracellular delivery of ASOs. Cationic lipids have a variation in transfection efficiency based upon the target sites as well as inducing toxicity. Electroporation technique seems to be highly effective in introducing ASO in cells in vitro; however, it requires specialized sophisticated instruments and expertise and thus makes the process cumbersome (Márquez-Jurado et al. 2018).

Some investigations revealed the direct delivery of ASO through normal saline without the need for lipid. Mukherjee et al. (2014) developed ASOs against insulin-like growth factor–II (IGF-II), whose overexpression is evidenced in HCC and in preneoplastic hepatic foci for the treatment of HCC.

In the investigation, HCC was developed in Sprague Dawley rats by administering diethyl nitrosamine (DENA) as initiator and 2-acetylaminofluorene (2-AAF) as a promoter. Intravenous administration of ASOs suspended in normal saline showed that ASOs against IGF-II has significant curative potential against HCC. Thus, ASOs offer significant promise as powerful therapeutic weapons for specific targeting for radical improvements in HCC. Furthermore, their less or nontoxic nature augments the therapeutic response. However, very few ASOs have been translated into the clinical trial stages. Thus, ASOs-mediated therapeutic response should be investigated more extensively. Much sincere and delicate effort is warranted for proper designing of ASOs in increasing number to combat growing incidence of cancer and other diseases which need genetic manipulation.

6.3.8 RNA Interference (RNAi): Tools for Post-transcriptional Gene Silencing

The concept behind post-transcriptional gene silencing is to block an endogenous gene by the introduction of homologous double-stranded RNA (dsRNA) transgene or virus. The term RNA interference (RNAi) was denoted by Fire and Mello in 1998 upon conducting a study where they injected both sense and antisense strands into the nematode *Caenorhabditis elegans*. Results of this study revealed that dsRNA formed by both sense and antisense strands were found to be more powerful than antisense alone to block the target gene. RNAi is a cellular process present in all eukaryotic microorganisms as an innate defense mechanisms. Upon entering cells, dsRNA is processed by the enzyme dicer, resulting in the formation of duplexes with 3′ overhangs known as siRNA at the starting stage. In the entering stage, helicase enzyme separates two strands of siRNA from each other. The sense strands are degraded by endogenous nuclease enzyme and antisense strands bind with the RNA-induced silencing complex (RISC) followed by catalysis and cleavage of mRNA of the diseased gene by the enzyme slicer (Devi 2006). Thus, the expression of the diseased gene is suppressed, and the process is known as post-transcriptional gene silencing (PTGS).

Unlike siRNA, short hairpin RNA (shRNA) is synthesized in the nucleus. In the nucleus, they are processed by a complex known as Rnase-III family, Drosha and double-stranded RNA binding protein (DGCR8). The partially processed shRNA known as pre-shRNA is transported to cytoplasm by exportin5/RanGTPase. In the cytoplasm, it undergoes final processing leading to the formation of double-stranded siRNA responsible for the destruction of mRNA of the diseased gene as mentioned before. Thus RNAi through siRNA has enormous potential to combat malignancy in a safe and effective manner. Their in vivo delivery to the diseased sites as well as their stability in physiological fluid are two vital parameters governing enormous hope for the therapeutic success of siRNA (Mansoori et al. 2014).

Different chemical modifications in the constituent purine/pyrimidine bases of mRNA or modifications at phosphate backbone and at sugar moiety have been attempted to increase the in vivo stability of siRNA. Examples of some of the chemical modifications at the backbone are phosphothionate, borophosphothionates, 4-thioribonucleosides, phosphorothioates, 2 deoxy-2 fluorouridine, 2-O-methyl, 2-O-(2-methoxyethyl), and locked nucleotides. Modifications should be done in such a way that it will not affect specific regions responsible for gene silencing activity (Shen et al. 2018).

The delivery systems for siRNA are broadly classified into two: viral vectors and nonviral vectors. Among the viral vectors, lentiviruses (LVs), adenoviruses (AVs), and adeno-associated viruses (AAVs) are popularly exploited for the delivery of siRNA. However, the biosafety of viral vectors due to immunogenicity and insertional mutagenesis is a serious concern (Márquez-Jurado et al. 2018). Therefore, different nonviral vectors have also been explored for the delivery of siRNA. Nonviral vectors are broadly of three different types: (i) lipid-based vectors, (ii) nonlipid organic-based vectors, and (iii) nonlipid inorganic-based vectors. Nonviral vectors offer certain potential advantages over viral vectors, namely, biocompatibility, low or nontoxicity, stability, capability to escape endosomal degradation, and ease of production. The major drawback of nonviral vectors is that they are often less efficient compared to their viral counterparts.

Different types of lipid carriers utilized for siRNA delivery fall broadly under four categories such as, lipoplexes, lipopolyplexes, stable nucleic-acid-lipid particles (SNALPs), and membrane/core nanoparticles (MCNPs). Furthermore, lipid carriers mimic the phospholipid composition of membrane, which accelerates the cellular uptake of siRNA (Márquez-Jurado et al. 2018).

Lipoplexes are made up of multiple bilayers of cationic lipids. However, cationic lipids have a strong drawback of having cytotoxicity. Therefore, several neutral lipids are also attempted to develop siRNA-loaded lipopolyplex due to biocompatibility and ability of neutral lipids to provide superior pharmacokinetic profile of siRNA as compared to cationic lipids. The backbones of lipopolyplexes are lipid and polymer. Outer lipid layers enhance the penetration of lipopolyplex inside the cells whereas natural polymeric inner core encapsulates siRNA in a superior way. The outer layer of SNALP, on the other hand, is composed of neutral lipids while its inner layer is composed of cationic lipids. siRNA is loaded into the inner layer for the attraction between positively charged lipid and negatively charged siRNA (Oliveira et al. 2006).

siRNA is loaded into the inner core of MCNPs composed of inorganic nanoparticles, especially calcium phosphate because of its biocompatibility and sensitivity to acidic pH to release the loaded siRNA. The inner core is surrounded by lipid bilayer, as lipid-like molecules have the ability for cellular permeability for the delivery of siRNA. Among the nonlipid organic-based nanovectors, chitosan-based nanovectors have attracted significant attention due to their positive charge, low cytotoxicity, and nonimmunogenicity. However, certain disadvantages of chitosan are an obstacle as a delivery carrier, as mentioned below:

(i) Variability in composition and molecular weight.
(ii) pH of the surroundings has a strong influence on the positive charge of chitosan,

therefore in vivo efficacy of chitosan carrier is still skeptic.

Dendrimer, another popularly explored nonlipid base nanovector for the delivery of siRNA, offers significant promise due to its biocompatibility and nonimmunogenicity. Among the different types of dendrimers, amine-terminated polyamidoamine (PAMAM) and polypropyleneimine (PPI) have been most successfully investigated for the delivery of siRNA due to their pH sensitivity, leading to rapid intracellular delivery of siRNA (Marquez et al. 2018).

Branched and linear polyethyleneimine (PEI)-based nanovectors offer significant promise for the intracellular delivery of siRNA due to their ability to release nucleic acids by a proton-sponge effect caused by cationic polymer coated on the nanoparticles promoting the osmotic swelling of endosomes, resulting in the disruption of the endosomal membrane leading to the release of the loaded DNA. Furthermore, the proton-sponge effect helps the nanovector to escape lysosomal degradation. However, the main disadvantage of PEI is its poor biodegradation, leading to significantly high toxicity.

Gold nanoparticles (AuNPs) belong to the class of nonlipid base nanovectors that have been tried for use in drug delivery of siRNA due to their certain positive features such as nontoxicity, inertness, biocompatibility, and flexibility to functionalize with different modifications to enhance the cellular delivery of siRNA.

Supraparamagnetic iron oxide nanoparticles (SPIONs) have attracted considerable interest for the delivery of siRNA due to biodegradability, biocompatibility, and nontoxicity properties. Further, their ability to noninvasively detect cancer cells help to deliver siRNA to target sites. In addition, mesoporous silica nanoparticles, cell-penetrating peptides, and nanogels are also currently being exploited for the delivery of siRNA.

Despite the enormous future potential of siRNA as anticancer chemotherapeutics, sincere efforts are needed to address numerous important issues related to siRNA for rapid acceleration in their translation in the service to humankind as mentioned below:

(i) The role of innate defense machinery (a naturally occurring siRNA generating system) has strong integration with administered siRNA, causing therapeutic response
(ii) Their delivery especially to the target sites to avoid off-target silencing
(iii) Pharmacokinetics and stability which are essential in governing their in vivo efficacy.

6.4 Disease-Based Targeting

6.4.1 Diabetes and Drug Targeting

In recent times, researchers are involved in the discovery of single-stranded noncoding microRNAs (miRNAs) which opened a new window for treatment of diabetes. Poy et al. (2009) first identified miR375 that has a negative impact on glucose-stimulated insulin secretion whereas its antagonist increases insulin secretion. They suggested that miRNA not only regulates the insulin secretion but also has a pivotal role in pancreatic β-cell development (Poy et al. 2009). miRNA also functions in the pathway of insulin signaling in different tissues. The complication of diabetes in different organs such as eye, kidney, and foot can be controlled by miRNA. Diabetic cardiomyopathy is associated with the levels of different miRNAs. Inhibition of such miRNA can alter the conditions of the cardiac system. Apart from diabetic cardiomyopathy, miRNA also has a crucial role in diabetic neuropathy, diabetic retinopathy, and diabetic neuropathic osteoarthropathy. Reports from different researchers altogether suggest that miRNA-mediated regulation is a possible therapeutic approach in the management of diabetes. Regulation of certain miRNAs can be helpful in tuning glucose homeostasis (Kumar et al. 2012).

6.4.2 Central Nervous System and Drug Targeting

Systemic treatment strategies in neurological disorders such as Parkinson's disease and brain tumors require transport of the drug across the blood-brain barrier (BBB) to reach the central nervous systems (CNS). BBB is composed of brain capillary endothelial cells (BCECs, its chief component), pericytes, astrocytes foot process, and nerve endings terminating at the capillary surfaces. BCECs differ from other endothelial cells present in the rest of the body due to the absence of fenestrations, presence of much extensive tight junctions (TJs), and thinly dispersed or scattered pinocytic vesicular transport. The BBB plays a dual role as a transport barrier and a physiological barrier due to the presence of BCECs, TJs, membrane transporters, and vascular trafficking mediated by BCECs. Generally, BBB allows transport of molecules whose molecular weight is less than 400 kDa and primarily lipophilic. Therefore, nanocarrier-mediated transport of therapeutics, especially macromolecular therapeutics and siRNA, has been attempted for the treatment of various CNS disorders and glioblastoma. Furthermore, ligand-mediated active targeting of nanocarriers has also been explored by targeting proteins overexpressed in various disorders/diseases of the CNS, leading to penetration of nanocarriers into the brain through various mechanisms, such as transporter-mediated transcytosis and receptor-mediated endocytosis. For example, selectins, inflammatory cell adhesion molecule –I (ICAM-1), vascular endothelial adhesion molecule-I (VCAM-I), and matrix metalloproteinase (MMP) functionalized nanocarriers have been explored for the treatment of neuronal injury after reperfusion in brain ischemia and neuronal injury associated with ischemic conditions. Receptors for advanced glycation end products (RAGE) in BCECs regulate transport of amyloid-β-peptide from blood to brain and it is implicated in oxidative stress and neuroinflammation. About 2.5 times higher expression of RAGE is seen in Alzheimer's disease. Therefore, therapeutic strategies have been developed to target RAGE based on siRNA. Similarly, peptide-, transferrin-, and aptamer-mediated active targeting has been attempted for the treatment of glioblastoma. However, toxicity, the level of expression of target proteins, and stability are crucial factors among the various other factors governing the success of active-targeting nanotherapeutics.

Nanoliposomes have been widely investigated for their capabilities to transport drugs of either types – hydrophobic or hydrophilic – across the blood-brain barrier (BBB). However, sometimes nanoliposomes cannot bring the desired quantity of drug into the brain across the BBB. In one effort, we used a brain lipid along with its usual composition of nanoliposomes (phospholipid and cholesterol) (Satapathy et al. 2016). Incorporation of brain phospholipid into the constituents of nanoliposomes shows a remarkable increase of the drug-carrier into the brain across the BBB (Fig. 6.2).

This shows an incredible nonconventional drug targeting approach into the brain crossing the BBB. Satapathy et al. (2016) reported a quite uncommon targeting strategy for the treatment of glioblastoma and it seems to be very promising. They incorporated 1,2-distearoryl–sn-glycero-3-phosphoethanolamine (DSPE) as one of the constituents of nanoliposomes as DSPE that constitutes 45% of all phospholipids in the brain. Thus, it accelerates the transport of nanoliposomes across the BBB to reach the brain for superior therapeutic outcomes. Further, this targeting strategy was found to be the least toxic and economic due to the enrichment of nanoliposomal formulation by the endogenous component of brain lipids. In conclusion, this type of innovative, simple targeting strategy will accelerate the development of potential therapeutic weapons for significant improvements in glioma and other CNS disorders, and the study is a classical example of nonconventional drug targeting.

6.4.3 Peripheral Nerves and Drug Targeting

Due to the wide distribution of peripheral nerves in our body and various common peripheral nerve-related diseases and disorders in humans, targeted delivery is highly desired. Neuronal damage is mostly signifying partial damage of only one or few numbers of neuron of the entire system (Bronzino 1995). Selective permeability

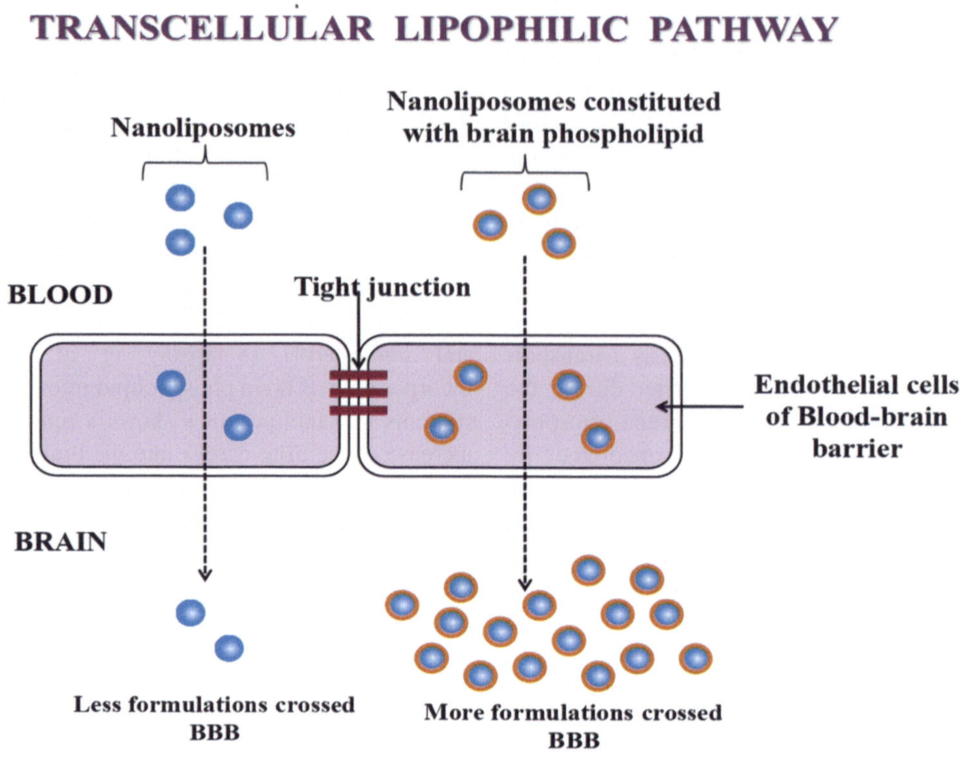

Fig. 6.2 Transcellular delivery of brain-phospholipid-coated nanoliposomes in comparison to noncoated nanoliposomes through the blood brain barrier

through the blood-nerve barrier (BNB) causes very limited access to the drug in the peripheral nerves. However, nerves in the peripheral nervous system (PNS) involve most of the inflammatory and infectious neuropathies which are difficult to treat, and successful noninvasive targeting is hardly reported. The proper delivery of the drug at its therapeutic level is highly essential for symptomatic relief and neuronal regenerations. One of the approaches for this delivery strategy is the use of natural toxins, as they have the ability to bind the nervous system and can be manipulated for targeting peripheral neuropathy if the toxicity, inflammatory, and immunogenic complications can be avoided. In that case, cell-penetrating peptide or inactive form of holotoxins can be chosen for targeting the PNS (Surana et al. 2018). Tetanus toxin as a vector targets the ganglioside GT1b receptor on the presynaptic terminals of peripheral nerves and helps in targeting peptide cargo. This is due to the retrograde transport of the peptide by tetanus toxin from neuromuscular joint to cell body or motor and sensory neurons. Another 12-aminoacid peptide with C-terminal binding domain as tetanus toxin, Tet 1 shows similar affinity towards ganglioside GT1b (Liu et al. 2016). Botulinum toxin showed that retrograde trafficking of BoNT/A, a botulinum neurotoxin, to the motor neurons in mice models was effective over neuropathic pain (Restani et al. 2012). Cholera toxin specificity towards ganglioside GM1 was recently exploited to target mesoporous silicone nanoparticles (MSNPs) to motor neurons (Porras et al. 2018). Nonreplicating herpes simplex virus (HSV)-based vectors transduce neurons in the dorsal root ganglion to deliver encephalin successfully to combat neuronal pain and are effective over progressive sensory neuropathy caused by toxins, chemotherapeutic drugs, or diabetes (Kanda et al. 2017). However, inflammatory and immunogenic complications are key limitations of the processes, and alternative methods are needed to be established. One of such less toxic approach is tagging local anesthetic. Due to their hydrophobic nature, local anesthetics can diffuse the BNB and can access motor and sensory axons (Angelova and Angelov 2017). As intraneuronal injection causes several side-effects like longer nerve block and even apoptosis, injury, or long-term neurological dysfunction, some other approaches, like sustained release liposome formulation of bupivacaine (Santamaria et al. 2017), have been considered. For infectious neuropathy, it is essential to treat the infection as well as providing anti-inflammatory protection. But most antiviral drugs are unable to cross the BNB because of their hydrophilic nature. One of the recent breakthroughs is the dual delivery of antiviral and anti-inflammatory drugs in a single liposomal carrier for the application of infectious neuropathy. Sengupta et al. (2018) have investigated the application of procaine (hydrophobic anti-inflammatory moiety) for peripheral nerve targeting of a nanoliposomal formulation containing a broad-spectrum antiviral drug ribavirin (hydrophilic). These nanocarriers delivered drug successfully at the PNS in vivo in rats and proved to reduce neuronal excitation of the nerve as well as antiviral protection to the PNS, to combat diseases such as herpes, hydrophobia, etc. Thus, incorporation of a special chemical in the chemical constituents of drug-loaded nanocarriers can also assist to transport a drug cargo to a desired target site in the body. As mentioned above (Sengupta et al. 2018), procaine conjugation in the nanocarrier helps for the delivery of drug to peripheral nerves (Fig. 6.3).

Drug targeting to peripheral nerves has lots of significance as many viruses reside in the peripheral nerves at the initial stage of infections and even at the later stage of infections also. Transportation of drugs to the PNS with a desirable drug concentration often remains unsuccessful, causing rapid progression of diseases. Examples of such viruses are herpes simplex virus, Rabies viruses responsible for causing hydrophobia in humans, etc. Many other diseases occur due to the problems associated with the PNS. Examples of such diseases are gout, arthritis, etc. The above study shows procaine helps to bring the formulation to the PNS to release an antiviral drug ribavirin. Furthermore, procaine suppresses excitation of peripheral nerve to show a dual drug effect. This is another example of nonconventional drug targeting.

6.4.4 Lungs and Drug Targeting

Carcinoma and fungal infections in lungs are very difficult to treat resulting in severe fatal consequences, because maintaining the concentration of drugs in lungs, especially in the lower

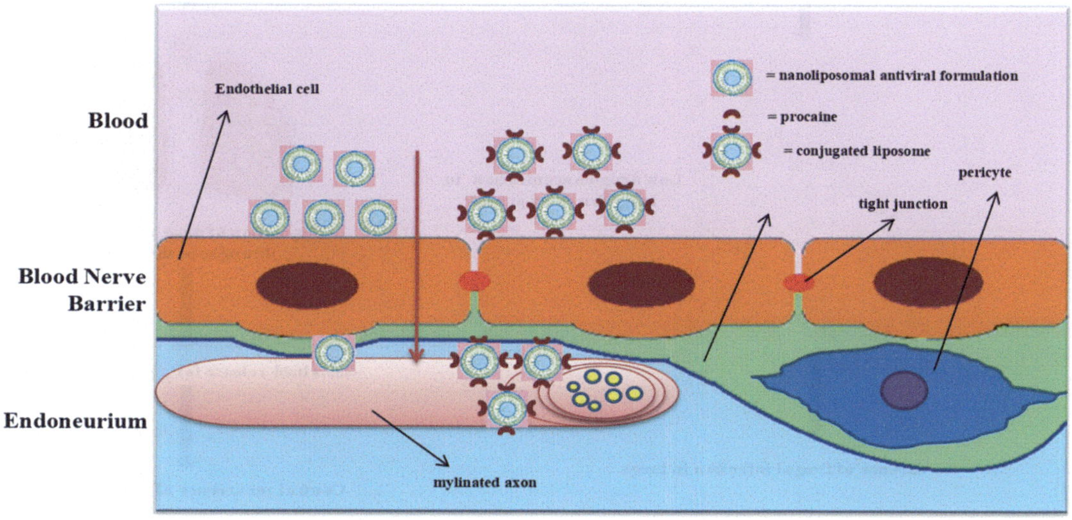

Fig. 6.3 Peripheral nerve targeting by local anesthetic conjugation

respiratory tract, is a herculean task due to high blood turnover in lungs, resulting in rapid removal. Therefore, different nanocarrier-mediated passive targeting and ligand-functionalized nanocarrier-mediated active targeting have been developed to achieve adequate drug concentration for therapeutic response for prolonged periods. Even gene silencing approaches through siRNA therapeutics have been explored for superior therapeutic outcome by site-specific blocking of expressions of oncogenes responsible for lung cancer. However, their delivery to and retention in target sites in lungs is the real challenging issue.

Different devices can also deliver the formulations to a target site for providing sustained drug action for a prolonged periods in a more localized way, and thereby enable more drug targeting at the localized tissue. Delivery of antifungal drug in nanocarriers or mucoadhesive polymer-coated nanocarriers into the lungs by DPI/nebulizer can provide prolonged drug action all through the lungs (Sinha et al. 2013; Das et al. 2015; Paul et al. 2018) and this can be a unique example of nonconventional drug targeting with a highly efficacious site-specific drug delivery management. In case of lung fungal infection, drug delivery by other routes is unable to manage persistent desirable drug concentration in lungs due to very rapid turnover of blood in lungs. A high amount of antifungal drug should be maintained in the blood for a long period to provide drug in the upper, middle, and lower part of the pulmonary tissues to kill fungi and fungal spores (Fig. 6.4) (Das et al. 2015; Paul et al. 2018). Since almost all available antifungal drugs are highly toxic in nature, they cannot be used for a prolonged period with a high blood level, as this may cause survival of spores and recurrence of the diseases.

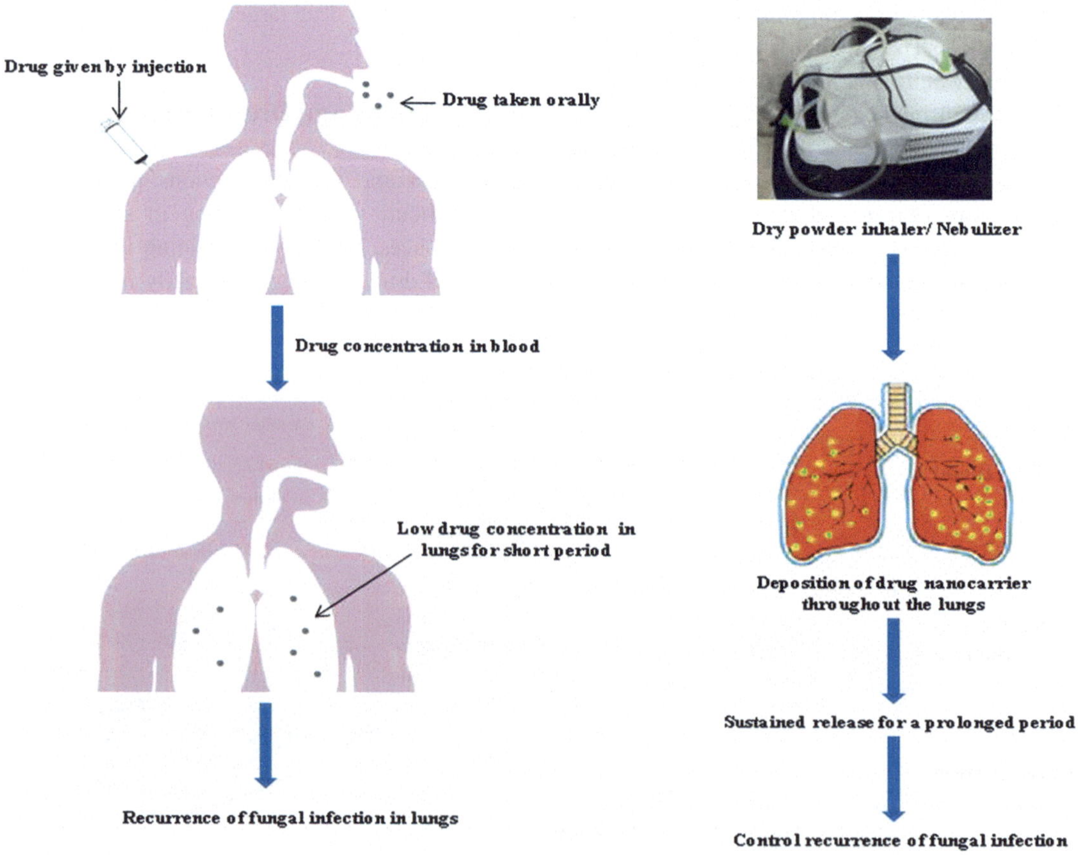

Fig. 6.4 Comparison of pulmonary route with oral/parenteral route for controlling fungal infection in lungs

6.5 Conclusion

Growing incidences of fatality associated with metabolic disorders and/or fungal/viral infections at some specific sites in the body necessitate the rapid development of potential target-specific therapeutic weapons in the near future. Despite several efforts for the development of site-specific targeting strategies, very little target-specific therapeutics are available so far and it seems to be inadequate to combat such diseases. Numerous drawbacks associated with conventional drug targeting approaches are probably the prime reasons for such poor translation of therapeutic outcomes from bench to bedside. The alleviated toxicity at the normal/healthy cells by the existing modes of therapies sometimes leading to even death of the patients should not be ignored. Therefore, a great amount of attention has been shifted towards nonconventional modes of drug targeting for radical improvement in the development of site-specific therapeutics. Furthermore, different innovative techniques or technologies such as nanorobots and nanocrystals may be extensively explored for the development of site-specific therapeutics. In the near future, the biomedical field may experience a radical improvement in the quality and quantity of site-specific therapeutics for a significant improvement in the quality of life.

References

Accardo A, Mannucci S, Nicolato E, Vurro F, Diaferia C, Bontempi P, Marzola P, Morelli G (2019) Easy formulation of liposomal doxorubicin modified with a bombesin peptide analogue for selective targeting of GRP receptors overexpressed by cancer cells. Drug Deliv Transl Res 9:215–226

Ahmedah H, Patterson L, Shnyder S, Sheldrake H (2017) RGD-binding integrins in head and neck cancers. Cancers 9:56–72

Ai J, Xu Y, Li D, Liu Z, Wang E (2012) Folic acid as delivery vehicles: targeting folate conjugated fluorescent nanoparticles to tumors imag¬ing. Talanta 101:32–37

Angelova A, Angelov B (2017) Dual and multi-drug delivery nanoparticles towards neuronal survival and synaptic repair. Neural Regen Res 12:886–889

Araújo F, Shrestha N, Gomes MJ, Herranz-Blanco B, Liu D, Hirvonen JJ, Granja PL, Santos HA, Sarmento B (2016) In vivo dual-delivery of glucagon like peptide-1 (GLP-1) and dipeptidyl peptidase-4 (DPP4) inhibitor through composites prepared by microfluidics for diabetes therapy. Nanoscale 8:10706–10713

Azhdarzadeh M, Atyabi F, AtaSaei A, Varnamkhasti BS, Omidi Y, Fateh M et al (2016) Theranostic MUC1aptamer targeted gold coated super paramagnetic iron oxide nano particles for magnetic resonance imaging and photo thermal therapy of colon cancer. Colloids Surf B: Biointerfaces 143:224–232

Åkerman ME, Chan WC, Laakkonen P, Bhatia SN, Ruoslahti E (2002) Nanocrystal targeting in vivo. Proc Natl Acad Sci 99:12617–12621

Bronzino JD (ed) (1995) The biomedical engineering handbook, R. F. Valentini. CRC, Boca Raton

Calzolari A, Oliviero I, Deaglio S, Mariani G, Biffoni M, Sposi NM, Malavasi F, Peschle C, Testa U (2007) Transferrin receptor 2 is frequently expressed in human cancer cell lines. Blood Cells Mol Dis 39:82–91

Cardarelli PM, Quinn M, Buckman D, Fang Y, Colcher D, King DJ, Bebbington C, Yarranton G (2002) Binding to CD20 by anti-B1 antibody or F (ab') 2 is sufficient for induction of apoptosis in B-cell lines. Cancer Immunol Immunother 51:15–24

Cerchia L, Ducongé F, Pestourie C, Boulay J, Aissouni Y, Gombert K, Tavitian B, De Franciscis V, Libri D (2005) Neutralizing aptamers from whole-cell SELEX inhibit the RET receptor tyrosine kinase. PLoS Biol 3:e123

Chen S, Zhao X, Chen J, Kuznetsova L, Wong SS, Ojima I (2010) Mechanism-based tumor-targeting drug delivery system. Validation of efficient vitamin receptor-mediated endocytosis and drug release. Bioconjug Chem 21:979–987

Chen C, Ke J, Zhou XE, Yi W, Brunzelle JS, Li J, Yong EL, Xu HE, Melcher K (2013) Structural basis for molecular recognition of folic acid by folate receptors. Nature 500(7463):486–489

Cheung A, Bax HJ, Josephs DH, Ilieva KM, Pellizzari G, Opzoomer J, Bloomfield J, Fittall M, Grigoriadis A, Figini M, Canevari S (2016) Targeting folate receptor alpha for cancer treatment. Oncotarget 7:52553–52574

Chittasupho C, Jaturanpinyo M, Mangmool S (2013) Pectin nanoparticle enhances cytotoxicity of methotrexate against HepG2 cells. Drug Deliv 20:1–9

Cilek A, Celebi N, Tırnaksız F, Tay A (2005) A lecithin-based microemulsion of rh-insulin with aprotinin for oral administration: investigation of hypoglycemic effects in non-diabetic and STZ-induced diabetic rats. Int J Pharm 298:176–185

Das PJ, Paul P, Mukherjee B, Mazumder B, Mondal L, Baishya R, Debnath MC, Dey KS (2015) Pulmonary delivery of voriconazole loaded nanoparticles providing a prolonged drug level in lungs: a promise for treating fungal infection. Mol Pharm 12:2651–2664

Devi GR (2006) siRNA-based approaches in cancer therapy. Cancer Gene Ther 13(9):819–829

Dong L, Zhou H, Zhao M, Gao X, Liu Y, Liu D, Guo W, Hu H, Xie Q, Fan J, Lin J, Wu W (2018) Phosphorothioate-modified AP613-1 specifically targets GPC3 when used for hepatocellular carcinoma cell imaging. Mol Ther Nucleic Acids 13:376–386

Fan X, Guo Y, Wang L, Xiong X, Zhu L, Fang K (2016) Diagnosis of prostate cancer using anti-PSMA aptamer A10-3.2-oriented lipid nanobubbles. Int J Nanomedicine 11:3939–3950

Ghosh MK, Patra F, Ghosh S, Hossain CM, Mukherjee B (2014) Antisense oligonucleotides directed against insulin-like growth factor-II messenger ribonucleic acids delay the progress of rat hepatocarcinogenesis. J Carcinog. 13:2. Published online 2014 Feb 7. https://doi.org/10.4103/1477-3163.126761

Guo Y, Zhang Y, Li J, Zhang Y, Lu Y, Jiang X, He X, Ma H, An S, Jiang C (2015) ACS Appl Mater Interfaces 7:5444–5553

Hicke BJ, Marion C, Chang YF, Gould T, Lynott CK, Parma D, Schmidt PG, Warren S (2001) Tenascin-C aptamers are generated using tumor cells and purified protein. J Biol Chem 276:48644–48654

Holgado E, Perez-Garcia J, Gion M, Cortes J (2018) Is there a role for immunotherapy in HER2-positive breast cancer? NPJ Breast Cancer 4:21–23

Hong S, Zhang X, Chen J, Zhou J, Zheng Y, Xu C (2013) Targeted gene silencing using a follicle-stimulating hormone peptide-conjugated nanoparticle system improves its specificity and efficacy in ovarian clear cell carcinoma in vitro. J Ovarian Res 6:80–88

Jain K, Kesharwani P, Gupta U, Jain NK (2012) A review of glycosylated carriers for drug delivery. Biomaterials 33:4166–4186

Kamei N, Aoyama Y, Khafagy ES, Henmi M, Takeda-Morishita M (2015) Effect of different intestinal conditions on the intermolecular interaction between insulin and cell-penetrating peptide penetratin and on its contribution to stimulation of permeation through intestinal epithelium. Eur J Pharm Biopharm 94:42–51

Kaminski MS, Estes J, Zasadny KR, Francis IR, Ross CW, Tuck M, Regan D, Fisher S, Gutierrez J, Kroll S, Stagg R (2000) Radioimmunotherapy with iodine 131I tositumomab for relapsed or refractory B-cell non-Hodgkin lymphoma: updated results and long-term follow-up of the University of Michigan experience. Blood 96:1259–1266

Kanda H, Liu S, Kanao M, Yi H, Iida T, Huang W, Kunisawa T, Lubarsky DA, Hao S (2017) Gene therapy with HSV encoding p55TNFR gene for HIV neuropathic pain: an evidence-based mini-review. Transl Perioper Pain Med 2:24–32

Karra N, Nassar T, Ripin AN, Schwob O, Borlak J, Benita S (2013) Antibody conjugated PLGA nanoparticles for targeted delivery of paclitaxel palmitate: efficacy and biofate in a lung cancer mouse model. Small 9(24):4221–4236

Kiaris H, Schally AV, Nagy A, Szepeshazi K, Hebert F, Halmos G (2001) A targeted cytotoxic somatostatin (SST) analogue, AN-238, inhibits the growth of H-69 small-cell lung carcinoma (SCLC) and H-157 non-SCLC in nude mice. Eur J Cancer 37:620–628

Kim J-W, Tchernyshyov I, Semenza GL, Dang CV (2006) HIF-1-mediated expression of pyruvate dehydrogenase kinase: A metabolic switch required for cellular adaptation to hypoxia. Cell Metab 3(3):177–185

Kinesh VP, Neelam DP, Bhavesh SB, Pragna KS (2010) Novel approaches for oral delivery of insulin and current status of oral insulin products. Int J Pharm Sci Nanotechnol 3:1057–1064

Kumar M, Nath S, Prasad HK, Sharma GD, Li Y (2012) MicroRNAs: a new ray of hope for diabetes mellitus. Protein Cell 3:726–738

Kumar S, Ahsan SM, Kumar JM, Kondapi AK, Rao NM (2017) Overcoming blood brain barrier with a dual purpose temozolomide loaded lactoferri nanoparticles for combating glioma (SERP-17-12433). Sci Rep 7:6602–6613

Ladju RB, Pascut D, Massi MN, Tiribelli CSC (2018) Aptamer: a potential oligonucleotide nanomedicine in the diagnosis and treatment of hepatocellular carcinoma. Oncotarget 9:2951–2961

Langert KA, Von Zee CL, Stubbs EB Jr (2013) Tumour necrosis factor α enhances CCL2 and ICAM-1 expression in peripheral nerve microvascular endoneurial endothelial cells. ASN Neuro 5:AN20120048

Leamon CP, Low PS (2001) Folate-mediated targeting: from diagnostics to drug and gene delivery. Drug Discov Today 6:44–51

Lee S, Ashizawa AT, Kim KS, Falk DJ, Notterpek L (2013) Liposomes to target peripheral neurons and Schwann cells. PLoS One 8:e78724

Lepenies B, Lee J, Sonkaria S (2013) Targeting C-type lectin receptors with multivalent carbohydrate ligands. Adv Drug Deliv Rev 65:1271–1281

Li N, Larson T, Nguyen HH, Sokolov KV, Ellington AD (2010) Directed evolution of gold nanoparticle delivery to cells. Chem Commun 46:392–394

Li M, Zhang W, Wang B, Gao Y, Song Z, Zheng QC (2016) Ligand-based targeted therapy: a novel strategy for hepatocellular carcinoma. Int J Nanomedicine 11:5645–5669

Li L, Jiang G, Yu W, Liu D, Chen H, Liu Y, Tong Z, Kong X, Yao J (2017) Preparation of chitosan-based multifunctional nanocarriers overcoming multiple barriers for oral delivery of insulin. Mater Sci Eng C 70:278–286

Liu JK, Teng Q, Garrity-Moses M, Federici T, Tanase D, Imperiale MJ et al (2005) A novel peptide defined through phage display for therapeutic protein and vector neuronal targeting. Neurobiol Dis 19:407–418

Liu M, Zhang J, Zhu X, Shan W, Li L, Zhong J, Zhang Z, Huang Y (2016) Efficient mucus permeation and tight junction opening by dissociable "mucus-inert" agent coated trimethyl chitosan nanoparticles for oral insulin delivery. J Control Release 222:67–77

Lo A, Lin CT, Wu HC (2008) Hepatocellular carcinoma cell-specific peptide ligand for targeted drug delivery. Mol Cancer Ther 7(3):579

Lucock M (2000) Folic acid: nutritional biochemistry, molecular biology, and role in disease processes. Mol Genet Metab 71:121–138

Lynn RC, Poussin M, Kalota A, Feng Y, Low PS, Dimitrov DS, Powell DJ (2015) Targeting of folate receptor β on acute myeloid leukemia blasts with chimeric antigen receptor–expressing T cells. Blood 125:3466–3476

Mallikaratchy P, Tang Z, Kwame S, Meng L, Shangguan D, Tan W (2007) Aptamer directly evolved from live cells recognizes membrane bound immunoglobin heavy mu chain in Burkitt's lymphoma cells. Mol Cell Proteomics 6:2230–2238

Mansoori B, Shotorbani SS, Baradaran B (2014) RNA interference and its role in cancer therapy. Adv Pharm Bull 4:313–321

Marinelli S, Vacca V, Ricordy R, Uggenti C, Tata AM, Luvisetto S, Pavone F (2012) The analgesic effect on neuropathic pain of retrogradely transported botulinum neurotoxin A involves Schwann cells and astrocytes. PLoS One 7:e47977

Márquez-Jurado S, Nogales A, Ávila-Pérez G, Iborra F, Martínez-Sobrido L, Almazán F (2018) An alanine-to-valine substitution in the residue 175 of Zika virus NS2A protein affects viral RNA synthesis and attenuates the virus in vivo. Viruses 10(10):547

Millotti G, Laffleur F, Perera G, Vigl C, Pickl K, Sinner F, Bernkop-Schnürch A (2014) In vivo evaluation of thiolated chitosan tablets for oral insulin delivery. J Pharm Sci 103:3165–3170

Minshull J, Hunt T (1986) The use of single-stranded DNA and RNase H to promote quantitative 'hybrid arrest of translation' of mRNA/DNA hybrids in reticulocyte lysate cell-free translations. Nucleic Acids Res 14(16):6433–6451

Mone AP, Cheney C, Banks AL, Tridandapani S, Mehter N, Guster S, Lin T, Eisenbeis CF, Young DC, Byrd JC (2006) Alemtuzumab induces caspase-independent cell death in human chronic lymphocytic leukemia cells through a lipid raft-dependent mechanism. Leukemia 20:272–279

Monforte V, Ussetti P, Gavaldà J, Bravo C, Laporta R, Len O, García-Gallo CL, Tenorio L, Solé J, Román A (2010) Feasibility, tolerability, and outcomes of nebulized liposomal amphotericin B for Aspergillus infection prevention in lung transplantation. J Heart Lung Transplant 29:523–530

Moosavian SA, Abnous K, Akhtari J, Arabi L, Gholamzade Dewin A, Jafari M (2018) 5TR1 aptamer-PEGylated liposomal doxorubicin enhances cellular uptake and suppresses tumour growth by targeting MUC1 on the surface of cancer cells. Artif Cells Nanomed Biotechnol 46:2054–2065

Mukherjee B, Patra F, Ghosh M, Ghosh S, Hossain CM (2014) Antisense oligonucleotides directed against insulin-like growth factor-II messenger ribonucleic acids delay the progress of rat hepatocarcinogenesis. J Carcinogenesis 13(1):2

Nagesh PKB, Johnson NR, Boya VKN, Chowdhury P, Othman SF, Sharghi VK, Hafeez BB (2016) PSMA targeted docetaxel-loaded superparamagnetic iron oxide nanoparticles for prostate cancer. Colloids Surf B Biointerfaces 144:8–20

Ohhara Y, Fukuda N, Takeuchi S, Honma R, Shimizu Y, Kinoshita I, Dosaka-Akita H (2016) Role of targeted therapy in metastatic colorectal cancer. World J Gastrointest Oncol 8:642–655

Oliveira S, Storm G, Schiffelers RM (2006) Targeted Delivery of siRNA. J Biomed Biotechnol 2006:1–9

Pandit N, Joshi T (2015) A review on novel approaches for oral delivery of insulin. J Drug Deliv Ther 5:61–70

Paul P, Sengupta S, Mukherjee B, Shaw TK, Gaonkar RH, Debnath MC (2018) Chitosan-coated nanoparticles enhanced lung pharmacokinetic profile of voriconazole upon pulmonary delivery in mice. Nanomedicine 13:501–520

Pitari GM, Di Guglielmo MD, Park J, Schulz S, Waldman SA (2001) Guanylyl cyclase C agonists regulate progression through the cell cycle of human colon carcinoma cells. Proc Natl Acad Sci 98:7846–7851

Porras G, Durfee MP, Gregory PN, Sieck AM, Brinker GC, Mantilla CB (2016) A novel approach for targeted delivery to motoneurons using cholera toxin-B modified protocells. J Neurosci Methods 273:160–174

Porras MA, Durfee P, Giambini S, Sieck GC, Brinker CJ, Mantilla CB (2018) Uptake and intracellular fate of cholera toxin subunit b-modified mesoporous silica nanoparticle-supported lipid bilayers (aka protocells) in motoneurons. Nanomedicine 14:661–672

Poy MN, Hausser J, Trajkovski M, Braun M, Collins S, Rorsman P, Zavolan M, Stoffel M (2009) miR-375 maintains normal pancreatic α- and β-cell mass. Proc Natl Acad Sci U S A 106:5813–5818

Quinn T, Zhang X, Miao Y (2010) Targeted melanoma imaging and therapy with radiolabeled alpha-melanocyte stimulating hormone peptide analogues. G Ital Dermatol Venereol 145:245–258

Restani L, Giribaldi F, Manich M, Bercsenyi K, Menendez G, Rossetto O et al (2012) Botulinum neurotoxins A and E undergo retrograde axonal transport in primary motor neurons. PLoS Pathog 8:e1003087

Russell-Jones G, McTavish K, McEwan J, Rice J, Nowotnik D (2004) Vitamin-mediated targeting as a potential mechanism to increase drug uptake by tumours. J Inorg Biochem 98:1625–1633

Sano K, Takayama T, Murakami K, Saiki I, Makuuchi M (2003) Overexpression of retinoic acid receptor alpha in hepatocellular carcinoma. Clin Cancer Res 9:3679–3683

Santamaria CM, Woodru A, Yang R, Kohane DS (2017) Drug delivery systems for prolonged duration local anesthesia. Mater Today (Kidlington) 20:22–31

Satapathy BS, Mukherjee B, Baishya R, Debnath MC, Dey NS, Maji R (2016) Lipid nanocarrier-based transport of docetaxel across the blood brain barrier. RSC Adv 6(88):85261–85274

Sauer RS, Krug SM, Hackel D, Staat C, Konasin N, Yang S, Niedermirtl B, Bosten J, Günther R, Dabrowski S, Doppler K (2014) Safety, efficacy, and molecular mechanism of claudin-1-specific peptides to enhance blood–nerve–barrier permeability. J Control Release 185:88–98

Schmidt K, Moser C, Hellerbrand C, Zieker D, Wagner C, Redekopf J, Schlitt HJ, Geissler EK, Lang SA (2015) Targeting fibroblast growth factor receptor (FGFR) with BGJ398 in a gastric cancer model. Anticancer Res 35:6655–6665

Sengupta S, Paul P, Mukherjee B, Gaonkar RH, Debnath MC, Chakraborty R, Khatun N, Roy S (2018) Peripheral nerve targeting by procaine-conjugated ribavirin-loaded dual drug nanovesicle. Nanomedicine (Lond) 13:3009–3023

Sharkey RM, Karacay H, Goldenberg DM (2010) Improving the treatment of non-Hodgkin lymphoma with antibody-targeted radionuclides. Cancer 116:1134–1145

Shen F, Wu M, Ross JF, Miller D, Ratnam M (1995) Folate receptor type. Gamma. Is primarily a secretory protein due to lack of an efficient signal for glycosylphosphatidylinositol modification: protein characterization and cell type specificity. Biochemistry 34:5660–5665

Shen Y, Li X, Dong D, Zhang B, Xue Y, Shang P (2018) Transferrin receptor 1 in cancer: a new sight for cancer therapy. Am J Cancer Res 8:916–931

Sheng J, He H, Han L, Qin J, Chen S, Ru G, Li R, Yang P, Wang J, Yang VC (2016) Enhancing insulin oral absorption by using mucoadhesive nanoparticles loaded with LMWP-linked insulin conjugates. J Control Release 233:181–190

Shijie Xu, Fangbo Cui, Huang Dafu, Zhang Dinghu, Zhu Anqing, Sun Xia, Cao Yiming, Sheng Ding et al (2019) PD-L1 monoclonal antibody-conjugated nanoparticles enhance drug delivery level and chemotherapy efficacy in gastric cancer cells. Int J Nanomedicine 14:17–32

Sinha B, Mukherjee B, Pattnaik G (2013) Poly-lactide-co-glycolide nanoparticles containing voriconazole for pulmonary delivery: in vitro and in vivo study. Nanomedicine 9:94–104

Song N, Zhao L, Zhu M, Zhao J (2019) Recent progress in LyP-1-based strategies for targeted imaging and therapy. Drug Deliv 26:363–375

Staat C, Coisne C, Dabrowski S, Stamatovic SM, Andjelkovic AV, Wolburg H, Engelhardt B, Blasig IE (2015) Mode of action of claudin peptidomimetics in the transient opening of cellular tight junction barriers. Biomaterials 54:9–20

Su FY, Lin KJ, Sonaje K, Wey SP, Yen TC, Ho YC, Panda N, Chuang EY, Maiti B, Sung HW (2012) Protease inhibition and absorption enhancement by functional nanoparticles for effective oral insulin delivery. Biomaterials 33:2801e11

Sun T, Wu H, Li Y, Huang Y, Yao L, Chen X, Han X, Zhou Y, Du Z (2017) Targeting transferrin receptor delivery of temozolomide for a potential glioma stem cell-mediated therapy. Oncotarget 8:74451–74465

Surana S, Tosolini AP, Meyer IFG, Novoselov SS, Schiavo G (2018) The travel diaries of tetanus and botulinum neurotoxins. Toxicon 147:58–67

Taghdisi SM, Abnous K, Mosaffa F, Behravan J (2010) Targeted delivery of daunorubicin to T-cell acute lymphoblastic leukemia by aptamer. J Drug Target 18:277–281

Toporkiewicz M, Meissner J, Matusewicz L, Czogalla A, Sikorski AF (2015) Toward a magic or imaginary bullet? Ligands for drug targeting to cancer cells: principles, hopes, and challenges. Int J Nanomedicine 10:1399–1414

van der Velden VH, te Marvelde JG, Hoogeveen PG, Bernstein ID, Houtsmuller AB, Berger MS, van Dongen JJ (2001) Targeting of the CD33-calicheamicin immunoconjugate Mylotarg (CMA-676) in acute myeloid leukemia: in vivo and in vitro saturation and internalization by leukemic and normal myeloid cells. Blood 97:3197–3204

Varshosaz J, Hassanzadeh F, Sadeghi H, Ghelich Khan Z, Rostami M (2013) Retinoic acid decorated albumin-chitosan nanoparticles for targeted delivery of doxorubicin hydrochloride in hepatocellular carcinoma. J Nanomater 2013:1–12

Watts JK, Corey DR (2012) Gene silencing by siRNAs and antisense oligonucleotides in the laboratory and the clinic. J Pathol 226:365–379

Wang C, Su L, Wu C, Wu J, Zhu C, Yuan G (2016) RGD peptide targeted lipid-coated nanoparticles for combinatorial delivery of sorafenib and quercetin against hepatocellular carcinoma. Drug Dev Ind Pharm 42(12):1938–1944

Wearley LL (1991) Recent progress in protein and peptide delivery by noninvasive routes. Crit Rev Ther Drug Carrier Syst 8:331–394

Woitiski CB, Carvalho RA, Ribeiro AJ, Neufeld RJ, Veiga F (2008) Strategies toward the improved oral delivery of insulin nanoparticles via gastrointestinal uptake and translocation. BioDrugs 22:223e37

Yang H, Sun X, Liu G, Ma R, Li Z, An Y, Shi L (2013) Glucoseresponsive complex micelles for self-regulated release of insulin under physiological conditions. Soft Matter 9:8589e99

Yao VJ, D'Angelo S, Butler KS, Theron C, Smith TL, Marchiò S, Gelovani JG, Sidman RL, Dobroff AS, Brinker CJ, Bradbury ARM, Arap W, Pasqualini R (2016) Ligand-targeted theranostic nanomedicines against cancer. J Control Release 240:267–286

Youn YS, Chae SY, Lee S, Kwon MJ, Shin HJ, Lee KC (2008) Improved peroral delivery of glucagon-like peptide-1 by site-specific biotin modification: design, preparation, and biological evaluation. Eur J Pharm Biopharm 68(3):667–675

Zhang B, Zhang Y, Wang J, Zhang Y, Chen J, Pan Y, Ren L, Hu Z, Zhao J, Liao M, Wang S (2007) Screening and identification of a targeting peptide to hepatocarcinoma from a phage display peptide library. Mol Med 13:246–254

Zhang G, Han B, Lin X, Wu X, Yan H (2008) Modification of antimicrobial peptide with low molar mass poly (ethylene glycol). J Biochem 144:781–788

Zhang J, Jia X, Lv XJ, Deng YL, Xie HY (2010) Fluorescent quantum labelled aptamer bioprobes specifically targeting mouse liver cancer cells. Talanta 81:505–509

Zhong Y, Meng F, Deng C, Zhong Z (2014) Ligand-directed active tumor targeting polymeric nanoparticles for cancer chemotherapy. Biomacromolecules 15:1955–1969

Zhuo Z, Yu Y, Wang M, Li J, Zhang Z, Liu J, Wu X, Lu A, Zhang G, Zhang B (2017) Recent advances in SELEX technology and aptamer applications in biomedicine. Int J Mol Sci 18(10):2142

Zwanziger D, Hackel D, Staat C, Böcker A, Brack A, Beyermann M, Rittner H, Blasig IE (2012) A peptidomimetic tight junction modulator to improve regional analgesia. Mol Pharm 9:1785–1794

Recent Developments and Challenges in Nanoformulations Targeting Various Ailments of the Colon

7

Nidhi Mishra, Samipta Singh, Priyanka Maurya, Raquibun Nisha, and Shubhini A. Saraf

Abstract

The oral route of drug administration is the most preferred and patient-compliant route. When a drug is required to be delivered to the colon, special attention is required as the colon is the distal-most part of the gastrointestinal system. Also, a drug has to face a wide range of pH conditions before reaching the colon as it varies significantly, starting from 1.2 to 2.0 (acidic) in the stomach, 4.5–6.8 in the small intestine and 7–7.4 (basic) in the colon. Therefore, targeted approaches are required to protect a drug from the variations it has to face/deal with in the gastric milieu in order to reach the colon. Though targeting to the colon is tedious, it has its own advantages as the enzymatic activity in the colon is less, the residence time is more and bioavailability of drugs enhances significantly. Targeting of proteins and peptides can also be done easily to the colon as their structure remains integrated due to minimum enzymatic activity.

In recent years, the advancement in nanotechnology has tremendously helped target drugs to the colon. The nanoformulations target the drugs to the colon by using simple approaches that may be based on size, pH sensitivity, surface charges, polymers used, ligand-receptor interactions, etc., and are thus useful in enhancing the cell specificity.

The nanoparticles conjugated with ligands like peptides, carbohydrates, antibodies, aptamers, etc. act as new-generation therapies for various colon-associated diseases. These conjugated nanoparticles are beneficial in recognizing and targeting the desired site at cellular as well as molecular levels.

The upcoming outlook of the targeted nanoparticles stands dazzling as many promising nanoformulations targeting various colon-associated ailments are under preclinical and clinical trials and will soon be available in the market.

In this chapter, we will discuss the anatomy of the colon and the associated diseases, the factors that influence the delivery of a drug to the colon, the various strategies for colon targeting, types of nanoformulations used for colon targeting and the role and mechanism of nanoformulations in colon targeting, as well as existing nanoformulations for colon targeting.

Keywords

Colon-specific targeting · Colon anatomy · Nanoparticles · Active targeting · Passive targeting

N. Mishra · S. Singh · P. Maurya · R. Nisha
S. A. Saraf (✉)
Department of Pharmaceutical Sciences, Babasaheb Bhimrao Ambedkar University, Lucknow, India

S. Talegaonkar, M. Rai (eds.), *Nanoformulations in Human Health*, https://doi.org/10.1007/978-3-030-41858-8_7

7.1 Introduction

The application of particulate drug delivery to the medical arena has tremendous potential in the successful development of a variety of healthcare-related products. This has helped to develop dosage forms that can effectively treat various severe diseases minimizing side effects (Tao and Desai 2003). The use of a particulate delivery system is an effective and promising concept to deliver a drug in its original form at the required site, thus, enhancing its bioavailability and maximizing its beneficial effects (Allémann et al. 1998).

Targeting of drugs can be the answer for the treatment of various colonic diseases such as colon carcinoma, chronic inflammatory diseases, Crohn's disease and amoebiasis. The milieu of the colonic region is less intimidating with lesser miscellany in terms of bacterial flora and intensity of activity than stomach or small intestinal region (Vaidya et al. 2015). It has a physiological pH between 6.5 and 7.5, less protein and peptide enzyme concentrations and activity, and there are about 400 kinds of beneficial microbial flora. Thus, the colon is attracting interest as a site for various drug molecules (Dong et al. 2015).

If the drugs are delivered directly to the colon, without being absorbed in the upper gastrointestinal (GI) tract a higher concentration of the drug will reach the colon. The colon is considered an ideal site for drug delivery because of longer retention time (up to 5 days), minimum enzymatic activity and least fluctuation in pH.

Two routes can be used for drug delivery to the colon: oral route and rectal route. Among these two, the oral route is a vastly preferred route for drug delivery to the colon as it offers less pain than injection using a needle and syringe. Also side effects and risk of infections reduce in the oral route (Lee et al. 2004). Oral dosage forms also offer industrial advantage for their easy manufacture and design compared to other dosage forms. Sterilization is also not of prime importance in such dosage forms.

Drug delivery through the rectal route is challenging as the route itself is quite inconvenient, secondly the drug distribution depends totally on the spreadability and retention time of the dosage form.

An ideal colon-specific drug delivery system (CDDS) should be formulated keeping in mind the physical and chemical properties of the drug chosen, dosage form, factors influencing GI transit time and interactions between GIT and drug.

Orally administered drugs, however, can be ineffective due to the variations in pH it has to face in the gastric milieu. Therefore, the oral CDDS formulations must guarantee that it degrades neither in the acidic conditions of the stomach nor in the upper part of the intestine. This has been made possible by utilizing approaches that aim at delaying drug release until the delivery system reaches the colon (Xing et al. 2003).

Nanotechnology is of much interest to many pharmaceutical scientists, and nanoformulations hold incredible possibilities for delivering drugs to the target site.

However, a clear understanding is required of the interactions between nanomaterials and the biological environment of the body, possibilities of targeting cell-surface receptors, drug release mechanisms, drug administration regimes, drug-dosage form stability and molecular mechanisms involved in the pathobiology of the disease.

Several functionalized and nonfunctionalized nano-based drug delivery systems have been formulated to target various colonic diseases. Here, we cover various strategies, disease-specific receptors, nanoformulations and functionalization of nanoformulation with targeting moieties utilized to target them. The aim of the chapter is to familiarize the readers with the gastrointestinal system with emphasis on the anatomy of the colon, the various ailments associated with the colon and the treatment approaches for ailments thereof via nanotechnology and colon targeting.

7.2 Anatomy of the Colon

The oral cavity is the site from where the external substances like food, drugs, xenobiotics, etc. enter the body. The alimentary canal is a complex system of tubes within tubes extending from the oral cavity to the rectum. The alimentary canal or the gastrointestinal tract (GIT) begins from the oral cavity and further comprises of the oesophagus, stomach, small intestine, cecum, large intestine,

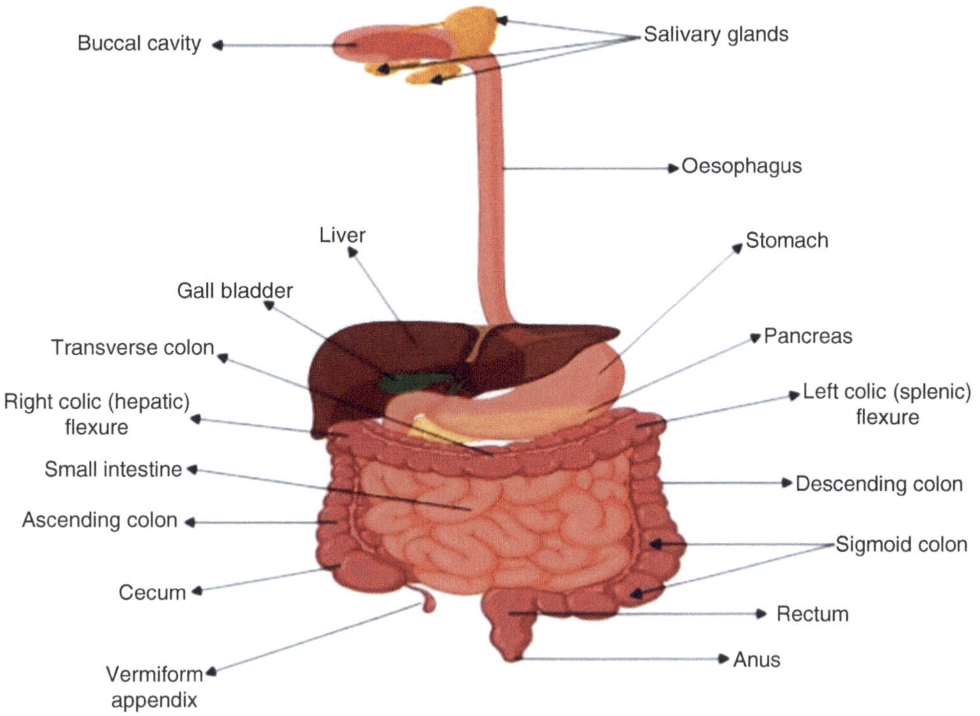

Fig. 7.1 Anatomy of the digestive tract

colon and rectum. The GIT contains smooth and/or striated muscles along the walls to propel the ingested food. The length of the GIT varies greatly among different species with the shortest in carnivores and the longest, most complex in herbivores (Moran 2006). The anatomy of the digestive tract is shown in Fig. 7.1.

In this chapter, we will discuss the colon and its parts in detail since it is a prerequisite to understanding the various aspects of colon-targeted delivery. The discussion of other elements of the GIT is beyond the scope of this chapter.

The colon serves as a reservoir for the liquids emptied from the small intestine. Starting from lower right-hand side of the abdomen and ending towards its lower left-hand side, the large intestine forms a horseshoe-like structure surrounding the coiled small intestine. It has a much larger diameter than the small intestine, but its length is about one-quarter of the small intestine. The large intestine is about 5–6 feet (1.5 m) long and about 7.5 cm wide. Figure 7.2 shows the length (diameter) and pH variation in the gastrointestinal tract.

The primary functions of the colon are water absorption, maintaining osmotic balance, regulation of electrolyte levels in blood and storage of faecal material. The walls of the large intestine secrete mucus, which helps in the lubrication of the contents, thereby facilitating their easy transport throughout. Each day about 1.5–2 litres of chyme (partially digested food) moves down the ileocecal valve (separating the small and large intestine) into the colon. This chyme is condensed to 150 ml after water absorption. The remaining indigestible food constituents along with dead mucosal cells and bacteria constitute the faeces.

Numerous beneficial bacteria are present in the colon which help in the synthesis of essential vitamins like niacin (nicotinic acid), thiamine (vitamin B_1), vitamin K and other vitamins necessary for various metabolic activities.

The large intestine can be divided into: (i) cecum, (ii) ascending colon, (iii) transverse colon, (iv) descending colon, (v) sigmoid colon, (vi) rectum, (vii) anal canal and (viii) anus. The large intestine begins with the cecum, which

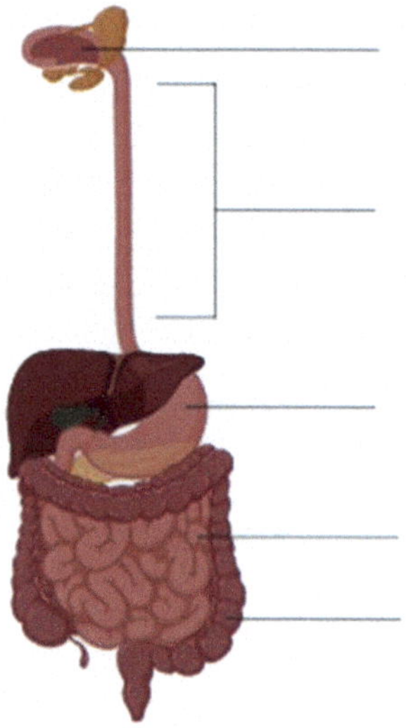

Diameter(cms)	pH	Average gastric residence time (hrs.)
10	6.8	-
2-4	-	-
15	1.4-2.1(fasted state) 2-5 (fed state)	2-6
3-5	4.4-6.4	3±1
3-9	5.4-7.4	upto 48

Fig. 7.2 Length (diameter) and pH variation in the gastrointestinal tract

resembles a sac with a closed end occupying the right iliac fossa. The cecum opening from ileum is guarded by the ileocecal sphincter (formed by circular muscle fibres of the ileum and cecum). The ascending colon outspreads from the cecum to the hepatic flexure located underneath the right lobe of the liver. Located at the level of the tenth rib, the transverse colon ascends across the abdomen towards its left side to the bend termed as the splenic flexure. The colon passes inferiorly down to the iliac crest to the left side of the posterior abdominal wall in the form of the descending colon, just in front of the left kidney. The sigmoid colon consists of iliac and pelvic parts. The iliac colon begins from the left crest of the ilium and ends at the inner border of the psoas muscle.

The pelvic colon lies in the lower part of the pelvis (true part) and forms a loop-like structure that first reaches the right side of the pelvis and then bends back and, at the midline, turns downwards, where it becomes the rectum.

The layers that make up the wall of the colon are the taeniae, haustra and appendices epiploicae. The taeniae consist of three longitudinal groups of muscle fibres which are each 1 cm wide, situated at equal distances all around the colon. The taeniae being shorter leads to the formation of circular troughs of changing depth called haustra, or sacculations. The appendices epiploicae are collections of fatty tissue beneath the covering membrane. Two rows of these tissues exist on the ascending and descending colon while one row is present on the transverse colon.

Crypts creased with mucous glands and goblet cells line the interior surface of the colon. The large intestine is devoid of villi and plicae circulares, which are a feature of the small intestine. The compartmentalization of lumen and its contents is the result of colonic contractions (Phillips 1984; Grand et al. 1976; Moran 2006; Jayasekeran et al. 2013; Gelberg 2014; Mahadevan 2017).

7.2.1 Blood and Nerve Supply

The large intestine is richly supplied with blood by the branches of the superior and inferior mesenteric arteries (branches of the abdominal aorta) and the hypogastric branch of the internal iliac artery. The blood vessels form a continuous row of arches to drain the venous blood in the large intestine. This is further drained into the superior and inferior mesenteric veins, which join with the splenic vein to form the portal vein.

7.2.2 Contractions and Motility

The contractions and propulsions ensure the mixing of colonic contents as well as a good time of contact with the mucosa.

Motility of the colon is enhanced by the mastication and by the presence of fat, bile acids and the hormones gastrin and cholecystokinin, but the role of unabsorbed bile salts is yet unclear.

The hormones secretin, glucagon and vasoactive intestinal peptide act to suppress the colonic propulsions and contractions (Mike and Kano 2013; Moulari et al. 2014; Vdoviaková et al. 2016).

7.3 Diseases Associated with the Colon

The major diseases affecting the colon are discussed in this section.

7.3.1 Inflammatory Bowel Diseases

Inflammatory bowel diseases (IBD) have an effect on a multitude of people worldwide. IBD is a chronic disease, characterized by persistent or recurring inflammation in the small intestine and colonic region. It is further classified into two types: (a) Crohn's disease (CD) (b) ulcerative colitis (UC)).

The symptoms of IBD are periodic abdominal pain, vomiting, fever, bloody stool, diarrhoea and weight loss. These symptoms, if left untreated, may affect the quality of life of the patient and even enhance the risk of colorectal cancer. The major cause of intestinal inflammation in IBD occurs due to disturbances in synthesis and release of anti-inflammatory cytokines, including interleukins (IL-4, IL-10, and IL-11) or transforming growth factor (TGF)-β, as well as proinflammatory cytokines, such as tumor necrosis factor α (TNF-α), interferons (IFN-γ, IL-1β, IL-6 and IL-12). Enhanced levels of free radicals or reactive oxygen species (ROS) cause tissue damage, which again leads to intestinal inflammation (Dinesen and Travis 2007; Jodeleit et al. 2018).

Crohn's disease is an inflammatory bowel disease that causes inflammatory conditions in the gastric lining, which leads to abdominal pain, fatigue, diarrhoea, loss in weight and deficiency of nutrients.

The conventional therapy for IBD advocates administration of nonsteroidal anti-inflammatory drugs, drug that suppresses the immune response of an individual, corticosteroids, etc. which results in several side effects. Nanotechnology can play an important role in making the drugs to reach the colon, enhancing local drug delivery, thereby minimizing the side effects and management and treatment of IBD more efficiently (Philip and Philip 2010).

7.3.2 Colon Cancer

Colon cancer, commonly known as colorectal cancer or large bowel cancer refers to cancerous growth in the colon, rectum, or cecum (Wong et al. 2011). Colon cancer is one of the leading causes of cancer morbidity and mortality among men and women worldwide. The incidences of colon cancer have risen in recent years due to change in people's lifestyles and dietary habits (Verghese et al. 2006).

Colorectal cancer is the third most common type of cancer in men and women in the Western world. Almost 60% of cases are encountered in developed countries. In India, the annual incidence rates for colon cancer in men and women are 4.4 and 3.9 per 100,000, respectively.

Importantly, colon cancer is one of the most curable forms of cancer, when detected early, 90% of the patients can be cured (Elzagheid et al. 2006; Atlanta 2015).

7.3.3 Irritable Bowel Syndrome

Irritable Bowel Syndrome (IBS) is a disorder related to intestinal muscle functioning which may also involve constipation, diarrhoea or both, along with pain, cramps and bloating. The symptoms of IBS closely resemble conditions like cancer, diverticulitis, depression, etc. therefore proper diagnosis is needed. Along with medical attention, mental health counselling and stress reduction can help relieve symptoms in patients.

Also, increasing the amount of liquids and bulk-forming foods that enable softening of stools may provide relief.

7.3.4 A Few Other Colon-Related Diseases

7.3.4.1 Constipation

A condition when typically less than three to four bowel movements occur in a week with hard, dry, small and painful stools is called constipation.

7.3.4.2 Diverticulosis and Diverticulitis

Formation of many tiny pockets (diverticula) in the sigmoid colon and anorectal region due to straining during bowel movement is called as diverticulosis. Usually diverticula are pea-sized but size may increase if the GIT wall is pressurized by gas, liquid or faecal matter. The rupture of the diverticulum is known as diverticulitis. This rupture leads to infection in the surrounding area, which may cause tenderness, abdominal pain or colonic obstruction.

7.3.4.3 Anal Fissure

Small wear and tear in the lining of the anus due to hard, dry stool, diarrhoea or inflammation is termed as anal fissure.

7.3.4.4 Bowel Incontinence

It is the inability to control gas or stool release due to weakened anal muscles. Childbirth, nerve/muscle injury, old age, etc. may be possible reasons.

7.3.4.5 Colon Polyps

Growths on the inner lining of colon are called as polyps. These polyps may turn cancerous if not treated.

7.3.4.6 Rectal Bleeding

It is a symptomatic problem when bleeding occurs from one or more parts of the GIT. The site of bleeding can be known by examining the colour of the blood. The more the bright red the blood nearer to the anus is the site of bleeding and vice versa.

7.3.4.7 Haemorrhoids

The condition of swelled veins around the anal cavity is termed as haemorrhoids. Severe forms of haemorrhoids are known as piles.

7.3.4.8 Peritonitis

Peritonitis occurs due to bacterial or fungal infection, which results in inflamed peritoneum (tissue lining inner wall of the abdomen).

7.3.4.9 Ulcer

Ulcers can occur in any part of the GIT but the most severe condition of ulceration occurs when a wound forms in the lining of the stomach or duodenum.

7.3.4.10 Hernias

Hernias commonly occur in the abdomen due to pushing of an organ into the muscle or tissue that holds it in place (Irving and Catchpole 1992; Bratten and Jones 2006).

7.4 Strategies for Colon-Specific Systems

The rational design of colon-specific system is enabled through numerous strategies such as macro-, micro-, and nanoparticles. Various biochemical, physiological and molecular factors like microfold cells, pH environment, the release of reactive oxygen species, receptor upregulation, GI tract, etc. play a dominant role in oral drug administration. In a specific example, nanomaterials designed for IBD treatments and colon cancers have discrete physiological features. In the normal course, colorectal cancer cells destroy various layers: muscularis, submucosa and serosa. Epithelial-enhanced permeability and retention (eEPR) remains valuable in maintaining a large number of nanoparticles, and an enormous concentration of ROS will produce cancerous conditions. The pathophysiological functions indicate the strong expression of transmembrane glycoprotein and the immune globulin molecules that act as a potential target for therapeutics (Lu et al. 2016). A number of design strategies for achieving colon-targeted drug delivery have been summarized and numerous physiopathological characteristics of colon sites are outlined.

7.4.1 Size-Dependent Nanodelivery Systems

NPs demonstrate superior residence time in inflamed colonic regions, thus proving beneficial in colon therapy. NPs of range <100 nm drastically enhance the delivery index and selectivity into the colitis tissue by mediating a better eEPR effect (Collnot et al. 2012; Bo Xiao and Merlin 2012). The small size of the particles causes privileged uptake of the nanomaterials by the immune cells that produce a better response to the inflammatory conditions (Lamprecht et al. 2005). Hasty carrier elimination can be avoided by nanodelivery systems. In contrast to conventional formulations, NPs provide added advantage of enhanced local tissue concentration, which proves beneficial in the treatment of IBD and associated diseases (Beloqui et al. 2013). In the GIT, it undergoes internalization by endocytosis or paracellular transport into the epithelial cells. M cells, specialized differentiated epithelial cells, are preferentially involved in the re-uptake of NPs through the process known as transcytosis. Translocation of NPs occurs by persorption through gaps in the villi (Pichai and Ferguson 2012). Microparticulates have lesser efficacy than NPs due to increased targeting and bioavailability as a result of small size and increased surface area. The physiological barriers play a significant role in retaining the formulation in the target area. The inflamed tissues retain almost threefold concentration of NPs when compared to normal skin (Talaei et al. 2013; Lautenschläger et al. 2014).

7.4.2 Surface Functionalized Nanodelivery Systems

The development of the localized colon drug delivery system (CDDS) results in higher concentrate in the colon and lesser systemic side effects. Gastrointestinal tract (GIT)-specific drug delivery approach is found to be very useful for ulcerative colitis, gastroenteritis, gastric ulceration, infectious diarrhoea, gastrointestinal (GI) stromal tumors, Crohn's disease, amoebiasis, colonic cancer therapeutics and local treatment of colonic ulceration. CDDS not only transports the drugs to the colon but also is an important tool to protect gene products (which get degraded in the stomach or small intestine) or acid labile drugs from adverse conditions. Colon holds the advantage of reduced enzyme and P-glycoprotein activity, thus, absorption of numerous drugs (e.g. simvastatin) is better in the colon than in the small intestine and stomach, irrespective of the fact that the colon has a lower epithelial surface area (Krishna et al. 2009). All these factors stimulated interest in targeted delivery of drug molecules and gene products to the colon's surface.

Modification with hyaluronic acid (HA), chitosan (CS)–Carboxymethyl Starch (CMS), near-IR (NIR) fluorescent human serum albumin (HSA), etc. stabilized the sustained and targeted drug delivery, improved the therapeutic efficacy, enhanced bioavailability and ensured superior anticancer activity.

Naeem et al. (2018) developed dual-functional Eudragit® (E) FS30D/PLGA nanoparticles (PNPs) and delivered cyclosporine-A to the colon for the amelioration of murine experimental colitis. These dual-functional nanoparticles avoided burst release of the drug in the stomach, exhibited its slow and incomplete release at the ileum and colonic pH, followed by a sustained release of cyclosporine-A, thus delivering a sufficient amount of cyclosporine-A to the disease-affected colon (Naeem et al. 2018).

7.4.3 pH-Sensitive Polymer-Coated Drug Delivery System

The polymer that has specific solubility at colonic pH can shield the formulation in the stomach, and proximal small intestine, solubilizing and dissolving only in the colon (Jain 2017). The ileum and colon have higher pH than other gastrointestinal regions (Bratten and Jones 2006);

thus, a dosage form disintegrating at higher pH, preferentially, has the potential for colonic delivery. The easiest way to achieve this is to coat the dosage forms with a pH-sensitive biocompatible polymer (Karn et al. 2011). An additional enteric coating protects the API from the harsh GI environment (such as bile acids, gastric juices, microbial degradation, etc.). It creates an extended and delayed-release profile of drug to specific GI regions. The first coating is an acid-soluble polymer and the outer coating is an enteric polymer (Chourasia and Jain 2004). The core of formulation comprises the API and excipients. When the drug passes through the GI tract, the formulation does not degrade or release in the stomach due to enteric coating, and the enteric coating dissolves in the small intestine, where the pH is above 6. When the drug reaches the colon, the bacteria enzymatically degrade the polysaccharides into organic acid. This lowers the pH of the surrounding system and causes the dissolution of the surrounding system which is acid-soluble coating, and subsequently the drug releases (Singh et al. 2018). The most commonly used pH-dependent coating polymers for oral delivery are methacrylic acid copolymers (Eudragit®).

Eudragits® can be manipulated to alter the pH at which they are soluble by simply changing the composition of attached side groups in their molecular structures. When drug release is required within pH 6–7, then a combination of Eudragit L100 and Eudragit S100 is utilized in suitable ratios as they dissolve at pH 6 and 7, respectively.

The delayed release of drugs is achieved by incorporation into a pH-sensitive polymer that protects it from the low pH of the stomach and high enzymatic activity of the small intestine. As higher pH is encountered, such polymers break down to release the drug in the colon, thereby ensuring colon targeted drug delivery (Das et al. 2010; Kumar et al. 2010; Leuva et al. 2012).

Recently, Ahmadi et al., (2019) co-delivered doxorubicin hydrochloride and Hydroxytyrosol to HT-29 colon cancer cells using a pH-responsive nanocarrier. It resulted in more than 94% cellular uptake and high apoptosis on HT-29 cancer cells in comparison to free drugs (Ahmadi et al. 2019). Using water-in-oil emulsion technique, Couce et al., (2019) coated dexamethasone-loaded chitosan beads with a pH-dependent poly (acrylic acid)/poly (vinyl pyrrolidone) complex to deliver dexamethasone to the colon. It was found to be effective with reduced side effects and loss of drug (García et al. 2019).

7.4.4 Delayed Release Drug Delivery System

This approach is entirely based on the gastric transit time (~ 5 hr) from mouth to colon. For colon delivery, the reported transit time for small intestine is ~3 hr to 4 hr, which is based on the size of the formulation administered and gastric motility (Ratnaparkhi et al. 2013). The release of drug from the system depends on either swelling or osmosis or a combination of both. It is not affected by any means by intestinal microbial flora or pH. Pulsincap®, a newly developed device fabricated for this approach, has been strategically designed for producing a lag time for a predetermined interval. The transit from the mouth to the colon is fixed at a lag time of 5 hr and is fairly constant, not being affected by the type of formulation. For the management of colon-related diseases, for example ulcerative colitis and irritable bowel syndrome (IBS), these time-dependent systems are not appropriate to deliver the drug to the specific sites of the colon. Due to the little variability in the transmit time in the intestine (3 ± 1 hr), these time-release systems are more successful in colon delivery rather than the stomach. After gastric emptying, the release of the drug begins at a predetermined interval, and therefore the pH-sensing function would probably diminish the disparity in the gastric residence time (Philip and Philip 2010).

7.4.5 Microbially Triggered System

When the drug is completely absorbed before reaching the colon, it imposes a great challenge to the therapeutic efficacy and the microbial triggered delivery system remains a boon for specific targeting to the colon. In this approach, the drug is released alongside the degradation of polysaccharides by the gut microflora, such as Enterobacteria, Clostridia, Bacteroides, Bifidobacteria, Enterococci, Ruminococcus and Eubacteria. The microflora produces several imperative biodegradable enzymes such as xylosidase, deaminase, arabinosidase, nitroreductase, glucoronidase, urea dehydroxylase and galactosidase due to the process of fermentation. The drug is usually administered in enteric-coated formulations and when it reaches the intestine, it gets degraded into nascent forms and eventually releases the drug in the local milieu. The same approach may be employed for specific release to the stomach (Vagare 2015).

A specific example quoted by Zhang et al. involved modulation of colonic tumorigenesis by several dietary factors such as sodium butyrate, high-fat diet, dihydromyricetin and cholic acid through gut microfloral interaction and host chloride channels. It was perceived that diets high in fat and low in fibre presented a high CRC risk and strong evidence of the theory that colonic tumorigenesis is associated with the alteration of chloride ion channels. Dihydromyricetin showed an acute reduction in susceptibility to tumorigenesis and considerably advanced the gut dominant microbes in mice (Mishra et al. 2019, Zhang et al. 2018).

7.4.6 Redox-Sensitive Polymer Coating

Under homeostatic conditions, a balance subsists between ROS formation and ant-oxidant molecules that scavenge the ROS. A high quantity of ROS is released when the inflammatory process is activated. When the balance is lost in the due course, an enormous concentration of ROS results and the antioxidant capacity gets lost. These cause a state of oxidative stress which produces stern cellular injuries and precipitates a large number of diseases. For example, investigation of models of ulcerative colitis demonstrated a 100-fold enhancement of ROS concentrations in the mucosal tissues and therefore can be correlated with the progression of the disease (Simmonds et al. 1992). Similarly, IBD tissues have analogous higher ROS concentrations. Utilizing the thioketal-sensitive polymers, coated formulations are developed that ultimately get dissolved locally (Talaei et al. 2013). Abnormally high concentrations of ROS lead to complete dissolution of polymer and provide specific activity. Enhanced redox nanoparticles are taken up by ROS-treated epithelial colonic cells more rapidly than ROS-untreated cells. In colitis-induced mice model, similar observations have been observed and a significant reduction of ROS is indirectly observed (Vong et al. 2015a). In a study, the combination of irinotecan along with redox nanoparticles drastically progressed the therapeutic index and reduces side effects considerably (Gao et al. 2014; Vong et al. 2015b).

Based on 4-amino thiophenol-carboxymethyl inulin (ATP-CMI) conjugate for budesonide (BDS) delivery, Sun and co-workers developed redox-sensitive nanoparticles for treating IBD. BDS-loaded ATP-CMI nanoparticles have been seen to accrue in inflamed sites, and improved intracellular drug delivery was detected. This type of system holds promise for the treatment of IBD (Sun et al. 2018).

7.4.7 Osmotic Controlled Systems

In the due course of study, for delayed or pulsed delivery, a well-established mechanism has evolved. As a result of augmentation in diffusion of water into the osmotic layer, an osmotic gradient occurs. In the formulation development, both the drug and the osmogen are compressed directly to form a "core," which is further enclosed in a polymeric membrane, which allows sustained release. The geometry acquires a hole as that area is weaker in comparison to other places, and hence facilitates rapid access of fluids situated in the intestinal milieu, which leads to drug release with the driving force via a constant zero-order release (Kumar et al. 2010). OROS-CT, a specifically designed engineered system (enteric-coated hard gelatin capsule) comprising of a semipermeable membrane, is regulated by osmotic pressure. When the pH is basic, the system dissolves in the intestine region and permits penetration of fluid. The content swells and facilitates the drug to force out of the system. The capsule consists of

5–6 components as well as individual layers of enteric coating to bypass the corrosive acidic pH in the stomach region. The system covers an osmotic push section as well as a drug section. When water enters, it swells and transforms into a gel through the orifice, it reaches the next drug compartment through the membrane. First-order release of drug is possible through this system. This system may be further modified in a rational manner to induce a lag time between the drug release and the dissolution profile of the enteric coating (Amidon et al. 2015).

7.4.8 Pressure-Controlled Drug-Delivery System (PCDS)

The principle of PCDS exclusively lies on the lumen pressure disparity between the large and small intestine. The drug present in the specially designed water-insoluble polymer-coated capsule expels out into the colonic milieu due to the increase in the localized pressure. This modified system is composed of ethyl-cellulose-coated gelatine capsules along with an internally engineered suppository base that swiftly dissolves at body temperature. The mechanism involved enhancement of viscosity as a result of rapid absorption of water from the intestinal content, which drives out the drug content from the concocted formulation. However, augmentation of viscosity beyond a critical limit forces the reabsorption of water, which often leads to high site-specific delivery due to amplified colonic pressure (Rangari and Puranik 2015).

7.4.9 Enzyme Sensitive

By the emerging applications of enzyme-responsive nanomaterials, a stimuli-sensitive approach has been fabricated by researchers. Enzymes play a dominant function in the physiological and biochemical processes, in expressing therapeutic targeting, diagnostics and drug release, in addition to the pathophysiology of several diseases, they play a key role in the progression. A considerable application in the vibrant area of nanomedicine has been taken into account while experimenting with the development of controlled drug release formulations based on enzyme-responsive systems. Azoreductase remains a vital enzyme that has received adequate attention in the recent era. It is produced in the colon by the microbial flora and is known to have multiple applications in the treatment of diseases restricted to the colon (Rao and Khan 2013).

Rao et al. fabricated an azoreductase-responsive system through amphiphilic diblock copolymer and azobenzene linkage via a covalent coupling. Through the atom transfer radical polymerization-based macro-initiator approach, the azobenzene-linked poly (ethylene glycol)-b-poly (styrene) amphiphilic copolymer was prepared. The micellar constitution disassembles into two different segments: poly(ethylene glycol) segment and poly(styrene) segment, when exposed to the azoreductase enzyme. Due to the selectivity and sensitivity of the azoreductase system, the recently developed azoreductase-responsive drug delivery systems have great pharmacotherapeutics in the chronic treatment of diseases of colonic origin (Rao and Khan 2013).

In biological detection as well as in drug delivery, smart biomaterials such as enzyme-sensitive amphiphilic polymers have found immense applications. Novel fluorescent amphiphilic copolymer probes containing azo-tetraphenylethylene bridges have been fabricated by Yuan et al. for azoreductase-triggered release. For colonic conditions, amphiphilic block copolymers have numerous applications in the controlled release of the drug and also in biosensing. During drug release, for polymer micelles, a reduction-triggered drug release was confirmed through fluorescence (Yuan et al. 2019).

7.4.10 CODES™

For circumventing the probable troubles associated with the time-dependent drug delivery system, microbial-triggered drug delivery system and pH-dependent drug delivery system, CODES™ was designed rationally for inimitable colon-targeted drug delivery systems. This is a combination of all three systems stated above. The uniquely fabricated system involves the application of lactulose, which activates drug release into the colon region. In the administration of this system, the enteric-coated approach is utilized, which protects the drug from the acid environment. The engineered material is followed by an acid-soluble coating that protects from the environment of the small intestine. Ultimately, in the colon region, the lactulose gets degraded and the drug gets released eventually (Talaei et al. 2013).

7.5 Types of Nanoformulations for Colon Targeting

The ideal range of nanoparticles suitable for colon targeting lies between 200 and 500 nm. Various types of nanoparticles are used for drug delivery and targeting. For all practical purposes, nanoparticles can be categorized as particulate systems, vesicular systems, gel systems, and others. Figure 7.3 shows different types of nanoformulation for colon drug delivery.

7.5.1 Particulate Nanosystems

7.5.1.1 Polymeric Nanoparticles

These are the most suitable and common types of nanoparticles used for colon drug delivery. Various natural and synthetic polymers are used in formulating polymeric nanoparticles. Natural polymers like pectin, chitosan, chondroitin sulphate, alginate, ethylcellulose, etc. and synthetic polymers like eudragit RS, eudragit S-100, polymethacrylates, etc. are used in the preparation of such nanoparticles.

Almost every colon-associated disease has been targeted using polymeric nanoparticles. These nanoparticles can be simply prepared by

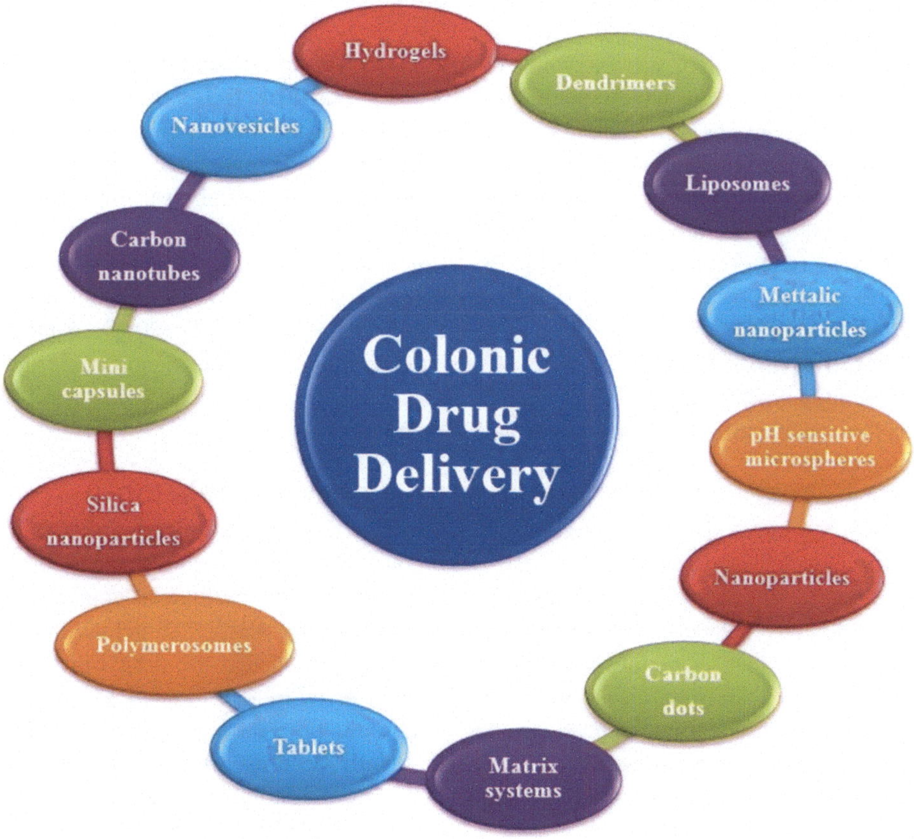

Fig. 7.3 Types of nanoformulations for colon drug delivery

using techniques like polymerization, solvent evaporation, solvent displacement, desolvation, ionic gelation, etc.

7.5.1.2 Nanospheres

Nanospheres are solid particles with a matrix, generally ranging from 10 to 200 nm. They act as good carriers for both hydrophilic and hydrophobic drugs, enzymes, proteins, genes, etc. They tend to increase drug circulation time.

Nanospheres can be prepared using simple methods like polymerization, nanoprecipitation method, solvent evaporation, salting out, desolvation and ionic gelation (Guterres et al. 2007; Makhlof et al. 2009; Zhang et al. 2015).

Budesonide nanospheres for IBD (colon-specific targeting) have been successfully designed by Makhlof et al. 2009 (Makhlof et al. 2009).

7.5.1.3 Nanocapsules

Nanocapsules can be defined as nano-sized polymeric shells that encapsulate the drug in their core. These nanocapsules are easily surface-modified by decorating their surface with cell surface receptors or antibodies which specifically bind to a target-specific site.

Nanocapsules have been used to target colon-specific diseases like inflammatory bowel disease (IBD), which includes ulcerative colitis (UC) and Crohn's disease (CD) (Feng et al. 2016a, b; Kshirsagar et al. 2012).

7.5.1.4 Metallic Nanoparticles

The most common type of metallic nanoparticles used for colon-specific drug delivery are gold and silver nanoparticles.

Silver nanoparticles act as good carriers to deliver the drug to target sites, therefore are also being used in colon delivery (Satapathy et al. 2013).

Gold nanoparticles are used as drug delivery carriers for both active as well as passive targeting. It is reported that cisplatin-loaded gold nanoparticles were able to reduce colorectal-cancer-related fibroblasts and also prevented the expression of profibrotic signals like CTGF, TGF-β1, VEGF in-vivo via Akt signalling pathway (Zhao et al. 2018).

7.5.1.5 Solid Lipid Nanoparticles (SLNs) and Nanostructured Lipid Carriers (NLCs)

SLNs are alternative drug carrier systems to other novel delivery approaches such as emulsions, liposomes, and polymeric nanoparticles as they are used to incorporate both hydrophilic and hydrophobic drugs easily. They also provide increased physical stability, low cost and easy scale-up (Chandran et al. 2018; Üner and Yener 2007).

Cholesteryl butyrate (Cb) has been extensively investigated as butyrate SLN formulation in several in vitro and in vivo studies as an anti-cancer agent and anti-inflammatory agent, respectively. SLNs also have applications in targeting IBD and colon cancers (Dianzani et al. 2017). NLCs are the next generation of SLNs, which have been beneficial as they overcome the innate drawbacks of SLNs, such as transition of lipids and subsequent expulsion of drugs. The inclusion of a liquid lipid makes this possible.

7.5.1.6 Mesoporous Silica Nanoparticles (MSNs)

MSNs are nano-sized porous structures with a solid framework and large surface area. MSNs resemble a honeycomb structure. They have an active surface which enables ease of surface functionalization as different functional groups can be attached easily for targeting drug to specific sites (Bharti et al. 2015). 5-fluorouracil-based mesoporous silica nanoparticles have been formulated by Kumar et al. 2017 for colon cancer targeting (Kumar et al. 2017).

7.5.1.7 Quantum Dots (QDs)

Quantum dots are nano-drug carriers with optical properties through which they can act as luminescent probes for biological applications. QDs entrap drug by various strategies like coupling and adsorption, also the drug can be dispersed and dissolved to load in them. Quantum dots are not used in the treatment of cancers but they have efficiently been used in the diagnosis of cancer, including colon cancer (Park et al. 2014; Zhao and Zhu 2016; Pardo et al. 2018).

7.5.2 Vesicular Nanosystems

7.5.2.1 Liposomes

Liposomes are spherical vesicles with an external hydrophobic phospholipid layer, which forms an internal hydrophilic compartment. Liposomes are prepared basically by two approaches, one is through a mechanical procedure which utilizes organic solvents, and another is via removal of surfactant from a phospholipid surfactant mixture. The factors to be kept in mind while preparing liposomes are: type and quantity of phospholipid, the ionic charge of the surfactant and also the charge of aqueous media as a whole (Akbarzadeh et al. 2013; Alavi et al. 2017).

Liposomes play a significant role in colon targeting. Usually, coated liposomes are used for colon targeting to ensure that their degradation is prevented in upper the GIT and they reach the colon. The natural polymers used for coating are chitosan and pectin, while Eudragit is the main synthetic polymer that is often used.

Advancement has been made to deliver the liposomes to the colon by attaching antibodies to its surface, such as monoclonal antibodies. Such liposomes are termed as immunoliposomes. These utilize the concept of active targeting and hence prove to be more efficient (Garg et al. 2009; Gupta et al. 2013; Alavi et al. 2017).

7.5.2.2 Niosomes

Niosomes are relatively more stable vesicles as compared to liposomes, fabricated from non-ionic surfactants (e.g. alkyl ester and alkyl ether) and cholesterol and are suitable carriers for amphiphilic as well as lipophilic drugs (Goudanavar and Joshi 2012; Ag Seleci et al. 2016; Yeo et al. 2017).

Though niosomes are not often used as drug delivery carriers for colon targeting, Capacitabine niosomes have been reported in treating colorectal cancers (Anbarasan et al. 2013).

7.5.2.3 Phytosomes

Phytosomes are vesicular drug delivery systems that carry plant-derived bioactives by encapsulating them in their core. These micelle structures conjugate the targeting proteins as surface decorations (Azeez et al. 2018). Many natural bioactives are used in the treatment of colon-associated diseases. Phytosomes of silibinin have been formulated to check therapeutic efficacy against colorectal cancers(Velmurugan et al. 2010).

7.5.2.4 Sphingosomes

Sphingosomes are bilayered vesicles that enclose an aqueous volume within the lipid bilayer. These are more stable vesicular systems than liposomes and niosomes and also circumvent their drawbacks, as sphingosomes have increased in vivo circulation time and high tumor loading efficacy. Sphingosomes find place as agents in colon tumor therapy (Jadhav et al. 2012; Lankalapalli and Damuluri 2012; Kamboj et al. 2013).

7.5.2.5 Virosomes

A virosome is an artificial vesicular drug delivery vector composed of a phospholipid bilayer and has viral surface proteins but lacks the multiplication ability. They encapsulate macromolecules and introduce them into the cell cytoplasm using their tendency to cross cell membranes. Virosomes find application in cancer therapy and are also helpful in colon cancer therapy (Saga and Kaneda 2013; Liu et al. 2015).

7.5.2.6 Bilosomes

Bilosomes are bilayer vesicles fabricated from non-ionic surfactants and bile salts that function as membrane-stabilizing agents for the vesicles in the GIT (Wilkhu et al. 2013; Aburahma 2016).

The advanced form of bilosomes used are probilosomes and surface-engineered bilosomes. Bilosomes find application in inflammatory bowel disease and colon tumors (Elnaggar 2015; Wilkhu et al. 2013).

7.5.3 Other Nanosystems

7.5.3.1 Micelles

Micelles are core-shell assemblies of a lipid/polymer monolayer with polar hydrophilic head outwards and non-polar hydrophilic tail inwards towards the centre.

Polymeric micelles are used in tumor targeting as they are nano-sized and have a hydrophilic outer layer, which helps in increasing the circulation time of the formulation. Also, accumulation in tumor cells is enhanced by their enhanced permeability and retention (EPR) effect. Thus, the efficacy of the drug improves and its systemic toxicity reduces (Gou et al. 2011; Yang et al. 2015; Ma et al. 2016).

Polymeric micelles have their application in tumor targeting. Colon tumors have also been targeted via polymeric micelles.

7.5.3.2 Dendrimers

Dendrimers are branched globular macromolecules synthetically designed to enhance the solubility of drug molecules. Their highly branched structure makes them a good carrier for delivery of gene and drug moieties. Dendrimers find application in colon-associated diseases like IBD and colorectal cancers (Abderrezak et al. 2012; Stanczy et al. 2012; Mignani and Majoral 2013; Xie et al. 2015).

7.5.3.3 Carbon Nanotubes

Carbon nanotubes (CNTs) are nano-sized cylindrical allotropes of carbon with unique mechanical, geometrical and electrical properties. They have good thermal conductivity, stiffness and strength. Based on their structure they are categorized into two: single-walled nanotubes (SWNTs) and multi-walled nanotubes (MWNTs). Carbon nanotubes, a novel drug delivery system, find application in colon cancer treatment (Rastogi et al. 2014; Zhou et al. 2014; DineshKumar et al. 2015; Prajapati et al. 2019).

7.5.3.4 Graphene Oxides

Graphene oxide forms a solitary sheet of sp^2 hybridized carbon atoms arranged in a honeycomb geometry. These structures contain abundant functional groups on their edges (hydrophilic groups like carbonyl, carboxyl) and basal planes (hydrophobic groups like phenol, hydroxyl and epoxide), which make them a suitable carrier for both hydrophilic as well as hydrophobic drugs. Graphene oxides are not only promising drug carriers for the advancement of novel anticancer therapies but they also exhibit their own inhibitory effects on tumor cells (Zhang et al. 2017a). Functionalized graphene oxide nanocarriers have been developed for colon cancer targeting, for example, aminated graphene oxide nanocarriers developed by Krasteva et al. 2018 (Krasteva et al. 2019).

7.5.3.5 Nanosponges

Nanosponges are miniature porous dosage forms having a three-dimensional mesh-like structure made up of polymers. This mesh-like structure forms perforated insoluble nanoparticles that are capable of being loaded with a drug of choice. The resultant nanoparticles may be crystalline, amorphous or spherical. The release of drug through nanosponges may depend on the swelling properties of the polymer used.

Nanosponges may be used as carriers for lipophilic and lipophobic or hydrophilic drugs. The major method of preparation of nanosponges is solvent method, emulsion solvent diffusion method and ultrasound-assisted synthesis. Nanosponges find application in cancer therapy such as breast cancer and colon cancer (Vishwakarma et al. 2014; Shivani and Poladi 2015).

7.5.3.6 Nanofibres

Nanofibres represent a new group of drug delivery carriers. They are nanosized fibres prepared using various biodegradable polymers like keratin, collagen, silk fibroin, cellulose, gelatin, poly(lactic acid) (PLA), poly(lactic-co-glycolic acid) (PLGA), poly(ethylene-co-vinyl acetate) (PEVA), sodium alginate and chitosan.

They can be made by using methods such as extrusion, phase separation, stencil synthesis, electro-spinning, flocculation or self-assembly and so on. Nanofibres have been developed for inflammatory colon diseases and colon cancer (Shen et al. 2011; Širc et al. 2012; Akhgari et al. 2013; Wang et al. 2015; Yang et al. 2018).

7.5.3.7 Nanoglobular Systems; Self-Nano-Emulsifying Drug Delivery System (SNEDDS)

Self-nano-emulsifying drug delivery systems (SNEDDSs) are an isotropic mixture of drugs, lipids and surfactants and/or cosurfactants that form a nanoemulsion when introduced in aqueous media even by mild agitation (in vivo peristalsis provides such agitation). SNEDDS are prepared by simply mixing the desired oil, surfactant/co-surfactant and water in the composition range obtained after plotting the ternary phase diagram (TPD) (Seo et al. 2013; Mohd et al. 2015; Izham et al. 2019; Kazi et al. 2019). Bruceine SNEDDS were formulated by Dou et al. (2018), for the treatment of ulcerative colitis by improving their oral bioavailability (Gaikwad et al. 2017; Dou et al. 2018).

7.5.3.8 Nanogels

Nanogels are hydrogel-based porous nanoparticles, which thereby act as carriers for drug targeting. Nanogels, when prepared with functionalized nanoparticles, can be made responsive to certain stimuli like pH, temperature and other biological phenomena. Nanogels can be utilized for targeting drugs to tumor cells, including colon cancer (Ashwanikumar et al. 2012; Neamtu et al. 2017; Zhang et al. 2017a, b).

7.6 Targeting Approaches (Active) and Their Molecular Mechanism in Colon Targeting

Site-specific drug delivery to colon has several advantages, for example rapid onset of action, reduction of the drug dose, minimization of harmful side effects, etc. Different approaches for colon targeting includes chemical manipulation of a drug molecule to produce prodrugs, or making a drug delivery system with special polymers to make the system pH-dependent, time-dependent and/or bacterially biodegradable, etc. (discussed in detail in section 7.4) or modify them in a way that will enable active targeting (Sardo et al. 2019) .

Active targeting approach relies on disease-induced changes in the expression or overexpression of specific-receptors, proteins or adhesion molecules on top of the cell membranes of the tissue that is affected by disease. Many researches opting this approach use the parenteral route to target conditions such as cancer, infection or an inflammatory condition (Hua et al. 2015) . Figure 7.4 shows the targeting approaches of nanoformulation in colon drug delivery.

To create a targeted nanoparticle it is necessary to tag its surface with a molecule that will specifically bind to a cell-surface receptor characteristic of a pathology, or at least overexpressed in comparison to normal tissues, or even any extracellular molecule of interest (Sousa et al. 2019).

Table 7.1 enlists numerous active targeting approaches against colon cancer via nanoformulation approaches.

The ligands explored so far include the following:

A. *Aptamers:* Aptamers are oligonucleotides from DNA or RNA. They are usually single-stranded, non-immunogenic and of small size (from 20 to 50 nucleotides) and have elevated affinity and specificity towards their target molecule. They can be conjugated to a chemotherapeutic agent, nanoparticles, siRNA and solid-phase interphases for various therapeutic or diagnostic uses (Morita et al. 2018; Urmann et al. 2017).
B. *Antibodies*: Monoclonal antibodies (Mabs) were the first ones to be shown to bind with specific tumor antigens and were preferably used because of their high affinity, specificity and versatility. Antibodies have also been engineered to obtain a compact and multivalent structure, such as single-chain Fv antibody fragments (scFv), mini bodies, bispecific, diabodies, tribodies, etc. Antibody-conjugated nanoparticles have the desirable properties to overcome several conditions or barriers (Cardoso et al. 2012).
C. *Carbohydrate/lectin*: discussed in Sect. 7.6.1.
D. *Other Ligands*: Other than carbohydrate, aptamers, antibodies, ligands for example folate, peptides, hyaluronic have also been explored to bind to their specific receptors.

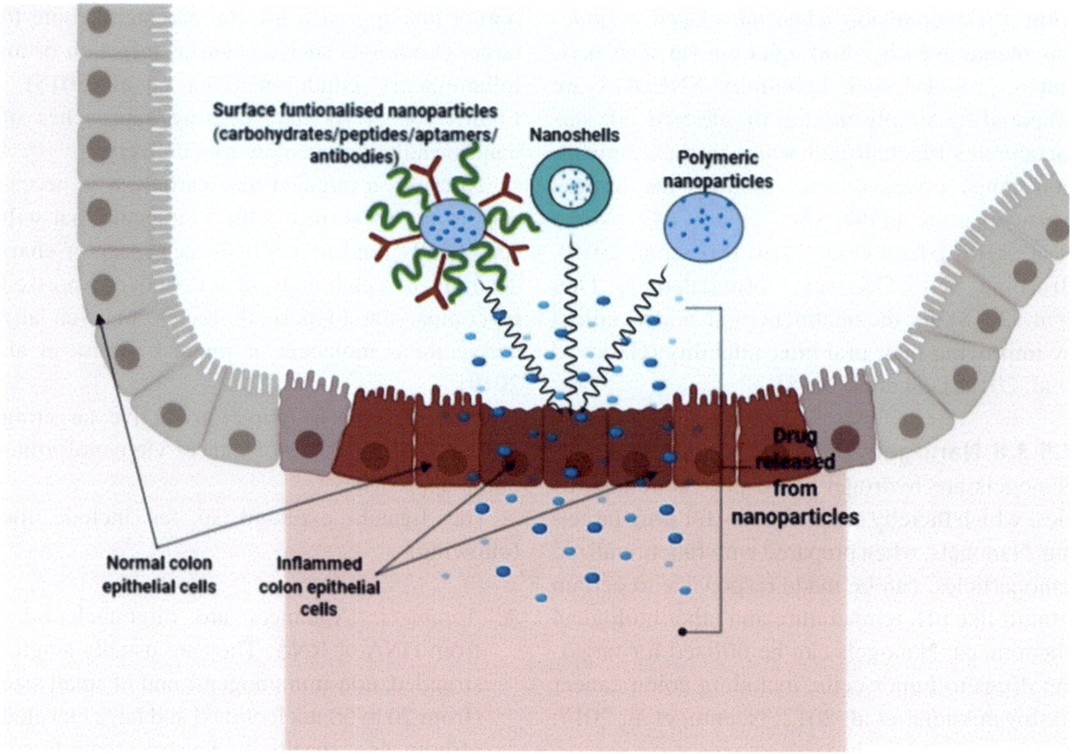

Fig. 7.4 Targeting approaches of nanoformulation in colon drug delivery

7.6.1 Targeting Inflammatory Bowel Disease

Inflammatory bowel disease is a term defining the group of colonic diseases, namely ulcerative colitis and Crohn's disease. Both have many similar clinical features, such as being characterized by relapsing cycles and remitting mucosal inflammation. Certain factors that are suggested to play a role in causing diseases are genetics, microbiome, environmental stress and immune dysfunction. The therapies for both Crohn's disease and ulcerative colitis include aminosalicylates, antibiotics, immune-suppressive agents and steroids. Monoclonal antibodies and peptides are capable of being used as specific targeting moieties, but their oral administration requires further formulation design to avoid encounters such as degradation by stomach acid and enzymes. Mannose receptors and galactose-type lectin receptors are overly expressed by activated macrophages under inflammatory conditions. Other targets for inflamed colon tissue are transferrin receptors, epithelial CD98 (a glycoprotein heterodimer) etc. (Hua et al. 2015). Each target for specific colon inflammatory diseases are described below.

7.6.1.1 Targeting Ulcerative Colitis

Targeting the cells affected by ulcerative colitis can be done by suppressing glucose (Jodeleit et al. 2018) or by host-directed therapy by targeting interleukin-13 (Hoving 2018). Such an approach hardly finds application in gastro intestinal tract as antibodies degrade in intestinal fluid due to pH-dependant denaturation or proteolysis (Moulari et al. 2014). The most common active targeting approaches for ulcerative colitis are discussed next.

Targeting CD44

Epithelial cells of colon and macrophages are strongly implicated in the inflammatory process

Table 7.1 Numerous targeting approaches against colon cancer via nanoformulation approaches

Targeting moiety	Nanoformulation	Drug	Approach/targeted	Outcome	References
Asiatic acid	Pegylated liposomes	Doxorubicin	Attenuating stroma collagen Cell line: SW620 Model: Xenograft mice (SW620)	Enhanced intratumor drug exposure	Fang et al. (2019)
Peptides (BR2 and CyLoP1)	PEGylated PAMAM dendrimers	7-Ethyl-10-hydroxy-camptothecin	Receptor not specified Cell lines: C26 Model: Mice bearing C26 tumor	Higher accumulation on tumor	Mahmoudi et al. (2019)
Folic acid	Nanoliposomes	5-fluorouracil	Receptor: Folate Cell line: Caco-2	Higher anti-tumor efficiency	Handali et al. (2019)
Jacalin	Pectin-gold nanoparticles	Inositol hexaphosphate	Targeted: antigenic disaccharides (overexpressed in most tumor) Cell line: HCT-15, NCM460 (M1) Model: 1,2-dimethylhydrazine (DMH) induced tumor model (M2)	Significant apoptotic effects in time and dose dependent manner. Restored several parameters that were distorted by DMH	Arya et al. (2019a, b)
Galactose	Chitosan-functionalized mesophoroussilica nanoparticles	5-fluorouracil	Targeted: galactin receptor Cell line: SW620	Higher cytotoxicity	Liu et al. (2018)
Transferrin	Poly(butylene adipate)/ terephthalate nanoparticles	5-fluorouracil	Targeted: transferrin receptors Cell line: HT-59	More cytotoxic effects compared to 5-fluorouracil and non-targeted nanoparticles	Varshosaz et al. (2017)
L-carnitine	PLGA nanoparticles	5-fluorouracil	Targeted: to transporter OCTN2 and ATB^{0+} Cell line: Caco-2 Model: 3D-spheroid model of tumor growth	Increase in uptake efficiency and cytotoxicity Enhanced antitumor efficacy	Kou et al. (2017)
Chondroitin sulphate	Polymeric nanoparticles	Camptothecin (CPT)	Targeted: CD44 Cell line: CT-26 Model: Tumor bearing BALB/c mice (CT-26)	Excellent in vitro colon cancer targeting capacity Improved anti-colon cancer activities compared to non-targeted NPs Favourable blood compatibility	Zu et al. (2019)
EpCAM	Mesophorous silica nanoparticles	Doxorubicin hydrochloride	Targeted: EpCAM Cell lines: SW620	Increased binding (to EpCAM positive cells) Enhanced cellular uptake Increased cytotoxicity and significant inhibition effects on SW620	Xie et al. (2016)
EpCAM	PLGA-lecithin-curcumin-PEG nanoparticles	Curcumin	Targeted: EpCAM Cell lines: HT29	Increased binding to HT29 colon cancer cells Enhancement in cellular uptake. Improvement in cytotoxicity toward HT29 cells Increased bioavailability of delivered CUR compared to that of free CUR in vivo	Li et al. (2014)
MUC1 aptamer	Superparamagnetic iron oxide nanoparticles	–	Targeted: MUC-1 Cell line: HT-29	Efficient delivery of NPs to the target cell line	Azhdarzadeh et al. (2016)

of colitis and CD44 is a transmembrane glycoprotein and is overexpressed on their surface. Hyaluronic acid is a biocompatible polysaccharide, and functionalization of nanoparticles with hyaluronic acid can increase cellular uptake of nanoparticles via hyaluronic acid-mediated endocytosis. Xiao et al. (2017) applied the same strategy and formulated hyaluronic acid-modified lysine-proline-valine nanoparticles and found the nanoparticles to be nontoxic, biocompatible with intestinal cells and enabled both mucosal healing as well as inflammatory relief in ulcerative colitis. After incorporating these nanoparticles into chitosan/alginate gel and administering it orally in mice, prevention of mucosal damage down-regulation of TNF-α and therapeutic efficacy was established to be stronger in hyaluronic acid nanoparticles than non-modified ones. This approach enabled therapeutic agents release into the colonic lumen, nanoparticles penetration into the colitis tissues and internalization. The strategy also proved to be efficient when Xiao et al., functionalized PLGA nanoparticles with hyaluronic acid (Xiao et al. 2015, 2017) .

Targeting Lectins/Carbohydrate Receptors

Melo-Junior et al. (2004) reported binding site alteration in ulcerative-colitis-affected tissue compared to healthy tissue. Wheat germ agglutinin (WGA), Lotus tetragonolobus agglutinin (LTA), etc. were used as histological markers. It presented a recognition pattern for affected tissues. There was a difference in carbohydrate expression. N-acetyl glucosamine, mannosidase and galactose were either not present or not available in normal tissues whereas L-fucose was present in the intestinal crypts of normal glands. There was elevated expression of N-acetylglucosamine and L-fucose in gland cells and inflammatory cells, respectively, in ulcerative colitis (Melo et al. 2004). Moulari et al. (2014) decorated PLGA nanoparticles with wheat germ agglutinin and peanut agglutinin due to their good resistance to acidic pH and enzymatic degradation and low cytotoxicity. Wheat germ agglutinin provided non-specific binding to the mucosa throughout the GIT whereas peanut agglutinin was a good candidate for specific targeting to the inflamed tissue. There was an enhanced therapeutic efficacy in the case of lectin-decorated nanoparticles (Moulari et al. 2014). In severe ulcerative colitis, lectin peanut binds to the N-acetyl-D-galactosamine that is overexpressed in the cells. It binds to the glycocalyx and/or apical region of columnar cells, crypt goblet cells and total cytoplasm of “regenerative or hyperplastic” epithelium, whereas in normal colon, it binds to the supranuclear (SN) portion of the goblet and columnar cells (Cooper et al. 1987).

Targeting Integrins

Integrins are the cell surface heterodimeric proteins, which are therapeutic targets. Integrins are highly expressed in human intestinal inflammation. β-7 integrins (α4β7and αEβ7) have been the potential targets for treating ulcerative colitis and have been targeted by the use of a monoclonal antibody etrolizumab (Stefanich et al. 2011; Goodman and Picard 2012) . Rodriguez-Nogales et al. (2016) functionalized silk-fibroin nanoparticles with RGD peptide and there was an improvement in the anti-inflammatory effects in trinitrobenzene sulfonic acid-induced experimental colitis in rats (Nogales et al. 2016).

C5a

C5a is a receptor that has found a role in inflammation, C5a-aptamer-conjugated nanoparticles have found to cause an improvement in colitis (Li et al. 2017) .

7.6.1.2 Targeting Crohn’s Disease

Too much tumor necrosis factor (TNF) or inappropriate production of TNF provokes chronic inflammation such as Crohn’s disease. A PEGylated Antibody’s fragment (Fab’s) of a humanized anti-TNF-α MAB (Certolizumapegol (CDP870) has shown clinical response and remission in Crohn’s disease in Phase III trials.

PEGylation enhances the half-life and reduces the frequent dosing requirement (Dinesen and Travis 2007). a4bx and a5b1 can be the integrin targets for Crohn's disease and can be targeted by TRK-170 and ATN-161, respectively (Stoeltzing et al. 2003; Goodman and Picard 2012; Sugiura et al. 2013).

7.6.1.3 Targeting Colorectal Cancer (CRC)

Numerous targeting approaches against colon cancer via nanoformulation approaches are mentioned in Table 7.1.

Cell-Adhesion Protein Carcinoembryonic Antigen (CEA)

These are also known as CEACAM5; CD66e. In healthy cases, the colon cells express this antigen through the apical side only, but once the tumorigenic course starts, basal lamina in the tissue does not remain defined anymore, cells start losing polarity and finally CEA is expressed in the entire surface. Targeting this antigen can be carried out by modifying the drug-loaded nanoparticles with a specific monoclonal antibody or a suitable aptamer (Sousa et al. 2019).

Tumor-Associated Glycoprotein-72 (TAG-72)

The overexpression of this membrane mucin is correlated with increased invasion and metastasis and advanced stage of the tumor. TAG-72 can be targeted by functionalizing the nanoparticles with antibodies (B72.3 and CC49), a variable heavy-chain domain of a heavy-chain antibody (VHH), etc. (Xu et al. 2010).

Folate Receptor-α (FRα)

This is a protein which is overly expressed on most cancer cell surfaces. However, its percentage in a normal cell membrane is limited. The receptor provides the folic acid to cancer cells for their need to biosynthesize DNA and RNA. The dissociation constant of the folate receptor and folic acid is about 0.1–1 nM. These receptors can be targeted by functionalizing the nanoparticles with folic acid (Silindir-Gunay et al. 2019; Soleymani et al. 2019).

CD44

CD44 has more than 20 isoforms, of which, CD44v6 is considered to be a molecular biomarker of breast and colorectal cancers. When a ligand like adaptor protein or cytoskeletal elements binds to the intracellular domains of CD44 receptor, conformational changes takes place that activate various pathways leading to cellular proliferation, adhesion, migration and invasion. This can be targeted by conjugating the drug-loaded nanoparticles with ligands such as hyaluronic acid, chondroitin sulfate, osteopontin, serglycin and fibrinb (Basakran 2015; Chen et al. 2018).

Epithelial Growth Factor Receptor (EGFR)

It is also called human EGF receptor (HER) or c-ernB1, and has an intrinsic protein tyrosine kinase activity. It is expressed in 60–80% colorectal cancers. The mechanisms by which it promotes tumorigenesis are diverse. Using nanoparticles, it is most commonly targeted by modifying nanoparticles with antibodies (Pabla et al. 2015).

Serum Carbohydrate Antigen 19-9 (CA 19-9)

The elevated serum concentration of this tumor marker is observed in metastatic colon cancer (Vukobrat-Bijedic et al. 2013; Yu et al. 2013). Specificity to detect CA 19-9 in colorectal cancer is 96%, but sensitivity lies only around 23%. Its elevated level is strongly related to poor projection in nodal-positive CRC after adjuvant chemotherapy completion, but not found useful in the case of nodal negative CRC. This antigen can be embattled by modifying nanoparticles with ligands such as L-fucose (Yu et al. 2017).

Alpha Fetoprotein (AFP)

Limited cases have been reported with AFP overexpressing colon cancer. The AFP-producing CRC are generally linked with poor prognosis due to frequent blood-borne metastases (Fu et al. 2006; Yachida et al. 2003).

Vascular Endothelial Growth Factor Receptor (VEGFR)

This is a significant angiogenic factor linked to the progression of tumor and its metastasis in many hematopoietic and solid malignancies. VEGF receptor-1 (VEGFR-1) or Flt-1is a receptor with high affinity for VEGF, and is found to be expressed in all colorectal cancer cell lines as described by Fan et al. (2005). Using nanoparticles, they can be targeted by modifying nanoparticles with polyclonal antibodies (Fan et al. 2005).

Transferrin Receptor Protein 1 (TfR1)

It is overexpressed in many types of cancers, but for colon cancer, more studies are needed (Shen et al. 2018).

Tyrosine Kinase Receptor c-MET

c-MET (mesenchymal-epithelial transition factor) is made active by hepatocyte growth factor and decides the course of numerous biological developments, such as cell scattering, survival and proliferation. Through various mechanisms, the genetic alteration of c-Met takes place, which is associated with the progression of colorectal cancer and its metastasis. It has also been shown that attribution to tumorigenesis and therapeutic resistance development also goes to crosstalk between various cell surface receptor and c-Met (Qamsari et al. 2017).

Epithelial Cell Adhesion Molecule (EpCAM)

It is a membranous glycoprotein (molecular weight: 40 kDa) that is coded by the GA733-2 gene.

EpCAM is overexpressed in many colorectal cancers. It is involved in many signal transductions. It can support cell motility and is associated with the proliferation of cells, their migration and invasion. EpCAM is targeted most commonly by modifying the nanoparticles with EpCAM aptamers (Li et al. 2014; Xie et al. 2016).

Death Receptor 5 (DR-5)

This is a cell-surface receptor which is overexpressed in patients suffering from stage II or stage III colorectal cancer. DR4 and DR5 receptors are found in cells of various human tissues and are also detected in some tumor cell lines, such as HeLa, Jurkat, Ramos, Colo205, etc. Identification of the death and cysteine-rich domains of DR4 and DR5 is 64% and 66%, respectively. Using nanoparticle approach, these receptors can be targeted by modifying them with Mabs (Ukrainskaya et al. 2017; Sousa et al. 2019).

7.7 Existing Nanoformulations for Colon Targeting

The nanoformulations that have been formulated for colon targeting are listed in Table 7.2.

Table 7.2 Existing nanoformulations for colon targeting

Existing nanoformulations	Polymer	Drug	Method	Route	Advantages	Toxicity study/ Cytotoxicity	Target	Reference
Co-polymeric hydrogels	Methacrylic acid (MAA) and itaconic acid (IA) through ethylene glycol dimethacrylate (EGDMA)	5-fluorouracil (5-FU) and leucovorin calcium (LV)	Aqueous-based free radical polymerization	Oral	Exhibited higher swelling and release at higher ph 7.4 compared to lower ph 1.2	Acute oral toxicity study on rabbits	Colon cancer	Abdullah et al. (2019)
Liposomes	1,2- dipalmitoyl-sn-glycero-3-phosphocholine (DPPC), N-(Carbonyl-methoxypolyethylenglycol-2000)-1,2-distearoyl-sn-glycero-3-phosphoethanolamine (Na salt) (MPEG-2000-DSPE), cholesterol (CHOL)	5-fluorouracil (5-FU)	Lipid film hydration	Parenteral	Formulation exhibited strong and similar inhibitory effect as that of 5-FU	C26 cells cultivated in monoculture as well as in co-culture with murine peritoneal macrophages	Colo-rectal cancer	Achim et al. (2017)
Nanoparticles	PLGA	Curcumin	Single emulsion solvent evaporation	Parenteral	Formulation possesses higher cellular uptake than native curcumin solution	Cellular uptake	Colon cancer	Akl et al. (2016)
pH sensitive microspheres	Hydrolyzed polyacrylamide-g-carboxymethylcellulose sodium (paam-g-Na CMC) co-polymer	Capecitabine	Co-polymer synthesized through free radical polymerisation	Oral	pH sensitive targeting to colon	–	Colon cancer	Alange et al. (2017)
Nanoparticles	PLGA	Budenoside	Oil in water emulsion evaporation technique	Parenteral	Efficient targeting	–	Inflammatory bowel disease	Ali et al. (2016)
Matrix	Chitosan PLGA	SN-38(7-ethyl-10-hydroxy camptothecin)	Single emulsion method	Parenteral	Targeted delivery to integrin overexpressed cancer cells	Cytotoxicity	Colon adenocarcinoma	Alibolandi et al. (2018)
Polymersomes	PEG-PLGA	Camptothecin	–	Parenteral	Increase in therapeutic index of camptothecin	Cytotoxicity HT29, C26 and CHO cell line	Colon adenocarcinoma	Alibolandi et al. (2017a)
Dendrimers	Polyamidoaminedendrimer generation 5 (PAMAM G5)	Camptothecin and anti-nucleolinaptamer AS1411	Two step reaction through EDC/NHS	Parenteral (i.v.)	Selective delivery to nucleolin-positive colorectal cancer cells, growth inhibition and increased the cellular uptake	Cytotoxicity HT29, C26 and CHO cell line	Colorectal cancer	Alibolandi et al. (2017b)

(continued)

Table 7.2 (continued)

Existing nanoformulations	Polymer	Drug	Method	Route	Advantages	Toxicity study/ Cytotoxicity	Target	Reference
Tablets	Pluronic F-127 and PEG 6000	Fluticasone propionate	Press coated tablets	Oral	Colonic drug delivery with improved dissolution	–	Crohn's disease and Ulcerative colitis	Al-Zheery and Kamal (2016)
Liposome	Leptin-derived peptide (LP16, 91–110 of Leptin,), Mal-PEG2000-DSPE	Pegylated liposomal doxorubicin(PLD, Doxil®)	Post-insertion method	Parenteral	Increased therapeutic efficacy of LP16 peptide	C26 cell line	Colon carcinoma	Amiri Darban et al. (2018)
Magnetic nanoparticles	Tetraethylorthosilicate (TEOS),	Epirubicin	Modified co- precipitation method, Alkaline hydrolysis	Parenteral	Low systemic toxicity and high tumor cell uptake	C26 cell line	Colorectal cancer	Ansari et al. (2018)
Hydrogel bead	Portulaca mucilage	5-fluorouracil	Ionotropic gelation	Oral	Sustained release of up to 16 hr in colon	HT-29 cell line	Colon cancer	Asnani and Kokare (2018)
Nanoparticles	MUC1 aptamer	Epirubicin	–	Parenteral	Significant inhibition of tumor growth as compared to epirubicin alone. Also showed synergistic effect.	MCF-7 and CHO cells	Colon cancer	Bahreyni et al. (2019)
Hydrogel	Poly(methoxyl ethylene glycol-caprolactone)-acryloyl Chloride (MPEG-PCL-AC) copolymers	5 aminosalicylic acid	Free radical polymerisation	Oral	Effective oral colon targeting system	–	Ulcerative colitis	Bai et al. (2016)
Polymerosomes	Chitosan	Quantum dots	Crosslinking	Parenteral	Effective delivery in lymph nodes	Colon cancer grafted mice	Colon cancer	Bakalova et al. (2015)
Hydrogels	Methacrylic acid and chondroitin sulphate	Oxaliplatin	Free radical polymerisation	–	Nontoxic to biological systems	Toxicity study on rabbits	Colorectal cancer	Barkat et al. (2017)
Nanoparticles	Thiourea, Boron-doped p-Si (100) chip	Silica nps	Galvanostaticanodization of porous silicon layer	–	Time dependent uptake	Caco-2 and CCD cells	EGFR overexpression in cancer cells	Behray et al. (2016)
Nanocapsules	Poly-L-glutamic acid sodium salt, PGA and Poly-L- lysine hydrobromide, PLL.	Camptothecin	Encapsulation	–	Similar activity of free and encapsulated drug provides for an alternative delivery.	CT26-CEA and 4T1	Colon cancer and mammary carcinoma	Bzowska et al. (2018)
Nanoparticles	PLGA, YI peptide	Paclitaxel	Emulsion solvent evaporation method	Parenteral	Tumor microenvironment targeting	HT-26 colorectal tumor-bearing mice	Colon cancer	Cao et al. (2018)
Microcapsules	Alginate, Chitosan	Interlukin 1 Ra (IL1-Ra)	Single-step electrospraying	Oral	Oral delivery of proteins	–	DSS induced colitis	Cao et al. (2019)

Nanovesicles	PEG, Chitosan, Nutriose, soy phosphatidylcholine	Quercetin	–	–	Synergistic effects due to quercetin, chitosan and nutriose	–	Chronic intestinal inflammatory diseases	Castangia et al. (2015)
Nanoparticles	Poly(N-isopropylacrylamide) and hyaluronic acid	Doxorubicin	Inverse mini-emulsion and click chemistry	–	Twice active against cancer cells than healthy fibroblasts	HT29 and NIH 3T3	Colon adenocarcinoma	Cerroni et al. (2015)
Nanoparticles	Calcium carbonate and MUC1-Dimer aptamers as targeting agents	Epirubicin (Epi) and melittin (Mel)	Water in oil emulsion method	–	Better control of tumor growth and synergistic effect due to co-delivery of Epi and Mel	MCF7 and C26	Colorectal cancer	Yazdian-Robati et al. (2019)
3WJ RNA nanoparticles	Epcam19 aptamers as targeting ligands	D5Dtarget sirna	Bottom up approach	–	Significant suppression of xenograft tumor growth in mice bearing HCA-7 tumors	HCA-7	Colon cancer	Xu et al. (2019)
Hydrogel	Tragacanth gum, Itaconic acid,	Ciprofloxacin	Graft polymerisation	–	pH sensitive release up to colon	–	Colon	Verma (2019)
Nonpolymer, pH-sensitive carbon dots (PSCDS)	Citric acid (CA) and 1-(3-aminopropyl) imidazole	Doxorubicin	One spot synthesis	–	Drug released 7 times more than control	HCT-116 (human colon cancer), PANC-1 (human pancreatic cancer), and SKBR-3 (human breast cancer)	Colon cancer	Seo et al. (2019)
Liposome	1, 2–Distearoyl–sn–glycero-3-phosphocholine (DSPC)	5-FU, apigenin	Modified thin film hydration method	–	Passive targeting and synergistic effect leads to higher anti-neoplastic and anti-tumorigenic effect	Nude mice tumor xenograft model, HT 29 cells	Colorectal cancer	Sen et al. (2019)
Minicapsules	1,2-dipalmitoyl-sn-glycero-3-phosphocholine(DPPC)	HBsAg	Solvent evaporation technique	Oral	Formulation induced significant mucosal immunity	Bone marrow-derived DCS (BMDCS)	Colon targeting	Sahu et al. (2019)

(continued)

Table 7.2 (continued)

Existing nanoformulations	Polymer	Drug	Method	Route	Advantages	Toxicity study/ Cytotoxicity	Target	Reference
Pegylated multi-walled carbon nanotubes	Hyaluronic acid	Gemcitabine	Synthesis	–	Increased survival rate show MWCNT are safe and effective	HT-29	Colon cancer	Prajapati et al. (2019)
Nanoparticles	Chitosan, chondroitin sulphate (CS)-modified PLGA	10-Hydroxy camptothecin (HCPT),	Solvent evaporation	–	Efficacy of chondroitin sulphate as CD44 targeting agent, maintains body weight reduces tumor nodules	C26 cells	Colon cancer	Liu et al. (2019)
Co-polymeric hydrogels	Methacrylic acid (MAA) and itaconic acid (IA) through ethylene glycol dimethacrylate (EGDMA)	5-fluorouracil (5-FU) and leucovorin calcium (LV)	Aqueous-based free radical polymerization	Oral	Exhibited higher swelling and release at higher ph 7.4 as compared to lower ph 1.2.	Acute oral toxicity study on rabbits.	Colon cancer	Abdullah et al. (2019)
Liposomes	1,2- dipalmitoyl-sn-glycero-3-phosphocholine (DPPC), N-(Carbonyl-methoxypolyethylenglycol-2000)-1,2-distearoyl-sn-glycero-3-phosphoethanolamine (Na salt) (MPEG-2000-DSPE), cholesterol (CHOL)	5-fluorouracil (5-FU)	Lipid film hydration	Parenteral	Formulation exhibited strong and similar inhibitory effect as that of 5-FU	C26 cells cultivated in monoculture as well as in co-culture with murine peritoneal macrophages.	Colo-rectal cancer	Achim et al. (2017)
Nanoparticles	PLGA	Curcumin	Single emulsion solvent evaporation	Parenteral	Formulation possesses higher cellular uptake than native curcumin solution	Cellular uptake	Colon cancer	Akl et al. (2016)
pH sensitive microspheres	Hydrolyzed polyacrylamide-g-carboxymethylcellulose sodium (paam-g-Na CMC) co-polymer	Capecitabine	Co-polymer synthesized through free radical polymerisation	Oral	pH sensitive targeting to colon	–	Colon cancer	Alange et al. (2017)
Nanoparticles	PLGA	Budenoside	Oil in water emulsion evaporation technique	Parenteral	Efficient targeting	–	Inflammatory bowel disease	Ali et al. (2016)
Matrix	Chitosan PLGA	SN-38(7-ethyl-10-hydroxy camptothecin)	Single emulsion method	Parenteral	Targeted delivery to integrin overexpressed cancer cells	Cytotoxicity	Colon adenocarcinoma	Alibolandi et al. (2018)

Polymersomes	PEG-PLGA	Camptothecin	–	Parenteral	Increase in therapeutic index of camptothecin	Cytotoxicity HT29, C26 and CHO cell line	Colon adenocarcinoma.	Alibolandi et al. (2017a)
Dendrimers	Polyamidoaminedendrimer generation 5 (PAMAM G5)	Camptothecin and anti-nucleolinaptamer AS1411	Two step reaction through EDC/NHS	Parenteral (i.v.)	Selective delivery to nucleolin-positive colorectal cancer cells, growth inhibition and increased the cellular uptake	Cytotoxicity HT29, C26 and CHO cell line	Colorectal cancer	Alibolandi et al. (2017b)
Tablets	Pluronic F-127 and PEG 6000	Fluticasone propionate	Press coated tablets	Oral	Colonic drug delivery with improved dissolution	–	Crohn's disease and vlcerative colitis	Al-Zheery and Kamal (2016)
Liposome	Leptin-derived peptide (LP16, 91–110 of Leptin,), Mal-PEG2000-DSPE	Pegylated liposomal doxorubicin(PLD, Doxil®)	Post-insertion method	Parenteral	Increased therapeutic efficacy of LP16 peptide	C26 cell line	Colon carcinoma	Amiri Darban et al. (2018)
Magnetic nanoparticles	Tetraethylorthosilicate (TEOS),	Epirubicin	Modified co- precipitation method, Alkaline hydrolysis	Parenteral	Low systemic toxicity and high tumor cell uptake	C26 cell line	Colorectal cancer	Ansari et al. (2018)
Hydrogel bead	Portulaca mucilage	5-fluorouracil	Ionotropic gelation	Oral	Sustained release of up to 16 hr in colon	HT-29 cell line	Colon cancer	Asnani and Kokare (2018)
Nanoparticles	MUC1 aptamer	Epirubicin	–	Parenteral	Significant inhibition of tumor growth as compared to epirubicin alone. Also showed synergistic effect.	MCF-7 and CHO cells	Colon cancer	Bahreyni et al. (2019)
Hydrogel	Poly(methoxyl ethylene glycol-caprolactone)-acryloyl Chloride (MPEG-PCL-AC) copolymers	5 aminosalicylic acid	Free radical polymerisation	Oral	Effective oral colon targeting system	–	Ulcerative colitis	Bai et al. (2016)
Polymerosomes	Chitosan	Quantum dots	Crosslinking	Parenteral	Effective delivery in lymph nodes	Colon cancer grafted mice	Colon cancer	Bakalova et al. (2015)
Hydrogels	Methacrylic acid and chondroitin sulphate	Oxaliplatin	Free radical polymerisation	–	Nontoxic to biological systems	Toxicity study on rabbits	Colorectal cancer	Barkat et al. (2017)

(continued)

Table 7.2 (continued)

Existing nanoformulations	Polymer	Drug	Method	Route	Advantages	Toxicity study/ Cytotoxicity	Target	Reference
Nanoparticles	Thiourea, Boron-doped p-Si (100) chip	Silica NPs	Galvanostaticanodization of porous silicon layer	–	Time dependent uptake	Caco-2 and CCD cells	EGFR overexpression in cancer cells	Behray et al. (2016)
Nanocapsules	Poly-L-glutamic acid sodium salt, PGA and Poly-L- lysine hydrobromide, PLL.	Camptothecin	Encapsulation	–	Similar activity of free and encapsulated drug provides for an alternative delivery	CT26-CEA and 4T1	Colon cancer and mammary carcinoma	Bzowska et al. (2018)
Nanoparticles	PLGA, YI peptide	Paclitaxel	Emulsion solvent evaporation method	Parenteral	Tumor microenvironment targeting	HT-26 colorectal tumor-bearing mice	Colon cancer	Cao et al. (2018)
Microcapsules	Alginate, Chitosan	Interlukin 1 Ra (IL1-Ra)	Single-step electrospraying	Oral	Oral delivery of proteins	–	DSS-induced colitis	Cao et al. (2019)
Nanovesicles	PEG, Chitosan, Nutriose, soy phosphatidylcholine	Quercetin	–	–	Synergistic effects due to quercetin, chitosan and nutriose	–	Chronic intestinal inflammatory diseases	Castangia et al. (2015)
Nanoparticles	Poly(N-isopropylacrylamide) and hyaluronic acid	Doxorubicin	Inverse mini-emulsion and click chemistry	–	Twice active against cancer cells than healthy fibroblasts	HT29 and NIH 3T3	Colon adenocarcinoma	Cerroni et al. (2015)
Nanoparticles	Calcium carbonate and MUC1-Dimer aptamers as targeting agents	Epirubicin (Epi) and melittin (Mel)	Water in oil emulsion method	–	Better control of tumor growth and synergistic effect due to co-delivery of Epi and Mel	MCF7 and C26	Colorectal cancer	Yazdian-Robati et al. (2019)
3WJ RNA nanoparticles	Epcam19 aptamers as targeting ligands	D5Dtarget sirna	Bottom up approach	–	Significant suppression of xenograft tumor growth in mice bearing HCA-7 tumors	HCA-7	Colon cancer	Xu et al. (2019)
Hydrogel	Tragacanth gum, Itaconic acid,	Ciprofloxacin	Graft polymerisation	–	pH sensitive release up to colon	–	Colon	Verma et al. (2019)

Nonpolymer, pH-sensitive carbon dots (PSCDS)	Citric acid (CA) and 1-(3-aminopropyl) imidazole	Doxorubicin	One spot synthesis	–	Drug released 7 times more than control	HCT-116 (human colon cancer), PANC-1 (human pancreatic cancer), and SKBR-3 (human breast cancer)	Colon cancer	Seo et al. (2019)
Liposome	1, 2–Distearoyl–sn–glycero-3-phosphocholine (DSPC)	5-FU, apigenin	Modified thin film hydration method	–	Passive targeting and synergistic effect leads to higher anti-neoplastic and anti-tumorigenic effect	Nude mice tumor xenograft model, HT 29 cells	Colorectal cancer	Sen et al. (2019)
Minicapsules	1,2-dipalmitoyl-sn-glycero-3-phosphocholine(DPPC)	HBsAg	Solvent evaporation technique	Oral	Formulation induced significant mucosal immunity	Bone-marrow-derived DCS (BMDCS)	Colon targeting	Sahu et al. (2019)
Pegylated multi-walled carbon nanotubes	Hyaluronic acid	Gemcitabine	Synthesis	–	Increased survival rate show MWCNT are safe and effective	HT-29	Colon cancer	Prajapati et al. (2019)
Nanoparticles	Chitosan, chondroitin sulphate (CS)-modified PLGA	10-Hydroxy camptothecin (HCPT),	Solvent evaporation	–	Efficacy of chondroitin sulphate as CD44 targeting agent, maintains body weight reduces tumor nodules	C26 cells	Colon cancer	Liu et al. (2019)

7.8 Conclusion

The colon is an intricate but highly suitable site for targeting drugs for localized as well systemic effects. Even highly degradable drugs like proteins and peptides can be targeted to the colon. Nanoparticle approach for drug targeting forms one of the hopeful, up-and-coming approaches for targeting drugs to colon as they decrease the amount of drug required for therapeutic action, thereby minimizing the toxicity and reducing the side effects.

Thus far, several strategies using nanoparticles have been designed to target colon by both active and passive means. Despite this, millions die from colonic diseases. This may be due to the unavailability of nanoformulated products in the market or the higher cost at which these are produced. Even though we have attained many advances in nanotechnology, conventional dosage forms remain the most utilized for colonic diseases and a cure eludes the target group. Approaches like particle size, surface decoration with ligands, aptamers, carbohydrates, antibodies, various materials as design strategy for targeting, pH sensitivity, microbially triggered systems, redox-sensitive polymers coatings, enzyme sensitive, those that use smart polymer technology, and so on are all systems that can be used for the alleviation of colonic disease-related suffering. Hence, we need to take steps to translate the scope of these nanosystems from bed to bench side. The promise to significantly, prevent, treat and cure colon diseases is one that should enable many such products to be available for patients in the near future.

References

Abderrezak A, Bourassa P, Mandeville J-S, Sedaghat-Herati R, Tajmir-Riahi H-A (2012) Dendrimers bind antioxidant polyphenols and cisplatin drug. PLoS One 7(3):e33102–e33102. https://doi.org/10.1371/journal.pone.0033102

Abdullah O, Usman Minhas M, Ahmad M, Ahmad S, Ahmad A (2019) Synthesis of hydrogels for combinatorial delivery of 5-fluorouracil and leucovorin calcium in colon cancer: optimization, in vitro characterization and its toxicological evaluation. Polym Bull 76(6):3017–3037. https://doi.org/10.1007/s00289-018-2509-5

Aburahma MH (2016) Bile salts-containing vesicles: promising pharmaceutical carriers for oral delivery of poorly water-soluble drugs and peptide/protein-based therapeutics or vaccines. Drug Deliv 23(6):1847–1867. https://doi.org/10.3109/10717544.2014.976892

Achim M, Tomuță I, Muntean D, Porfire A, Tefas LR, Patras, Licarete E, Costel M (2017) Optimization and in vitro evaluation of 5-fluorouracil – loaded long – circulating liposomes. Farmacia 65(1):82–91

Ag Seleci D, Seleci M, Walter J-G, Stahl F, Scheper T (2016) Niosomes as nanoparticular drug carriers: fundamentals and recent applications. J Nanomater 2016:7372306

Ahmadi E, Zarghami N, Asghari Jafarabadi M, Alizadeh L, Khojastehfard M, Rahmati Yamchi M, Salehi R (2019) Enhanced anticancer potency by combination chemotherapy of HT-29 cells with biodegradable, pH-sensitive nanoparticles for co-delivery of hydroxytyrosol and doxorubicin. J Drug Deliv Sci Technol 51. https://doi.org/10.1016/j.jddst.2019.03.003

Akbarzadeh A, Rezaei-Sadabady R, Davaran S, Joo SW, Zarghami N, Hanifehpour Y et al (2013) Liposome: classification, preparation, and applications. Nanoscale Res Lett 8(1):102

Akhgari A, Heshmati Z, Makhmalzadeh BS (2013) Indomethacin electrospun nanofibers for colonic drug delivery: preparation and characterization. Adv Pharm Bullet 3(1):85

Akl MA, Kartal-Hodzic A, Oksanen T, Ismael HR, Afouna MM, Yliperttula M et al (2016) Factorial design formulation optimization and in vitro characterization of curcumin-loaded PLGA nanoparticles for colon delivery. J Drug Deliv Sci Technol 32:10–20. https://doi.org/10.1016/j.jddst.2016.01.007

Alange VV, Birajdar RP, Kulkarni RV (2017) Novel spray dried pH-sensitive polyacrylamide-grafted-carboxymethylcellulose sodium copolymer microspheres for colon targeted delivery of an anti-cancer drug. J Biomater Sci Polym Ed 28(2):139–161. https://doi.org/10.1080/09205063.2016.1257083

Alavi M, Karimi N, Safaei M (2017) Application of various types of liposomes in drug delivery systems. Adv Pharm Bullet 7(1):3

Ali H, Weigmann B, Collnot EM, Khan SA, Windbergs M, Lehr CM (2016) Budesonide loaded PLGA nanoparticles for targeting the inflamed intestinal mucosa--pharmaceutical characterization and fluorescence imaging. Pharm Res 33(5):1085–1092. https://doi.org/10.1007/s11095-015-1852-6

Alibolandi M, Rezvani R, Farzad SA, Taghdisi SM, Abnous K, Ramezani M (2017a) Tetrac-conjugated polymersomes for integrin-targeted delivery of camptothecin to colon adenocarcinoma in vitro and in vivo. Int J Pharm 532(1):581–594. https://doi.org/10.1016/j.ijpharm.2017.09.039

Alibolandi M, Taghdisi SM, Ramezani P, Hosseini Shamili F, Farzad SA, Abnous K, Ramezani M (2017b) Smart AS1411-aptamer conjugated pegylated PAMAM dendrimer for the superior delivery of camptothecin to colon adenocarcinoma in vitro and in vivo. Int J Pharm 519(1–2):352–364. https://doi.org/10.1016/j.ijpharm.2017.01.044

Alibolandi M, Amel Farzad S, Mohammadi M, Abnous K, Taghdisi SM, Kalalinia F, Ramezani M (2018) Tetrac-decorated chitosan-coated PLGA nanoparticles as a new platform for targeted delivery of SN38. Artif Cells Nanomed Biotechnol 46(sup2):1003–1014. https://doi.org/10.1080/21691401.2018.1477789

Allémann E, Leroux J-C, Gurny R (1998) Polymeric nano-and microparticles for the oral delivery of peptides and peptidomimetics. Adv Drug Deliv Rev 34(2–3):171–189

Al-Zheery WH, Kamal BA (2016) Formulation and evaluation of fluticasone propionate colon targeted tablet. Int J Pharm Sci Rev Res 41(2):322–329

Amidon S, Brown JE, Dave VS (2015) Colon-targeted oral drug delivery systems: design trends and approaches. AAPS PharmSciTech 16(4):731–741

Amiri Darban S, Nikoofal-Sahlabadi S, Amiri N, Kiamanesh N, Mehrabian A, Zendehbad B et al (2018) Targeting the leptin receptor: to evaluate therapeutic efficacy and anti-tumor effects of Doxil, in vitro and in vivo in mice bearing C26 colon carcinoma tumor. Colloids Surf B: Biointerfaces 164:107–115. https://doi.org/10.1016/j.colsurfb.2018.01.035

Anbarasan B, Rekha S, Elango K, Shriya B, Ramaprabhu S (2013) Optimization of the formulation and in-vitro evaluation of Capecitabine Niosomes for the treatment of Colon Cancer. Int J Pharm Sci Res 4(4):1504

Ansari L, Jaafari MR, Bastami TR, Malaekeh-Nikouei B (2018) Improved anticancer efficacy of epirubicin by magnetic mesoporous silica nanoparticles: in vitro and in vivo studies. Artif Cells Nanomed Biotechnol 46(sup2):594–606. https://doi.org/10.1080/21691401.2018.1464461

Arya M, Mishra N, Singh P, Tripathi CB, Parashar P, Singh M, ... & Saraf SA. (2019a) In vitro and in silico molecular interaction of multiphase nanoparticles containing inositol hexaphosphate and jacalin: Therapeutic potential against colon cancer cells (HCT-15). J Cell Physiol 234(9):15527–15536

Arya M, Singh P, Tripathi CB, Parashar P, Singh M, Kanoujia J et al (2019b) Pectin-encrusted gold nanocomposites containing phytic acid and jacalin: 1, 2-dimethylhydrazine-induced colon carcinogenesis in Wistar rats, PI3K/Akt, COX-2, and serum metabolomics as potential targets. Drug Deliv Transl Res 9(1):53–65

Ashwanikumar N, Kumar NA, Nair SA, Kumar GV (2012) Methacrylic-based nanogels for the pH-sensitive delivery of 5-fluorouracil in the colon. Int J Nanomedicine 7:5769

Asnani GP, Kokare CR (2018) In vitro and in vivo evaluation of colon cancer targeted epichlorohydrin crosslinked Portulaca-alginate beads. Biomol Concepts 9(1):190–199. https://doi.org/10.1515/bmc-2018-0019

Atlanta G (2015) Cancer facts and figures. name of press, pace of publication, page range ??

Azeez NA, Deepa VS, Sivapriya V (2018) Phytosomes: emergent promising nano vesicular drug delivery system for targeted tumor therapy. Adv Nat Sci Nanosci Nanotechnol 9(3):033001

Azhdarzadeh M, Atyabi F, Saei AA, Varnamkhasti BS, Omidi Y, Fateh M et al (2016) Theranostic MUC-1 aptamer targeted gold coated superparamagnetic iron oxide nanoparticles for magnetic resonance imaging and photothermal therapy of colon cancer. Colloids Surf B: Biointerfaces 143:224–232

Bahreyni A, Alibolandi M, Ramezani M, Sarafan Sadeghi A, Abnous K, Taghdisi SM (2019) A novel MUC1 aptamer-modified PLGA-epirubicin-PβAE-antimir-21 nanocomplex platform for targeted co-delivery of anticancer agents in vitro and in vivo. Colloids Surf B: Biointerfaces 175:231–238. https://doi.org/10.1016/j.colsurfb.2018.12.006

Bai XY, Yan Y, Wang L, Zhao LG, Wang K (2016) Novel pH-sensitive hydrogels for 5-aminosalicylic acid colon targeting delivery: in vivo study with ulcerative colitis targeting therapy in mice. Drug Deliv 23(6):1926–1932. https://doi.org/10.3109/10717544.2014.996924

Bakalova R, Lazarova D, Nikolova B, Atanasova S, Zlateva G, Zhelev Z, Aoki I (2015) Delivery of size-controlled long-circulating polymersomes in solid tumours, visualized by quantum dots and optical imaging in vivo. Biotechnol Biotechnol Equip 29(1):175–180. https://doi.org/10.1080/13102818.2014.984894

Barkat K, Ahmad M, Minhas MU, Khalid I (2017) Oxaliplatin-loaded crosslinked polymeric network of chondroitin sulfate-co-poly(methacrylic acid) for colorectal cancer: its toxicological evaluation. J Appl Polym Sci 134(38). https://doi.org/10.1002/app.45312

Basakran NS (2015) CD44 as a potential diagnostic tumor marker. Saudi Med J 36(3):273

Behray M, Webster CA, Pereira S, Ghosh P, Krishnamurthy S, Al-Jamal WT, Chao Y (2016) Synthesis of diagnostic silicon nanoparticles for targeted delivery of Thiourea to epidermal growth factor receptor-expressing cancer cells. ACS Appl Mater Interfaces 8(14):8908–8917. https://doi.org/10.1021/acsami.5b12283

Beloqui A, Coco R, Alhouayek M, Solinís MÁ, Rodríguez-Gascón A, Muccioli GG, Préat V (2013) Budesonide-loaded nanostructured lipid carriers reduce inflammation in murine DSS-induced colitis. Int J Pharm 454(2):775–783

Bharti C, Nagaich U, Pal AK, Gulati N (2015) Mesoporous silica nanoparticles in target drug delivery system: a review. Int J Pharm Investig 5(3):124–133. https://doi.org/10.4103/2230-973X.160844

Bratten J, Jones MP (2006) New directions in the assessment of gastric function: clinical applications of physiologic measurements. Dig Dis 24(3–4):252–259

Bzowska M, Karabasz A, Szczepanowicz K (2018) Encapsulation of camptothecin into pegylated polyelectrolyte nanocarriers. Colloids Surf A Physicochem

Eng Asp 557:36–42. https://doi.org/10.1016/j.colsurfa.2018.05.070
Cao D, Liang L, Xu Y, Sun J, Lei M, Wang M et al (2018) Tumor associated macrophages and angiogenesis dual-recognizable nanoparticles for enhanced cancer chemotherapy. Nanomedicine 14(3):651–659. https://doi.org/10.1016/j.nano.2017.12.018
Cao J, Cheng J, Xi S, Qi X, Shen S, Ge Y (2019) Alginate/chitosan microcapsules for in-situ delivery of the protein, interleukin-1 receptor antagonist (IL-1Ra), for the treatment of dextran sulfate sodium (DSS)-induced colitis in a mouse model. Eur J Pharm Biopharm 137:112–121. https://doi.org/10.1016/j.ejpb.2019.02.011
Cardoso MM, Peca IN, Roque ACA (2012) Antibody-conjugated nanoparticles for therapeutic applications. Curr Med Chem 19(19):3103–3127
Castangia I, Nácher A, Caddeo C, Merino V, Díez-Sales O, Catalán-Latorre A et al (2015) Therapeutic efficacy of quercetin enzyme-responsive nanovesicles for the treatment of experimental colitis in rats. Acta Biomater 13:216–227. https://doi.org/10.1016/j.actbio.2014.11.017
Cerroni B, Pasale SK, Mateescu A, Domenici F, Oddo L, Bordi F, Paradossi G (2015) Temperature-tunable nanoparticles for selective biointerface. Biomacromolecules 16(6):1753–1760. https://doi.org/10.1021/acs.biomac.5b00268
Chandran SP, Nachinmuthu KP, Natarajan SB, Inamdar MG, Shahimi MS (2018) Papain loaded solid lipid nanoparticles for colorectal cancer therapy. Curr Cancer Therapy Rev 14(1):75–87
Chen C, Zhao S, Karnad A, Freeman JW (2018) The biology and role of CD44 in cancer progression: therapeutic implications. J Hematol Oncol 11(1):64
Chourasia M, Jain S (2004) Polysaccharides for colon targeted drug delivery. Drug Deliv 11(2):129–148
Collnot E-M, Ali H, Lehr C-M (2012) Nano-and microparticulate drug carriers for targeting of the inflamed intestinal mucosa. J Control Release 161(2):235–246
Cooper H, Farano P, Coapman R (1987) Peanut lectin binding sites in colons of patients with ulcerative colitis. Arch Pathol Lab Med 111(3):270–275
Das S, Deshmukh R, Jha A (2010) Role of natural polymers in the development of multiparticulate systems for colon drug targeting. Syst Rev Pharm 1(1):79
Dianzani C, Foglietta F, Ferrara B, Rosa AC, Muntoni E, Gasco P et al (2017) Solid lipid nanoparticles delivering anti-inflammatory drugs to treat inflammatory bowel disease: effects in an in vivo model. World J Gastroenterol 23(23):4200
Dinesen L, Travis S (2007) Targeting nanomedicines in the treatment of Crohn's disease: focus on certolizumab pegol (CDP870). Int J Nanomedicine 2(1):39
Dineshkumar B, Krishnakumar K, Bhatt AR, Paul D, Cherian J, John A, Suresh S (2015) Single-walled and multi-walled carbon nanotubes based drug delivery system: cancer therapy: a review. Indian J Cancer 52(3):262–264. https://doi.org/10.4103/0019-509x.176720
Dong R, Wang M, Dong F (2015) The new progress and outlook of oral colon-specific drug delivery system for treating cancer. Int J Adv Med Sci 3:25–32
Dou Y-X, Zhou J-T, Wang T-T, Huang Y-F, Chen VP, Xie Y-L et al (2018) Self-nanoemulsifying drug delivery system of bruceine D: a new approach for anti-ulcerative colitis. Int J Nanomedicine 13:5887
Elnaggar YSR (2015) Multifaceted applications of bile salts in pharmacy: an emphasis on nanomedicine. Int J Nanomedicine 10:3955–3971. https://doi.org/10.2147/IJN.S82558
Elzagheid A, Ålgars A, Bendardaf R, Lamlum H, Ristamaki R, Collan Y et al (2006) E-cadherin expression pattern in primary colorectal carcinomas and their metastases reflects disease outcome. World J Gastroenterol: WJG 12(27):4304
Fan F, Fan F, Wey JS, MF MC, Belcheva A, Liu W, Bauer TW, Somcio RJ, Wu Y, Hooper A, Hicklin DJ, Ellis LM (2005) Expression and function of vascular endothelial growth factor receptor-1 on human colorectal cancer cells. Oncogene 24:2647–2653. https://doi.org/10.1038/sj.onc.1208246
Fang L, Kong S-S, Zhong L-K, Wang C-M, Liu Y-J, Ding H-Y et al (2019) Asiatic acid enhances intratumor delivery and the antitumor effect of pegylated liposomal doxorubicin by reducing tumor-stroma collagen. Acta Pharmacol Sin 40(4):539
Feng B, Zhou F, Wang D, Xu Z, Yu H, Li Y (2016a) Gold nanomaterials for treatment of metastatic cancer. Sci China Chem 59(8):984–990. https://doi.org/10.1007/s11426-016-5593-0
Feng M, Zhong L-X, Zhan Z-Y, Huang Z-H, Xiong J-P (2016b) Resveratrol treatment inhibits proliferation of and induces apoptosis in human colon cancer cells. Med Sci Monit 22:1101
Fu K, Kobayashi A, Saito N, Sano Y, Kato S, Ikematsu H et al (2006) Alpha-fetoprotein-producing colon cancer with atypical bulky lymph node metastasis. World J Gastroenterol 12(47):7715–7716. https://doi.org/10.3748/wjg.v12.i47.7715
Gaikwad NM, Shaikh KS, Chaudhari PD (2017) Development and evaluation of a system for colonic delivery of budesonide. Indian J Pharma Educ Res 51(4):551–561
Gao F, Yuan Q, Gao L, Cai P, Zhu H, Liu R et al (2014) Cytotoxicity and therapeutic effect of irinotecan combined with selenium nanoparticles. Biomaterials 35(31):8854–8866
García-Couce J, Bada-Rivero N, López Hernández OD, Nogueira A, Caracciolo PC, Abraham GA et al (2019) Dexamethasone-loaded chitosan beads coated with a pH-dependent interpolymer complex for colon-specific drug delivery. Int J Polym Sci 2019:4204375
Garg A, Tisdale AW, Haidari E, Kokkoli E (2009) Targeting colon cancer cells using PEGylated liposomes modified with a fibronectin-mimetic peptide. Int J Pharm 366(1–2):201–210

Gelberg HB (2014) Comparative anatomy, physiology, and mechanisms of disease production of the esophagus, stomach, and small intestine. Toxicol Pathol 42(1):54–66

Goodman SL, Picard M (2012) Integrins as therapeutic targets. Trends Pharmacol Sci 33(7):405–412

Gou M, Men K, Shi H, Xiang M, Zhang J, Song J et al (2011) Curcumin-loaded biodegradable polymeric micelles for colon cancer therapy in vitro and in vivo. Nanoscale 3(4):1558–1567. https://doi.org/10.1039/C0NR00758G

Goudanavar PS, Joshi VG (2012) Development and targeting efficiency of irinotecan engineered proniosomes. Trop J Pharm Res 11(1):1–8

Grand RJ, Watkins JB, Torti FM (1976) Development of the human gastrointestinal tract: a review. Gastroenterology 70(5):790–810

Gupta AS, Kshirsagar SJ, Bhalekar MR, Saldanha T (2013) Design and development of liposomes for colon targeted drug delivery. J Drug Target 21(2):146–160

Guterres SS, Alves MP, Pohlmann AR (2007) Polymeric nanoparticles, nanospheres and nanocapsules, for cutaneous applications. Drug Target Insights 2:117739280700200002

Handali S, Moghimipour E, Kouchak M, Ramezani Z, Amini M, Angali KA et al (2019) New folate receptor targeted nano liposomes for delivery of 5-fluorouracil to cancer cells: strong implication for enhanced potency and safety. Life Sci 227:39–50

Hoving JC (2018) Targeting IL-13 as a host-directed therapy against ulcerative colitis. Front Cell Infect Microbiol 8:395

Hua S, Marks E, Schneider JJ, Keely S (2015) Advances in oral nano-delivery systems for colon targeted drug delivery in inflammatory bowel disease: selective targeting to diseased versus healthy tissue. Nanomedicine 11(5):1117–1132. https://doi.org/10.1016/j.nano.2015.02.018

Irving M, Catchpole B (1992) ABC of colorectal diseases. Anatomy and physiology of the colon, rectum, and anus. Br Med J 304(6834):1106

Izham M, Nadiah M, Hussin Y, Aziz MNM, Yeap SK, Rahman HS et al (2019) Preparation and characterization of self nano-emulsifying drug delivery system loaded with Citraland its antiproliferative effect on colorectal cells in vitro. Nano 9(7):1028

Jadhav SM, Morey P, Karpe M, Kadam V (2012) Novel vesicular system: an overview. J Appl Pharm Sci 2(1):193–202

Jain A (2017) Colon targeting using pH sensitive materials. Adv Res Gastroenterol Hepatol 8:1–3

Jayasekeran V, Holt B, Bourke M (2013) Normal adult colonic anatomy in colonoscopy. Video J Encycl GI Endosc 1(2):390–392

Jodeleit H, Al-Amodi O, Caesar J, Villarroel Aguilera C, Holdt L, Gropp R et al (2018) Targeting ulcerative colitis by suppressing glucose uptake with ritonavir. Dis Model Mech 11(11):dmm036210. https://doi.org/10.1242/dmm.036210

Kamboj S, Saini V, Magon N, Bala S, Jhawat V (2013) Vesicular drug delivery systems: a novel approach for drug targeting. Brain 1:11

Karn PR, Vanić Z, Pepić I, Škalko-Basnet N (2011) Mucoadhesive liposomal delivery systems: the choice of coating material. Drug Dev Ind Pharm 37(4):482–488

Kazi M, Al-Swairi M, Ahmad A, Raish M, Alanazi FK, Khan AA et al (2019) Evaluation of self-nanoemulsifying drug delivery system (SNEDDS) for poorly water-soluble talinolol: preparation, in vitro and in vivo assessment. Front Pharmacol 10:459

Kou L, Yao Q, Sivaprakasam S, Luo Q, Sun Y, Fu Q et al (2017) Dual targeting of l-carnitine-conjugated nanoparticles to OCTN2 and ATB0,+ to deliver chemotherapeutic agents for colon cancer therapy. Drug Deliv 24(1):1338–1349

Krasteva N, Keremidarska-Markova M, Hristova-Panusheva K, Andreeva T, Speranza G, Wang D et al (2019) Aminated graphene oxide as a potential new therapy for colorectal cancer. Oxidative Med Cell Longev 2019:3738980

Krishna R, Garg A, Jin B, Keshavarz SS, Bieberdorf FA, Chodakewitz J, Wagner JA (2009) Assessment of a pharmacokinetic and pharmacodynamic interaction between simvastatin and anacetrapib, a potent cholesteryl ester transfer protein (CETP) inhibitor, in healthy subjects. Br J Clin Pharmacol 67(5):520–526

Kshirsagar SJ, Bhalekar MR, Patel JN, Mohapatra SK, Shewale NS (2012) Preparation and characterization of nanocapsules for colon-targeted drug delivery system. Pharm Dev Technol 17(5):607–613

Kumar M, Ali A, Kaldhone P, Shirode A, Kadam V (2010) Report on pharmaceutical approaches to colon targeted drug delivery systems. J Pharm Res 3(3):470–473

Kumar B, Kulanthaivel S, Mondal A, Mishra S, Banerjee B, Bhaumik A et al (2017) Mesoporous silica nanoparticle based enzyme responsive system for colon specific drug delivery through guar gum capping. Colloids Surf B: Biointerfaces 150:352–361

Lamprecht A, Yamamoto H, Takeuchi H, Kawashima Y (2005) Nanoparticles enhance therapeutic efficiency by selectively increased local drug dose in experimental colitis in rats. J Pharmacol Exp Ther 315(1):196–202

Lankalapalli S, Damuluri M (2012) Sphingosomes: applications in targeted drug delivery. Int J Pharm Chem Biol Sci 2:507–516

Lautenschläger C, Schmidt C, Fischer D, Stallmach A (2014) Drug delivery strategies in the therapy of inflammatory bowel disease. Adv Drug Deliv Rev 71:58–76

Lee C-M, Kim D-W, Lee H-C, Lee K-Y (2004) Pectin microspheres for oral colon delivery: preparation using spray drying method andin vitro release of indomethacin. Biotechnol Bioprocess Eng 9(3):191–195

Leuva V, Patel B, Chaudhary D, Patel J, Modasiya M (2012) Oral colon-specific drug delivery system. J Pharm Res 5(4):2293–2297

Li L, Xiang D, Shigdar S, Yang W, Li Q, Lin J et al (2014) Epithelial cell adhesion molecule aptamer functionalized PLGA-lecithin-curcumin-PEG nanoparticles for targeted drug delivery to human colorectal adenocarcinoma cells. Int J Nanomedicine 9:1083

Li Z, Wang X, Chen M, Wang Y, Sun R, Qu H et al (2017) Effectiveness of C5a aptamers in a TNBS-induced colitis mouse model. Exp Ther Med 14(6):6119–6124

Liu H, Tu Z, Feng F, Shi H, Chen K, Xu X (2015) Virosome, a hybrid vehicle for efficient and safe drug delivery and its emerging application in cancer treatment. Acta Pharma 65(2):105116. https://doi.org/10.1515/acph-2015-0019

Liu W, Zhu Y, Wang F, Li X, Liu X, Pang J, Pan W (2018) Galactosylated chitosan-functionalized mesoporous silica nanoparticles for efficient colon cancer cell-targeted drug delivery. R Soc Open Sci 5(12):181027–181027. https://doi.org/10.1098/rsos.181027

Liu ZL, Li LF, Xia SS, Tian HP, Yan ZH, Zhang GJ et al (2019) Chondroitin sulfate modification enhances the targeting and therapeutic effect of nanomedicine on AOM/DSS-induced mouse colon cancer. J Drug Deliv Sci Technol 52:1–7. https://doi.org/10.1016/j.jddst.2019.04.010

Lu L, Chen G, Qiu Y, Li M, Liu D, Hu D et al (2016) Nanoparticle-based oral delivery systems for colon targeting: principles and design strategies. Sci Bullet 61(9):670–681

Ma ZG, Ma R, Xiao XL, Zhang YH, Zhang XZ, Hu N et al (2016) Azo polymeric micelles designed for colon-targeted dimethyl fumarate delivery for colon cancer therapy. Acta Biomater 44:323–331. https://doi.org/10.1016/j.actbio.2016.08.021

Mahadevan V (2017) Anatomy of the caecum, appendix and colon. Surgery (Oxford) 35(3):15–120

Mahmoudi A, Jaafari MR, Ramezanian N, Gholami L, Malaekeh-Nikouei B (2019) BR2 and CyLoP1 enhance in-vivo SN38 delivery using pegylated PAMAM dendrimers. Int J Pharm 564:77–89

Makhlof A, Tozuka Y, Takeuchi H (2009) pH-sensitive nanospheres for colon-specific drug delivery in experimentally induced colitis rat model. Eur J Pharm Biopharm 72(1):1–8

Melo-Júnior MR, Telles A, Albuquerque FE, Pontes-Filho NT, Carvalho LB Jr, Beltrão EI (2004) Altered lectin-binding sites in normal colon and ulcerative colitis. Jornal Brasileiro de Patologia e Medicina Laboratorial 40(2):123–125

Mignani S, Majoral J-P (2013) Dendrimers as macromolecular tools to tackle from colon to brain tumor types: a concise overview. New J Chem 37(11):3337–3357. https://doi.org/10.1039/C3NJ00300K

Mike M, Kano N (2013) Reappraisal of the vascular anatomy of the colon and consequences for the definition of surgical resection. Dig Surg 30(4–6):383–392

Mishra N, Arya M, Gupta KP, Saraf SA (2019) Optimization of inositol hexaphosphate colon targeted formulation for anticarcinogenic marker modulation. AAPS PharmSciTech 20(8):319

Mohd AB, Sanka K, Bandi S, Diwan PV, Shastri N (2015) Solid self-nanoemulsifying drug delivery system (S-SNEDDS) for oral delivery of glimepiride: development and antidiabetic activity in albino rabbits. Drug Deliv 22(4):499–508

Moran E Jr (2006) Anatomy, microbes, and fiber: small versus large intestine. J Appl Poult Res 15(1):154–160

Morita Y, Leslie M, Kameyama H, Volk DE, Tanaka T (2018) Aptamer therapeutics in cancer: current and future. Cancers 10(3):80. https://doi.org/10.3390/cancers10030080

Moulari B, Béduneau A, Pellequer Y, Lamprecht A (2014) Lectin-decorated nanoparticles enhance binding to the inflamed tissue in experimental colitis. J Control Release 188:9–17

Naeem M, Bae J, Oshi MA, Kim M-S, Moon HR, Lee BL et al (2018) Colon-targeted delivery of cyclosporine a using dual-functional Eudragit® FS30D/PLGA nanoparticles ameliorates murine experimental colitis. Int J Nanomedicine 13:1225

Neamtu I, Rusu AG, Diaconu A, Nita LE, Chiriac AP (2017) Basic concepts and recent advances in nanogels as carriers for medical applications. Drug Deliv 24(1):539–557

Pabla B, Bissonnette M, Konda VJ (2015) Colon cancer and the epidermal growth factor receptor: current treatment paradigms, the importance of diet, and the role of chemoprevention. World J Clin Oncol 6(5):133–141. https://doi.org/10.5306/wjco.v6.i5.133

Pardo J, Peng Z, Leblanc R (2018) Cancer targeting and drug delivery using carbon-based quantum dots and nanotubes. Molecules 23(2):378

Park Y, Ryu Y-M, Jung Y, Wang T, Baek Y, Yoon Y et al (2014) Spraying quantum dot conjugates in the colon of live animals enabled rapid and multiplex cancer diagnosis using endoscopy. ACS Nano 8(9):8896–8910

Philip AK, Philip B (2010) Colon targeted drug delivery systems: a review on primary and novel approaches. Oman Med J 25(2):79

Phillips S (1984) Functions of the large bowel: an overview. Scand J Gastroenterol Suppl 93:1–12

Pichai MV, Ferguson LR (2012) Potential prospects of nanomedicine for targeted therapeutics in inflammatory bowel diseases. World J Gastroenterol: WJG 18(23):2895

Prajapati SK, Jain A, Shrivastava C, Jain AK (2019) Hyaluronic acid conjugated multi-walled carbon nanotubes for colon cancer targeting. Int J Biol Macromol 123:691–703. https://doi.org/10.1016/j.ijbiomac.2018.11.116

Rangari Nalanda T, Puranik Prashant K (2015) Review on recent and novel approaches to colon targeted drug delivery systems. Int J Pharm Pharma Res 3(1):167–186

Rao J, Khan A (2013) Enzyme sensitive synthetic polymer micelles based on the azobenzene motif. J Am Chem Soc 135(38):14056–14059. https://doi.org/10.1021/ja407514z

Rastogi V, Yadav P, Bhattacharya SS, Mishra AK, Verma N, Verma A, Pandit JK (2014) Carbon nanotubes: an emerging drug carrier for targeting cancer cells. J Drug Deliv 2014:670815

Ratnaparkhi Mukesh P, Somvanshi Fattesingh U, Pawar Sham A, Chaudhari Shilpa P, Gupta Jyoti P, Budhavant Kalyani A (2013) Colon targeted drug delivery system. IJPRR 2(8):33–42

Rodriguez-Nogales A, Algieri F, Laura de Matteis A, Perez JG-M, Vezza T, de la Fuente JM et al (2016) Intestinal anti-inflammatory effects of RGD-functionalized silk fibroin nanoparticles in trinitrobenzenesulfonic acid-induced experimental colitis in rats. Int J Nanomedicine 11:5945

Safaie Qamsari E, Safaei Ghaderi S, Zarei B, Dorostkar R, Bagheri S, Jadidi-Niaragh F et al (2017) The c-Met receptor: implication for targeted therapies in colorectal cancer. Tumor Biol 39(5):1010428317699118

Saga K, Kaneda Y (2013) Virosome presents multimodel cancer therapy without viral replication. Biomed Res Int:764706–764706. https://doi.org/10.1155/2013/764706

Sahu KK, Kaurav M, Pandey RS (2019) Chylomicron mimicking solid lipid nanoemulsions encapsulated enteric minicapsules targeted to colon for immunization against hepatitis B. Int Immunopharmacol 66:317–329. https://doi.org/10.1016/j.intimp.2018.11.041

Satapathy SR, Mohapatra P, Preet R, Das D, Sarkar B, Choudhuri T et al (2013) Silver-based nanoparticles induce apoptosis in human colon cancer cells mediated through p53. Nanomedicine 8(8): 1307–1322

Sen K, Banerjee S, Mandal M (2019) Dual drug loaded liposome bearing apigenin and 5-fluorouracil for synergistic therapeutic efficacy in colorectal cancer. Colloids Surf B: Biointerfaces 180:9–22. https://doi.org/10.1016/j.colsurfb.2019.04.035

Seo YG, Kim DH, Ramasamy T, Kim JH, Marasini N, Oh Y-K et al (2013) Development of docetaxel-loaded solid self-nanoemulsifying drug delivery system (SNEDDS) for enhanced chemotherapeutic effect. Int J Pharm 452(1–2):412–420

Seo J, Lee J, Lee CB, Bae SK, Na K (2019) Nonpolymeric pH-sensitive carbon dots for treatment of tumor. Bioconjug Chem 30(3):621–632. https://doi.org/10.1021/acs.bioconjchem.8b00813

Shahdadi Sardo H, Saremnejad F, Bagheri S, Akhgari A, Afrasiabi Garekani H, Sadeghi F (2019) A review on 5-aminosalicylic acid colon-targeted oral drug delivery systems. Int J Pharm 558:367–379. https://doi.org/10.1016/j.ijpharm.2019.01.022

Shen X, Yu D, Zhu L, Branford-White C, White K, Chatterton NP (2011) Electrospun diclofenac sodium loaded Eudragit® L 100-55 nanofibers for colon-targeted drug delivery. Int J Pharm 408(1–2): 200–207

Shen Y, Li X, Dong D, Zhang B, Xue Y, Shang P (2018) Transferrin receptor 1 in cancer: a new sight for cancer therapy. Am J Cancer Res 8(6):916–931

Shivani S, Poladi KK (2015) Nanosponges-novel emerging drug delivery system: A review. Int J Pharm Sci Res 6(2):529

Silindir-Gunay M, Karpuz M, Ozturk N, Ozer AY, Erdogan S, Tuncel M (2019) Radiolabeled, folate-conjugated liposomes as tumor imaging agents: formulation and in vitro evaluation. J Drug Deliv Sci Technol 50:321–328

Simmonds NJ, Allen RE, Stevens TR, Niall R, Van Someren M, Blake DR, Rampton DS (1992) Chemiluminescence assay of mucosal reactive oxygen metabolites in inflammatory bowel disease. Gastroenterology 103(1):186–196

Singh CK, Saxena S, Yadav M, Samson AL (2018) A review on novel approaches for colon targeted drug delivery systems. PharmaTutor 6(7):11–22

Širc J, Hobzová R, Kostina N, Munzarová M, Juklícková M., ... & Michálek, J. (2012) Morphological characterization of nanofibers: methods and application in practice. J Nanomater 1212:1–15

Soleymani J, Hasanzadeh M, Somi MH, Shadjou N, Jouyban A (2019) Highly sensitive and specific cytosensing of HT 29 colorectal cancer cells using folic acid functionalized-KCC-1 nanoparticles. Biosens Bioelectron 132:122–131

Sousa AR, Oliveira MJ, Sarmento B (2019) Impact of CEA-targeting nanoparticles for drug delivery in colorectal cancer. J Pharmacol Exp Therap 118:254441

Stanczyk M, Dziki A, Morawiec Z (2012) Dendrimers in therapy for breast and colorectal cancer. Curr Med Chem 19(29):4896–4902

Stefanich E, Danilenko D, Wang H, O'Byrne S, Erickson R, Gelzleichter T et al (2011) A humanized monoclonal antibody targeting the β7 integrin selectively blocks intestinal homing of T lymphocytes. Br J Pharmacol 162(8):1855–1870

Stoeltzing O, Liu W, Reinmuth N, Fan F, Parry GC, Parikh AA et al (2003) Inhibition of integrin alpha-5beta1 function with a small peptide (ATN-161) plus continuous 5-FU infusion reduces colorectal liver metastases and improves survival in mice. Int J Cancer 104(4):496–503. https://doi.org/10.1002/ijc.10958

Sugiura T, Kageyama S, Andou A, Miyazawa T, Ejima C, Nakayama A et al (2013) Oral treatment with a novel small molecule alpha 4 integrin antagonist, AJM300, prevents the development of experimental colitis in mice. J Crohns Colitis 7(11):e533–e542. https://doi.org/10.1016/j.crohns.2013.03.014

Sun Q, Luan L, Arif M, Li J, Dong Q-J, Gao Y et al (2018) Redox-sensitive nanoparticles based on 4-aminothiophenol-carboxymethyl inulin conjugate for budesonide delivery in inflammatory bowel diseases. Carbohydr Polym 189:352–359

Talaei F, Atyabi F, Azhdarzadeh M, Dinarvand R, Saadatzadeh A (2013) Overcoming therapeutic obstacles in inflammatory bowel diseases: a comprehensive review on novel drug delivery strategies. Eur J Pharm Sci 49(4):712–722

Tao SL, Desai TA (2003) Microfabricated drug delivery systems: from particles to pores. Adv Drug Deliv Rev 55(3):315–328

Ukrainskaya VM, Stepanov AV, Glagoleva IS, Knorre VD, Belogurov AA Jr, Gabibov AG (2017) Death receptors: new opportunities in cancer therapy. Acta Nat 9(3):55–63

Üner M, Yener G (2007) Importance of solid lipid nanoparticles (SLN) in various administration routes and future perspectives. Int J Nanomedicine 2(3):289

Urmann K, Modrejewski J, Scheper T, Walter JG (2017) Aptamer-modified nanomaterials: principles and applications. BioNanoMaterials 18:1–2

Vagare RS (2015) Microbial triggered colon targeted compression coated tablets of tenoxicam: formulation and evaluation. J Drug Deliv Therap 5(1):75–81

Vaidya A, Jain S, Agrawal RK, Jain SK (2015) Pectin–metronidazole prodrug bearing microspheres for colon targeting. J Saudi Chem Soc 19(3):257–264

Varshosaz J, Riahi S, Ghassami E, Jahanian-Najafabadi A (2017) Transferrin-targeted poly(butylene adipate)/terephthalate nanoparticles for targeted delivery of 5-fluorouracil in HT29 colorectal cancer cell line. J Bioact Compat Polym 32(5):503–527. https://doi.org/10.1177/0883911517690756

Vdoviaková K, Petrovová E, Maloveská M, Krešáková L, Teleky J, Elias MZJ, Petrášová D (2016) Surgical anatomy of the gastrointestinal tract and its vasculature in the laboratory rat. Gastroenterol Res Pract 2016:1–12

Velmurugan B, Gangar SC, Kaur M, Tyagi A, Deep G, Agarwal R (2010) Silibinin exerts sustained growth suppressive effect against human colon carcinoma SW480 xenograft by targeting multiple signaling molecules. Pharm Res 27(10):2085–2097

Verghese M, Rao D, Chawan C, Walker L, Shackelford L (2006) Anticarcinogenic effect of phytic acid (IP6): apoptosis as a possible mechanism of action. LWT-Food Sci Technol 39(10):1093–1098

Verma C, Negi P, Pathania D, Sethi V, Gupta B (2019) Preparation of pH-sensitive hydrogels by graft polymerization of itaconic acid on tragacanth gum. Polym Int 68(3):344–350. https://doi.org/10.1002/pi.5739

Vishwakarma A, Nikam P, Mogal R, Talele S (2014) Review on nanosponges: a benefication for novel drug delivery. Int J PharmTech Res 6:11–20

Vong LB, Mo J, Abrahamsson B, Nagasaki Y (2015a) Specific accumulation of orally administered redox nanotherapeutics in the inflamed colon reducing inflammation with dose–response efficacy. J Control Release 210:19–25

Vong LB, Yoshitomi T, Matsui H, Nagasaki Y (2015b) Development of an oral nanotherapeutics using redox nanoparticles for treatment of colitis-associated colon cancer. Biomaterials 55:54–63

Vukobrat-Bijedic Z, Husic-Selimovic A, Sofic A, Bijedic N, Bjelogrlic I, Gogov B, Mehmedovic A (2013) Cancer antigens (CEA and CA 19-9) as markers of advanced stage of colorectal carcinoma. Med Arch (Sarajevo, Bosnia and Herzegovina) 67(6):397401. https://doi.org/10.5455/medarh.2013.67.397-401

Wang X, Yu D-G, Li X-Y, Bligh SA, Williams GR (2015) Electrospun medicated shellac nanofibers for colon-targeted drug delivery. Int J Pharm 490(12):384–390

Wilkhu JS, McNeil SE, Anderson DE, Perrie Y (2013) Characterization and optimization of bilosomes for oral vaccine delivery. J Drug Target 21(3):291–299. https://doi.org/10.3109/1061186X.2012.747528

Wong TW, Colombo G, Sonvico F (2011) Pectin matrix as oral drug delivery vehicle for colon cancer treatment. AAPS PharmSciTech 12(1):201–214

Xiao B, Merlin D (2012) Oral colon-specific therapeutic approaches toward treatment of inflammatory bowel disease. Expert Opin Drug Deliv 9(11):1393–1407

Xiao B, Han MK, Viennois E, Wang L, Zhang M, Si X, Merlin D (2015) Hyaluronic acid-functionalized polymeric nanoparticles for colon cancer-targeted combination chemotherapy. Nanoscale 7(42):17745–17755. https://doi.org/10.1039/c5nr04831a

Xiao B, Xu Z, Viennois E, Zhang Y, Zhang Z, Zhang M et al (2017) Orally targeted delivery of tripeptide KPV via hyaluronic acid-functionalized nanoparticles efficiently alleviates ulcerative colitis. Mol Ther 25(7):1628–1640

Xie J, Wang J, Chen H, Shen W, Sinko PJ, Dong H et al (2015) Multivalent conjugation of antibody to dendrimers for the enhanced capture and regulation on colon cancer cells. Sci Rep 5:9445–9445. https://doi.org/10.1038/srep09445

Xie X, Li F, Zhang H, Lu Y, Lian S, Lin H et al (2016) EpCAM aptamer-functionalized mesoporous silica nanoparticles for efficient colon cancer cell-targeted drug delivery. Eur J Pharm Sci 83:28–35

Xing L, Dawei C, Liping X, Rongqing Z (2003) Oral colon-specific drug delivery for bee venom peptide: development of a coated calcium alginate gel beads-entrapped liposome. J Control Release 93(3):293–300

Xu JS, Huang J, Qin R, Hinkle GH, Povoski SP, Martin EW, Xu RX (2010) Synthesizing and binding dual-mode poly (lactic-co-glycolic acid)(PLGA) nanobubbles for cancer targeting and imaging. Biomaterials 31(7):1716–1722

Xu Y, Pang L, Wang H, Xu C, Shah H, Guo P et al (2019) Specific delivery of delta-5-desaturase siRNA via RNA nanoparticles supplemented with dihomo-γ-linolenic acid for colon cancer suppression. Redox Biol 21. https://doi.org/10.1016/j.redox.2018.101085

Yachida S, Fukushima N, Nakanishi Y, Akasu T, Kitamura H, Sakamoto M, Shimoda T (2003) Alpha-fetoprotein-producing carcinoma of the colon: report of a case and review of the literature. Dis Colon Rectum 46(6):826–831. https://doi.org/10.1007/s10350-004-6663-5

Yang X, Li Z, Wang N, Li L, Song L, He T et al (2015) Curcumin-encapsulated polymeric micelles suppress the development of colon cancer in vitro and in vivo. Sci Rep 5:10322–10322. https://doi.org/10.1038/srep10322

Yang Y-Y, Liu Z-P, Yu D-G, Wang K, Liu P, Chen X (2018) Colon-specific pulsatile drug release provided by electrospun shellac nanocoating on hydrophilic amorphous composites. Int J Nanomedicine 13:2395

Yazdian-Robati R, Arab A, Ramezani M, Rafatpanah H, Bahreyni A, Nabavinia MS et al (2019) Smart aptamer-modified calcium carbonate nanoparticles for controlled release and targeted delivery of epirubicin and melittin into cancer cells in vitro and in vivo. Drug Dev Ind Pharm 45(4):603–610. https://doi.org/10.1080/03639045.2019.1569029

Yeo PL, Lim CL, Chye SM, Ling APK, Koh RY (2017) Niosomes: a review of their structure, properties, methods of preparation, and medical applications. Asian Biomed 11(4):301–314

Yu H, Son G-M, Joh Y-G (2013) The clinical significance of preoperative serum levels of carbohydrate antigen 19-9 in colorectal cancer. J Korean Surg Soc 84(4):231–237

Yu Z, Chen Z, Wu J, Li Z, Wu Y (2017) Prognostic value of pretreatment serum carbohydrate antigen 19-9 level in patients with colorectal cancer: a meta-analysis. PLoS One 12(11):e0188139

Yuan X, Wang Z, Li L, Yu J, Wang Y, Li H et al (2019) Novel fluorescent amphiphilic copolymer probes containing azo-tetraphenylethylene bridges for azoreductase-triggered release. Mater Chem Front 3(6):1097–1104

Zhang P, Qiao Z-A, Dai S (2015) Recent advances in carbon nanospheres: synthetic routes and applications. Chem Commun 51(45):9246–9256

Zhang B, Yan Y, Shen Q, Ma D, Huang L, Cai X, Tan S (2017a) A colon targeted drug delivery system based on alginate modificated graphene oxide for colorectal liver metastasis. Mater Sci Eng C Mater Biol Appl 79:185–190. https://doi.org/10.1016/j.msec.2017.05.054

Zhang Q, Colazo J, Berg D, Mugo SM, Serpe MJ (2017b) Multiresponsive nanogels for targeted anticancer drug delivery. Mol Pharm 14(8):2624–2628

Zhang Y, Kang C, Wang X l, Zhou M, Chen M t, Zhu X h et al (2018) Dietary factors modulate colonic tumorigenesis through the interaction of gut microbiota and host chloride channels. Mol Nutr Food Res 62(5):1700554

Zhao M-X, Zhu B-J (2016) The research and applications of quantum dots as nano-carriers for targeted drug delivery and cancer therapy. Nanoscale Res Lett 11(1):207

Zhao X, Pan J, Li W, Yang W, Qin L, Pan Y (2018) Gold nanoparticles enhance cisplatin delivery and potentiate chemotherapy by decompressing colorectal cancer vessels. Int J Nanomedicine 13:6207

Zhou M, Peng Z, Liao S, Li P, Li S (2014) Design of microencapsulated carbon nanotube-based microspheres and its application in colon targeted drug delivery. Drug Deliv 21(2):101–109. https://doi.org/10.3109/10717544.2013.834413

Zu M, Ma L, Zhang X, Xie D, Kang Y, Xiao B (2019) Chondroitin sulfate-functionalized polymeric nanoparticles for colon cancer-targeted chemotherapy. Colloids Surf B Biointerfaces 177:399–406. https://doi.org/10.1016/j.colsurfb.2019.02.031

Nose to Brain Drug Delivery for the Treatment of Epilepsy

8

Pratishtha, Samriddhi Srivastava, and Swati Gupta

Abstract

Drug delivery is basically the process of transferring a drug entity or formulation to the desired target following administration via various routes in the human body. In this chapter we will be focusing on nose to brain drug delivery. Nose to brain drug delivery, as the title indicates, is delivering a drug or targeting the drug to brain via the nasal route. This technique is noninvasive and relies on the highly permeable nasal mucosa, which allows rapid drug absorption. Drug enters the brain from the olfactory region bypassing the blood-brain barrier. The blood-brain barrier has tight junctions that allows only a specific amount and a specific size of drug particles to enter or pass through to provide a desired therapeutic effect in brain. Nanoparticles of size below 100 nm may only pass through blood-brain barrier and have been used in the form of various formulations for the treatment of different neurological diseases. In recent years, nanoformulations are widely being used for the treatment of CNS diseases. Epilepsy is a chronic neurodegenerative disease with recurrent seizure episodes affecting nervous system and it is a life-threatening disease that requires immediate treatment. Current conventional therapy has limited bioavailability via oral, intravenous, and rectal administration. To overcome these limitations, nose to brain delivery using nanoformulations has shown promising results for the treatment of this disease.

Keywords

Intranasal · Drug absorption · Blood brain barrier · Nanoparticles · Nanoformulations · CNS · Epilepsy

8.1 Introduction

Neurological diseases or disorders are hazardous to humankind, difficult to treat, and treatments are time consuming. Therefore, after years of hard work, researches and scientists have provided physicians and medicinal practitioners a feasible route of administration, i.e., the intranasal (IN) route targeting brain for the treatment of central nervous system (CNS) disorders or diseases. Drug delivery directly to the brain has always been challenging in the medical world (Tiwari et al. 2012). In the case of conventional dosage forms, drug has to pass through various barriers such as first pass metabolism where most of the drug either degrades or gets modified/

Pratishtha · S. Srivastava · S. Gupta (✉)
Amity Institute of Pharmacy, Amity University Uttar Pradesh, Sector 125, Noida, India

S. Talegaonkar, M. Rai (eds.), *Nanoformulations in Human Health*,
https://doi.org/10.1007/978-3-030-41858-8_8

altered. Also, there are chances for the drug to interact with enzymes, proteins, or receptors present in the GI route. Thus, it is strenuous to achieve the desired therapeutic effect for the treatment of CNS diseases. Considering these drawbacks of conventional strategies for delivering drug to brain, nose to brain drug delivery system serves as an effective and more convenient way to treat CNS diseases. The blood-brain barrier (BBB) acts as a potent guard and prevents approximately 90% of molecules (drug, bacteria, viruses, other foreign substances present in blood stream) from crossing it. In other words, the BBB is selectively permeable in order to protect brain from hazardous substances (Mittal et al. 2014). Certain physicochemical properties, such as molecular weight less than 600 Daltons (Da), partition coefficient in the range of 1.5–2.7 (approx.), and lipophilicity may enhance the chance of drug permeation. This route is viable in treatment of various neurological disorders, i.e., epilepsy, Parkinson's disease, Alzheimer's disease, meningitis, etc.

For chronic and acute treatment, the intranasal route shows promising results. Intranasal drug delivery shows alternative route to parenteral, delivering drugs rapidly into the central nervous system as it allows delivery directly to the brain. Intranasal drug delivery follows three pathways: olfactory, systemic, and trigeminal pathways. The trigeminal pathway transmits sensory information to the CNS from the nasal cavity, eyelids, or cornea via maxillary nerve, ophthalmic nerve, and mandibular nerve. The mandibular division spreads to teeth and lower jaw, with no neural input from the trigeminal pathway into the nasal cavity (Clossen and Reddy 2017).

Intranasal route using colloidal carriers such as nanoemulsions, microemulsions, nanoparticles, lipid nanoparticles, in situ gels, etc., is a promising route being investigated for the treatment of CNS and brain disorders, including epilepsy.

8.2 Nasal Anatomy

The nasal mucosa only allows smaller particles to absorb, which then can permeate through the blood-brain barrier. Thus, the nasal route may be used to target the brain to treat CNS diseases. Various components of the nasal cavity and their functions are captured in Table 8.1.

8.3 Blood-Brain Barrier

In 1885, the German scientist Paul Ehlrich observed after administering vital dye to adult animal by parenteral route that the dye had stained all the organs in that animal except the brain and the central nervous system. Ehlrich thought the reason behind the unstained CNS were the different affinities to bind.

In 1898, Bield and Kraus suggested the existence of a barrier at the level of the cerebral vessels. In 1900, Lewandowsky coined the term Blood-Brain Barrier (BBB) to explain his observations. Lewandowsky observed no physiological or therapeutic effect of cholic acid or sodium ferrocyanide when given intravenously but observed neurological symptoms after administering the same (i.e., cholic acid or sodium ferrocyanide) intraventrically (Ribatti et al. 2006).

The BBB is formed by a number of endothelial cells, which are connected to each other forming tight junctions and restricting entry of foreign particles into the brain. It consists of highly specialized capillaries. Drugs that are found to be highly lipid soluble can permeate through the BBB rather than water-soluble drugs (Daneman and Prat 2015). Examples of drugs that can cross the BBB are: dopamine, donepezil, rivastigmine, etc. The nasal route, with the help of the olfactory region, allows drugs to enter the CNS by crossing the BBB.

Mechanism for drug absorption via the BBB (Fig. 8.1):

(a) Paracellular transport: In this process, drug molecules pass through the BBB in between the tight junctions of the endothelial cells acting as guards for the brain. This process does not require energy or carrier. This process is dependent on the concentration gradient.
(b) Transcellular transport: In this process, drug molecules pass through the endothelial cell in order to bypass the BBB. It is also called a carrier-mediated process or transport.

Table 8.1 Brief description of the nasal anatomy

S. No.	Name	Anatomy	Function	Reference
1.	Nasal bone	They are of four types and make two joints at cranium and facial each to provide structure to the nose. The upper part of the bone is attached to cartilage	It binds with cartilage to provide shape to the individual's nose, allow the passage of air to pass for respiration and to protect the nose	Tiwari et al. (2012)
2.	Nasal mucosa	The nasal mucosa has the largest surface area within nasal cavity and it connects with the external skin of nose. The outermost layer consists of epithelium cells called as nasal epithelium. Other layers of the nasal mucosa are Stratified squamous epithelium and Pseudostratified columnar ciliated epithelium	Allows the absorption of drugs and restrict the entry of larger particles. It is responsible for filtering the air and allowing only filtered air to breath	Gong (2012)
3.	Olfactory sensory neuron	They are the sensory receptors that are found in nasal epithelium and sends sensory signals to central nervous system after detecting odors	Help in detecting odor and sending signals to CNS	Gong (2012)
4.	Olfactory bulb	Glomeruli are present at the surface covering olfactory bulb	Help sensory neurons for signaling CNS	Mori (2009)
5.	Olfactory epithelium	Consists of various epithelium cells lining olfactory region.	Restrict entry of foreign particles	Leinders-Zufall and Ma (2009)
6.	Nasal valve	They are mobile part of nose that can open and close in order to control the flow of air. They consist of cartilage and erectile tissues within the nasal cavity	Help in regulating air flow and fluid/liquid flow by opening and closing of valves	Eduardo Nazareth Nigro et al. (2009)
7.	Turbinates (superior, middle and inferior)	They are thin bones like sausage and are covered by mucus membrane	They filter, humidify and warm the air we breathe	Măru et al. (2015)
8.	Nasopharynx	Epithelial layer lining muscle and fascia forming a cuboidal cavity	Allow to breathe in and out	Baines (2014)
9.	Septum	Present in nasal cavity allowing the separation of left and right airways	Separating left and right airways	East (2019)
10.	Palate (soft and hard)	They consist of fibres	Soft palate is responsible for closing of the nasal mucosa	–
11.	Uvula	Muscular tissues, serous and sero-mucous altogether create uvula.	It is responsible for producing and may help in speech	Finkelstein et al. (1992)
12.	Cilia	Small hair-like structure present in nasal cavity	Restrict entry of larger particles, such as dust by moving back and forth by air flow while respiring	–
13.	Glomerular	Lining the surface of olfactory bulb	Act as protective layer above Olfactory bulb	–
14.	Axon	It is part of neuron and also known as nerve fibre	Help in nervous system transmission	Ghaffarieh and Levin (2012)
15.	Vestibule	Squamous epithelium lining vestibules containing sweat glands, sebaceous glands and vibrissae glands	Filter air to breath	–

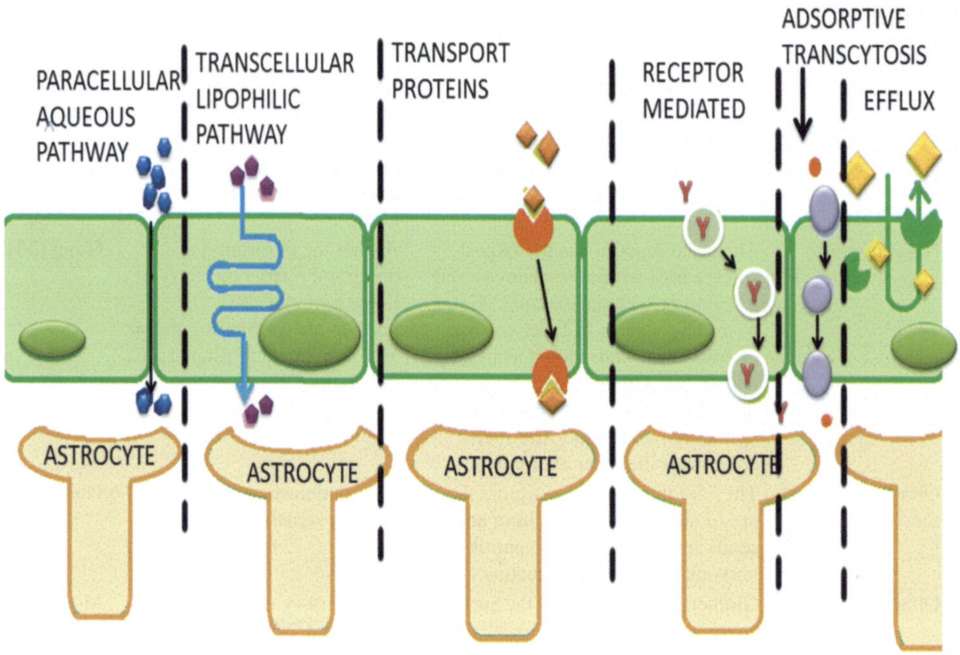

Fig. 8.1 Various absorption pathways associated with blood-brain barrier

Carriers are present at the surface of the BBB to allow molecules to attach to them and then these carriers transport these molecules to the other side of the barrier.

(c) Receptor-mediated transport: This process is somewhat similar to carrier-mediated transport. In this process receptors present on the BBB will bind to specific molecules only (may change or modify molecules structure) and transfer the molecules across the BBB for therapeutic actions in order to treat neurodegenerative diseases. This transport system does not depend on the concentration gradient.

(d) Efflux: It is not the transport system but it is also an important mechanism that plays an effective role in the BBB. This mechanism acts by throwing out unwanted molecules that somehow manage to enter the endothelial cells (Abbott and Friedman 2012).

8.4 Drug Transport to Brain

Drug transported by the nasal cavity is a potential route for nanocarriers or therapeutic modalities by passing the blood-brain barrier and by noninvasive administration. Drug is transported by three pathways, namely olfactory, trigeminal, and systemic pathways. The transport mechanism from nose to brain delivery is shown in Fig. 8.2 (Selvaraj et al. 2018).

8.4.1 Olfactory Pathway

Therapeutic substance once executed via nose navigate to olfactory epithelium, also known as olfactory mucosa. Transduction is carried out due to the presence of olfactory epithelium neurons or receptors. Transcellular or paracellular mechanism is responsible for the transport of molecules to the olfactory receptors. Paracellular transport is achieved by the virtue of the nasal epithelium as well as with tight junctions, adherent junctions, and desmosomes and at the interval of epithelium cells. Drug elements accompanied with axon and by the route of nerve bundle move across the cribriform plate and reach the surface of the brain through the olfactory bulb. Drug may enter the cerebrospinal fluid (CSF) and the olfactory bulb from olfactory nerves. With the mixing of interstitial fluid in the brain, drug can be scat-

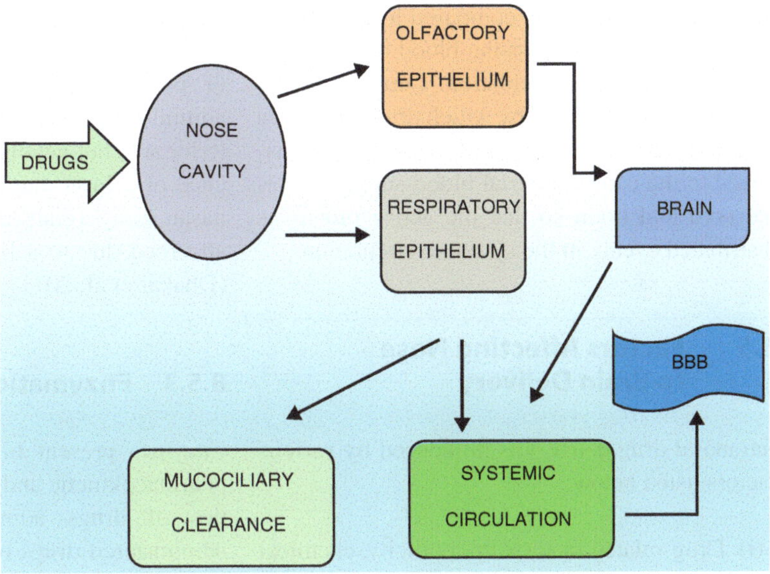

Fig. 8.2 Mechanism of drug absorption in nose to brain delivery

tered from the CSF to the brain. In the brain, there are two olfactory pathways, namely, extraneuronal pathway and intraneuronal pathway. The extraneuronal pathway involves transport by the virtue of perineural channels, which cause the element of drug to reach the brain in a few minutes. In the case of the intraneuronal pathway, which involves transport by the virtue of axonal transport, the drug reaches different parts of the brain, such as the cerebellum, cortex, cerebrum, and deeper areas of the brain, in hours to days.

8.4.2 Trigeminal Pathway

The trigeminal nerve pathway is linked to the appendage part of the brain, like the medulla, spinal cord, and the pons. The mechanism of drug transport through the trigeminal pathway is by intracellular or endocytosis transport from the nasal route. This pathway is classified into three sections: mandibular, ophthalmic, and maxillary. In nose to brain drug delivery, only the ophthalmic and maxillary sections play an important role. Neurons present in the ophthalmic and maxillary sections directly reach the nasal mucosa. Segments from the ophthalmic part move to anterior nose and to the back of the nasal mucosa but the maxillary part moves to the turbinate of the nasal mucosa. Drug reaches the branches of the trigeminal nerves after diffusion through the nasal mucosa in the olfactory and respiratory regions and through the medium of the brain stem it is carried to the axonal route. From nasal cavity, therapeutic compounds can be delivered to the forebrain through a part of the trigeminal nerve that involves passage through the cribriform plate. In the transportation through mucosa, several mechanisms are involved after crossing the nasal mucosa. These mechanisms are transcellular, paracellular, receptor-mediated transport, transcytosis, and carrier-mediated transport.

8.4.3 Systemic Pathways

Blood circulation also contributes to the process of uptake of drug via the nasal route into the brain. Respiratory epithelium has a rich vasculature than olfactory mucosa, therefore a fraction of drug gets absorbed into the system circulation. The respiratory segment is composed of a mixture of fenestrated and continuous epithelium, which let the transfer of large or small molecules into blood circulation and finally cross the blood-brain barrier into the CNS. Large molecules and hydrophilic molecules have difficulty entering the systemic circulation compared to small molecules which easily cross the blood brain barrier and reach systemic circulation. Counter current exchange is the process by which drug molecules entering into the nasal blood vessels get transferred to the carotid arterial blood supply to spinal cord and brain so that the active moiety is distributed evenly in the systemic circulation.

8.5 Factors Affecting Nose to Brain Delivery

Intranasal drug delivery is influenced by various factors listed below:

(i) Drug-related factors: lipophilicity, chemical form, polymorphism, partition coefficient and pKa, solubility, and dissolution of drug
(ii) Formulation-related factors: pH or mucociliary irritancy, osmolality, viscosity, molecular weight
(iii) Biological factors: nasal blood flow, mucociliary clearance, and enzymatic activity in the nose

8.5.1 Lipophilicity

Permeation of compounds through the nasal mucosa increases on increasing the lipophilicity of the molecule. Lipophilic compounds can cross biological barriers as they are able to cross the lipid bilayer of the cell membrane, and get scattered into the cell. The nasal mucosa has a hydrophilic character, but mucosae are lipophilic in nature and the barrier of the membrane is maintained by lipids. Therefore, lipophilic compounds tend to be well absorbed in the nasal mucosa rather than hydrophilic compounds (ChitraKarthikeyini and Kavitha 2016).

8.5.2 Mucociliary Clearance

Absorption is reduced due to mucociliary clearance as the drug administered through the nasal cavity undergoes elimination after 15–30 min, and this reduces the residence time of the drug in the nasal mucosa. Drug is retained in the anterior or posterior part of the nasal mucosa when administered. Nasal drops are retained in the posterior area but get eliminated rapidly due to presence of a large number of ciliated cells, while, nasal spray retained in the anterior area gets absorbed due to a less number of ciliated cells (Dhakar et al. 2011).

8.5.3 Enzymatic Activity

Enzymes present in the nasal cavity alter the pharmacokinetic and pharmacodynamics properties of drugs administered nasally. Nasally administered drugs bypass hepatic and gastrointestinal metabolism. Due to the presence of the enzyme cytochrome P450-dependent esterase, acid phosphates, oxidoreductase, monoxegenase, hydrolases, and lactate dehydrogenase, drugs may get metabolized in the lumen of the nasal cavity. Proteolytic enzymes like aminopeptidases or proteases are the major barriers for peptide drug delivery through the nasal cavity. Cytochrome P450 acts against drugs like cocaine, alcohols, nicotine, decongestants, and progesterone (Dhakar et al. 2011).

8.5.4 Drug Solubility and Dissolution Rate

Drug dissolution rate and solubility is an important factor for drug absorption, as like various dosage forms, nasal drug absorption also takes place after drug dissolution. Prior to absorption, the drug particles in the nasal cavity need to be dissolved, as no absorption will take place if particles are not dissolved (ChitraKarthikeyini and Kavitha 2016).

8.5.5 Partition Coefficient and pKa

The permeation through the biomembrane is affected not only by lipophilicity or hydrophilicity of the drug but also due to drug present in uncharged form. This uncharged form depends upon partition coefficient or pKa of the drug at the absorption site. According to pH-partition theory, nonionized drug is more permeable than ionized drug. Ionization degree is the major factor for the nasal absorption of weak electrolytes. To optimize systemic absorption, pH of the cavity and partition coefficient of drug should be considered. To reduce nasal irritation, pH should be around 4.5–6.5. In the nasal secretion, lysozyme is found, which destroys bacteria only at acidic pH. Therefore, acidic pH should be maintained in the range of 4.5–6.5, otherwise lysozyme gets inactivated and the nasal cavity becomes prone to microbial infection.

8.5.6 Molecular Weight

Drug molecules having molecular size more than 300D have highly sensitive permeation. Peptides and protein compounds like insulin have low bioavailability when administered via the intranasal route because of high molecular weight and hydrophilicity. Molecules having a molecular weight more than 1000D have a low absorption rate (Dhakar et al. 2011).

8.5.7 Nasal Blood Flow

For drug absorption, the nasal mucosa is optimal as it has a large surface area and it is supplied with a rich vasculature. Drug absorption is enhanced by blood flow rate as more drug reaches the systemic circulation by passing through the membrane. Vasodilation and vasoconstriction regulate the blood flow and rate and the extent of drug absorbed, as most drugs are absorbed by diffusion, the concentration gradient has to be maintained by blood flow (Dhakar et al. 2011).

8.5.8 Osmolality

Nasal absorption decreases due to hypertonic and hypotonic solutions, which hinder the cilia movement. Therefore, nasal formulation must be isotonic in nature. Isotonic formulation can be achieved by the addition of isotonic excipients such as dextrose, glycose, sodium chloride, and glycerin (Dhakar et al. 2011).

8.5.9 Viscosity

Drug absorption increases with the increase in viscosity, as contact time between drug and the nasal mucosa gets increased. However, at high viscosity, the permeability of drug alters due to impact on mucociliary clearance and normal ciliary beating. Viscosity of the solution produces a longer therapeutic duration of nasal formulations (ChitraKarthikeyini and Kavitha 2016).

8.6 Understanding Epilepsy

According to the International League Against Epilepsy (ILAE) (2014), "epilepsy is a disease characterized by an enduring predisposition to generate Epileptic seizures and by the neurobiological, cognitive, psychological and social consequences of this condition."

In the early eighteenth century, epilepsy was thought to be caused due to internal dysfunction of the brain affecting other organs in the process. The explanation of the modern epileptology was given by Tissot, whose work also explained different types of epilepsies. In the early eighteenth century some research papers were published by physicians of French medical school. Those papers were published by Jean-Etienne Dominique Esquirol (1772–1840), Calmeil (1798–1895), and Maisonneuve (1745–1826). Maisonneuve emphasized on significations of epileptic patient's hospitalization. He explained the idiopathic and sympathetic epilepsies in his work. Whereas Jean-Etienne Dominique Esquirol had described the difference between petite and grand mal and he also studied systematically insanity and epilepsy. In the mid nineteenth century, there were publications by prestigious physicians on epileptogenesis and taxonomy and etiology of epilepsy in 1852 and 1867 by Theodore Herpin (1799–1865), in 1854 by Louis

J. F. Delasiauve, in 1861 by John Russell Reynolds (1828–1896), and in 1881 by Sir William Richard Gowers (1845–1915).

In 1903, a Swedish physician Lundborg was the first to explain that epilepsy could be hereditary. A prominent book named *The Borderlands of Epilepsy* was published in 1907 by Gower. The book described narcolepsy, vertigo, migraine, etc. In 1920, *Epilepsy from the Standpoint of Physiology and Treatment* was published by Lennox (1884–1964) and Cobb (1887–1968), describing ketogenic diet (i.e., low-carbohydrates diet), effects of the amount of oxygen present in brain on seizures, etc. The proof that the origination site of psychomotor seizures is the temporal lobe was provided by Jasper (1906–1999) and Kershmann in 1941 after the claim of a German-American psychologist Kluver (1897–1979) and an American neuropathologist Bucy, who are famous for discovering the Kluver-Bucy Syndrome in the 1940s. Kluver and Bucy described the chances for change in the behavior of monkeys caused by lesions in the temporal bone. In 1969, James Kiffin Penry (1929–1996) published his research article describing epilepsy mechanism, treatment for epilepsy, drugs used in treating epilepsy, mode of action of antiepileptic drugs, etc. (Magiorkinis et al. 2014).

8.7 Neurobiology of Epilepsy

The interference in the mode of action maintaining a steady state between excitation and inhibition causes seizures. Mechanisms that promote excitation get inhibited after disruption of the mechanism causing seizures. The nervous system is a function of its ionic milieu, the chemical and electrical gradients that create the setting for electrical activity (seizures) (Schmidt and Moore 1995). Seizure hinders this potential of resting membrane and may inhibit excessive discharge. Transmembrane gradient change can also be led by seizures due to excessive discharge, causing increase in extracellular potassium and eventually depolarizing neurons. The mechanism of ionic basis can also lead to seizure. For example, a dysfunction of the sodium channel in the cell membrane can reduce the threshold, and mutation in subunits of the sodium channel depending on voltage can also lead to epilepsy. Disruption of mechanism leads to increased inhibition of neuron to reach close to their firing threshold and prevents seizure. Temporal lobe epilepsy (TLE) is a good example of epilepsy. In patients having TLE, the injury may not show any confirmation of overt seizure, but later on recurrent seizures may occur.

8.8 Causes of Epilepsy

Epilepsy can be caused due to following conditions:

(a) *Cerebrovascular disease:* Epilepsy can occur due to the presence of cerebrovascular diseases. The stroke site's size and number of lesions can be responsible for epilepsy (Liu et al. 2016). Possibilities for epilepsy to arise increase with conditions like ischemic stroke, hemorrhagic stroke, stroke lesions getting stimulated mechanically, and formation of glial scar (Huang et al. 2014). Some of these conditions have been deliberated below:
   - *Ischemic stroke:* Ischemic strokes have complications, such as hemorrhagic transformation. That can be associated with thrombolytic therapy leading to epilepsy (Zhang et al. 2014). Elderly patients have chances of having thrombolytic stroke due to the presence of cardiovascular diseases. Therefore, such patients are more susceptible to epilepsy. Numerous other factors such as smoking, depression, diabetes, hypertension, alcohol consumption, coronary heart disease, etc., can lead to ischemic stroke and may contribute to epilepsy.
   - *Hemorrhagic stroke:* Hemorrhagic stroke can more likely lead to epilepsy compared to ischemic stroke due to the involvement of cerebral cortex carrying lesions. These lesions hinder the cerebral cortex causing intracranial bleeding and venous injury that enhance the possibility of epilepsy.

(b) *Small vessel and multivascular disease:* Radiographic evidence prove that high blood pressure, coronary arterial disease, peripheral arterial disease and high cholesterol associated with large and small vessels, and multivascular diseases activate epilepsy. Lacunar infracts and leukoaraiosis diseases (multivascular diseases) cause epilepsy and can be more crucial when they are associated with impaired cognition.
(c) *Alzheimer's disease:* Alzheimer's is a neurodegenerative disease. Patients with dementia are reported to be affected more by epilepsy.
(d) *Tumor*: Tumor increases the possibility for developing epilepsy (symptomatic and all other epilepsies).

Other major causes of epilepsy are:

- Lack of oxygen during child birth.
- Injury of head either during birth or due to accident may lead to epilepsy in the childhood or even in the adulthood.
- Tuberous sclerosis.
- Epilepsy can be genetic.
- Infectious diseases such as meningitis or encephalitis.
- Increase or decrease in sodium or potassium can lead to epilepsy due to dysfunction of sodium or potassium channels present in the cell membrane.

8.9 Conventional Treatment

Antiepileptic drug (AED) therapy has been the backbone for the treatment of most epilepsy patients. Such a therapy has four goals: to reduce the frequency of the seizures or to eliminate seizures to maximum degree, to elude the side effects occurring due to long-term medication, to maintain normal life, and to restore patient's psychological or vocational activities.

AEDs should be introduced early to prevent seizures. The possibility of seizure varies amongst patients, depending on the type of epilepsy or correlated with neurological conditions or medical problems. The ideal characteristics of AED should be to stop seizures and at the same time avoiding occurrence of adverse effects. Currently AED are not able to stop seizures completely and also induce adverse effects, varying from minimal impairment of CNS to death. (Mittal et al. 2014). A classification of antiepileptic drugs is given in Table 8.2.

There has been rapid expansion in the type and number of available antiepileptic drugs for over the last two decades, but there is also increase in unwanted adverse effects. Approximately 75% of seizures are controlled through conventional treatment with AEDs, but nonconventional medical treatment also plays a major role in controlling seizures, like surgery, nonstandard medical treatment, dietary approaches, and nonpharmacological medication with minimum toxicity. A list of nonconventional treatment for epilepsy is given in Table 8.3 (Kneen and Appleton 2006).

Table 8.2 Classification of antiepileptic drugs

S. No	Class	Drugs
1	Barbiturate	Phenobarbitone
2	Deoxybarbiturate	Primidone
3	Hydantoin	Phenytoin Fosphenytoin
4	Iminostilbene	Carbamezapine Oxcarbazepine
5	Succinimide	Ethosuximide
6	Aliphatic carboxylic acid	Valproic acid [sodium valproate]
7	Benzodiazepines	Clonazepam Diazepam Lorazepam Clobazam
8	Phenyltriazine	Lamotrigine
9	Cyclic gaba analogues	Gabapentin Pregabalin
10	Newer drugs	Topiramate Zonisamide Levetricetam Vigabatrin Tiagabine Lacosamide

Table 8.3 Classification of nonconventional treatment for epilepsy

Non-conventional treatment for epilepsy	
Non-AED medical treatment	*Non-pharmacological treatment*
Steroids	Exercise
Vitamins	Avoid excessive alcohol
Intravenous immunoglobulins	Avoid sleep deprivation
Melatonin	
Dietary treatment	*Psychological treatment*
Ketogenic diet	Avoid psychiatric co-morbidity
Oligoantigenic diet	Yoga
Surgery treatment	*Alternative treatment*
Lesional surgery	Herbal medicine
Specific surgical techniques	Homeopathy
Palliative surgery	Aromatherapy

8.10 Nanoformulations for the Treatment of Epilepsy

8.10.1 Colloidal Carriers

Colloidal carriers are the delivery systems formulated for targeted, controlled, and sustained release of drug. Nanoparticles, niosomes, liposomes, etc., serve as colloidal carriers. They provide easy access to lipid-soluble drugs to pass through biological membranes due to their lipophilicity (lipophilic bilayer either encapsulating drug molecule or drug dispersed through lipophilic media), and are target specific.

Colloidal carriers are the most important vehicles employed for successful transport of loaded drugs. Colloidal carriers are drug vectors, which secrete, retain, and transport or deliver the drug within or surrounding the target. Colloidal carriers not only transfer the drug to the desired site and enhance drug therapeutic effect but also decrease the amount of drug and also minimize toxic effects. A classification of colloidal carrier systems is given in Fig. 8.3.

8.10.2 Nanogels

Nano gels are a 3D network of hydrogel materials in a nanoscale size. They have a swellable network and are cross-linked and can hold a large volume of water. They are prepared by synthetic polymers or biopolymers or both. Their physicochemical properties can be modified by changing their properties, such as size, charge, porosity, degradability, amphiphilicity, and softness. They are composed of a core-shell structure with cross-links and have different shapes for structural integrity. Nanogels are biocompatible, hydrophilic, and have a high drug loading capacity. Hence, they are useful for targeted delivery. They exhibit stimuli-responsive behavior, which protects the drug from degradation, making them useful for biomedical treatments such as drug delivery and diagnostic tools, etc. They have a high drug loading capacity because when nanogels swell, the inner space becomes available for drug loading. The swelling capacity is influenced by various factors, such as chemical structure of the polymer matrix, charge density, external triggers, and the degree of cross-linking. For optimum drug loading, their capacity to swell and collapse is important. They are easily permeated to various physiological barriers. They are small in size, making them optimum for delivering drug to target site and enhancing cellular uptake. Drug release through nanogels is determined by the degree of gel cross-linking, degradation of gel network, interaction of drug with polymers, and molecular weight of the polymer. Nanogels can be used to deliver hydrophilic and hydrophobic drugs. They can bypass the blood-brain barrier, and therefore are used to treat brain diseases. Nanogels are more effective because of reduced toxicity, high drug loading capacity, release of drug in a controlled manner at the target site, and enhanced cellular uptake. Materials used in the preparation of nanogels can lead to loss of epithelial cell, loss of ciliary cells, and shrinkage of the mucosal layer (Aderibigbe 2018).

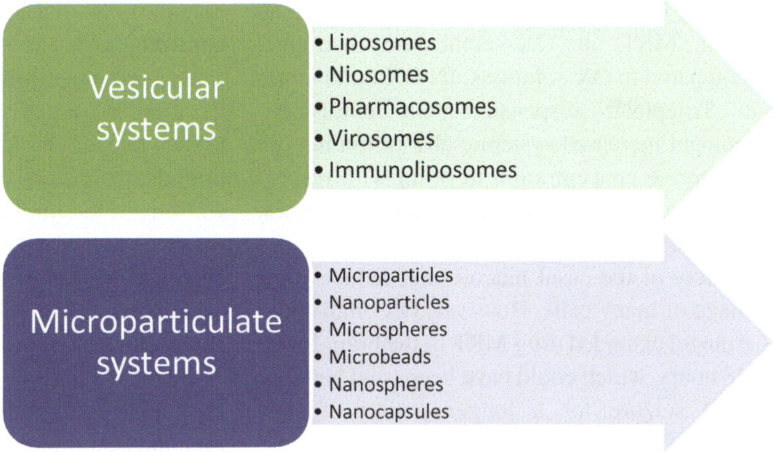

Fig. 8.3 Classification of colloidal carriers

Omar et al. prepared carbamazepine [CBZ]-loaded oil-in-water nanogel, which was characterized for various parameters like oil droplet size, in vitro drug release of CBZ, mucoadhesion, and CBZ uptake by phosphatidylcholine liposome for in vitro model of olfactory cells. Swiss albino mice were used to determine the anticonvulsant activity of nasal nanogel by inducing convulsions chemically and electrically. The in vitro release of CBZ from nanogel was found to be low, yet drug uptake from the liposome membrane was found to be 65% in 1 hour. The onset time of convulsion in chemically convulsive mice was prolonged which also protected the animals from two electric shocks along with decreased side effects of conventional CBZ following treatment with developed nanogel (Omar et al. 2012).

8.10.3 Liposomes

Liposomes are composed of unilamellar or multilamellar vesicles enclosing the central aqueous compartment. Liposomes are biocompatible and biodegradable and have the ability to encapsulate drugs with diverse lipophilicity and molecular weight. They are mostly preferred in antiepileptic drug delivery systems. They are ideal nanocarriers due to their ability to alter the surface characteristics, membrane fluidity, and dimensions. Liposome carriers have reduced enzymatic degradation and enhanced bioavailability across the cellular membrane. By the use of glycolipids, polyethylene glycols, and variation in vesicle size and enhanced surface lipophilicity, the half-lives of liposomes can be modified. For optimal drug delivery, immunoliposomes are the best strategy. They are formulated by fusion with polyethylene glycol [PEG] and stabilized with monoclonal antibody. Immunoliposomes deliver drug at four times more than the PEG-liposomes. Certain limitations of liposomal delivery have been noted, including rapid clearance from blood through RES, fast metabolic degradation of phospholipids, and low stability after extended release. Also compared to other nanocarriers, it fails in continuous delivery of drug. Drawbacks of liposomes-AED are overcome by improving stability and shelf-life (Jabir et al. 2015).

Recently, Zaafarany et al prepared emulsomes consisting of enclosed lipid core which was stabilized by phospholipids (PC) bilayers and tween 80 coating. The antiepileptic drug Oxcarbazepine [OX] was entrapped in emulsomes, localized in a poly(lactic acid co-glycolic acid)–poly(ethylene glycol)–poly(lactic acid co-glycolic acid) (PLGA-PEG-PLGA) triblock thermogel copolymer. Drug release was found to be retarded, and the mean residence time (MRT) was found to be increased in rats when OX emulsomes were incorporated in the thermogel. In vitro sustained drug release was found to be about 81.1% from OX emulsomes and 53.5% from OX emulsomes-thermogel within 24 hours. The pharmacokinetic study in rats showed systemic transport of drug OX after nasal administration with a higher uptake of OX emulsomes in the brain tissue and highest MRT in OX emulsomes-thermogel as compared to OX-solutions, IN OX-emulsomes and Trileptal® suspension. OX emulsome-thermogel increased systemic absorption but did not increase concentration in brain with respect to Cmax and AUC compared to OX emulsomes. The PLGA-PEG-PLGA can be used to enhance the safety of the nasal mucosa and reduce nasal damage of many cells. However, OX emulsome-thermogel extended drug MRT in the brain for up to 48 hours, which could have been used better to control seizure for a longer period of time (El-Zaafarany et al. 2018).

Jian-sheng liu et al. developed a nanoscale delivery system to improve brain penetration and solubility of Lamotrigine (LTG), an antiepileptic drug. LTG loaded polymeric micelles were prepared by loading LTG in Pluronic® P123 (P123/LTG). The encapsulation efficiency was found to be 98.07%, particle size was 18.73 nm and drug loading was 5.63%. The solubility of drug LTG in polymeric micelles (P123/LTG) was increased to 2.17 mg/mL. Drug showed sustained release properties from an in vitro release study of P123/LTG. After IV administration in rats, drug loaded with polymeric micelles was accumulated more in brain than free drug at 0.5, 1, and 4 hours. By incorporating P-gp substrate in P123, micelles showed higher penetration by crossing the blood brain barrier in vitro and in vivo. Hence P123 micelles showed better targeted delivery of antiepileptic drugs in the treatment of epilepsy (Liu et al. 2014).

8.10.4 Solid-Lipid Nanoparticles

Solid-lipid nanoparticles (SLNs) are colloidal drug carriers for intravenous application. They are submicron particles ranging from 10 to 1000 nm. SLNs are made up of solid lipids which are scattered in water or aqueous surfactant. To overcome any disadvantage solid lipid is combined with liquid lipid. Solid-lipid nanoparticles have various advantages, such as controlled release of drug over long periods of time, biocompatibility, improved stability, sterilization by autoclaving or gamma radiation, better release kinetics of encapsulated compounds, increased bioavailability, chemical protection of labile compounds, ease of manufacturing, avoidance of organic solvents, high and long-term stability, ease of industrial scale production, relatively cheaper and stable. For prolonged release or protection of drug from chemical degradation, solid-lipid nanoparticles are a proven better alternative delivery system than the traditional oil-in-water emulsion. SLNs have lower toxicity and relatively low cost excipients, as solvents are not used in the preparation process. Further, as SLNs are prepared by simple process of high-pressure homogenization, they have high chances of large-scale production. SLNs provide protection to drug against chemical degradation, as there is no or less water to the inner core of lipid particles compared to liposomes. SLNs can be delivered through various routes such as parenteral, nasal, rectal, ophthalmic and topical. Antiepileptic drugs loaded in SLNs may show high efficacy for the treatment of epilepsy by their ability to cross blood brain barrier (Costa et al. 2019).

Nair Rahul, et al. prepared aqueous solution of SLNs containing chitosan by incorporating the antiepileptic drug Carbamazepine (CBZ). The preparation of SLNs of chitosan-CBZ showed high encapsulation efficiency and high drug stability. The drug showed a controlled release pattern for a prolonged period of time. The antiepileptic activity of SLNs of chitosan-CBZ showed better results compared to standard CBZ. Time for onset of convulsion in controlled group was less than in the standard group, i.e., 28 ± 1.195 and 58.17 ± 6.67 min respectively. An in vitro model showed 66.7% of drug release in 24 hours. Solid-lipid chitosan-CBZ showed improved antiepileptic activity as compared to standard CBZ in the treatment of seizures (Nair et al. 2012).

8.10.5 Nanoemulsions

Nanoemulsions are water-in-oil (W/O) or oil-in-water (O/W) emulsions with two immiscible liquids dispersed and stabilized by the addition of surfactants. The mean diameter of a nanoemulsion droplet is about 100 nm to 300 nm. Nanoemulsions are white to milky white in appearance as they are smaller than the wavelength of visible light. They can be formulated in various formulations such as liquid, creams, spray, gels, or foams. They can be formulated as various dosage forms such as parenteral, ocular, oral, in addition to nasal. Nanoemulsions have a high surface area due to small droplet size and long-term stability. The latter is attributed to small droplet size, which reduces destabilization phenomena, such as coalescence, sedimentation, and creaming. Drug problems such as lack of solubility and stability in certain environments can be solved by formulating nanoemulsions. When drug comes in contact with the aqueous environment, which is dissolved in oily phase, the hydrophobic drug is released from nanoemulsion and nanoprecipitation occurs. Particles with high surface area are formed by improving the drug solubility rate according to Noyes-Whitney equation. Advantages of nanoemulsions are increased solubility, reduced irritation, reduced toxicity, effective penetration of drug, and protection from hydrolysis and oxidation. The advantage of delivering antiepileptic drugs in the form of nanoemulsion is that it can easily penetrate the blood-brain barrier even if the drug has low bioavailability. Nanoemulsion is prepared by spontaneous emulsification process (Bonferoni et al. 2019).

Patel, et al. developed carbamazepine (CMP)-loaded microemulsion (CMPME) and mucoadhesive CMPME (CMPMME) for intranasal delivery for the treatment of epilepsy. Swiss albino rats were used to determine drug distribution in the brain. The CMPME was stable and crystal clear, with a size of 34.11 ± 1.41 nm. Brain/blood ratio of intranasal CMPMME was found to be 2-3 folds higher than that of intravenous CMPME indicating larger extent of CMP distribution inbrain. Drug targeting efficacy and direct drug transport were found to be higher in intranasallly administered CMPMME as compared to intravenous CMP. It was found that CMPMME-loaded drug had higher uptake in brain. CMPMME showed a better result in the treatment of epilepsy (Patel et al. 2014).

8.10.6 Nanostructured Lipid Carriers

Nanostructured lipid carriers (NLCs) are the second-generation of lipid-based nanocarriers. They are formed by mixing liquid lipids and solid lipids. They have an unstructured matrix due to the different moieties of the NLC constituents. They are designed to overcome the limitations of SLNs. Due to improper crystal structure, they have a high drug loading capacity. Furthermore, chances of drug expulsion can be avoided during storage and manufacturing by lipid crystallization. They have high drug solubility in lipid matrix and show a more controllable release matrix than SLNs. They have a lower melting point than SLNs; they are solid at body temperature. Furthermore, because of their imperfect crystalline structure and unstructured matrix, they have high drug dissolution and payload in the liquid part of NLCs. NLCs show less gelation in preparation and storage than SLNs. Hydrophobic and hydrophilic drugs can be loaded in NLCs with a wide range of drug-loading properties. They can be surface-modified. The chemical and physical properties of NLCs are stable. As NLCs have liquid lipids, by increasing the liquid lipid the solubility of drug can be increased and encapsulation of drug enhanced compared to SLNs (Ghasemiyeh and Mohammadi-Samani 2018).

Eskandari et al. conducted a study by incorporating valproic acid (VPA) in NLCs for the treatment of epilepsy. Six groups of rats with each group containing six animals were used, each animal received VPA-NLC intranasally or intraperitoneally. Maximal electric shock was used to examine brain responses. The hind limb tonic extension: flexion inhibition was determined at different time intervals: 15, 30, 60, 90, and 120 minutes. By using gas chromatography, drug concentration in plasma and brain was determined. The particle size, percent drug loading and percent drug release of the NLCs was found

Table 8.4 Various nanoformulations for antiepileptic drugs

S. No.	Name of drug	Formulation	Reference
1.	Gabapentine	Nanoparticles	Wilson et al. (2014)
2.	Lamotrigine	Pluronic 123 micelles, lipid nanoparticles	Liu et al. (2014)
3.	Carbamazepine	Solid lipid nanoparticles	Nair et al. (2012)
4.	Oxcarbazepene	PLGA nanoparticles	Lopalco et al. (2015)
5.	Valproic acid	Nanoparticles, nano-structured lipid carrier	Varshosaz et al. (2010), Hamidi et al. (2012)
6.	Diazepam	Solid lipid nanoparticles	Abdelbary and Fahmy (2009)
7.	Ethosuximide	Chitosan nano-carrier	Hsiao et al. (2012)
8.	Acetazolamide	Nanoparticles	–

to be 154 ± 64 nm, 47 ± 0.8% and 75 ± 1.9% respectively after 21 days. After treatment via intranasal route, in vitro studies showed difference between protective effects of NLCs VPA and control group at 15, 30, 90, and 120 minutes. Treatment via the intraperitoneal route showed positive result for protective effects of NLCs VPA and control group. Brain/plasma drug concentration ratio was found to be higher following intranasal administration of NLCs VPA as compared to intraperitoneal administration. Hence, intranasal administration of NLCs VPA provided better protection from seizures (Eskandari et al. 2011). Various nanoformulations of antiepileptic drugs are summarized in Table 8.4.

8.11 Toxicological Studies

Formulations need enhanced drug absorption in nose to brain delivery of drug in order to achieve the desired therapeutic effect for treatment of brain- or CNS-related diseases. It can be achieved by the addition of some mucoadhesive excipients to enhance the adhesive property of the formulation. These mucoadhesive excipients allow the formulation containing the drug molecule to adhere to the mucous membrane for a longer period of time, thereby helping in slow release of the drug and providing more time for the drug to be absorbed by the membrane. Gelling agents can also be used for this effect. Nanoformulations are prepared to achieve smaller particle size of the drug's formulation to enable access to the formulation through BBB. Improvement or increase in the adhesiveness of the formulation may cause toxicity or adverse effect on the mucous membrane, such as ciliotoxicity, shrinking of the mucous layer, or may affect the mucociliary clearance and respiratory system. Therefore, it is recommended to evaluate all formulations (drug or active ingredient, all excipients, final formulation, etc.) because certain effects of toxicity might be challenging to treat afterwards. For example, once the mucous layer shrinks it cannot be repaired. Therefore, special precautions are taken during preparation of such formulations. Biodegradable studies, drug compatibility studies with excipients, in vivo studies on laboratory animals, mucociliary clearance studies, etc., are also performed for the detection of toxicity and effect of formulation (Costa et al. 2019). Some clinical trials on nose to brain delivery of antiepileptic drugs are listed in Table 8.5.

Table 8.5 Clinical trial on nose to brain delivery of antiepileptic drug

S. No	Drug	Product name	Company	Phase	Study Result	Status
1	Midazolam	–	–	Pre-clinical	Comparison between IN-MDZ and IV-MDZ for status epilectus showed IN-MDZ was better in controlling seizures than IV-MDZ	Complete
2	Oxcarbazepine	–	–	III	Able to treat uncontrollable focal seizures in children	Complete
3	Eslicarbazepine acetate	I – Zebinix II – Aptiom	I – Eisai co. Ltd II – Sunovion Pharmaceuticals Inc.	III	Partial-onset seizures were treated with long-term monotherapy -Uncontrollable focal seizures were well tolerated and effective in patients Tested for refractory partial seizure as an adjunct therapy	Complete
4	Brivaracetam	Briviact	Approved by FDA	III	To treat safety and efficacy for adjunctive i.v. and bolos antiepileptic therapy in patients and with partial- onset seizures	Ongoing
5	Cenobamate	YKP3089	S K Pharmaceuticals	II III	Patients with photosensitive epilepsy showed efficacy and were tolerated. Adjunctive therapy for partial seizure in patients was conducted Adjunctive therapy for patients having partial seizure is being conducted for drug safety and efficacy	Complete Ongoing
6	Verapamil	–	–	II	Children and adult with Dravet Syndrome showed adjunctive therapy for seizures	Complete
7	Diazepam	NRL-1	Neurelis Inc.	I	Healthy volunteers showed tolerability for the drug	Complete
8	Midazolam	USL261	Upsher smith laboratories	III	Outpatient treatment for patients having seizure cluster	Recruiting
9	Diazepam	Plumiaz™	Neuronex Acorda	I	Tolerability, safety, efficacy of nasal spray in healthy volunteers	Ongoing
10	Diazepam	Plumiaz™	Neuronex Acorda	II	Patients experiencing a seizure episode, single dose through nasal spray was studied	Complete
11	Diazepam	Plumiaz™	Neuronex Acorda	II	To examine tolerability, efficacy and bioavailability of nasal gel, rectal and nasal spray	Recruiting

Charalambous et al. (2019), Aboutabl (n.d.), Kaur et al. (2016)

8.12 Conclusion

Nose-to-brain delivery is considered an evolving approach to overcome the BBB. Intranasal (IN) delivery of antiepileptic drug delivery systems (AEDs) has been recommended and explored by various researchers. The 3N rule combining nose, nanomedicine, and neurotherapeutics is the impending solution to accomplish the above-mentioned goal. The large number of in vivo studies published over the last few years on IN delivery of AEDs indicates the growing interest in this route. Nanomedicine represents a captivating strategy to overcome some of the major limitations, combined with the IN route of administration as investigated in preclinical studies. Some of the nanoformulations are also under clinical trials. These novel substitutes to traditional oral and intravenous delivery methods will definitely lead to more effective treatments for epilepsy patients in the future.

References

Abbott NJ, Friedman A (2012) Overview and introduction: the blood-brain barrier in health and disease: blood-brain barrier in health and disease. Epilepsia 53:1–6. https://doi.org/10.1111/j.1528-1167.2012.03696.x

Abdelbary G, Fahmy RH (2009) Diazepam-loaded solid lipid nanoparticles: design and characterization. AAPS PharmSciTech 10:211–219. https://doi.org/10.1208/s12249-009-9197-2

Aboutabl (n.d.) Antiepileptic drugs: progress and development [WWW Document]. URL http://www.epj.eg.net/article.asp?issn=1687-4315;year=2018;volume=17;issue=3;spage=129;epage=140;aulast=Aboutabl. Accessed 11.1.19

Aderibigbe BA (2018) In situ-based gels for nose to brain delivery for the treatment of neurological diseases. Pharmaceutics 10. https://doi.org/10.3390/pharmaceutics10020040

Baines SJ (2014) Chapter 51 - Pharynx, in: Langley-Hobbs, S.J., Demetriou, J.L., Ladlow, J.F. (Eds.), Feline Soft Tissue and General Surgery. W.B. Saunders, pp.617–633. https://doi.org/10.1016/B978-0-7020-4336-9.00051-2

Bonferoni MC, Rossi S, Sandri G, Ferrari F, Gavini E, Rassu G, Giunchedi P (2019) Nanoemulsions for "nose-to-brain" drug delivery. Pharmaceutics 11:84. https://doi.org/10.3390/pharmaceutics11020084

Charalambous M, Volk HA, Tipold A, Erath J, Huenerfauth E, Gallucci A, Gandini G, Hasegawa D, Pancotto T, Rossmeisl JH, Platt S, De Risio L, Coates JR, Musteata M, Tirrito F, Cozzi F, Porcarelli L, Corlazzoli D, Cappello R, Vanhaesebrouck A, Broeckx BJG, Van Ham L, Bhatti SFM (2019) Comparison of intranasal versus intravenous midazolam for management of status epilepticus in dogs: a multi-center randomized parallel group clinical study. J Vet Intern Med. https://doi.org/10.1111/jvim.15627

ChitraKarthikeyini S, Kavitha K (2016) Nasal drug delivery-a pre hospital therapy in status epilepsy-review. IOSR J Pharm Biol Sci 11:39

Clossen BL, Reddy DS (2017) Novel therapeutic approaches for disease-modification of epileptogenesis for curing epilepsy. Biochim Biophys Acta Mol basis Dis 1863:1519–1538. https://doi.org/10.1016/j.bbadis.2017.02.003

Costa C, Moreira JN, Amaral MH, Sousa Lobo JM, Silva AC (2019) Nose-to-brain delivery of lipid-based nanosystems for epileptic seizures and anxiety crisis. J Control Release 295:187–200. https://doi.org/10.1016/j.jconrel.2018.12.049

Daneman R, Prat A (2015) The blood–brain barrier. Cold Spring Harb Perspect Biol 7. https://doi.org/10.1101/cshperspect.a020412

Dhakar RC, Maurya SK, Tilak V, Gupta K (2011) A review on factors affecting the design of nasal drug delivery system. Int J Drug Deliv 3. https://doi.org/10.5138/ijdd.v3i2.214

East C (2019) 17 - Crooked Nose, in: Frame JD, Bagheri SC, Smith DJ, Khan HA (Eds.), Aesthetic Surgery Techniques. Content Repository Only!, London, pp. 133–136. https://doi.org/10.1016/B978-0-323-41745-7.00017-5

Eduardo Nazareth Nigro C, Faria de Aguiar Nigro J, Mion O, Mello J (2009) Nasal Valve: Anatomy and physiology. (15)30795–3. https://doi.org/10.1016/S1808-8694

El-Zaafarany GM, Soliman ME, Mansour S, Cespi M, Palmieri GF, Illum L, Casettari L, Awad GAS (2018) A tailored thermosensitive PLGA-PEG-PLGA/Emulsomes composite for enhanced oxcarbazepine brain delivery via the nasal route. Pharmaceutics 10. https://doi.org/10.3390/pharmaceutics10040217

Eskandari S, Varshosaz J, Minaiyan M, Tabbakhian M (2011) Brain delivery of valproic acid via intranasal administration of nanostructured lipid carriers: in vivo pharmacodynamic studies using rat electroshock model. Int J Nanomedicine 6:363–371. https://doi.org/10.2147/IJN.S15881

Finkelstein Y, Meshorer A, Talmi YP, Zohar Y, Brenner J, Gal R (1992) The riddle of the uvula. Otolaryngol.--Head Neck Surg. Off. J. Am. Acad. Otolaryngol.-Head Neck Surg. 107, 444–450. https://doi.org/10.1177/019459989210700318

Ghasemiyeh P, Mohammadi-Samani S (2018) Solid lipid nanoparticles and nanostructured lipid carriers as novel drug delivery systems: applications, advantages and disadvantages. Res Pharm Sci 13:288–303. https://doi.org/10.4103/1735-5362.235156

Ghaffarieh A, Levin LA (2012) Chapter One - Optic Nerve Disease and Axon Pathophysiology, in: Goldberg JL, Trakhtenberg EF (Eds.), International Review of Neurobiology, Axon Growth and Regeneration: Part 1. Academic Press, pp. 1–17. https://doi.org/10.1016/B978-0-12-398309-1.00002-0

Gong Q (2012) Culture of Mouse Olfactory Sensory Neurons. Curr. Protoc. Neurosci. Editor. Board Jacqueline N Crawley Al CHAPTER, Unit3.24. https://doi.org/10.1002/0471142301.ns0324s58

Hamidi M, Azadi A, Mohamadi-Samani S, Rafiei P, Ashrafi H (2012) Valproate-loaded hydrogel nanoparticles: preparation and characterization. J Appl Polym Sci 124:4686–4693. https://doi.org/10.1002/app.35527

Hsiao M-H, Larsson M, Larsson A, Evenbratt H, Chen Y-Y, Chen Y-Y, Liu D-M (2012) Design and characterization of a novel amphiphilic chitosan nanocapsule-based thermo-gelling biogel with sustained in vivo release of the hydrophilic anti-epilepsy drug ethosuximide. J Control Release 161:942–948. https://doi.org/10.1016/j.jconrel.2012.05.038

Huang L, Wu Z-B, ZhuGe Q, Zheng W, Shao B, Wang B, Sun F, Jin K (2014) Glial scar formation occurs in the human brain after ischemic stroke. Int J Med Sci 11:344–348. https://doi.org/10.7150/ijms.8140

Jabir N, Tabrez S, Firoz CK, Zaidi S, Baeesa S, Gan S, Shakil S, Kamal M (2015) A synopsis of nano-technological approaches toward anti-epilepsy therapy: present and future research implications. Curr Drug Metab 16:336–345. https://doi.org/10.2174/138920021566614112514260

Kaur H, Kumar B, Medhi B (2016) Antiepileptic drugs in development pipeline: a recent update. eNeurologicalSci 4:42–51. https://doi.org/10.1016/j.ensci.2016.06.003

Kneen R, Appleton RE (2006) Alternative approaches to conventional antiepileptic drugs in the management of paediatric epilepsy. Arch Dis Child 91:936–941. https://doi.org/10.1136/adc.2005.080002

Leinders-Zufall T, Ma M (2009) Olfactory Epithelium, in: Squire, L.R. (Ed.), Encyclopedia of Neuroscience. Academic Press, Oxford, pp. 113–118. https://doi.org/10.1016/B978-008045046-9.01684-3

Liu J-S, Wang J-H, Zhou J, Tang X-H, Xu L, Shen T, Wu X-Y, Hong Z (2014) Enhanced brain delivery of lamotrigine with Pluronic® P123-based nanocarrier. Int J Nanomedicine 9:3923–3935. https://doi.org/10.2147/IJN.S62263

Liu S, Yu W, Lü Y (2016) The causes of new-onset epilepsy and seizures in the elderly. Neuropsychiatr Dis Treat 12:1425–1434. https://doi.org/10.2147/NDT.S107905

Lopalco A, Ali H, Denora N, Rytting E (2015) Oxcarbazepine-loaded polymeric nanoparticles: development and permeability studies across in vitro models of the blood-brain barrier and human placental trophoblast [WWW Document]. Int J Nanomedicine. https://doi.org/10.2147/IJN.S77498

Magiorkinis E, Diamantis A, Sidiropoulou K, Panteliadis C (2014) Highights in the history of epilepsy: the last 200 years [WWW Document]. Epilepsy Res Treat. https://doi.org/10.1155/2014/582039

Măru N, Rusu MC, Săndulescu M (2015) Variant anatomy of nasal turbinates: supreme, superior and middle conchae bullosae, paradoxical superior and inferiorturbinates, and middle accessory turbinate. Romanian J. Morphol. Embryol. Rev. Roum. Morphol. Embryol. 56, 1223–1226.

Mittal D, Ali A, Md S, Baboota S, Sahni JK, Ali J (2014) Insights into direct nose to brain delivery: current status and future perspective. Drug Deliv 21:75–86. https://doi.org/10.3109/10717544.2013.838713

Mori K (2009) Olfactory Bulb Mapping, in: Squire, L.R. (Ed.), Encyclopedia of Neuroscience. Academic Press, Oxford, pp. 71–75. https://doi.org/10.1016/B978-008045046-9.01688-0

Nair R, Kumar AC, Priya VK, Yadav CM, Raju PY (2012) Formulation and evaluation of chitosan solid lipid nanoparticles of carbamazepine. Lipids Health Dis 11:72. https://doi.org/10.1186/1476-511X-11-72

Omar S, Hanan R, Kamal ET (2012) Carbamazepine mucoadhesive nanoemulgel (MNEG) as brain targeting delivery system via the olfactory mucosa. Drug Deliv 19:58–67. https://doi.org/10.3109/10717544.2011.644349

Patel R, Patel M, Kashyap B, Patel BG, Gaikwad RV (2014) Microemulsion-based drug delivery system for transnasal delivery of Carbamazepine: preliminary brain-targeting study. Drug Deliv 23:1–7. https://doi.org/10.3109/10717544.2014.908980

Ribatti D, Nico B, Crivellato E, Artico M (2006) Development of the blood-brain barrier: a historical point of view. Anat Rec B New Anat 289:3–8. https://doi.org/10.1002/ar.b.20087

Schmidt WK, Moore HP (1995) Ionic milieu controls the compartment-specific activation of proopiomelanocortin processing in AtT-20 cells. Mol Biol Cell 6:1271–1285

Selvaraj K, Gowthamarajan K, Karri VVSR (2018) Nose to brain transport pathways an overview: potential of nanostructured lipid carriers in nose to brain targeting. Artif Cells Nanomed Biotechnol 46:2088–2095. https://doi.org/10.1080/21691401.2017.1420073

Tiwari G, Tiwari R, Sriwastawa B, Bhati L, Pandey S, Pandey P, Bannerjee SK (2012) Drug delivery systems: an updated review. Int J Pharm Investig 2:2. https://doi.org/10.4103/2230-973X.96920

Varshosaz J, Eskandari S, Tabakhian M (2010) Production and optimization of valproic acid nanostructured lipid carriers by the Taguchi design. Pharm Dev Technol 15:89–96. https://doi.org/10.3109/10837450903013568

Wilson B, Lavanya Y, Priyadarshini SRB, Ramasamy M, Jenita JL (2014) Albumin nanoparticles for the delivery of gabapentin: preparation, characterization and pharmacodynamic studies. Int J Pharm 473:73–79. https://doi.org/10.1016/j.ijpharm.2014.05.056

Zhang J, Yang Y, Sun H, Xing Y (2014) Hemorrhagic transformation after cerebral infarction: current concepts and challenges. Ann Transl Med 2. https://doi.org/10.3978/j.issn.2305-5839.2014.08.08

9 Recent Advances in Nanocarrier-Based Brain-Targeted Drug Delivery for Effective Treatment of Central Nervous System Disorders

Amita Sarwal, Gurpreet Singh, Priya Prasad, Sachin Sharma, and Waseem Ali

Abstract

One of the main obstacles for the effective treatment of CNS disorders is the incapability of drug molecules to cross the blood-brain barrier (BBB). Conventional drug delivery systems are having limited adequacy to assess the restrictions posed by the imperative blood-brain barrier. Numerous drugs designed for the treatment of various disorders are unable to permeate the BBB. This hampers their ability to effectively reach in the brain. Most of the drugs are given in high doses to provide adequate concentration in the brain. Complicated dosage regimens along with the systemic side effects reduce patient compliance, leading to the failure for the efficient disease management. A large number of delivery systems and target systems have been investigated to improve drug bioavailability and enhance drug accumulation at the targeted area in order to minimize systemic side effects, as well as to improve compliance. Nanotechnological approaches involve various nano-sized carrier systems, which promotes the brain availability of therapeutic agents for the effective management of neurodegenerative disorders. Over the conventional approaches, nanotechnological approaches have various promising strategies to cross blood-brain barrier and increase the bioavailability of therapeutics in the brain. This chapter elaborates upon the current and future utility of nano-drug delivery systems for the treatment of various CNS disorders.

Keywords

Blood-brain barrier · Magnetic nanoparticles · Solid lipid nanoparticles · Liposomes · Nanoemulsion

9.1 Introduction

Due to the severe impact on patients' long-term health, the growing incidence of CNS diseases and dementia is considered a major challenge in human health management. Health agencies and scientific reports have revealed that about 1.5 million people have CNS disorders and 11% of serious diseases are brain disorders (Silva 2005; Soni et al. 2016). Different drugs and therapeutic agents demonstrated not only effi-

A. Sarwal (✉) · G. Singh · P. Prasad · S. Sharma · W. Ali
University Institute of Pharmaceutical Sciences, UGC-Centre of Advanced Studies, Panjab University, Chandigarh, India

S. Talegaonkar, M. Rai (eds.), *Nanoformulations in Human Health*, https://doi.org/10.1007/978-3-030-41858-8_9

cacy but also shortcomings depending on the disease conditions of the individual patient. Therefore, there is a persistent demand for new therapies to develop better treatments for CNS diseases; however, the systematic implementation of such therapies poses significant challenges (Vinogradov 2010). The blood-brain barrier (BBB) and blood-cerebrospinal fluid barrier (BCSFB) inhibit site-specific therapeutic delivery, thus reducing their effectiveness against targeted diseases. The BBB can also reduce the concentration of a drug that enters the target site, thus increasing the ability to treat the target disease. The high-dose requirements of these drugs have intensified the need to develop nano-enabled drug delivery systems (DDSs) (Vashist et al. 2018), which have many advantages over conventional drugs and DDSs (Vashist et al. 2017). Such DDSs can noninvasively bypass the BBB. They can also easily modify their structure to encapsulate the desired drug, making it ideal for the treatment of CNS diseases.

The term "nanotechnology" comprises all the systems, as represented in Fig. 9.1, and materials having novel and improved physical, chemical, and biological properties, attributed to the nanoscale size range (Leyva-Gomez et al. 2015). Nanotechnology has been applied to improve the treatment of CNS disorders (Leyva-Gomez et al. 2015). Nanotechnology can be modulated to obtain preferred pharmacokinetics profiles, drug targeting to the specific site of action (Cupaioli et al. 2014). The major merits of using nanotechnology drug delivery systems include site-specific delivery for targeted action in the CNS, improved drug penetration, enhanced brain availability, and therapeutic performance of CNS drugs. The nanoparticles (NPs) intended for drug delivery of therapeutic agents are usually solid colloidal particles ranging from size 1 to 1000 nm (Fernandes et al. 2010; Md et al. 2015). NPs can

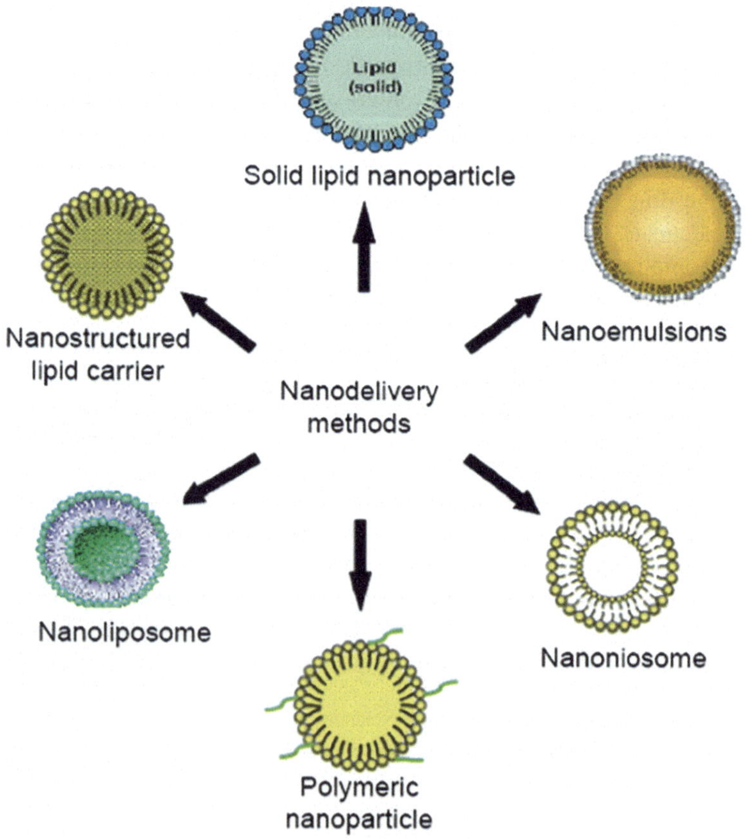

Fig. 9.1 Several different techniques that are currently under considerations for the nanodelivery to the brain

be thermoprotective for such as proteins, peptides, or DNA and can also be modified to execute site-specific drug targeting. Also, these systems can be used to maintain therapeutically desirable drug concentrations in plasma by increasing the half-life, solubility, and permeability of drugs.

9.2 BBB in a Normal Healthy Brain Condition

The BBB is a specific arrangement of fine endothelial cells which is imperative for providing basic supplements for normal working of brain and restrains the entry of harmful substances from the blood to the brain as represented in Fig. 9.2. BBB serves as a hindrance which is made up of endothelial cells (ECs), in conjunction with pericytes, astrocytes, perivascular neurons, tight junctions, and basal layer which adds to the intricate structure of the BBB (Guerra et al. 2017; Komarova et al. 2017; Lécuyer et al. 2017; Dong 2018). The endothelial cells in the cerebrum are not designed in a manner that prohibits disseminating drug particles. Endothelial cells are connected through intersection, creating a ceaseless hindrance, which limit the infiltration of hydrophilic drug substances (Umlauf and Shusta 2019). The penetrability of the barrier chiefly is monitored through these intersections which have proteinaceous nature, for example, adherens junctions, tight junctions, and gap junctions (Komarova et al. 2017; Dong 2018). Adherens intersections basically control the penetrability of the endothelial boundary. Tight junctions assume an imperative part in supporting the penetrability obstruction of epithelial and endothelial cells, which control tissue homeostasis (Lécuyer et al. 2017). Rather than behaving as a permanent feature, the barrier is consistently adjusting because of different physiological changes occurring in the brain (Banks 2016; Komarova et al. 2017; Dong 2018).

Physiochemical properties of the drug molecules affect the passively diffusing particles.

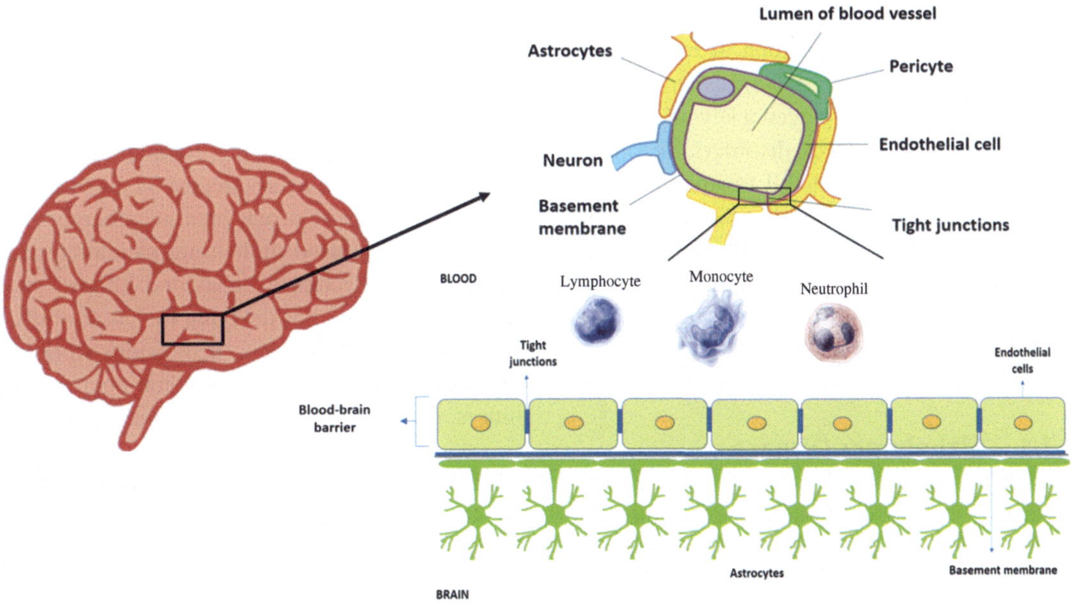

Fig. 9.2 Diagram of the various components of the neurovascular unit. The BBB mainly consists of the endothelial cells, connected by adherens and tight junctions (TJs) tightly; glial cells such as star-shaped astrocytes, having diverse functions such as axon pathfinding, neuronal synapse transmission, BBB regulation, and flow of blood; and other cells such as pericytes, found toward the outer surface of the blood vessels placed inside the basement membrane

Major factors impacting the penetration include the size, surface properties, lipophilicity, and charge on the surface of molecules. Physiological factors which can impact the BBB permeability includes action by enzymes, binding efficiency of molecule to the plasma protein, efflux transporters like P-glycoprotein (P-gp), and cerebrum blood flow (Banks 2009). Water-soluble molecules like proteins and peptides permeate into the brain through specific receptor-mediated transporters such as insulin transporter, transferrin transporter, and GLUT-1 (Ballabh et al. 2004). Transportation through receptor-specific mechanism has been widely examined for the drug's transport to the brain (Mäger et al. 2017).

9.3 CNS Disorders and Pharmacotherapy

Healthcare statistics conclude that the prevalence of CNS diseases, including neuroinfections and neurocognitive disorders, is increasing rapidly throughout the globe (Albert 2007; Brew and González-Scarano 2007; Hirtz et al. 2007; Nair et al. 2016; World Health Organization 2016) with a global economic burden of 6–8% due to neurological disorders. Advances in existing medical therapies have played a key role in treating and controlling CNS disorders, leading to higher survival rates, but full treatments remain lacking for most CNS disorders, including Alzheimer's disease (AD), Parkinson's disease (PD), depression, Huntington disease, and epilepsy (Kaushik et al. 2014, 2016a, b; Ruiz et al. 2015; Nair et al. 2016).

9.3.1 Alzheimer's Disease

Alzheimer's disease (AD) is one of the most severe neurological problems among the older population, with more than US$ 600 billion of socioeconomic burden (Kaushik et al. 2016a, b). AD is a brain disorder that results from the brain's diminished ability to repair neurons, resulting in loss of memory, changes of mood, depression, and anxiety (Kaushik et al. 2016a, b). There is a lack of AD-specific therapeutic agents at the moment, and this condition is therefore hard to treat and difficult to deal. Smart diagnostic sensing systems have been developed to monitor AD development under therapy (Kaushik et al. 2016a, b, c).

In 1906, a German neuropathologist, Alois Alzheimer, first described Alzheimer's disease (AD). At the beginning of the twenty-first century, Alzheimer's disease (AD) was identified as the most common form of dementia among geriatric individuals. In 2016, it was estimated that over 47.5 million people worldwide are diagnosed with dementia. The estimate is expected to rise to 75.6 million by 2030. (Chisholm et al. 2016). AD is a neurodegenerative disorder that usually occurs in adulthood. Various other mental capacities are correlated with a gradual and rather permanent deterioration in memory. Throughout AD, neuronal disruption and weakening of neural connections in the brain's cerebral cortex region are associated with a major loss of brain mass (Perl 2010). It is among the main five most common causes of death in the US population. Rarely, it occurs in people in their 40s and 50s, but still it is an old-age disorder. Two neuropathological marks, i.e., extracellular Aβ plaques and intracellular Tau neurofibrillary tangles (NFTs), are characterized by AD.

Treatment of AD is quite complex, and it is unlikely to be successfully treated by any drug or other intervention. Current pharmacotherapeutic strategies are focused on helping patients retain mental abilities, control behavioral effects, and delay progression, thus delaying the onset of disease symptoms. All current medications work by monitoring the brain levels of some neurotransmitters, mainly acetylcholine and glutamate.

9.3.1.1 Conventional Pharmacotherapy of AD

The existing drugs used in the medication of AD can be categorized broadly as:

(a) Acetylcholinesterase inhibitors: rivastigmine, donepezil, galantamine, and tacrine
(b) NMDA antagonist (glutamate inhibitor): memantine

9.3.1.2 Nutraceuticals for AD

Nutraceutical agents, commonly referred to as medical foods, are noticed to be useful in improving the quality of life in patients with AD.

(a) Tramiprosate
It is a small mimetic compound of glycosaminoglycan that can be orally taken. This binds to soluble Aβ and inhibits the accumulation and eventual deposition of amyloid plaques.
(b) Phosphatidylserine
The main component of the membrane in the nerve cells is phosphatidylserine, a lipid compound. Not only does it provide nourishment to the brain, it can also increase brain function, alleviate mental pressure, and enhance intelligence, memory, and force of response. This is also often referred to as a "brain nutrient" (Amaducci et al. 1991).
(c) Axona
It is a dietary supplement used in Alzheimer's treatment (Henderson et al. 2009). Axona's active ingredient is caprylic acid. It is a great source of triglycerides, and from processed coconut oil, it could also be obtained. To form β-hydroxybutyrate, a ketone mass, caprylic acid undergoes hepatic metabolism. These ketone bodies represent brain cells as an alternate form of energy. It is used as an additional food in AD (Thaipisuttikul and Galvin 2012).

9.3.2 Parkinson's Disease (PD)

Parkinson's disease (PD) is the most common neurodegenerative disorder associated with age. This disease affects an individual's motor or cognitive ability due to the loss of midbrain's dopaminergic neurons (Newland et al. 2016). The lack of PD vaccines, drugs, or therapies makes it difficult to manage this disorder.

Neurodegenerative disease causing cognitive impairment affects 1–2% of the elderly and is mainly the result of a dopamine deficiency due to the loss of dopaminergic neurons in the substantia nigra pars compacta (SNpc) (Dauer and Przedborski 2003; Sarrafchi et al. 2016; Steger et al. 2016). However, ongoing research indicates that oxidative stress, mitochondrial dysfunction, and genetic factor might be the causative factors. Oxidative stress is the result of an imbalance among antioxidant activity and reactive oxygen species (ROS) production from enzymes such as tyrosine hydroxylase (TH) and monoamine oxidase (Hwang 2013). PD is generally treated through either surgical management or supplement drug therapy. The most common clinical approach for PD treatment is drugs like L-3,4-dihydroxyphenylalanine (levodopa, L-dopa), which is a dopamine analog. This approach is recognized as the gold standard in the treatment of PD. (Jadavji and Metz 2009; Abbruzzese et al. 2016).

A few drugs, mostly dopamine agonists, have been developed to treat PD, and they are recommended to be used based on various stages of PD symptoms. PD can be classified as motor or non-motor symptoms. Motor symptoms such as weakness, bradykinesia, and tremor are caused by the destruction of dopaminergic neurons and are considered to represent a progressively worst stage of PD (Seppi et al. 2011; Xia and Mao 2012). In the early stage of PD, non-motor symptoms such as olfactory problem, indigestion, anxiety, and rapid eye movement disorder occur. In its initial stage, non-motor symptoms could be used to locate PD (Chaudhuri et al. 2006; Seppi et al. 2011). L-Dopa, dopamine agonists (pramipexole, ropinirole, rotigotine, cabergoline, and pergolide), monoamine oxidase B inhibitors (selegiline and rasagiline), and catechol-O-methyltransferase inhibitors (entacapone and tolcapone) are generally used to treat motor symptoms. It may be enough to treat patients in the first year after PD has been identified. Due to the presence of motor fluctuation and dyskinesia, patients will need elevated doses and L-dopa levels (Antonini 2007; Morgan and Fox 2016). Paroxetine, citalopram, sertraline, fluoxetine, atomoxetine, nefazodone, pergolide, and omega-3 fatty acids for depression; methylphenidate and modafinil for fatigue; amantadine for pathological gambling; donepezil, galantamine, and memantine for dementia; and quetiapine for schizophrenia are used to treat non-motor symptoms.

9.3.3 Depression

According to the World Health Organization, depression is a disorder characterized by sadness, loss of interest, feelings of guilt, disturbed sleep and appetite, feelings of tiredness, and poor concentration. Depressive disorders can be long lasting and recurring, impairing an individual's ability to perform their daily activities. It is an intense and debilitating mental condition that occasionally prompts suicide or sudden passing because of unattended physical issues (Miller et al. 2014).

Almost one of every five individuals will encounter a noteworthy major depressive episode sooner or later in their lives (Kessler et al. 2003); in this, genes, psychosocial adversity in childhood, and progressing psychosocial stress may affect multiple neurobiological systems relevant to major depressive disorder. There are different types of depression ranging from mild to severe, such as mental depression, wherein patients experience various manifestations such as deception and hallucinations. Coexistence of other mental disorders such as anxiety, which includes severe phobias, social anxiety disorders, post-traumatic stress disorder (PTSD), and obsessive-compulsive disorder (OCD) makes its diagnosis complex.

Coincidence invented the first antidepressants, following concise clinical investigation that iproniazid demonstrates mood elevating response, a drug refined for the therapy of tuberculosis. Similarly, imipramine, which demonstrates antidepressant response, is a so-called antipsychotic drug. Based upon the above consideration a guiding plan was established for developing antidepressants drugs like Tricyclic antidepressant and monoamine oxidase inhibitors and to the pathological perception of depression (Yildiz et al. 2002; Jacobsen et al. 2012). Regulating the brain monoamine neurotransmission is the operating strategy of many of the available antidepressant drugs. Escalating the long-term monoamine synaptic concentration (norepinephrine, serotonin together with dopamine) is the underlying mechanism of these drugs. By adhering to the specific neurotransmitter transporter together with obstructing their reuptake by the presynaptic neuron by reversible or irreversible hindrance of MAO, monoamine-destructing enzyme, they attain this (Holtzheimer and Nemeroff 2008). To modify the neurotransmission, some of the antidepressants also operate on neurotransmitter receptors present at presynaptic as well as postsynaptic part. In the market atypical antidepressants are also appearing, and it comprises neurokinin 1 (NK-1) antagonist, GR antagonists, and antipsychotics together with melatonergic drugs (Brain and Cox 2006; Kasper and Hamon 2009; Šagud et al. 2011). As conferred, after medication with antidepressants, there is a time lag on the commencement of the response. Long-lasting neuronal reworking may influence transporters or receptors that modify the neurotransmission. Monotonous in modification such as axonal sprouting, synaptic plasticity, and neurite expansion, as well as advancement of cell endurance, is believed to result from the stimulation of the neurons by these drugs, accompanied by intricate cellular signal transaction system, including neurotrophins together with diverse transcription factors (Yildiz et al. 2002).

9.3.4 Huntington Disease (HD)

Huntington disease (HD) is an inherited autosomal dominant neurodegenerative disorder characterized by gradual motor, psychological, and cognitive impairment, leading to death within 15–20 years of diagnosis. The pathological mutation consists of an expanded CAG (cytosine-adenine-guanine) repeat on chromosome 4 in the huntingtin gene (HTT), encoding the huntingtin (htt) protein, resulting in an excessively long stretch of polyglutamine near this protein's N-terminus. The traditional clinical trial in HD is (1) a progressive motor disorder; (2) gradual cognitive disturbance with dementia; and (3) psychiatric conditions, including depression, anxiety, apathy, obsessive-compulsive behavior, outbursts, addictions, and sometimes insanity. A common feature is weight loss.

HD does not have any cure. In addition, there is no documented therapy that slows down clinical degeneration or decline rate. A major area of HD research is this unmet need. Many symptoms can be handled pharmacologically, while others can be managed only through nonpharmacological support measures. Conditions of HD vary in response to medication. Psychiatric symptoms may be the most resistant to pharmacotherapy. Chorea is the most readily reactive of the motor symptoms. The least responsive are cognitive symptoms and dementia. Most people with chorea are either unaware of their involuntary movements or are not affected by chorea. Reassurance and education (especially from family members) are crucial in these situations. When chorea requires treatment since it affects the quality of life, function, or well-being of a patient, it best responds to drugs that minimize neurotransmission of dopaminergic substances. Dopamine receptor antagonists have been prescribed more frequently in the past. Haloperidol, risperidone, and olanzapine are examples of this. These agents have the benefit of increasing depression treatment and helping with irritability, outbursts, and major depression.

As per the available current scenario, diseases of the central nervous system (CNS) are growing rapidly globally. The efficacy of therapeutic agents presently used in the treatment of CNS diseases is significant. Nevertheless, the failure of these medications to cross the blood-brain barrier (BBB) and the invasiveness of technology to achieve targeted drug delivery in disease-specific parts of the brain have hindered pain-free and full treatment of CNS diseases. The presence of the blood-brain barrier (BBB) remains a bottleneck in the brain delivery of CNS drugs and is one of the main factors behind therapy failure. Their capacity to cross this biological obstacle is a determining feature for the efficacy of central drugs. Because treatment efficiency with CNS drugs depends on the levels of drugs at the bio phase (brain), oral and parenteral therapies are restricted as they require the drug to cross the BBB. Given the abovementioned facts, there is an emerging need for efficient dosage forms that controllably release the drug straight into the brain, reducing its systemic exposure, adverse effects, and drug-drug interactions (DDIs), and eventually circumvent pharmacoresistance problems. Therefore, significant research attention is currently being given to the effective, noninvasive, and targeted delivery of drugs to the brain using nanocarriers. Here, we discuss developments in state-of-the-art personalized nanomedicine for the treatment of CNS disorders (with an emphasis on dementia), relevant problems, potential solutions, and prospects for individually tailored nano-enabled medicine.

But many of the advancements are still in the initial stages and in a range of animal models that require more detailed preclinical testing. Security, effectiveness, and regulatory issues are major issues in the clinic for the development of customized nanomedicine to treat CNS disorders.

9.4 Brain-Targeted Delivery of CNS Drugs

The presence of the blood-brain barrier (BBB) remains a bottleneck in the development of brain drugs and is one of the main factors behind therapy failure. Their capacity to cross this biological obstacle is a determining feature for the efficacy of central drugs. The BBB is complicated and involves endothelial cerebral cells that contain transmembrane efflux proteins, especially those of the ATB-binding cassette family, primarily P-glycoprotein (P-gp) and breast cancer resistance protein (BCRP) (Bicker et al. 2014). These carriers limit the transport of lipophilic compounds to the brain and are reported to be overexpressed in refractory patients' brains (Tang et al. 2017). Antidepressant drugs have currently been recognized as substrates, inhibitors, and inducers of P-gp, although their interaction with BCRP remains unknown at present (O'Brien et al. 2012). Because efficient treatment with antidepressant drugs depends on the levels of drugs at the biophase (brain), oral and parenteral therapies are restricted as they require the drug to cross the BBB.

9.5 Approaches to Deliver Drug Through the BBB

Various attempts have been tried to enhance the partitioning of various molecules through the barrier as represented in Fig. 9.3 . Some of the formulation approaches for brain-targeted delivery of CNS drugs are listed in Table 9.1.

9.5.1 Invasive Methods for Brain-Targeted Delivery

Drug molecules from blood circulation to the brain are restrained by the BBB. Hence, via various physical and pharmacological methods, we can momentarily open this barrier to increase the pore size. This momentary opening of the barrier can help in the penetration of various compounds or nanoparticles into the brain (Gao 2016) by intracerebroventricular and intrathecal infusion and alteration in tight junctions via receptor-mediated and focused ultrasound (FUS). Intrathecal implants deliver the drugs directly into the brain parenchymal space. The drugs can be administered by either direct injection via intrathecal catheter or by control release matrices and microencapsulated chemicals. The basic mechanism is diffusion. It is useful in the treatment of different CNS diseases, e.g., brain tumor and Parkinson's disease. In the case of intracerebroventricular infusion, pharmacological effect is seen if the target receptors of the drug are located near the ependymal surface of the brain. The drug is infused using an ommaya reservoir, a plastic reservoir and implanted subcutaneously in the scalp and connected to ventricles. In focused ultrasound (FUS) thermochemical stimulation of the blood vessels occurs through the stable expansion and contraction of microbubbles which results in transient opening of the BBB.

9.5.2 Nanocarriers: Nanotechnology-Mediated Noninvasive Brain-Targeted Delivery

The noninvasive method includes chemical, biological, colloidal, and intranasal methods. In this context, nanosystems are considered to be promising approach for the target-specific drug delivery to the brain.

With the beginning of nanotechnologies, nanoparticles have been projected as an alluring tool to possibly improve drug delivery across the

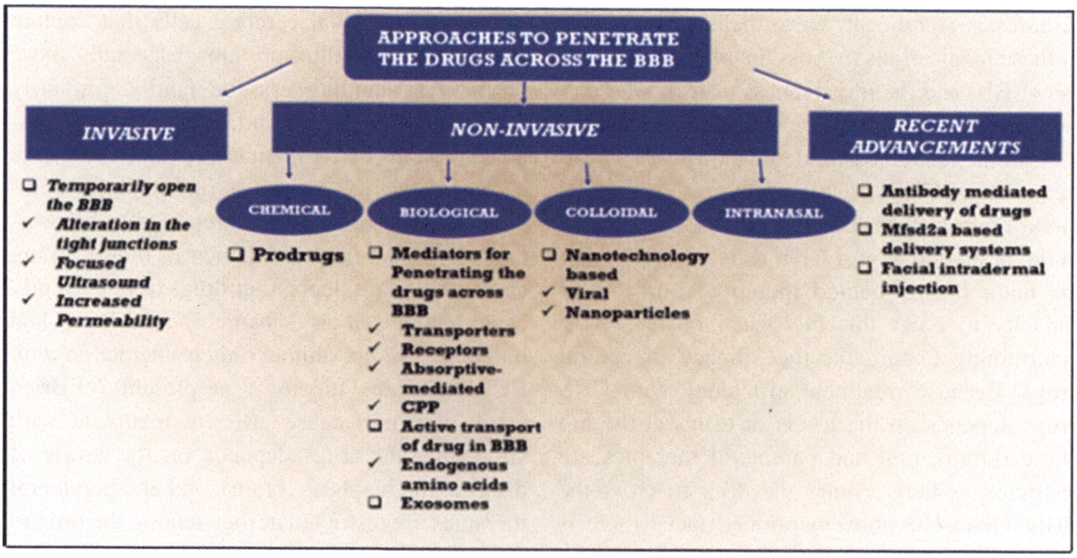

Fig. 9.3 Structural outline representing various approaches/strategies to deliver the drugs across the BBB

Table 9.1 Formulation approaches for brain-targeted delivery of CNS drugs

Drug	Dosage form	Relevant therapeutic outcomes	References
Levetiracetam	Thermoreversible gel	Noninvasive and safe intranasal administration route	Gonçalves et al. (2019)
Docetaxel	Liposome	Improved targeting ability and significantly increased brain concentration	Xiao et al. (2019)
Paclitaxel	Liposome	Superior targeting ability	Peng et al. (2018)
Desvenlafaxine SNRI	PLGA-chitosan nanoparticles	PLGA-CS NPs intranasal administration significantly enhances the level of monoamines in the brain in comparison with orally administered DVLF. It enhanced the pharmacokinetic profile of DVLF in brain	Tong et al. (2017)
Paroxetine SSRI	Nanoemulsion (O/W type)	Biochemical estimation results revealed that the prepared nanoemulsion was effective in enhancing the depressed levels of glutathione and decreasing the elevated levels of TBARS	Pandey et al. (2016)
Venlafaxine hydrochloride (VLF) SNRI	Alginate-chitosan nanoparticles (Alg-CS NPs)	VLF AG NPs intranasal treatment significantly improved the behavioral analysis parameters, i.e., swimming, climbing, and immobility in comparison to the VLF solution intranasal and VLF tablet oral	Haque et al. (2014)
Duloxetine SNRI	NLC	Intranasal administration exhibited about eight times higher concentration of DLX in the brain when compared with the intravenous administration of DLX solution	Alam et al. (2014)
Rivastigmine	Liposomes	Showed an enhanced ex vivo diffusion through goat nasal mucosa. Higher concentrations in the hippocampus, cortex, and olfactory region	Yang et al. (2013)
Levodopa	Polymeric nanoparticles	Improved uptake, avoid degradation of levodopa in peripheral circulation, enhanced residence	Sharma et al. (2013)

BBB. When nanoparticles are used for brain drug delivery, the first thing in mind should be the ability of the nanoparticles to cross the brain by themselves (Wohlfart et al. 2012). Nanoparticles offer several advantages as they can convey drug payloads, provide controlled drug release, and modify the pharmacokinetics of the drug.

Compared to conventional approaches used for brain delivery, NPs offer better tolerance and accurate targeting, leading to better therapeutic response at lower doses. This strategy demises the adverse effect, improves patient compliance, and treats the disease (Xie et al. 2019). In this context, nanosystems are considered to be promising approach for the target-specific drug delivery to the brain. Some of the formulations based on nanocarriers are listed in Table 9.2.

9.5.3 Types of Nanocarriers

9.5.3.1 Liposomes

Liposomes are tiny vesicles consisting of one or more bilayers of phospholipid containing an aqueous core. Their surface charge, size, lipid formation, and content of cholesterol can be adjusted to regulate the delivery of drugs and tissue uptake (Samad et al. 2007); therefore, apart from their low toxicity and capacity to supply both lipophilic and hydrophilic compounds, liposomes are likely the most well-studied and clinically acknowledged form of nanocarriers. Cationic, PEGylated, and immunoliposomal formulations are the most prevalent liposomal formulations for BBB (Garcia-Garcia et al. 2005). PEG grafted on the liposome surface allows them to avoid the reticuloendothelial system, thus extending their cir-

Table 9.2 List of nanocarriers used for CNS delivery

Drug	Technology	Indication	Therapeutic benefit	References
Methotrexate	Polymeric nanoparticle	Antitumor	Increased drug level in the brain and cerebrospinal fluids	Vakilinezhad et al. (2019)
Amphotericin	Liposome	Antifungal	Severalfold increase in brain uptake	Gao et al. (2019)
Doxorubicin	SLN	Antitumor	Improve the circulation time and brain accumulation	Stella et al. (2018)
Camptothecin	SLN	Antitumor	Drug release up to a week, highest enhancement in AUC was observed in the brain	Du et al. (2018)
Paclitaxel	SLN	Antitumor	Higher brain drug level	Xu et al. (2018)
Cisplatin	Liposome	Brain tumor	Increase drug concentration and cell killing in brain tumor-invaded area	Dou et al. (2017)
Stavudine	Liposome	Brain tumor	Reduce HIV-p24 levels in MT2 cells	Nayak et al. (2017)
Temozolomide	Polymeric nanoparticle	Antitumor	Enhance BBB uptake	Ananta et al. (2016)
Vincristine sulfate	Liposome	Brain tumor	Diffuse distribution and tissue binding	Deitcher et al. (2014)
Vasoactive intestinal peptide	Polymeric nanoparticle	Peptide hormone	Drug level in the brain increased by 5.6–7.7-fold	Xu et al. (2015)
Saquinavir	Nanoemulsion	Antiretroviral drug	Increased brain drug concentration	Vyas et al. (2008)

culation time and allowing them to slip past the BBB (Xiao et al. 2019).

Liposomes are designed to cross the BBB and deliver therapeutic molecules to the neurological disorder site only. Different mechanisms by which liposomes can reach the brain are:

1. Transport of liposomes via receptor-mediated transcytosis
2. Adsorption of endothelial cationic liposomes that increased the concentration of therapeutic molecules in brain cells
3. Antibody- or peptide-conjugated liposomes used to transport and target encapsulated drugs via transcytotic pathways into the brain
4. Efflux inhibition by combining liposomes with transporter-inhibitory compounds, such as PgP
5. BBB disruption

Liposomes, in addition, have the ability to revolutionize drug development for neurological disease treatment and/or diagnosis. In addition, liposomes are structures that are biocompatible and biodegradable, making them suitable for neuromedicine. Normally, liposomes increase the therapeutic index of new or proven medicines by enhancing the biological half-life and reducing their adverse effects. Liposomes can be an effective therapeutic method for the treatment and diagnosis of neurological disorders because of their ability to cross the BBB and deliver medications and/or contrast agents to the CNS effectively.

9.5.3.2 Polymeric Nanoparticles

Polymeric nanoparticles offer substantial drug delivery capacity to the CNS. Over the past 40 years, this technology has been rapidly expanding and is now prepared for clinical translation. Polymeric nanoparticles can supply not only traditional small molecular drugs but also proteins (Demento et al. 2009), nucleic acids (Woodrow et al. 2009), and diagnostic agents (Fahmy et al. 2007). Nanocarriers are colloidal systems containing a therapeutic agent, ranging in size from 1 to 300 nm. These can be made from a number of substances, including polymers, lipids, ceramics, and nanotubes of carbon. The systemic delivery of polymeric nanoparticles to the CNS is mainly based on their capacity for receptor-mediated transcytosis and adsorptive-mediated transcytosis through the BBB (Medina et al. 2019). This can be improved by adding cell-penetrating peptides and/or targeting ligands to the surface of the nanoparticles. Poly(butylcyanoacrylate) (PBCA) nanoparticles were the first nanoparticles based on polymer to be applied to the CNS(Kreuter et al. 1995).

Ideal polymer nanoparticles delivery system features:

1. Affordable and scalable
2. Biodegradable/biocompatible
3. Free from toxicity
4. Diameter less than 100 nm
5. Non-immunogenic

Today the most common polymers for controlled drug release applications are poly(D,L-lactide-co-glycolide) (PLGA), poly(aspartic acid), poly(e-caprolactone) (PCL), poly(lactic acid) (PLA), poly(butylcyanoacrylate) (PBCA), poly(glycolic acid) (PGA), and poly(amino acids), with PGA, PLA, and PLGA being the most commonly used in CNS drug delivery (Béduneau et al. 2007).

9.5.3.3 Solid Lipid Nanoparticles (SLNs)

Solid lipid nanoparticles (SLNs) are nanospheres made of solid biocompatible lipids with unique advantages for drug carriers: they can be used as carriers for crossing the BBB. SLNs consist of a solid hydrophobic core of lipids such as mono-, di-, and triglycerides or fatty acids with phospholipid coating monolayers (Kaur et al. 2008). Like polymeric nanoparticles, they can be controlled for release up to several weeks and can also be coated or grafted with drug targeting ligands (Kaur et al. 2008). They are also biodegradable and stable and under physiological conditions have a high drug loading capacity for both lipophilic and hydrophilic drugs (Yadav et al. 2014).

SLN provides a considerable improvement in the delivery of drugs via topical, oral, and parenteral routes. The encapsulation of drugs in SLN in particular can aid to:

1. Solve problems, because of their low water solubility
2. Safety against physical and chemical processes of degradation and evaporation
3. Provide slow release to the environment
4. Guide the trapped substance to a specific target

SLN is used to carry drugs to the CNS for different purposes; SLN can be used in general:

1. Used to stabilize molecules with physical or biological instability
2. Improved the bioavailability of a drug which is capable of crossing the BBB
3. Increased the permeation of a drug via the BBB

9.5.3.4 Magnetic Nanoparticles (MPs)

Magnetic nanoparticles most often consist of a core of iron oxide maghemite (γ-Fe_2O_3) or magnetite (Fe_3O_4). The core of iron oxide is a significant feature that allows motion in a magnetic field (Tomitaka et al. 2019). At present, magnetic nanoparticles are used for various in vivo and in vitro purposes such as:

1. Contrast agents for magnetic resonance imaging (Carvalho et al. 2014)
2. Cell labeling and separation (Ruan et al. 2011; Madsen et al. 2013)
3. Delivery of drug via magnetic targeting (Boyer et al. 2010; Halamoda Kenzaoui et al. 2013; Pilakka-Kanthikeel et al. 2013; Varallyay et al. 2013; Zhao et al. 2013; Shevtsov et al. 2014)

Magnetic nanoparticles can be coated with polymer; moreover, they can also be encapsulated in liposomes, resulting in magnetoliposomes (Saiyed et al. 2010; Carvalho et al. 2014; Ding et al. 2014).

In other words, this can be classified into two subdivisions: paramagnetic nanoparticles (PMNPs) and super-paramagnetic iron oxide nanoparticles (SPIONs). PMNPs are greater than 100 nm but still within the range of the nanometer, and SPIONs are smaller than 100 nm. SPIONs of less than 50 nm in size are also known as ultra-super paramagnetic iron oxide nanoparticles (USPIONs) (Boyer et al. 2010; Fan et al. 2013; Wadghiri et al. 2013). The physical properties of SPIONs are of great importance as they cause the particles to become magnetic with a strong magnetic sensitivity in the presence of an external magnet as opposed to the much poorer magnetic sensitivity of PMNPs with a larger diameter (Boyer et al. 2010). This feature makes SPIONs highly attractive for drug delivery purposes, as they are easier to attract to a magnet over long distances compared to PMNPs (Boyer et al. 2010). SPIONs are a suitable candidate for both targeting and biotherapeutic conjugation, as they can persist in tissues for long periods of time and are still biocompatible. Within liposomes, they can also be encapsulated (Wahajuddin 2012; Mok and Zhang 2013).

9.5.3.5 Nanoemulsion

Nanoemulsions (NEs) are water-in-oil (W/O) or oil-in-water (O/W) dispersions of two immiscible liquids with suitable surfactants (Comfort et al. 2015), with an average droplet diameter of 100 nm (Rodrigues et al. 2015). NEs are also referred to as miniemulsions, ultrafine emulsions, or submicron emulsions (Solans et al. 2005). NEs appear as transparent or clear to milky white. NEs can also be used to alleviate problems such as drug stability and solubility (pH, oxidation, hydrolysis, and mucosal enzyme degradation under physiological conditions) (Mahajan et al. 2014; Comfort et al. 2015). NEs can also be designed using various techniques which can be divided into two distinct categories: low-energy methods and high-energy methods. In the case of high-energy methods such as high-pressure homogenization and ultrasonication, small droplets are made up of a mechanical device that produces destructive forces breaking up oil and water phases to produce small oil droplets, a process which consumes significant energy (Bonferoni et al. 2019). Low-energy methods involve specific physicochemical processes such as the inversion temperature of the phase and the inversion of emulsion points to produce small droplets without significant energy consumption. The droplets are constituted in low-energy methods when the device undergoes a phase inversion in response to changes such as composition or temperature, thereby going through a low interfacial pressure state (Gupta et al. 2016).

9.6 Points of Concern

Nanoparticles have numerous merits like the tendency to cross the BBB noninvasively, better residence time in the systemic circulation, and quite limited commercial application. Toxicity due to overexposure to the nanoformulations containing polymers, lipids, etc., these excipients comprise the major percentage of the formulations; upon repeated dosing there can be chances of accumulation in the brain. Till date no conclusive evidence is available for the long-term toxic effects of nanoparticles in the brain. The scale-up of nanoformulation from lab scale to commercial scale is extremely intricate. Maintenance of the encapsulation efficiency rate is quite a tedious task. The formulation process optimization is also crucial for providing the clinical efficiency of the nanoformulations. The high cost of the scale-up and organic solvents used during the formulation of nanomedicines limits the process. Working for a cost-effective technique could be crucial for the realization of the commercial success.

9.7 Current Scenario for the Brain-Specific Delivery of Nanoparticles

Nanomedicine could be exploited in a diligent manner for the treatment of CNS diseases. In spite of numerous hurdles, nanomedicines are exhibiting its clinical presence. Nanotechnology can be applied to various complicated drugs. They are of great benefit to the BCS III and IV drugs which are really tough to formulate. A wide range of molecules along with polymers, peptides, and lipids have been encapsulated or conjugated with complicated pharmacological agents. Nanotechnology by virtue of its nanosize range has been found to have the utmost potential for treating the CNS diseases. Instead of all the progressive researches, brain-specific delivery through nanotechnology has not been taken up on the commercial front. Complicated federal regulations involved with nanotechnology are responsible for the low investment by the pharmaceutical industry. Drafting conclusive guidelines could prove to be a lease in resolving the treatment for the CNS disease.

Current update in targeted brain delivery includes antibody-mediated delivery of therapeutic agents and facial intradermal injection. Antibody-mediated delivery of therapeutic agents is an upcoming new trend and is successful in the treatment of CNS diseases such as Alzheimer's disease, multiple sclerosis, epilepsy, stroke, and neuro-inflammatory diseases. Facial intradermal injection is a method to bypass the BBB via trigeminal neural pathway. Trigeminal nerve communicates with the facial skin, facial muscles, meninges, and respiratory mucosa, and delivery through the facial skin is another method to cross the BBB.

9.8 Future Perspective

It should be recognized that nanotechnology is moving toward the production of safe and efficient nano-drugs capable of crossing BBB for the treatment of different CNS diseases. The noninvasive drug administration approach along with improved treatment and reduced side effects would greatly contribute to the advantages of crossing BBB provided by nanoparticulate systems. In this regard, the ability of different FDA-approved biodegradable polymers to deliver impermeable BBB drugs has been considered. Subsequent interventions will not only be helpful in minimizing successful therapeutic drug doses but may be also responsible for increasing the optimal blood retention time required for effective drug absorption. Nonetheless, as discussed, the systemic toxicity profile of nano-drugs should be considered seriously before the pharmaceutical industry moves toward their merchandizing. In fact, the level of damage caused by nano-drugs to the brain should be another important factor in the development of potential drugs to cross BBB. All of the above-listed apprehensions require extensive testing with advanced diagnostic techniques to assess the CNS-related toxicity of nano-drugs. Although the current state of nano-drug developments in the treatment of brain diseases is still under initial stages, recent promising advances in both research and clinical outcomes related to brain-oriented nanotherapeutics may provide safe and effective nano-drugs for the treatment of brain diseases in the years to come.

9.9 Conclusion

Nanotechnology has emerged as a topic of great interest over the past few decades. It comprises a wide range of highly advanced biomaterials and devices for targeted delivery of drugs, genes, or proteins. It also involves early diagnosis of diseases, leading to more effective treatment outcomes. Nanotechnology is immensely crucial for CNS disorders. Nanopharmaceuticals enhance the bioavailability, decrease toxicity, minimize non-specific interactions, and are able to permeate the BBB. It was optimistic that this scientific approach could be used for the treatment and diagnosis of CNS diseases. Using polymer-based technologies and nanomaterials, several nano-approaches focusing on enhanced drug administration for patients with CNS disorders are being investigated. Targeted nanotherapy and high-resolution imaging and modeling techniques help to understand the pathophysiology of CNS disorders, leading to new preventive approaches and treatments. It appears that nanointerventions during the course of time would improve the healthcare system drastically.

References

Abbruzzese G, Marchese R, Avanzino L, Pelosin E (2016) Rehabilitation for Parkinson's disease: current outlook and future challenges. Parkinsonism Relat Disord 22:S60–S64

Alam MI, Baboota S, Ahuja A, Ali M, Ali J, Sahni JK, Bhatnagar A (2014) Pharmacoscintigraphic evaluation of potential of lipid nanocarriers for nose-to-brain delivery of antidepressant drug. Int J Pharm 470(1–2):99–106

Albert SM (2007) Projecting neurologic disease burden: difficult but critical. Neurology 68(5):322–323, AAN Enterprises

Amaducci L, Crook T, Lippi A, Bracco L, Baldereschi M, Latorraca S, Piersanti P, Tesco G, Sorbi S (1991) Use of phosphatidylserine in Alzheimer's disease. Ann N Y Acad Sci 640(1):245–249

Ananta JS, Paulmurugan R, Massoud TF (2016) Tailored nanoparticle codelivery of antimiR-21 and antimiR-10b augments glioblastoma cell kill by temozolomide: toward a "personalized" anti-microRNA therapy. Mol Pharm 13:3164

Antonini A (2007) New strategies in motor parkinsonism. Parkinsonism Relat Disord 13:S446–S449

Ballabh P, Braun A, Nedergaard M (2004) The blood–brain barrier: an overview: structure, regulation, and clinical implications. Neurobiol Dis 16(1):1–13

Banks WA (2009) Characteristics of compounds that cross the blood-brain barrier. BMC Neurol 9(Suppl 1):S3. BioMed Central

Banks WA (2016) From blood–brain barrier to blood–brain interface: new opportunities for CNS drug delivery. Nat Rev Drug Discov 15(4):275

Béduneau A, Saulnier P, Benoit J-PJB (2007) Active targeting of brain tumors using nanocarriers. Biomaterials 28(33):4947–4967

Bicker J, Alves G, Fortuna A, Falcão A (2014) Blood–brain barrier models and their relevance for a successful development of CNS drug delivery systems: a review. Eur J Pharm Biopharm 87(3):409–432

Bonferoni MC, Rossi S, Sandri G, Ferrari F, Gavini E, Rassu G, Giunchedi P (2019) Nanoemulsions for "nose-to-brain" drug delivery. Pharmaceutics 11(2):84

Boyer C, Whittaker MR, Bulmus V, Liu J, Davis TP (2010) The design and utility of polymer-stabilized iron-oxide nanoparticles for nanomedicine applications. NPG Asia Mater 2(1):23

Brain SD, Cox HM (2006) Neuropeptides and their receptors: innovative science providing novel therapeutic targets. Br J Pharmacol 147(S1):S202–S211

Brew BJ, González-Scarano F (2007) HIV-associated dementia: an inconvenient truth. Neurology 68(5):324–325, AAN Enterprises

Carvalho A, Martins M, Corvo M, Feio G (2014) Enhanced contrast efficiency in MRI by PEGylated magnetoliposomes loaded with PEGylated SPION: effect of SPION coating and micro-environment. Mater Sci Eng C 43:521–526

Chaudhuri KR, Healy DG, Schapira AH (2006) Non-motor symptoms of Parkinson's disease: diagnosis and management. Lancet Neurol 5(3):235–245

Chisholm D, Sweeny K, Sheehan P, Rasmussen B, Smit F, Cuijpers P, Saxena S (2016) Scaling-up treatment of depression and anxiety: a global return on investment analysis. Lancet Psychiatry 3(5):415–424

Comfort C, Garrastazu G, Pozzoli M, Sonvico F (2015) Opportunities and challenges for the nasal administration of nanoemulsions. Curr Top Med Chem 15(4):356–368

Cupaioli FA, Zucca FA, Boraschi D, Zecca L (2014) Engineered nanoparticles. How brain friendly is this new guest? Prog Neurobiol 119:20–38

Dauer W, Przedborski S (2003) Parkinson's disease: mechanisms and models. Neuron 39(6):889–909

Deitcher OR, Glaspy J, Gonzalez R, Sato T, Bedikian AY, Segarini K, Silverman J, Deitcher SR (2014) High-dose vincristine sulfate liposome injection (Marqibo) is not associated with clinically meaningful hematologic toxicity. Clin Lymphoma Myeloma Leuk 14(3):197–202

Demento SL, Eisenbarth SC, Foellmer HG, Platt C, Caplan MJ, Saltzman WM, Mellman I, Ledizet M, Fikrig E, Flavell RA (2009) Inflammasome-activating nanoparticles as modular systems for optimizing vaccine efficacy. Vaccine 27(23):3013–3021

Ding H, Sagar V, Agudelo M, Pilakka-Kanthikeel S, Atluri VSR, Raymond A, Samikkannu T, Nair MP (2014) Enhanced blood–brain barrier transmigration using a novel transferrin embedded fluorescent magneto-liposome nanoformulation. Nanotechnology 25(5):055101

Dong X (2018) Current strategies for brain drug delivery. Theranostics 8(6):1481

Dou YN, Chaudary N, Chang MC, Dunnea M, Huang H, Jaffray DA, Milosevicg M, Allena C (2017) Tumor microenvironment determines response to a heat-activated thermosensitive liposome formulation of cisplatin in cervical carcinoma. J Control Release 262:182–119

Du Y, Ling L, Ismail M, He W, Xia Q, Zhou W, Yao C, Li X (2018) Redox sensitive lipid-camptothecin conjugate encapsulated solid lipid nanoparticles for oral delivery. Int J Pharm 549:352

Fahmy TM, Fong PM, Park J, Constable T, Saltzman WM (2007) Nanosystems for simultaneous imaging and drug delivery to T cells. AAPS J 9(2):E171–E180

Fan C-H, Ting C-Y, Lin H-J, Wang C-H, Liu H-L, Yen T-C, Yeh C-K (2013) SPIO-conjugated, doxorubicin-loaded microbubbles for concurrent MRI and focused-ultrasound enhanced brain-tumor drug delivery. Biomaterials 34(14):3706–3715

Fernandes C, Soni U, Patravale VJPR (2010) Nano-interventions for neurodegenerative disorders. Pharmacol Res 62(2):166–178

Gao H (2016) Progress and perspectives on targeting nanoparticles for brain drug delivery. Acta Pharm Sin B 6(4):268–286

Gao M, Hu P, Cai Z, Wu Y, Wang D, Hu W, Xu X, Zhang Y, Lu X, Chen D, Chen Z, Ma K, Wen J, Wang H, Huang C (2019) Identification of a microglial activation-dependent antidepressant effect of amphotericin B liposome. Neuropharmacology 151:33–44

Garcia-Garcia E, Andrieux K, Gil S, Couvreur P (2005) Colloidal carriers and blood–brain barrier (BBB) translocation: a way to deliver drugs to the brain? Int J Pharm 298(2):274–292

Gonçalves J, Bickera J, Gouvei F, Liberal J, Oliveirad RC, Alvesg G, Falcão A, Fortuna A (2019) Nose-to-brain delivery of levetiracetam after intranasal administration to mice. Int J Pharm 564:329–339

Guerra M, Blázquez J, Rodríguez E (2017) Blood–brain barrier and foetal-onset hydrocephalus, with a view on potential novel treatments beyond managing CSF flow. Fluids Barriers CNS 14(1):19

Gupta A, Eral HB, Hatton TA, Doyle PS (2016) Nanoemulsions: formation, properties and applications. Soft Matter 12(11):2826–2841

Halamoda Kenzaoui B, Angeloni S, Overstolz T, Niedermann P, Chapuis Bernasconi C, Liley M, Juillerat-Jeanneret L (2013) Transfer of ultrasmall iron oxide nanoparticles from human brain-derived endothelial cells to human glioblastoma cells. ACS Appl Mater Interfaces 5(9):3581–3586

Haque S, Md S, Sahni JK, Ali J, Baboota S (2014) Development and evaluation of brain targeted intranasal alginate nanoparticles for treatment of depression. J Psychiatr Res 48:1–12

Henderson ST, Vogel JL, Barr LJ, Garvin F, Jones JJ, Costantini LC (2009) Study of the ketogenic agent AC-1202 in mild to moderate Alzheimer's disease: a randomized, double-blind, placebo-controlled, multicenter trial. Nutr Metab 6(1):31

Hirtz D, Thurman D, Gwinn-Hardy K, Mohamed M, Chaudhuri A, Zalutsky R (2007) How common are the "common" neurologic disorders? Neurology 68(5):326–337

Holtzheimer PE, Nemeroff CB (2008) Novel targets for antidepressant therapies. Curr Psychiatry Rep 10(6):465–473

Hwang O (2013) Role of oxidative stress in Parkinson's disease. Exp Neurobiol 22(1):11–17

Jacobsen JP, Medvedev IO, Caron MG (2012) The 5-HT deficiency theory of depression: perspectives from a naturalistic 5-HT deficiency model, the tryptophan hydroxylase 2Arg439His knockin mouse. Philos Trans R Soc Lond B Biol Sci 367(1601):2444–2459

Jadavji N, Metz G (2009) Both pre-and post-lesion experiential therapy is beneficial in 6-hydroxydopamine dopamine-depleted female rats. Neuroscience 158(2):373–386

Kasper S, Hamon M (2009) Beyond the monoaminergic hypothesis: agomelatine, a new antidepressant with an innovative mechanism of action. World J Biol Psychiatry 10(2):117–126

Kaur IP, Bhandari R, Bhandari S, Kakkar V (2008) Potential of solid lipid nanoparticles in brain targeting. J Control Release 127(2):97–109

Kaushik A, Jayant RD, Sagar V, Nair M (2014) The potential of magneto-electric nanocarriers for drug delivery. Expert Opin Drug Deliv 11(10):1635–1646

Kaushik A, Jayant RD, Nair M (2016a) Advancements in nano-enabled therapeutics for neuroHIV management. Int J Nanomedicine 11:4317

Kaushik A, Jayant RD, Tiwari S, Vashist A, Nair M (2016b) Nano-biosensors to detect beta-amyloid for Alzheimer's disease management. Biosens Bioelectron 80:273–287

Kaushik A, Shah P, Vabbina PK, Jayant RD, Tiwari S, Vashist A, Yndart A, Nair M (2016c) A label-free electrochemical immunosensor for beta-amyloid detection. Anal Methods 8(31):6115–6120

Kessler RC, Berglund P, Demler O, Jin R, Koretz D, Merikangas KR, Rush AJ, Walters EE, Wang PS (2003) The epidemiology of major depressive disorder: results from the National Comorbidity Survey Replication (NCS-R). JAMA 289(23):3095–3105

Komarova YA, Kruse K, Mehta D, Malik AB (2017) Protein interactions at endothelial junctions and signaling mechanisms regulating endothelial permeability. Circ Res 120(1):179–206

Kreuter J, Alyautdin RN, Kharkevich DA, Ivanov AA (1995) Passage of peptides through the blood-brain barrier with colloidal polymer particles (nanoparticles). Brain Res 674(1):171–174

Lécuyer M-A, Saint-Laurent O, Bourbonnière L, Larouche S, Larochelle C, Michel L, Charabati M, Abadier M, Zandee S, Jahromi NH (2017) Dual role of ALCAM in neuroinflammation and blood–brain barrier homeostasis. Proc Natl Acad Sci 114(4):E524–E533

Leyva-Gomez G, Cortes H, Magana JJ, Leyva-Garcia N, Quintanar-Guerrero D, Floran B (2015) Nanoparticle technology for treatment of Parkinson's disease: the role of surface phenomena in reaching the brain. Drug Discov Today 20(7):824–837

Madsen SJ, Gach HM, Hong SJ, Uzal FA, Peng Q, Hirschberg H (2013) Increased nanoparticle-loaded exogenous macrophage migration into the brain following PDT-induced blood–brain barrier disruption. Lasers Surg Med 45(8):524–532

Mäger I, Meyer AH, Li J, Lenter M, Hildebrandt T, Leparc G, Wood MJ (2017) Targeting blood-brain-barrier transcytosis–perspectives for drug delivery. Neuropharmacology 120:4–7

Mahajan HS, Mahajan MS, Nerkar PP, Agrawal A (2014) Nanoemulsion-based intranasal drug delivery system of saquinavir mesylate for brain targeting. Drug Deliv 21(2):148–154

Md S, Mustafa G, Baboota S, Ali J (2015) Nanoneurotherapeutics approach intended for direct nose to brain delivery. Drug Dev Ind Pharm 41(12):1922–1934

Medina DX, Chung EP, Bowser R, Sirianni RW (2019) Lipid and polymer blended polyester nanoparticles

loaded with adapalene for activation of retinoid signaling in the CNS following intravenous administration. J Drug Delivery Sci Technol 52:927–933
Miller S, Dell'Osso B, Ketter TA (2014) The prevalence and burden of bipolar depression. J Affect Disord 169(2014):S3–S11
Mok H, Zhang M (2013) Superparamagnetic iron oxide nanoparticle-based delivery systems for biotherapeutics. Expert Opin Drug Deliv 10(1):73–87
Morgan JC, Fox SH (2016) Treating the motor symptoms of Parkinson disease. Continuum (Minneap Minn) 22(4):1064–1085
Nair M, Jayant RD, Kaushik A, Sagar V (2016) Getting into the brain: potential of nanotechnology in the management of NeuroAIDS. Adv Drug Deliv Rev 103:202–217
Nayak D, Boxi A, Ashe S, Thathapudi NC, Nayak B (2017) Stavudine loaded gelatin liposomes for HIV therapy: preparation, characterization and in vitro cytotoxic evaluation. Mater Sci Eng C 73:406–416
Newland B, Dunnett SB, Dowd E (2016) Targeting delivery in Parkinson's disease. Drug Discov Today 21(8):1313–1320
O'Brien FE, Dinan TG, Griffin BT, Cryan JF (2012) Interactions between antidepressants and P-glycoprotein at the blood–brain barrier: clinical significance of in vitro and in vivo findings. Br J Pharmacol 165(2):289–312
Pandey YR, Kumar S, Gupta BK, Ali J, Baboota S (2016) Intranasal delivery of paroxetine nanoemulsion via the olfactory region for the management of depression: formulation, behavioural and biochemical estimation. Nanotechnology 270:25102
Peng Y, Zhao Y, Chen Y, Yang Z, Zhang L, Xiao W, Yang J, Guo L, Wu Y (2018) Dual-targeting for brain-specific liposomes drug delivery system: synthesis and preliminary evaluation. Bioorg Med Chem 26:4677–4686
Perl DP (2010) Neuropathology of Alzheimer's disease. Mt Sinai J Med 77(1):32–42
Pilakka-Kanthikeel S, Atluri VSR, Sagar V, Saxena SK, Nair M (2013) Targeted brain derived neurotropic factors (BDNF) delivery across the blood-brain barrier for neuro-protection using magnetic nano carriers: an in-vitro study. PLoS One 8(4):e62241
Rodrigues RF, Costa IC, Almeida FB, Cruz RA, Ferreira AM, Vilhena JC, Florentino AC, Carvalho JC, Fernandes CP (2015) Development and characterization of evening primrose (Oenothera biennis) oil nanoemulsions. Rev Bras 25(4):422–425
Ruan J, Shen J, Wang Z, Ji J, Song H, Wang K, Liu B, Li J, Cui D (2011) Efficient preparation and labeling of human induced pluripotent stem cells by nanotechnology. Int J Nanomedicine 6:425
Ruiz A, Nair M, Kaushik A (2015) Recent update in NanoCure of NeuroAIDS. Sci Lett J 4:172
Šagud M, Mihaljević-Peleš A, Begić D, Vuksan-Ćusa B, Kramarić M, Živković M, Jakovljević MJPD (2011) Antipsychotics as antidepressants: what is the mechanism? Psychiatr Danub 23(3):302–307
Saiyed ZM, Gandhi NH, Nair MP (2010) Magnetic nanoformulation of azidothymidine 5′-triphosphate for targeted delivery across the blood–brain barrier. Int J Nanomedicine 5:157
Samad A, Sultana Y, Aqil M (2007) Liposomal drug delivery systems: an update review. Curr Drug Deliv 4(4):297–305
Sarrafchi A, Bahmani M, Shirzad H, Rafieian-Kopaei M (2016) Oxidative stress and Parkinson's disease: new hopes in treatment with herbal antioxidants. Curr Pharm Des 22(2):238–246
Seppi K, Weintraub D, Coelho M, Perez-Lloret S, Fox SH, Katzenschlager R, Hametner EM, Poewe W, Rascol O, Goetz CG (2011) The Movement Disorder Society evidence-based medicine review update: treatments for the non-motor symptoms of Parkinson's disease. Mov Disord 26(S3):S42–S80
Sharma S, Lohan S, Murthy RSR (2013) Formulation and characterization of intranasal mucoadhesive nanoparticulates and thermo-reversible gel of levodopa for brain delivery. Drug Dev Ind Pharm:1–10
Shevtsov MA, Nikolaev BP, Yakovleva LY, Marchenko YY, Dobrodumov AV, Mikhrina AL, Martynova MG, Bystrova OA, Yakovenko IV, Ischenko AM (2014) Superparamagnetic iron oxide nanoparticles conjugated with epidermal growth factor (SPION–EGF) for targeting brain tumors. Int J Nanomedicine 9:273
Silva GA (2005) Nanotechnology approaches for the regeneration and neuroprotection of the central nervous system. Surg Neurol 63(4):301–306
Solans C, Izquierdo P, Nolla J, Azemar N, Garcia-Celma MJ (2005) Nano-emulsions. Curr Opin Colloid Interface Sci 10(3–4):102–110
Soni S, Ruhela RK, Medhi B (2016) Nanomedicine in central nervous system (CNS) disorders: a present and future prospective. Adv Pharm Bull 6(3):319–335
Steger M, Tonelli F, Ito G, Davies P, Trost M, Vetter M, Wachter S, Lorentzen E, Duddy G, Wilson S (2016) Phosphoproteomics reveals that Parkinson's disease kinase LRRK2 regulates a subset of Rab GTPases. elife 5:e12813
Stella B, Peira E, Dianzani C, Gallarate M, Battaglia L, Gigliotti CL, Boggio E, Dianzani U, Dosio F (2018) Development and characterization of solid lipid nanoparticles loaded with a highly active doxorubicin derivative. Nanomaterials 8(2):110
Tang F, Hartz A, Bauer B (2017) Drug-resistant epilepsy: multiple hypotheses, few answers. Front Neurol 8:301
Thaipisuttikul P, Galvin JE (2012) Use of medical foods and nutritional approaches in the treatment of Alzheimer's disease. Clin Pract (Lond) 9(2):199
Tomitaka A, Kaushik A, Kevadiya B, Mukadam I, Gendelman HE, Khalili K, Liu G, Nair M (2019) Surface-engineered multimodal magnetic nanoparticles to manage CNS diseases. Drug Discov. Today 24(3):873–882
Tong G-F, Qin N, Sun L-W (2017) Development and evaluation of Desvenlafaxine loaded PLGA-chitosan

nanoparticles for brain delivery. Saudi Pharm J 25(6):844–851

Umlauf BJ, Shusta EV (2019) Exploiting BBB disruption for the delivery of nanocarriers to the diseased CNS. Curr Opin Biotechnol 60:146–152

Vakilinezhad MA, Amini A, Dara T, Alipour S (2019) Methotrexate and curcumin co-encapsulated PLGA nanoparticles as a potential breast cancer therapeutic system: in vitro and in vivo evaluation. Colloids Surf. B Biointerfaces 184:110515

Varallyay CG, Nesbit E, Fu R, Gahramanov S, Moloney B, Earl E, Muldoon LL, Li X, Rooney WD, Neuwelt EA (2013) High-resolution steady-state cerebral blood volume maps in patients with central nervous system neoplasms using ferumoxytol, a superparamagnetic iron oxide nanoparticle. J Cereb Blood Flow Metab 33(5):780–786

Vashist A, Kaushik A, Ghosal A, Nikkhah-Moshaie R, Vashist A, Jayant RD, Nair M (2017) Journey of hydrogels to nanogels: a decade after. In: Nanogels for biomedical applications, pp 1–8

Vashist A, Kaushik A, Vashist A, Bala J, Nikkhah-Moshaie R, Sagar V, Nair M (2018) Nanogels as potential drug nanocarriers for CNS drug delivery. Drug Discov Today 23(7):1436–1443

Vinogradov SVJN (2010) Nanogels in the race for drug delivery. Nanomedicine 5(2):165–168

Vyas TK, Shahiwala A, Amiji MM (2008) Improved oral bioavailability and brain transport of Saquinavir upon administration in novel nanoemulsion formulations. Int J Pharm 347:93–101

Wadghiri YZ, Li J, Wang J, Hoang DM, Sun Y, Xu H, Tsui W, Li Y, Boutajangout A, Wang A (2013) Detection of amyloid plaques targeted by bifunctional USPIO in Alzheimer's disease transgenic mice using magnetic resonance microimaging. PLoS One 8(2):e57097

Wahajuddin SA (2012) Superparamagnetic iron oxide nanoparticles: magnetic nanoplatforms as drug carriers. Int J Nanomedicine 7:3445

Wohlfart S, Gelperina S, Kreuter J (2012) Transport of drugs across the blood–brain barrier by nanoparticles. J Control Release 161(2):264–273

Woodrow KA, Cu Y, Booth CJ, Saucier-Sawyer JK, Wood MJ, Saltzman WM (2009) Intravaginal gene silencing using biodegradable polymer nanoparticles densely loaded with small-interfering RNA. Nat Mater 8(6):526

World Health Organization (2016) World health statistics 2016: monitoring health for the SDGs sustainable development goals. WHO Headquarters-Geneva, Switzerland

Xia R, Mao Z-H (2012) Progression of motor symptoms in Parkinson's disease. Neurosci Bull 28(1):39–48

Xiao W, Fu Q, Zhao Y, Zhang L, Yue Q, Hai L, Guo L, Wu Y (2019) Ascorbic acid-modified brain-specific liposomes drug delivery system with "lock-in" function. Chem Phys Lipids 224:104727

Xie J, Shen Z, Anraku Y, Kataoka K, Chen X (2019) Nanomaterial-Based Blood-Brain-Barrier (BBB) crossing strategies. Biomaterials 224:119491

Xu Z-R, Wang W-F, Liang X-F, Liu Z-H, Liu Y, Lin L, Zhu X (2015) Protective effects of poly (butyl) cyanoacrylate nanoparticles containing vasoactive intestinal peptide against 6-hydroxydopamine-induced neurotoxicity in vitro. J Mol Neurosci 55(4):854–864

Xu W, Bae EJ, Lee M-K (2018) Enhanced anticancer activity and intracellular uptake of paclitaxel-containing solid lipid nanoparticles in multidrug-resistant breast cancer cells. Int J Nanomedicine 13:7549–7563

Yadav P, Soni G, Mahor A, Alok S, Singh PP, Verma A (2014) Solid lipid nanoparticles: an effective and promising drug delivery system-A review. Int J Pharm Sci Res 5(4):1152

Yang Z-Z, Zhang Y-Q, Wang Z-Z, Wu K, Loud J-N, Qi X-R (2013) Enhanced brain distribution and pharmacodynamics of rivastigmine by liposomes following intranasal administration. Int J Pharm 452:344

Yildiz A, Gonul AS, Tamam L (2002) Mechanism of actions of antidepressants: beyond the receptors. Bull Clin Psychopharmacol 12:194–200

Zhao M, Li A, Chang J, Fu X, Zhang Z, Yan R, Wang H, Liang S (2013) Develop a novel superparamagnetic nano-carrier for drug delivery to brain glioma. Drug Deliv 20(3–4):95–101

Part III

Nanoformulations in Ocular Diseases

10 Application of Biocompatible Nanocarriers in Glaucoma: Challenges and Advances

Abhishek K. Sah, Nagendra Bhuwane, Ishwari Choudhary, Shweta Ramkar, and Preeti K. Suresh

Abstract

Glaucoma is a serious and complex eye disorder with worldwide occurrence in the aging societies and if left untreated at a precise time may lead to the irreversible loss of vision placing great financial burden on the patient and their families. It is a life-long disease that warrants individualized and multifaceted treatment approach. The standard treatment for glaucoma has been focused on the reduction of the intraocular pressure (IOP) by pharmaceutical and/or surgical means. Various conventional formulations are available in the market for the noninvasive and invasive delivery of drugs for the treatment of glaucoma, which include eye drops, eye ointment, periocular injections, etc. Eye drops are widely used for anterior segments application, being a convenient formulation; however, they are also associated with some limitations in terms of pharmacological profile, pharmacokinetic profile, dosing frequency, systemic untoward effect, and poor patient compliance. Low drug bioavailability due to transient contact time, rapid washout by tearing, nasolacrimal drainage are some of the major issues related to the ocular pharmacotherapy. To overcome these challenges, novel biocompatible nanocarriers have been widely explored and investigated for ophthalmic application. The nanocarriers for glaucoma treatment may have manifold advantages, viz., augment drug residence time on the ocular surface and concomitantly ocular bioavailability, and also enhance surgical success by optimization of postoperative scarring and endow a wider safety window. The novel carriers explored include nanoparticle, solid lipid nanoparticle (SLN), nanostructured lipid carrier (NLC), in situ gel, vesicular carrier, niosomes, mucoadhesive system among others. Additionally, biocompatible nanocarriers offer potential benefits like biodegradability, nontoxicity, self-degradability, protection of drug from degradation, controlled drug release, and site specific delivery. However, more studies are required to establish the cellular fate, clinical efficacy, and cytotoxicity of the nanocarriers. This chapter presents a broad overview of the application of biocompatible nanocarriers and reports the clinical findings and patents for the effective management of glaucoma.

A. K. Sah
Department of Pharmacy, Shri G. S. Institute of Technology & Science, Indore, Madhya Pradesh, India

N. Bhuwane · I. Choudhary · S. Ramkar
P. K. Suresh (✉)
University Institute of Pharmacy, Pandit Ravishankar Shukla University, Raipur, Chhattisgarh, India

S. Talegaonkar, M. Rai (eds.), *Nanoformulations in Human Health*,
https://doi.org/10.1007/978-3-030-41858-8_10

Keywords

Glaucoma · Biocompatible · Nanocarriers · Nanotechnology · Ocular drug delivery "biomaterial" · Ophthalmic

10.1 Introduction

Delivery of the drug to the ocular segments is one of the most challenging areas for the pharmaceutical scientist (Gonjari et al. 2010). The major ocular illnesses like glaucoma, conjunctivitis, inflammation, dry eye disease, and bacterial infection require timely dosing of the drug to the eye. The conventional ophthalmic formulations have the restricting limitation of low ocular bioavailability (< 1%). The major cause for the low bioavailability is the precorneal loss of the drug from the anterior segment of the eye, and this can be attributed to rapid tearing, nonproductive absorption, less residence time of the drug in the cul-de-sac, and low permeation profile of the drug to the corneal surface (Sah and Suresh 2017) (Fig. 10.1).

Presently, eye drops and ocular suspensions are the most popular and acceptable formulations to treat the ocular disorders due to convenience and ease of instillations. However, these conventional formulations have limited efficacy and may prove to be inefficient to combat the disease due to extensive loss of the drug by rapid tearing and drainage (Mysore et al. 1996). To overcome these limitations of the conventional formulations, novel nanocarriers have been explored and include polymeric nanoparticles, nanosuspensions, vesicular systems, dendrimers among others (Fig. 10.2). Other novel systems like ocular implants, hydrogels, ocular inserts, and in situ gels have also been investigated. Nanocarriers offer several benefits over the conventional formulations like improving drug bioavailability, avoid drug systemic toxicity, improving drug therapeutic efficacy, and better patient compliance (Wadhwa et al. 2010).

10.2 Glaucoma

Glaucoma is one of the major causes for the irreversible vision loss worldwide and thereby impinging on human health and economic growth. It is triggered by the elevation of the intraocular pressure (IOP) above the normal levels (Sah and Suresh 2017) (Fig. 10.3). Chronic glaucoma associated with open-angle glaucoma

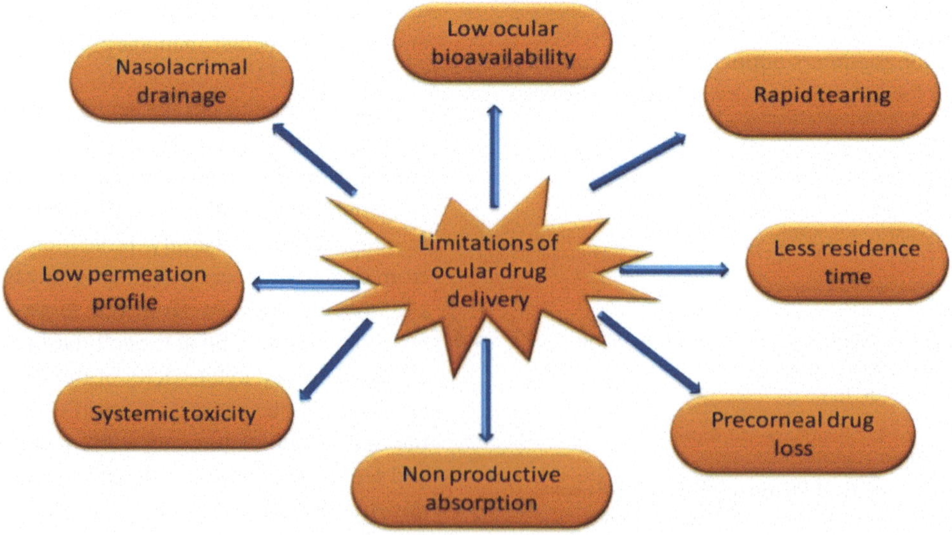

Fig. 10.1 Major constraints for the ocular drug delivery

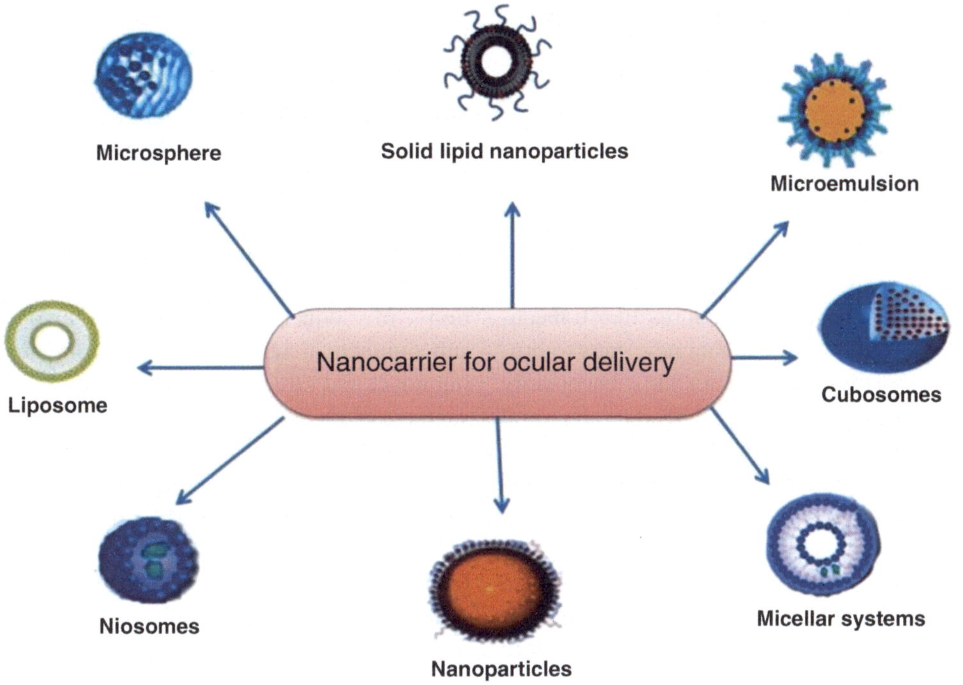

Fig. 10.2 Nanocarrier for ocular delivery of drugs/bioactives

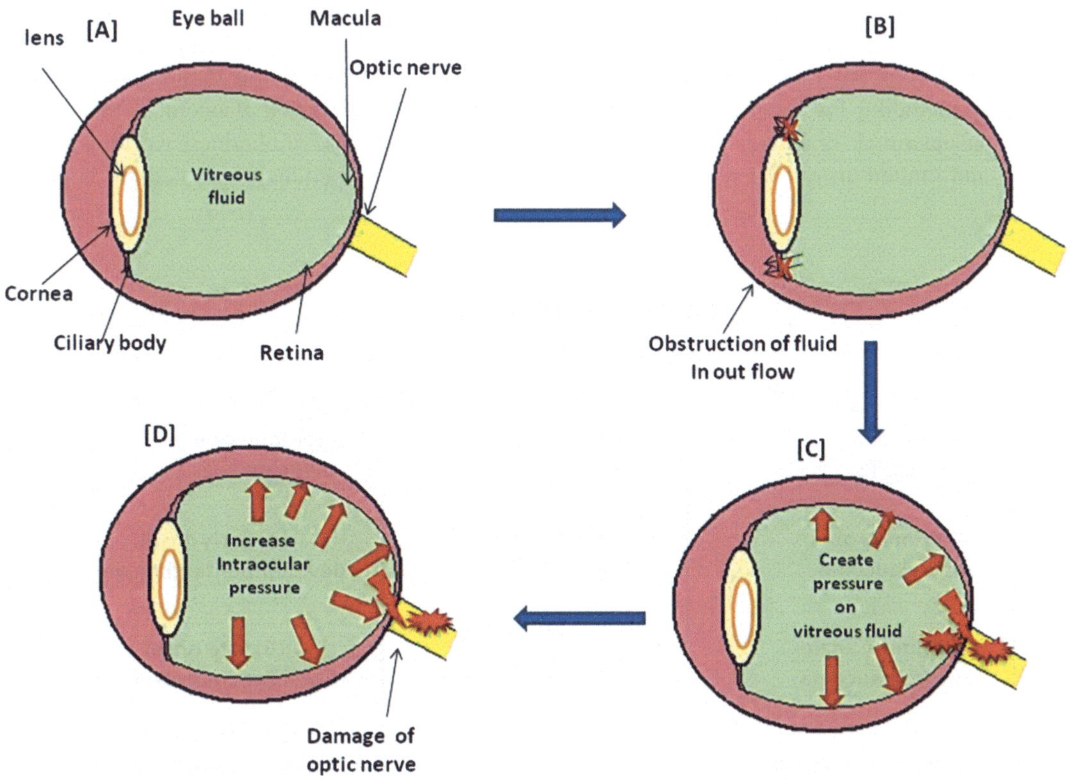

Fig. 10.3 Stages of development of glaucoma by increased intraocular pressure: (**a**) Normal eye ball, (**b**) obstruction in vitreous fluid flow by the ciliary body, (**c**) creation of pressure on vitreous fluid, (**d**) augmentation of intraocular pressure, damage to the optic nerve and loss of vision

(OAG) has been recognized as a major vision-related health problem worldwide and it is expected that by 2020; the number of glaucoma patients will be raised to approximately 79.6 million (Hashim Abu et al. 2014) and 111.8 million by 2040 globally(Tham et al. 2014).

Glaucoma can be corrected by either diminishing the production of aqueous humour (AH) or by augmenting the drainage of aqueous humor from the eye. Surgical procedures like trabeculectomy are employed to create new gaps to promote drainage of aqueous humor and subsequently lower IOP. But this process can lead to abnormal wound healing and scarring. Most of the current treatment strategies, such as medication or surgery, focus on lowering IOP. Increased IOP is not the only risk factor associated with glaucoma as downstream of IOP elevation, retinal ganglion cell degeneration leads to irreversible blindness in this disease (Ibrahim et al. 2013). Elevated IOP leads to the damage of the optic nerves and it promotes the irregular drainage of the ocular aqueous fluid (Hsiao et al. 2014).

Eye drops, suspension, and ointment are the preferred choices of treatment, but these conventional formulations are associated with inherent limitations including low ocular bioavailability (<1%), nasolacrimal drainage, drug systemic toxicity, and limited drug residence time in precorneal segments and poor patient compliance (Suresh and Sah 2014). To overcome these associated shortcomings, there is a strong need for novel biocompatible formulations which prolong drug release and improve drug therapeutic profile with enhanced patient compliance. Also, in the natural course, glaucoma progresses towards the degeneration of posterior segment. But the current drug treatments only aim towards the regulation of aqueous humor production or subconjunctival scarring and this call for devising novel and effective strategies for the anterior segment of the eye.

10.2.1 Classification of Glaucoma

Glaucoma has numerous types and basically it is classified into three types, primary, secondary, and developmental glaucoma (Fig. 10.4).

10.2.1.1 Primary Glaucoma

Primary open-angle glaucoma (POAG) is an asymptomatic optic neuropathic ocular disease characterized by enlarging optic disc cupping and visual field loss. World Health Organization (WHO) has reported that glaucoma is the second most common cause of blindness worldwide, and topical ocular hypertensive medication is effec-

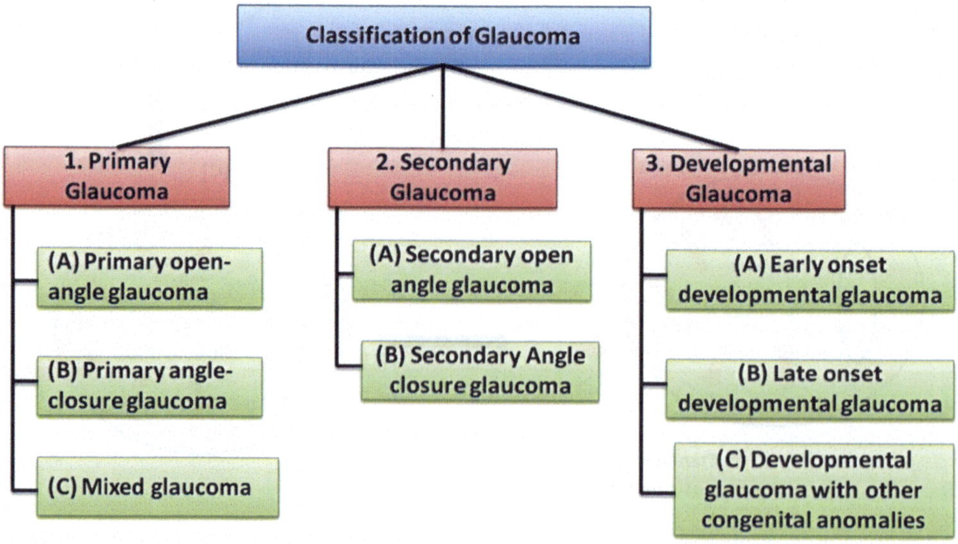

Fig. 10.4 The general classification of glaucoma

tive in delaying the onset of open-angle glaucoma in individuals with elevated ocular pressure (El-Saied et al. 2018).

Primary Open-Angle Glaucoma (POAG)

Primary open-angle glaucoma (POAG) comprises both conventional POAG and normal-tension glaucoma (NTG). Increased intraocular pressure (IOP) leads to the progression of POAG and weakening of optic nerve located in the posterior segments of the eye, and therefore, POAG and NTG cannot be differentiated. The normal limit of the IOP is in the range of 19.9–20.0 mmHg and ± 2 can be treated as the standard deviation for counting normal IOP. POAG is characterized by the chronic development of optic neuropathy. In this ocular disorder thinning of the optic disc margin and retinal nerve fiber occurs, while other disorders and congenital abnormalities are absent and the gonioscopy images also reveal normal anterior segments.

Patients with NTG have normal IOP with the progression and development of glaucomatous optic neuropathy. However, etiological response and finding conclude that factors free from IOP like circulatory injury may play a crucial role in the development of this type of glaucoma.

Primary Angle-Closure Glaucoma

Primary angle-closure glaucoma, the main cause of increment in the IOP is the closure of the angle of the anterior chamber. In this glaucoma, relative papillary block and plateau iris are involved as the main mechanism. Narrow angle eyes that progress angle closure but not develop glaucoma are specified as primary angle closure. This symptom in cases of the angles of anterior chamber express peripheral anterior synechiae, indicated the system of angle closure, however, avoid elevation of IOP or glaucomatous optic neuropathy (Guideline for Glaucoma 2006).

The primary angle-closure glaucoma with the relative papillary block is subdivided into the acute and chronic types. In the plateau iris glaucoma, there are morphological anomalies of iris root and the angle of anterior chamber closes due to the dilation of papillary without the block of iris. In this case, the optic neuropathy cannot be observed even though angle closure occurs. However, in the primary angle-closure glaucoma, there is combination of plateau iris mechanism along with the papillary block system (Guideline for Glaucoma 2006; Kitazawa 1996).

Mixed Glaucoma

This type of glaucoma is the combination of primary open-angle and primary closure glaucoma.

10.2.1.2 Secondary Glaucoma

In secondary glaucoma, the IOP is increased by other ocular medical conditions, systemic diseases, or even due to the use of certain drugs. This condition presents complexity in determining the morphological changes and various functional alterations due to glaucomatous optic neuropathy caused by another disease. Additionally, this glaucoma can be differentiated by numerous dimensions including etiology, mechanism for increasing IOP along with type of medication. This method of classification offers a few benefits but also pose limitations like dividing according to classification etiology, it becomes increasingly difficult to show the mechanism by which neovascular glaucoma starts as open-angle glaucoma and thereafter progress to angle-closure glaucoma. The differentiation according to mechanism for elevation of IOP is mostly considerable and beneficial as an aid to assessing the etiology and optimum medication. The most attention is needed in cases, when the circumstances having a similar etiology show contradictory mechanism for increasing IOP and/or the IOP increase occurs in one and the same eye. For the investigation of secondary glaucoma, gonioscopic examination of the eye is crucial to confirm the mechanism of increasing IOP (Guideline for Glaucoma 2006; Kitazawa et al. 2004).

Open-Angle Mechanisms in Secondary Glaucoma

It is generally described by resistance in an outflow of aqueous fluid between the trabecular meshwork and anterior chamber into the eye, and this irregularity of drainage is due to the fibrocascular membrane and conjunctival epithelium and as an upshot of pseudoexfoliative, inflammatory material, macrophages, and iris pigment deposition. Additionally, these elevations of IOP can also be due to the elevation of episcleral venous pressure along with increased pressure in the superior vena cava (Guideline for Glaucoma 2006).

Angle-Closure Mechanisms in Secondary Glaucoma

The angle closure in the secondary glaucoma is primarily because of the papillary block, and it occurs mostly due to swelling of the lens, luxation of the lens, and goniosynechiae (Guideline for Glaucoma 2006; Iwase et al. 2004). Another mechanism involved in the secondary glaucoma is the anterior movement of the intraocular lens and ciliary edema.

10.2.1.3 Developmental Glaucoma

The developmental or congenital glaucoma refers to glaucoma that is related to developmental anomalies that present at birth. Developmental glaucoma consists of three stages.

Early Onset Developmental Glaucoma

In this case of glaucoma, the congenital disorder is restricted to the trabecular meshwork. However, it is associated with mild hypoplasia as a consequence of progressive abnormality of iris. In addition, pathological condition like the increased diameter of cornea (normally referred as buphthalmos), corneal opacity can also recur.

Late Onset Developmental Glaucoma

This involves the hereditary disorders in the anterior segment of the angle, while the commencement of the glaucoma is delayed due to the minor abnormalities.

Developmental Glaucoma with Other Congenital Anomalies

This classification includes a wide range of medical condition like aniridia, Marfan syndrome, Axenfeld-Rieger syndrome, Peters' anomaly, Sturge-Weber syndrome, and neurofibroma (Guidelines for Glaucoma, 2006).

10.3 Glaucoma Therapies

The majority of work on glaucoma therapy is primarily focused on two strategies viz., delivery of hypotensive drugs and scar-inhibiting nucleotides. A number of hypotensive drugs like prostaglandin analogs (latanoprost, travoprost, unoprostone), beta blockers (metipranolol, timolol, propranolol), and carbonic inhibitors (acetazolamide, ethoxzolamide, methazolamide) have proven to be useful in reducing the production of aqueous humor Ong et al. 2013. Although topical eye drops are the most preferred for the application of drugs into the eye, these formulations have certain limitations, for example, approximately 95% of the drugs present in the drops is wasted due to the rapid tear drainage, metabolic degradation, corneal impermeability, or absorption via the conjunctiva. The existing ophthalmic formulation like solution, suspension, and ointment are no longer sufficient to combat the delivery barriers and achieve successful drug delivery in different ocular pathological conditions (Nair et al. 2015). Another serious issue that warrants urgent attention is that huge percent of the drug reaches the blood stream via conjunctival absorption and may be actively involved in triggering systemic side effects (Sah and Suresh 2017). The various conventional marketed products are enlisted in Table 10.1.

10.4 Biocompatible Nanocarriers for Ocular Application in Glaucoma

10.4.1 Nanoparticulate System

Polymeric colloidal particles with a diameter from 10 to 1000 nm have found wide application for ocular drug delivery (Ameeduzzafar et al. 2016).

Table 10.1 List of marketed product for the treatment of glaucoma

Brand name	Formulation	Composition	Manufacturer
Alpha Drops®	Eye drops	Apraclonidine 0.5%, Benzalconium chloride0.01%	Cipla
Alphagan® P	Eye drops	Brimonidine tartrate 0.1%, 0.15%	Allergan, Inc.
Azopt™	Suspension	Brinzolamide ophthalmic suspension 1%	Alcon Laboratories, Inc.
Betagan®	Eye drops	Levobunolol HCI 0.25%, 0.5%	Allergan, Inc.
Betoptic® S	Eye drops	Betaxolol HCI 0.25%, 0.5%	Alcon Laboratories, Inc.
Betimol®	Eye drops	Timolol hemihydrate 0.25%, 0.5%	Akorn Inc.
Careprost®	Eye solution	Bimatoprost 0.03%	Sun Pharma
Cosopt® Cosopt PF	Eye drops	Dorzolamide HCI & Timolol maleate	Akorn Inc.
Combigen®	Eye solution	Timolol maleate + brimonide tartrate	Allergan, Inc.
Combigan™	Eye solution	Brimonidine tartrate & Timolol maleate ophthalmic solution 0.2%/0.5%	Allergan, Inc.
Dorzox eye drop®	Eye drops	Dorzolamide 2%	Cipla
Diamox® Sequels®	Eye drops	Acetazolamide	Teva
Glucomol®	Eye drops	Timolol maleate 0.25% w/v	Allergan
Glucotim LA®	Eye drops	Timolol maleate 0.5% w/v	Centaur
Iopidine®	Eye drops	Apraclonidine HCI 0.5%, 1%	Alcon Laboratories, Inc.
Iotim®	Eye drops	Timolol maleate 0.25% w/v	FDC
Isopto® Carbacho	Eye drops	Carbachol 0.75%, 1.5%, 3%	Alcon Laboratories, Inc.
Isopto® Carpine	Eye drops	Pilocarpine HCI 1%, 2%, 4%	Alcon Laboratories
Iobrim®	Eye drops	Brimonide tartrate 0.2%	FDC
Istalol®	Eye solution	Timolol maleate ophthalmic solution 0.5%	Bausch & Lomb, Inc.
Lumigan®	Eye drops	Bimatoprost 0.01%, 0.03%	Allergan
Latocom®	Eye drops	Latanoprost 50mcg, Timolol 5 mg	Sun Pharma
Lupitors®	Eye drops	Travoprost 0.004%	Lupin
Neptazane®	Eye drops	Methazolamide	Fera Pharmaceuticals
9 PM Eye Drops®	Eye drops	Latanoprost 50 mcg/ml	Cipla
OptiPranolol®	Eye drops	Metipranolol 0.3%	Bausch & Lomb, Inc.
Ocupres®	Eye solution	Timolol 2.5 mg, 5 mg/ml	Cadila Pharma
Optipres eye drop®	Eye drop	Betaxolol 0.5%	Cipla
Pilocar®	Eye drop	Pilocarpine nit. 1%,2%,4%	FDC
Pilopine HS® Gel	Eye drops	Pilocarpine HCI gel 4%	Alcon Laboratories
Pilocarpine HCI Ophthalmic Solution USP	Eye drops	Pilocarpine HCI 1%, 2%, 4%	Bausch & Lomb, Inc.
Simbrinza™	Suspension	Brinzolamide/Bromonide tartrate 1%, 0.2%	Alcori
Simbrinza®	Eye drops	Brinzolamide & Brimonidine tartrate 1%/0.2%	Alcon Laboratories, Inc.
Travatan® Z	Eye drops	Travaprost 0.004%	Alcon Laboratories, Inc.
Timoptic in Ocudose (PF)	Eye solution	Timolol maleate Ophthalmic Solution 0.25%, 0.5% in Ocudose dispenser	Bausch & Lomb
Timoptic-XE®	Eye solution	Timolol maleate ophthalmic gel forming solution 0.25%, 0.5%	Bausch & Lomb
Timolo®	Eye solution	Timolol maleate 0.25%, 0.5%	Bell
Timoblu®	Eye drops	Timolol maleate 0.5% w/v	Lupin
Trusopt®	Eye drops	Dorzolamide HCI 2%	Merck & Co., Inc.
Timoptic-xe®	Ophthalmic gel	Timolol maleate 0.25%, 0.5%	Merck and Co, Inc.
Xalatan®	Eye drops	Latanoprost 0.005%	Pfizer
Xalacom®	Eye drops	Latanoprost 50mcg, timolol 5 mg	Pfizer
Zioptan™	Eye drops	Tafluprost ophthalmic solution 0.0015%	Akorn Inc.

Due to its nano size range, it assists in the capillary penetration and improving the uptake by the cells which translates into higher therapeutic concentration at the site of action. The nanoparticulates can be either nanospheres or nanocapsules depending upon the morphology and method of preparation. In case of nanospheres therapeutic agents are entrapped in the matrix structure within the particle. Likewise, in nanocapsules drug is present in the form of reservoir as a liquid or semi-solid core and encapsulated with solid surface. This colloidal dispersion has been extensively used for the ocular delivery of the drug due to its several benefits over the other carriers including improved durability, stability, enhanced bioavailability, sustained drug release at the site of action, low ocular irritation, and improved drug retentivity on to the precorneal surface (Ameeduzzafar et al. 2016). In this context, various polymers are being used for medical and pharmaceutical applications for the development of nanoparticle and these have been already approved by WHO and FDA. These polymers include polylactides (PLA), polyglycolides (PGA), and poly(lactide-co-glycolides) (PLGA) (Stevanovic and Uskokovic 2009). PLGA-based nanoparticles are most widely used due to their superior biocompatibility and biodegradability profiles (Zhao et al. 2014). For the ocular drug-delivery applications, polymer like polylactides, poly(D, L-lactides), poly-(D, L, lactide-co-glycolide) (PLGA) (Sah et al. 2017), e-caprolactone (Fessi et al., 1989; Aksungur et al. 2011; Gupta et al. 2011), polyacrylamide, and polycyanoacrylate and poly(methyl methacrylate) (Zimmer et al. 1991; Wenger et al., 2011) have been widely reported. Latanoprost acid (LA)-loaded controlled drug delivery system for the treatment of glaucoma has been reported. In this case, poly(lactide)/monomethoxy-poly(ethyleneglycol) (PLA-PEG) nanoparticles (NPs) were prepared by using an emulsification-solvent evaporation method. The prepared formulation NPs were in vitro characterized for the various parameters including particle size, zeta potential, drug entrapment efficiency (EE), and drug release. For the assessment of intraocular pressure (IOP), four groups of rabbits were taken (Giarmoukakis et al. 2013). In the Group A, LA-loaded nanoparticle (equivalent to 8.5 μg LA) was administered subconjunctivally into the normotensive rabbits. In group B, a plain drug solution of LA was administered. Likewise, dummy NPs were administered in Group C and Group D untreated served as control. The IOP was continuously assessed for 8 days by using tonometer (Tono-Pen XL®). Additionally, the quantification of LA in the aqueous humor (AH) was assessed by HPLC for 6 day post administration. The mean particle size and EE was found to be 80 nm and 18.3%. Drug-loaded NPs were found to have significantly IOP lowering effect on group A, while IOP level remained significantly lower than other groups throughout the experiment ($p = 0.04$). After the quantification of LA aqueous humor, the concentration was found to decrease with respect to time in group B, while in group A, it increased. The concentration of LA on sixth day was found to be quite higher in group A as compared to group B (344 ± 73.5 ng/ml and 228 ± 41.01 ng/ml), respectively, along with no ocular inflammation (Fig. 10.5). These results advocate that subconjunctival administration of LA-loaded nanoparticle provided sustained drug release in vivo and holds potential for the treatment of glaucoma (Giarmoukakis et al. 2013). Table 10.2 presents a summary of the studies with other nanocarriers for treatment of glaucoma.

10.4.2 Solid Lipid Nanoparticle (SLNs)

Solid lipid nanoparticle (SLNs) are the colloidal particles composed of lipids with the diameter falling in the size range of 10–1000 nm (Goyal et al. 2016). These colloidal particles show a solid state at normal body temperature as well as room temperature. SLNs circumvent the limitations associated with other colloidal particle and are, therefore, considered as promising substitutes for ocular delivery. The benefits of SLNs include very low irritation, high

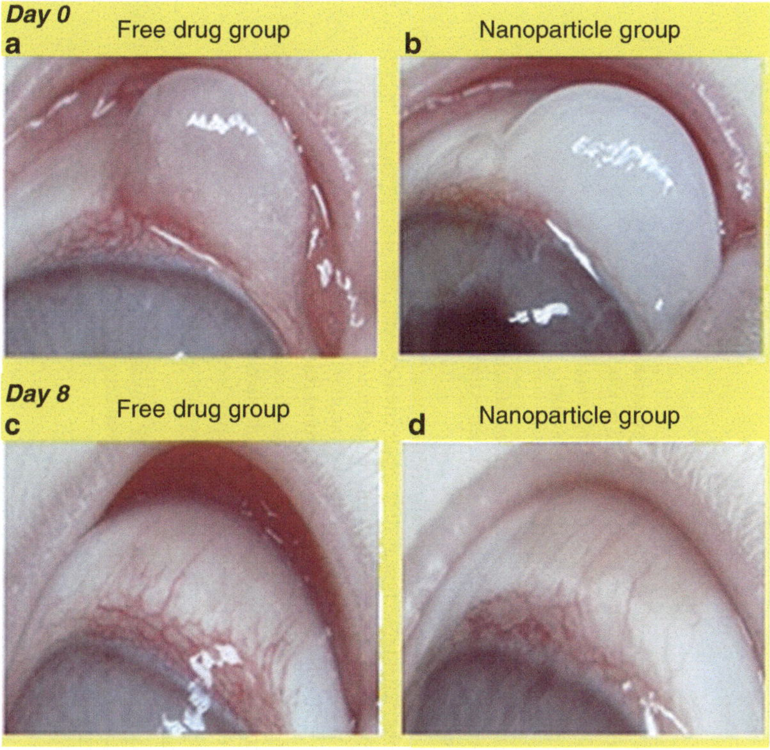

Fig. 10.5 Clinical assessment of LA-NPs after subconjunctival administration (**a**), (**b**) zero day, (**c**), (**d**) after eighth day. (Adapted from Giarmoukakis et al. 2013)

penetration profile into the deeper layer of ocular tissue among others. These features of SLNs contribute to potential enhancement in the therapeutic profile of the drug in the treatment of glaucoma. In this context, Li et al., reported the Methazolamide (MTA)-loaded SLNs for the ocular application for the treatment of glaucoma (Li et al. 2011). The nanocarrier was prepared by a modified emulsion-solvent evaporation technique and characterized for their physicochemical properties. The therapeutic potential of nanocarrier was assessed by intraocular pressure (IOP) lowering effect, and ocular irritation was evaluated by Draize test. Additionally, the in vivo studies showed improved therapeutic activity and prolonged drug release profile as compared with plain drug solution and marketed product. These results indicated that MTA-loaded SLNs would be a promising nanocarrier for ocular delivery in the treatment of glaucoma along with better patient compliance.

10.4.3 Nanostructured Lipid Carrier (NLC)

These types of biocompatible nanocarrier are the modified forms of the solid lipid nanoparticle (SLN) and consist of solid lipid outer membrane incorporated with liquid lipids. The availability of liquid lipid along with various types of fatty acid C chain developed NLC with less organized crystalline structure and consequently improved drug loading (DL) potential. In this context, Shrivastava et al., investigated timolol maleate (TM)- and brinzolamide (BRZ)-loaded nanostructured lipid carrier (NLC) for the effective treatment of glaucoma to improve the pharmacokinetic, permeation profile along with residence time on the precorneal segment Shrivastava et al. 2018. The novel formulation was developed by the melt emulsification method and characterized for various parameters including particle size, polydispersity index (PDI), entrapment efficiency (EE), drug loading (DL), in vitro drug

Table 10.2 Various drug-loaded nanocarriers for the treatment of glaucoma

Polymer/Lipid	Drug	Nanocarrier	Experimental model	Major outcomes	Reference
PLGA, lipid	Brinzolamide	LPNs	In vitro, In vivo	Sustained drug release profile, improved corneal permeation along with topical therapeutic effect as compared with marketed product (AZOPT®).	Zhou et al. (2019)
Bioadhesive, biocompatible materials	R-801 (a new drug molecule)	NPs	In vitro, In vivo	Improved encapsulation efficiency, prolonged corneal contact time, improved IOP lowering capacity along with safety profile	Ibrahim et al. (2019)
Flax seed gum, chitosan	Timolol maleate	Polymeric NPs	In vitro, In vivo	Improved bioadhesive profile, sustained drug release character, better corneal penetration profile as compared with marketed eye drop formulation, prolonged IOP lowering effect	Mittal and Kaur (2019)
Pluronic-F127 stabilized D-α-Tocopherol PEG	Curcumin	NPs	In vitro, In vivo	Improved drug solubility profile, better localization of nanocarrier with less than 20 nm size, significant protection against cobalt chloride-induced hypoxia and glutamate-induced toxicity, significant reduction in retinal ganglion cell loss as compared to control, improved neuroprotective therapy in glaucoma along with other eye diseases with neuronal pathology	Davis et al. (2018)
Gelatin	Timolol maleate	GNPs	In vitro, In vivo	Better IOP lowering effect along with sustained drug release, improved entrapment efficiency, better stability profile, and high bioavailability	Shokry et al. (2018)
–	Brimonidine	NLC, SLN	In vitro, In vivo	Better drug stability, improved permeation profile, better localization of NLC in anterior segment of the eye, sustained drug release along with high IOP lowering capacity.	Salamouni et al. (2018)
SPC, CTAB/DDAB	Carvedilol	NPs	In vitro, Ex vivo, In vivo	High corneal permeability coefficient, prolonged IOP lowering capacity up to 24 h as compared with carvedilol solution, improved drug bioavailability along with retinal atrophy of glaucomatous eyes	Hassan et al. (2018)
PLGA	Brinzolamide	NPs	In vivo	Prolonged drug release for the treatment of IOP	Salama et al. (2017)
Glycerol monooleate, poloxamer 407	Timolol maleate	Cubosomes	In vitro, Ex vivo, In vivo	Better physical stability along with high encapsulation efficiency, high penetration profile in the corneal tissue as compare with eye drop, longer retention time, high IOP lowering capacity as compared with commercial eye drop	Huang et al. (2017)
Phospholipid/ cholesterol	Acetazolamide	Hybridized vesicles	In vitro, In vivo	Improved IOP lowering potential as compared to the conventional liposomes	Naguib et al. (2017)
2-Hydroxy-propyl-b-cyclodextrin	Disulfiram	NPs	In vitro, In vivo	High stability profile, high antimicrobial activity against *E. coli,* high transcorneal penetration profile across excised rabbit corneas, high drug residence time on precorneal segments, better IOP lowering capacity as compared to plain drug solution, good tolerability in corneal epithelial cell	Nagai et al. (2015)

Chitosan, succinic anhydride (CSUC) Sodium tripolyphosphate (TPP)	Timolol maleate	NPs	In vitro	High drug entrapment efficiency, sustained drug release profile, improved therapeutic efficacy	Siafaka et al. (2015)
Softisan® 100, Didecyldimethyl-ammonium bromide	Melatonin	CSLN	In vitro, In vivo	Higher IOP lowering capacity of the formulation, sustained drug release, good stability	Leonardi et al. (2015)
PLGA	Dorzolamide	NPs	In vitro, In vivo	Prolonged drug release, improved precorneal permeation, and high concentration in aqueous humor. Significant reduction of IOP	Warsi et al. (2014)
DPPC	Timolol maleate	Liposome	In vitro	Sustained drug release as compared with plain liposome, improved bioavailability	Ong and Hui (2014)
Chitosan	Dorzolamide	In situ nanoparticle gel	In vitro, Ex vivo	Sustained drug release and better drug corneal retention profile as compared with marketed formulation, nonirritant property of the formulation	Katiyar et al. (2014)
Poly acrylic acid (carbopol C934P)	Timolol maleate and brimonidine tartrate	Stimuli-sensitive hydrogel	In vitro, In vivo	Prolonged drug release, high IOP lowering	Dubey and Prabhu (2014)
–	Timolol maleate and dorzolamide hydrochloride	Polymeric nanofiber patches	In vitro, In vivo	Better IOP lowering potential as compared to commercial eye drop	Gagandeepet al. (2014)
Glyceryl monoolein (GMO)	Pilocarpine nitrate	Liquid crystal nanoparticle	In vitro, In vivo	High encapsulation efficiency, sustained drug release profile for up to 8 h, ex vivo drug permeability was 2.05-fold higher than marketed eye drops, prolonged IOP lowering effect in experimental animal	Li et al. (2013)
PLGA,-poly (ethylenglycole) (PEG)	Melatonin	NPs	In vitro, In vivo	Sustained drug release, improved drug residence time on pre-corneal segment, better pharmacological profile	Musumeci et al. (2013)
Chitosan, 6-O-carboxymethyl (OCM-CS)	Dorzolamide hydrochloride	NPs	In vitro, In vivo	High entrapment efficiency, sustained drug release profile, higher bioavailability	Shinde et al. (2013)
Egg-phosphatidylcholine	Latanoprost	Liposomes	In vitro, In vivo	Improved drug-loading efficiency, improved stability of formualtion up to 6 months, sustained drug release profile along with better IOP lowering potential up to 90 days	Natrajan et al. (2012)
PLGA, PAMAM	Brimonidine and timolol maleate	Dendrimer hydrogel-PLGA-NPs	In vitro, In vivo	High cellular uptake, prolonged residence time on precorneal segment, sustained drug release up to 28–35 days in vitro, high IOP lowering capacity in normotensive adult Dutch-belted male rabbits, improved drug bioavailability in aqueous fluid and in cornea along with low dosing frequency	Yang et al. (2012)

(continued)

Table 10.2 (continued)

Polymer/Lipid	Drug	Nanocarrier	Experimental model	Major outcomes	Reference
Chitosan	Timolol maleate	Mucoadhesive film	In vitro, In vivo	Prolonged drug release profile along with IOP lowering potential	Fulgêncio et al. (2012)
Carbopol, cholesterol	Brimonidine tartrate	Nanovesicles	In vitro, In vivo	Improved drug entrapment efficiency, high stability profile at refrigerated temperature, better IOP lowering efficacy than marketed eye drops along with sustained drug release up to 7.5 h	Maiti et al. (2011)
Phospholipids, Polyethylene glycol 400	Methazolamide	SLNs	In vitro, In vivo	Higher therapeutic efficacy along with prolonged drug release profile as compared with plain drug solution and commercial eye drop at lower doses and better patient compliance	Li et al. (2011)
Ammonium sulfate	Timolol maleate	Liposomal-hydrogel	In vitro, In vivo	Enhanced drug permeability, prolonged drug residence time on precorneal segments, improved physical stability of the hydrogel formulation, improved bioavailability along with prolonged IOP lowering potential	Hui et al. (2011)

GNPs Gelatin Nanoparticles, *NPs* Nanoparticle, *PEG* Polyethylene glycol, *DPPC* 1,2-dipalmitoy-sn-glycero-3-phosphocholine, *PLGA* Poly (d, l-lactide-co-glycolide), *PEG* Poly(ethylene glycol), *PAMAM* Polyamidoamine, *CSLNs* Cationic solid lipid nanoparticle, *NLC* Nanostructured lipid carrier, *SLN* Solid lipid nanocarrier, *SPC* Soy phosphatidyl choline, *CTAB* Cetyltrimethylammonium bromide, *DDAB* Dimethyldidodecylammonium bromide, *LPNs* Lipid-polymer nanoparticles release, and ex vivo drug penetration studies. For the TM-loaded NLC particle size, PDI, EE, and DL of the optimized NLC were found to be 110.36 ± 0.47 nm, 0.24, 77.12 ± 0.64%, and 0.360 ± 0.01%. While for BRZ-loaded NLC, the EE and DL were found to be 70.73 ± 0.64% and 0.71 ± 0.02%, respectively. The in vitro drug release profile for the first 5 h exhibited initial burst release pattern of 34 ± 2.90% for TM and 38 ± 3.10% for BRZ followed by sustained drug release of 72.29 ± 5.90% and 70.08 ± 6.40% for TM and BRZ-NLC for 24 h. The ex vivo drug penetration profile for 24 h was found to be 72.30 ± 6.40% and 67.69 ± 6.50% for TM and BRZ, respectively. The clinical findings reported that there was significant improvement in the pharmacokinetic, therapeutic profile along with the permeation profile of the NLC as compared with their drug suspension. Some other NLC formulations studied are listed in Table 10.2.

10.4.4 In Situ Gel

Lai and Hsieh developed the biodegradable in situ gel formulation for intracameral administration of the antiglaucoma drug (Lai and Hsieh 2012). For the development of these formulations, aminated gelatin was grafted with carboxylic end-capped poly(N-isopropylacrylamide) (PN) using carbodiimide-mediated coupling reaction. Fourier transforms infrared (FTIR) spectroscopy were used for the conformation of chemical copolymer gelatin-g-PNIPAAm (GN). The stage of molar ratio for NH_2/COOH was 0.36, and the grafting ratio, grafting degree along with efficiency, weight ratio of PN to aminated gelatin was found to be 25.6, 18.6%, 52.6%, and 1.9, respectively. The GN exhibited improved thermal gelation capacity along with adherence, and it also demonstrated better transition features of the copolymer as compared with PN. In vitro cytocompatibility studies were conducted on the cell culture of anterior part of the eye. It was reported that in situ gels do not change production with small effect on inflammation. High encapsulation efficiency and cumulative drug release were also attained (approximately 62% and 95%, respectively) which attributed to initial rapid temperature triggered capture for pilocarpine following progressive degradation of gelatin network.

In vivo study was also performed for the assessment of IOP in established rabbit glaucoma model and pilocarpine-loaded GN displayed better ocular bioavailability and pharmacological effect as compared to eye drop or plain drug injection or drug-loaded PN. The various in situ gel formulations are listed in Table 10.2.

10.4.5 Vesicular Carrier

10.4.5.1 Niosomes

Niosomes are the vesicular drug-delivery carrier developed by self-assembly of nonionic amphiphiles in liquid media resulting in an enclosed bilayer arrangement. This bilayered vesicular system permits entrapment of hydrophilic as well as a lipophilic therapeutic agent either in the liquid film or in the lipid layer (Carafa et al. 1998). Additionally, sparingly soluble drugs can also be entrapped in the vesicular carriers (Arunothayanun et al. 2000). Vesicular carriers have been widely investigated for the ocular delivery owing to its special features like prolonged and controlled drug release in the ocular tissues along with protection from enzymatic drug degradation in the corneal segments (Kaur et al. 2004). Moreover, vesicular carrier facilitates drug transport across the corneal segment. Hashim et al., reported atenolol-loaded niosomal hydrogel for the ocular application in the treatment of glaucoma (Hashim Abu et al. 2014). The niosomes were prepared by film hydration technique using span 60 and cholesterol and followed by the in vitro characterization. The entrapment efficiency was found to be high at 80.7% with 2:1 molar ratio of span 60/cholesterol. Good stability profile of niosomes was found up to

3 months at 4 °C. Niosomal hydrogel composed of Carbopol 934P showed sustained drug release profile as compared to free drug solution and polymeric hydrogel. The IOP lowering potential of niosomal hydrogel was found to be high as compared with plain drug solution, and it was concluded that prepared atenolol-loaded niosomal hydrogel formulation could be promising carrier for ocular drug delivery in the treatment of glaucoma.

10.4.5.2 Liposomes

Liposomes are self-closed phospholipidic bilayers that have a spherical vesicular form and an aqueous core. They entrap mostly hydrophilic drug in the aqueous core and hydrophobic drug in the lipid bilayer system. These structures have been known for their large potential as drug carriers for optimized drug-delivery systems as well as for membranes model studies (Sah et al. 2018). These lipid carriers have several benefits over

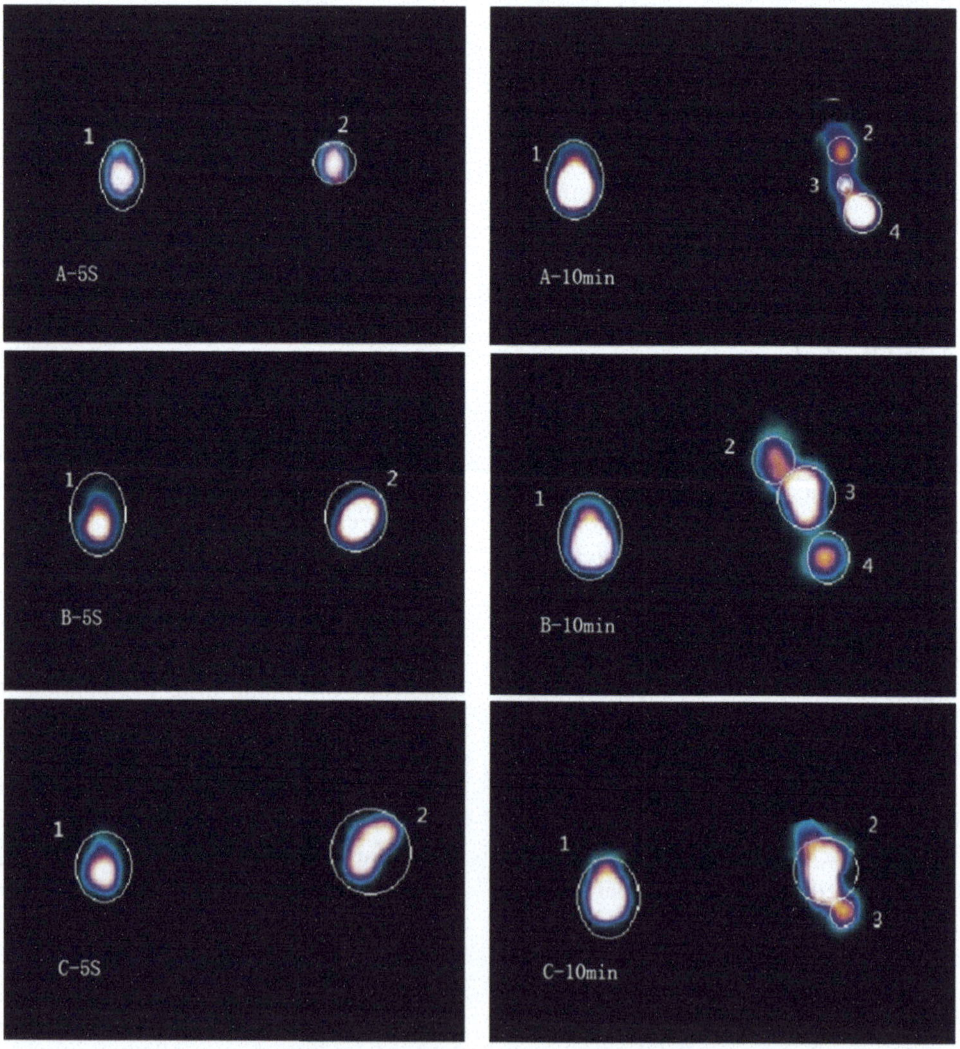

Fig. 10.6 Gamma scintigraphic study revealed improved drug retentivity profile on the precorneal surface as compared to commercial eye drops. Formulation labeled with 99mTc: (**a**) TM-CH-coated liposomes, (**b**) TM liposomes, (**c**) TM eye drops. RIO: 1—Reference spot, 2—Corneal surface, 3—Inner canthus, 4—Nasolacrimal duct. (Adapted from Tan et al. 2017)

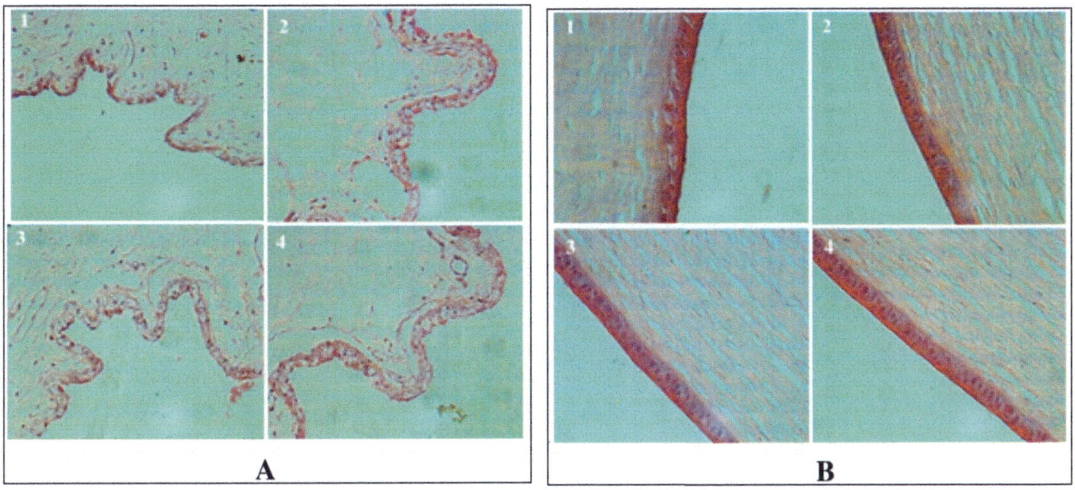

Fig. 10.7 Histopathological images of ocular tissue after treatment with different formulations for 7 days: (**a**) Conjunctiva, (**b**) Cornea: 1—TM eye drops, 2—TM liposomes, 3—TM—CH coated liposomes, 4—Control. (Adapted from Tan et al. 2017)

the other drug-delivery systems including high biocompatibility, high corneal penetration, prolonged clearance time, absence of immunogenicity, low toxicity and, therefore, it has been extensively investigated for ocular drug-delivery application (Ebrahim et al. 2005). Additionally, these carriers offer ease in local application and maintain high drug therapeutic activity. Other advantages include simple technology for liposomal preparation along with flexibility of its physical profile (Bourlais et al. 1998; Meisner and Mezei 1995). It is reported that liposomes composed of phospholipids and cholesterol are restricted by their clearance into the tear fluid applicable for negative charge and neutral liposomes. It has been also suggested that cationic liposomes have superior binding affinity to the corneal surface and improved precorneal retention of the drug and which may translate into improved drug absorption (Tan et al. 2017). Recently, timolol maleate-loaded chitosan-coated liposomes (TM-CHL) have been reported to improve the ocular permeation along with improved therapeutic profile (Tan et al. 2017). The mean particle size of the prepared formulation was found to be 150.7 nm with 75.83 ± 1.61% of entrapment efficiency. The formulation exhibited considerable mucin adhesion properties as compared to traditional eye drops. TM-CHL showed 3.18 fold more permeability coefficient and as a result significantly improved corneal permeation profile of the lipid carrier. Additionally, the gamma scintigraphic study revealed improved drug retentivity profile on precorneal surface as compared to commercial eye drop (Fig. 10.6). Also, no ocular irritation was evident in the corneal epithelial cells (Fig. 10.7), and therapeutic profile indicated that maximum reduction in IOP was produced by TM-CHL (19.67 ± 1.14) mmHg as compared with TM eye drops (23.80 ± 1.49) mmHg. The result gave an affirmation that CHL is a promising carrier for ocular drug delivery with improved therapeutic efficacy. The various patents of nanocarrier-based system for the treatment of glaucoma are listed in the Table 10.3.

Table 10.3 Some patents of nanocarriers for ocular delivery in the treatment of glaucoma

Patent No.	Assignee	Delivery system	Drug	Invention	Reference
WO2016048242 A1	Nanyang Technological University	Liposome	Timolol maleate	Timolol maleate-loaded liposomes for the management of glaucoma	Venkatraman et al. (2016)
US 2011/0206773 A1	Yale University; University of Iowa Research Foundation	Microparticle	–	Drug-loaded polymeric microparticle for the effective treatment of elevated intraocular pressure in the eye. The prepared formulation delivers the therapeutic agent for more than 14 days in experimental animal. The therapeutic agent improves in the optic nerve regeneration and effectively lowering the elevated intraocular pressure.	Lavik et al. (2011)
US 7,993,634 B2	Allergan, Inc., Irvine, CA (US)	Oil-in-oil emulsified implants/ microparticles	Prostamide	Fabrication of intraocular biocompatible implant consisting of o/w or microparticle, which included the prostamide as a biodegradable polymer for extended release in the treatment of glaucoma	Hughes et al. (2011)
US 2010/0104654 A1	Allergan, Inc., (US)	Biocompatible, bioerodible implant, microspheres	Latanoprost	Latanoprost-loaded intraocular implants along with microspheres for the ocular delivery in the treatment of glaucoma	Robinson et al. (2010)
US 7,589,057 B2	Allergan, Inc., Irvine, CA (US)	Microparticle	–	Biocompatible o/w emulsified microparticle for effective treatment of glaucoma comprising alpha-2 adrenergic receptor agonist as a therapeutic agent.	Chang et al. (2009)
US 2006/0182781 A1	Allergan, Inc., Irvine, CA (US)	Biocompatible microparticles	–	Biocompatible microparticle comprising active cyclic lipid along with biodegradable polymer for the effective treatment of glaucoma or AMD	Hughes et al. (2006)
US 2006/0246145 A1	Allergan, Inc., Irvine, CA (US)	Biocompatible microparticles	–	Biocompatible microparticle for the ophthalmic application in the treatment of glaucoma and age-related macular degeneration (AMD).	Chang et al. (2006)
US 6,369,116 B1	Oculex PharmaceuticalsInc., Sunnyvale, CA (US)	Implant	–	Ocular implant and method for improvement in wound healing and rescue the infection in glaucoma filtration surgery.	Wong et al. (2002)

10.5 Mucoadhesive System

Park et al. 2015 investigated brimonide-loaded mucoadhesive microparticle for ocular application in the treatment of glaucoma. The microparticles were adorned with nanostructured surface and comprised of poly(lactic-co-glycolic acid) as a diffusion wall material and polyethylene glycol (PEG) as a mucoadhesive polymer. The presence of PEG in the nanostructured surface of the microparticle showed 13-fold higher specific surface areas along with improved adherence profile on to the ocular mucous layer as compared with the conventional microparticle. The clinical finding reported that novel mucoadhesive microparticle improved the therapeutic profile of the drug and improved bioavailability ensuring better patient compliance as compared with the commercial eye drop. The other mucoadhesive carriers are listed in Table 10.2.

10.6 Current and Future Developments

Glaucoma is a vision-threatening disease that warrants life-long treatment and patient noncompliance can cause irreversible loss of vision. The various conventional formulation are available in the market but they fail to achieve their pharmacological potential and ensure better patient compliance. Advancements in the area of biocompatible nanocarriers like nanoparticles, solid lipid nanoparticles, nanolipidic carriers, vesicular systems, and hydrogels have shown encouraging results for the effective treatment of glaucoma. Recently, one of the researchers reported the development of noninvasive brimonidine tartrate (BT)-loaded poly(lactic-co-glycolic)acid (PLGA) microspheres incorporated in thermoresponsive hydrogels eye drop for the treatment of glaucoma (Fedorchak et al. 2017). These biocompatible nanocarriers can be used for the delivery of newer therapeutic agents including genes, antibodies, and bioactive proteins (Dewangan et al. 2018).

Moreover, the major challenges with the biocompatible nanocarriers that need to be addressed are the technical concerns like establishing safe manufacturing technologies and stability profile. The technological advancement in biocompatible nanocarrier has opened new avenues for improving ocular pharmacotherapy along with better patient compliance. However, more studies are required to establish the cellular fate, clinical efficacy, and cytotoxicity of the biocompatible nanocarriers.

Acknowledgments The authors are thankful to the Director, University Institute of Pharmacy, Pt. Ravishankar Shukla University, Raipur, India. Abhishek K. Sah is thankful to the Head, Department of Pharmaceutical Engineering and Technology, Indian Institute of Technology (Banaras Hindu University), Varanasi, India, and also thankful to the Science Engineering Research Board (SERB-DST), New Delhi, India, for National Postdoctoral Fellowship (NPDF) (PDF/2016/001909). The authors are also thankful to the Chhattisgarh Council of Science and Technology for MRP (1863/CCOST/MRP/2014).

Conflict of Interest The authors confirm that the content of this chapter has no conflict of interest.

References

Aksungur P, Demirbilek M, Denkbaş EB (2011) Development and characterization of Cyclosporine A loaded nanoparticles for ocular drug delivery: cellular toxicity, uptake and kinetic studies. J Control Release 151(3):286–294. https://doi.org/10.1016/j.jconrel.2011.01.010

Ameeduzzafar AJ, Fazil M, Qumbar M, Khan N, Ali A (2016) Colloidal drug delivery system: amplify the ocular delivery. Drug Deliv 23(3):700–716. https://doi.org/10.3109/10717544.2014.923065

Arunothayanun P, Bernard MS, Craig DQ, Uchegbu IF, Florence AT (2000) The effect of processing variables on the physical characteristics of non-ionic surfactant vesicles (niosomes) formed from a hexadecyl diglycerol ether. Int J Pharm 201:7–14. https://doi.org/10.1016/S0378-5173(00)00362-8

Bourlais CL, Acar L, Zia H, Sado PA, Needham T, Leverge R (1998) Ophthalmic drug delivery systems – recent advances. Prog Retin Eye Res 17:33–58. https://doi.org/10.1016/S1350-9462(97)00002-5

Carafa M, Santucci E, Alhaique F, Coviello T, Murtas E, Riccieri FM, Lucania G, Torrisi MR (1998) Preparation and properties of new unilamellar non-ionic/ionic surfactant vesicles. Int J Pharm 160:51–59. https://doi.org/10.1016/S0378-5173(97)00294-9

Chang J, Hughes P, Chang CM (2006) Methods for treating ocular conditions with cyclic lipid containing microparticles. US 2006/0246145 A1

Chang J, Beach N, Hughes P, Viejo A (2009) Oil-in-water method for making alpha-2 agonist polymeric drug delivery systems. US 7,589,057 B2

Davis BM, Pahlitzsch M, Guo L, Balendra S (2018) Topical curcumin nanocarriers are neuroprotective in eye disease. Sci Rep 8:1–13. https://doi.org/10.1038/s41598-018-29393-8

Dewangan HK, Pandey T, Maurya L, Singh S (2018) Rational design and evaluation of HBsAg polymeric nanoparticles as antigen delivery carriers. Int J Biol Macromol 111:804–812. https://doi.org/10.1016/j.ijbiomac.2018.01.073

Dubey A, Prabhu P (2014) Formulation and evaluation of stimuli-sensitive hydrogels of timolol maleate and brimonidine tartrate for the treatment of glaucoma. Int J Pharm Investig 4:112–118. https://doi.org/10.4103/2230-973X.138340

Ebrahim S, Peyman GA, Lee PJ (2005) Applications of liposomes in ophthalmology. Surv Ophthalmol 50:167–182. https://doi.org/10.1016/j.survophthal.2004.12.006

El-Saied SH, Zaky AG, El-Agha A, Ali AER (2018) Evaluation of topical monotherapy for early primary open angle glaucoma patient. Egypt J Hosp Med 70:403–408. https://doi.org/10.12816/0043477

Fedorchak MV, Conner IP, Schuman JS, Cugini A, Little SR (2017) Long term glaucoma drug delivery using a topically retained gel/microsphere eye drop. Sci Rep 7:1–11. https://doi.org/10.1038/s41598-017-09379-8

Fessi H, Puisieux F, Devissaguet JP, Ammoury N, Benita S (1989) Nanocapsule formation by interfacial polymer deposition following solvent displacement. Int J Pharm 55:R1–R4

Fulgêncio GDO, Viana FAB, Ribeiro RR, Yoshida MI, Faraco AG, Junior ADSC (2012) New mucoadhesive chitosan film for ophthalmic drug delivery of Timolol Maleate: in vivo evaluation. J Ocul Pharmacol Ther 28:1–11. https://doi.org/10.1089/jop.2011.0174

Gagandeep, Garg T, Malik B, Rath G, Goyal AK (2014) Development and characterization of nano-fiber patch for the treatment of glaucoma. Eur J Pharm Sci 53:10–16. https://doi.org/10.1016/j.ejps.2013.11.016

Giarmoukakis A, Labiris G, Sideroudi H, Tsimali Z, Koutsospyrou N, Avgoustakis K, Kozobolis V (2013) Biodegradable nanoparticles for controlled subconjunctival delivery of latanoprost acid: in vitro and in vivo evaluation. Preliminary results. Exp Eye Res 112:29–36. https://doi.org/10.1016/j.exer.2013.04.007

Gonjari ID, Karmarkar AB, Khade TS, Hosmani AH, Navale RB (2010) Use of factorial design in formulation and evaluation of ophthalmic gels of gatifloxacin: comparison of different mucoadhesive polymers. Drug Discov Ther 4(6):423–434

Goyal R, Macri LK, Kaplan HM, Kohn J (2016) Nanoparticles and nanofibers for topical drug delivery. J Control Release 240:77–92. https://doi.org/10.1016/j.jconrel.2015.10.049

Guidelines for Glaucoma, Japan Glaucoma Society, 2nd edn. Tokyo, Japan, September 2006, pp 13–18

Gupta H, Aqil M, Khar RK, Ali A, Bhatnagar A, Mittal G (2011) Biodegradable levofloxacine nanoparticles for sustained ocular drug delivery. J Drug Target 19:409–417. https://doi.org/10.3109/1061186X.2010.504268

Hashim Abu II, El-dahan MS, Yusif RM, Abd-Elgawad AE, Arima H (2014) Potential use of niosomal hydrogel as an ocular delivery system for atenolol. Biol Pharm Bull 37:541–551. https://doi.org/10.1248/bpb.b13-00724

Hassan DH, Abdelmonem R, Abdellatif MM (2018) Formulation and characterization of carvedilol leciplex for glaucoma treatment: in-vitro, ex-vivo and in-vivo study. Pharmaceutics 10:197–205. https://doi.org/10.3390/pharmaceutics10040197

Hsiao MH, Chiou SH, Larsson M, Hung KH, Wang YL, Liu CJL, Liu DM (2014) A temperature-induced and shear-reversible assembly of latanoprost-loaded amphiphilic chitosan colloids: characterization and in vivo glaucoma treatment. Acta Biomater 10:3188–3196. https://doi.org/10.1016/j.actbio.2014.03.016

Huang J, Peng T, Li Y, Zhan Z, Zeng Y, Huang Y, Pan X, Wu CY, Wu C (2017) Ocular cubosome drug delivery system for timolol maleate: preparation, characterization, cytotoxicity, ex vivo, and in vivo evaluation. AAPS PharmSciTech:1–8. https://doi.org/10.1208/s12249-017-0763-8

Hughes P, Viejo A, Chang-Lin JE, Welty DF, Ranch F (2006) Methods for treating ocular conditions with cyclic lipid containing microparticles. US 2006/0182781 A1

Hughes PM, Viejo A, Boix M, Sarrazin C, Do M (2011) Oil-in-oil emulsified polymeric implants containing a hypotensive lipid and related methods. US 7,993,634 B2

Hui ZH, Hua LQ, Jun YZ, San PW, Fang NS (2011) Novel ophthalmic timolol maleate liposomal-hydrogel and its improved local glaucomatous therapeutic effect in vivo. J Drug Deliv 18:502–510. https://doi.org/10.3109/10717544.2011.595839

Ibrahim MM, Jablonski MM (2019) The impact of R-801 nanoparticles as a long acting topical Glaucoma therapy. J Biomed Nanotechnol 15(9):1968–1981. https://doi.org/10.1166/jbn.2019.2817

Ibrahim MM, Abd-Elgawad AE, Soliman OA, Jablonski MM (2013) Novel topical ophthalmic formulations for management of glaucoma. Pharm Res 30:2818–2831. https://doi.org/10.1007/s11095-013-1109-1

Iwase A, Suzuki Y, Araie M, Shirato S, Kuwayama Y, Mishima HK et al (2004) Tajimi Study Group, Japan Glaucoma Society: the prevalence of primary openangle glaucoma in Japanese. The Tajimi Study. Ophthalmology 111:1641–1648

Katiyar S, Pandit J, Mondal RS, Mishra AK, Chuttani K, Aqil M, Ali A, Sultana Y (2014) In situ gelling dorzolamide loaded chitosan nanoparticles for the treatment of glaucoma. Carbohydr Polym 102:117–124. https://doi.org/10.1016/j.carbpol.2013.10.079

Kaur IP, Garg A, Singla AK, Aggarwal D (2004) Vesicular systems in ocular drug delivery: an overview. Int J Pharm 269:1–14. https://doi.org/10.1016/j.ijpharm.2003.09.016

Kitazawa Y (1996) Glaucoma clinic, 3rd edn. Kanehara Shuppan, Tokyo

Kitazawa Y, Shirato S, Araie M, Yamamoto T (2004) Glaucoma. Igaku Shoin, Tokyo

Lai JY, Hsieh AC (2012) A gelatin-g-poly(N-isopropylacrylamide) biodegradable in situ gelling delivery system for the intracameral administration of pilocarpine. Biomaterials 33:2372–2387. https://doi.org/10.1016/j.biomaterials.2011.11.085

Lavik E, Bertram J, Saluja S, Kuehn M, Kwon YH, Robinson R, Huang JJ (2011) Sustained delivery of drugs from biodegradable polymeric microparticles. US 2011/0206773 A1

Leonardi A, Bucolo C, Drago F, Salomone S, Pignatello R (2015) Cationic solid lipid nanoparticles enhance ocular hypotensive effect of melatonin in rabbit. Int J Pharm 478:180–186. https://doi.org/10.1016/j.ijpharm.2014.11.032

Li R, Jiang S, Liu D, Bi X, Wang F, Zhang Q, Xu Q (2011) A potential new therapeutic system for glaucoma: solid lipid nanoparticles containing methazolamide. J Microencapsul 28:134–141. https://doi.org/10.3109/02652048.2010.539304

Li J, Wu L, Wu W, Wang B, Wang Z, Xin H (2013) A potential carrier based on liquid crystal nanoparticles for ophthalmic delivery of pilocarpine nitrate. Int J Pharm 455:75–84. https://doi.org/10.1016/j.ijpharm.2013.07.057

Maiti S, Paul S, Mondol R, Ray S, Sa B (2011) Nanovesicular formulation of brimonidine tartrate for the management of glaucoma: in vitro and in vivo evaluation. AAPS PharmSciTech 12:1–9. https://doi.org/10.1208/s12249-011-9643-9

Meisner D, Mezei M (1995) Liposome ocular delivery systems. Adv Drug Deliv Rev 16:75–93. https://doi.org/10.1016/0169-409X(95)00016-Z

Mittal N, Kaur G (2019) Investigations on polymeric nanoparticles for ocular delivery. Adv Polym Technol:1–14. https://doi.org/10.1155/2019/1316249

Musumeci T, Bucolo C, Carbone C, Pignatello R, Drago F, Puglisi G (2013) Polymeric nanoparticles augment the ocular hypotensive effect of melatonin in rabbits. Int J Pharm 440:135–140. https://doi.org/10.1016/j.ijpharm.2012.10.014

Mysore N, Sood A, Venugopalan P, Vyas SP (1996) Controlled ocular drug delivery and vesicular system: an overview. Indian Drugs 33:431–442

Nagai N, Yoshioka C, Mano Y, Tnabe W, Ito Y, Okamoto N, Shimomura Y (2015) A nanoparticle formulation of disulfiram prolongs corneal residence time of the drug and reduces intraocular pressure. Exp Eye Res 132: 115–123. https://doi.org/10.1016/j.exer.2015.01.022

Naguib SS, Hathout RM, Mansour S (2017) Optimizing novel penetration enhancing hybridized vesicles for augmenting the in-vivo effect of an anti-glaucoma drug. Drug Deliv 24:99–108. https://doi.org/10.1080/10717544.2016.1233588

Nair RV, Nair SC, Anoop KR (2015) Ocular insert of Timolol Maleate using naturally occurring biodegradable polymer. J Chem Pharm Res 7(7):476–485

Natrajan JV, Ang M, Darwitan A, Chattopadhyay S, Wong TT, Venkatraman SS (2012) Nanomedicine for glaucoma: liposomes provide sustained release of latanoprost in the eye. Int J Nanomedicine 7:123–131. https://doi.org/10.2147/IJN.S25468

Ong, Hui LC (2014) Sustained delivery of timolol maleate from liposomal nanocarriers. Final Year Project (FYP). School of Materials Science and Engineering,Nanyang Technological University, NTU Library, Nanyang Avenue, Singapore

Ong FS, Kuo JZ, Wu WC, Cheng CY, Blackwell WLB, Taylor BL, Grody WW, Rotter JI, Lai CC, Wong TY (2013) Personalized medicine in ophthalmology: from pharmacogenetic biomarkers to therapeutic and dosage optimization. J Pers Med 3:40–69. https://doi.org/10.3390/jpm3010040

Park CG, Kim KY, Kim MJ, Park M, Kim MH, Lee SH, Choi SY, Lee WS, Chung YJ, Jung YE, Park KH, Choy YB (2015) Mucoadhesive microparticles with a nanostructured surface for enhanced bioavailability of glaucoma drug. J Control Release 220:180–188. https://doi.org/10.1016/j.jconrel.2015.10.027

Robinson MR, Liu H, Hughes PM, Spada LT, Ghebremeskel AN (2010) Prostaglandin and prostamide drug delivery systems and intraocular therapeutic uses thereof. US 2010/0104654 A1

Sah AK, Suresh PK (2017) Medical management of glaucoma: focus on ophthalmologic drug delivery systems of timolol maleate. Artif Cells Nanomed Biotechnol 45:448–459. https://doi.org/10.3109/21691401.2016.1160917

Sah AK, Suresh PK, Verma VK (2017) PLGA nanoparticles for ocular delivery of loteprednol etabonate: a corneal penetration study. Artif Cells Nanomed Biotechnol 45:1156–1164. https://doi.org/10.1080/21691401.2016.1203794

Sah AK, Vyas A, Suresh PK, Gidwani B (2018) Application of nanocarrier-based drug delivery system in treatment of oral cancer. Artif Cells Nanomed Biotechnol 46:650–657. https://doi.org/10.1080/21691401.2017.1373284

Salama HA, Ghorab M, Mahmoud AA, Abdel Hady M (2017) PLGA nanoparticles as subconjunctival injection for management of glaucoma. AAPS PharmSciTech 18:2517–2528. https://doi.org/10.1208/s12249-017-0710-8

Salamouni NSE, Farid RM, Kamel AHE, Gamal SSE (2018) Nanostructured lipid carriers for intraocular brimonidine localisation: development, in-vitro and in-vivo evaluation. J Microencapsul 35:102–113. https://doi.org/10.1080/02652048.2018.1425753

Shinde U, Ahmed MH, Singh K (2013) Development of dorzolamide loaded 6-O-carboxymethyl chitosan nanoparticles for open angle glaucoma. J Drug Deliv 2013:562727. https://doi.org/10.1155/2013/562727

Shokry M, Hathout MR, Mansour S (2018) Exploring gelatin nanoparticles as novel nanocarriers for Timolol Maleate: augmented in-vivo efficacy and safe histological profile. Int J Pharm 545:229–239. https://doi.org/10.1016/j.ijpharm.2018.04.059

Shrivastava N, Khan S, Baboota S, Ali J (2018) Fabrication and characterization of timolol maleate and brinzolamide loaded nanostructured lipid carrier system for ocular drug delivery. Curr Drug Deliv 15:829–839. https://doi.org/10.2174/1566523218666171129205626

Siafaka PI, Titopoulou A, Koukaras EN, Kostoglou M, Koutris E, Karavas E, Bikiaris DN (2015) Chitosan derivatives as effective nanocarriers for ocular release of timolol drug. Int J Pharm 495:249–264. https://doi.org/10.3390/molecules23092107

Stevanovic M, Uskokovic D (2009) Poly (lactide-co-glycolide)-based micro and nanoparticles for the controlled drug delivery of vitamins. Curr Nanosci 5:1–14. https://doi.org/10.2174/157341309787314566

Suresh PK, Sah AK (2014) Nanocarriers for ocular delivery for possible benefits in the treatment of anterior uveitis: focus on current paradigms and future directions. Expert Opin Drug Deliv 11:1747–1768. https://doi.org/10.1517/17425247.2014.938045

Tan G, Yu S, Pan H, Li J, Liu D, Yuan K, Yang X, Pan W (2017) Bioadhesive chitosan-loaded liposomes: a more efficient and higher permeable ocular delivery platform for timolol maleate. Int J Biol Macromol 94:355–363. https://doi.org/10.1016/j.ijbiomac.2016.10.035

Tham YC, Li X, Wong TY, Quigley HA, Aung T, Cheng CY (2014) Global prevalence of glaucoma and projections of glaucoma burden through 2040: a systematic review and meta-analysis. Ophthalmology 121:2081–2090. https://doi.org/10.1016/j.ophtha.2014.05.013

Venkatraman S, Boey Chiang Y, Boey F, Natarajan JV (2016). Sustained timolol maleate delivery from liposomes for glaucoma therapy and ocular hypertension. WO 2016048242 A1

Wadhwa S, Paliwal R, Paliwal SR, Vyas SP (2010) Hyaluronic acid modified chitosan nanoparticles for effective management of glaucoma: development, characterization, and evaluation. J Drug Target 18:292–302. https://doi.org/10.3109/10611860903450023

Warsi MH, Anwar M, Garg V, Jain GK, Talegaonkar S, Ahmad FJ, Khar RK (2014) Dorzolamide-loaded PLGA/vitamin E TPGS nanoparticles for glaucoma therapy: pharmacoscintigraphy study and evaluation of extended ocular hypotensive effect in rabbits. Colloids Surf B: Biointerfaces 122:423–431. https://doi.org/10.1016/j.colsurfb.2014.07.004

Wenger Y, Schneider RJ, Reddy GR, Kopelman R, Jolliet O, Philbert MA (2011) Tissue distribution and pharmacokinetics of stable plyacrylamide nanoparticles following intravenous injection in the rat. Toxicol Appl Pharmacol 251(3):181–190. https://doi.org/10.1061/j.taap.2010.11.017

Wong V, Park M, Peng L, Jose S (2002) Composition and method for treating glaucoma. US 6,369,116 B1

Yang H, Tyagi P, Kadam RS, Holden CA, Kompella UB (2012) Hybrid dendrimer hydrogel/PLGA nanoparticle platform sustains drug delivery for one week and antiglaucoma effects for four days following one-time topical administration. ACS Nano 6:7595–7606. https://doi.org/10.1021/nn301873v

Zhao L, Seth A, Wibowo N, Zhao CX, Mitter N, Yu C, Middelberg AP (2014) Nanoparticle vaccines. Vaccine 32:327–337. https://doi.org/10.1016/j.vaccine.2013.11.069

Zhou Y, Fang A, Wang F, Li H, Jin Q, Huang L, Fu C, Zeng J, Jin Z, Song X (2019) Core-shell lipid-polymer nanoparticles as a promising ocular drug delivery system to treat glaucoma. Chin Chem Lett. https://doi.org/10.1016/j.cclet.2019.04.048

Zimmer AK, Kreuter J, Robinson JR (1991) Studies on the transport pathway of PBCA NPs in ocular tissues. J Microencapsul 8:497–504. https://doi.org/10.3109/02652049109021873

11 Point-of-Care Nanoplatforms for Glaucoma and Age-Related Macular Degeneration: Clinical Implications and Emerging Concepts

Honey Goel, Richu Singla, and Ashok K. Tiwary

Abstract

This chapter focuses on current updates in the development of nanotechnology-based systems for the therapy of ocular disease. The aim of this chapter is to provide the perspective of nanotechnology and existing challenges in conditions of glaucoma and age-related macular degeneration (AMD) with deeper insights into clinical aspects and pathophysiological mechanisms. Topical drug delivery has been quite challenging for the ocular conditions especially in wet AMD, which mostly require intravitreal injections owing to the tear layer and the anatomy of the ocular surface. Sustained ocular therapies to both anterior and posterior segments of the eye have been made possible only with the significant contribution of nanotechnology. Nanotechnology-driven platforms (nanoscale formulations and smart coatings) offer just a minute fraction of nanotech's potential by plummeting the requirement for intravitreal injections and may lead to hassle-free therapeutic management of ophthalmic conditions like glaucoma and AMD. The intent behind this compilation of literature was to warrant the advances in basic and clinical research in ophthalmology, which may foster better understanding of the disease physiology by providing the impetus for better design and development of dosage froms for intractable ocular diseases such as glaucoma and AMD. Therefore, a comprehensive analysis of the impact of nanomedicine in pathological conditions like glaucoma and AMD has been undertaken in the present study to ensure better disease prevention, new diagnostic procedures, and novel drug treatments whose final endpoint may be preclinical or clinical testing.

Keywords

Glaucoma · Age-related wet macular degeneration (AMD) · Nanotechnology · Ocular drug delivery · Intraocular pressure (IOP)

H. Goel (✉)
University Institute of Pharmaceutical Sciences and Research, Baba Farid University of Health Sciences, Faridkot, India

R. Singla
Department of Microbiology, Viral Research Diagnostic Laboratory (VRDL), Guru Gobind Singh Medical College and Hospital, Baba Farid University of Health Sciences, Faridkot, India

A. K. Tiwary
Department of Pharmaceutical Sciences and Drug Research, Punjabi University, Patiala, India

S. Talegaonkar, M. Rai (eds.), *Nanoformulations in Human Health*,
https://doi.org/10.1007/978-3-030-41858-8_11

11.1 The Nano-State: Impact of Nanomedicine on Ocular Drug Delivery

It is no wonder these days why the "small" matters in pharmaceutical science. With the advent of nanotechnology, the fabrication of nanosystems has emerged as an effective tool to overcome the obstacles in the therapeutic management of ocular diseases and has reshaped the science of ophthalmology. The application of emerging nanotechnological strategies and nanoscience methods has been increasingly adopted for the management of ocular diseases by improving the drug delivery design (bioadhesive enhancement, sustainable release, stealth function, specifically targeted delivery, and stimuli-responsive release) and targeted approaches to both anterior and posterior segments of the eye (Weng et al. 2017). Nanotechnology-driven systems have the ability to deliver both ocular drugs (imagine prescribing eye drops to treat wet AMD) and delivering genes to the retina (in patients with retinitis pigmentosa) or eye tissue via corneal absorption, periocular injection, and intravitreal injection, for ocular disease therapy and diagnosis.

Advances have been carried out for encapsulating conventional drugs in order to broaden the treatment spectrum in ocular clinical settings by increasing bioavailability, decreasing toxicity, and better tissue adherence of the nanocarriers. Further, it is a well-debated argument that the majority of the preclinical studies in the ocular segment are highly focused on the drug targeting and therapeutic efficacy; however, it is warranted that more impetus should be laid on the biodistribution and fate of the nanocarriers as well as clearance from the ocular tissues.

11.2 Challenges in the Ocular Drug Delivery

Despite the enormous insufficiencies, the mainstay option of ocular therapy is a topical application on the ocular surface, which accounts for >90% of ophthalmic preparations in the global markets. Figure 11.1 highlights the anatomy of the eye, its protective mechanisms, and elimination processes such as tear turnover, nasolacrimal drainage, protein binding, systemic absorption, enzymatic degradation, and complex ocular barriers (corneal barrier, blood–aqueous barrier, and blood–retinal barrier) which pose major obstacles for the ineffective ocular drug delivery.

Further, the administration of any dosage form via topical mode occurs through anatomical (corneal or non-corneal routes) and physiological barriers (such as tear film). The cornea is a very tightly multilayered tissue in which corneal epithelium acts as a principal barrier due to the formation of high paracellular resistance by tight junctions. However, the other layers of the cornea (such as Bowman's membrane, stroma, Descemet's membrane, and endothelium) are more permeable to hydrophilic molecules (Sridhar 2018). Non-corneal route circumvents the cornea and encompasses movement across layers—conjunctiva and sclera, which are more suited for the permeation of large hydrophilic molecules (as these layers exhibit low expression of tight junction proteins with respect to corneal epithelium).

Furthermore, topical delivery to cornea becomes herculean task when it influences another physiological barrier, i.e., aqueous layer of the tear film, which rapidly washes away anything in an aqueous formulation, whereas mucus layer with sticky molecules (glycosylated mucins) arrests any foreign particles or pathogens progressing toward cornea, binds them, and prepares for its removal (Hodges and Dartt 2013). In the same way, the blood ocular barrier prevents systemically administered drugs from effective penetration. Further, topical application to the retina is totally ineffective; however, scientists have experimented with alternate modes of drug delivery that can overcome anatomical and physiological barriers presented by conventional routes. These include injections (such as intravitreal (commonly used in wet AMD) subconjunctival, retrobulbar and peribulbar, sub-tendon, and intracameral) through visible portions of the sclera targeting various sections of ocular structures by a trained specialist (Kwatra and Mitra 2013; Mandal et al. 2018).

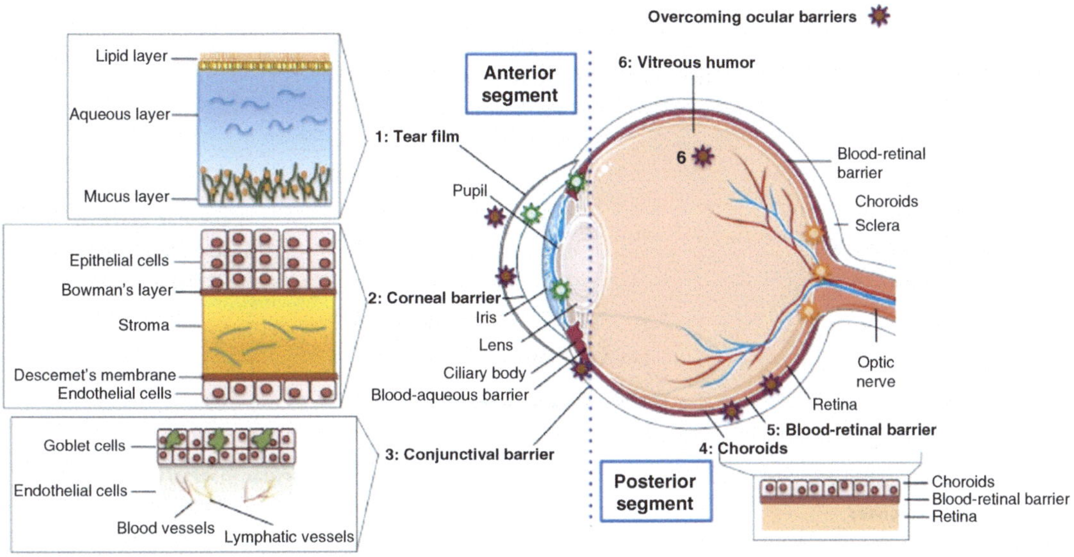

Fig. 11.1 Eye anatomy and various protective mechanisms, elimination processes, and ocular barriers. (Reproduced in original from with licenced permission from Elsevier)

Recently in 2019, Ozkan and Willcox elucidated the significant immunomodulatory role of ocular surface microbiota (low diversity microbiome) and its compositional changes in various ocular surface disorders such as blepharitis, trachoma, and dry eye. The study also revealed the role of the ocular and non-ocular microbiome in retinal diseases including AMD, glaucoma, uveitis, and diabetic retinopathy (Ozkan and Willcox 2019). Therefore, the key challenges of conventional drug delivery systems comprise of multiple drug administrations, dependency on caregivers for drug administration especially in pediatrics and geriatrics, patient-dependent dose precision, physiological barriers, poor bioavailability due to low corneal permeability, and drugs with shorter half-lives. Further, these challenges (such as the role of ocular microbiome in eye homeostasis) and requirements vary tremendously for the anterior and posterior ocular segments.

Nanotechnological approaches have provided a platform, not only to encase the existing drugs employing nanocarriers, they have also given a huge impetus in the efficient delivery of the next generation of medicine especially in ocular diseases. Nanosystems such as nanoparticles, nanocrystals, nanodiamonds, liposomes, dendrimers, nanoemulsions, and nanodevices (including nanoparticle composed contact lenses) have been developed to provide better tissue adherence, targeted drug release, noninvasive routes of administration with high patient compliance, higher solubility and bioavailability profiles, controlled rate of drug delivery, longer shelf life and duration of action, biocompatibility, biodegradability, stability, and minimal tissue toxicity as depicted in Fig. 11.2.

Hence, it can be postulated that nanoparticle based topical systems (eye drops/solutions) shall be able to penetrate through protective mucins in the tear film, into ocular surface tissue, via cornea into the anterior chamber. These systems also possess capacity of gene delivery and delivery of therapeutically active biomolecules to the posterior segment with enhanced residence time. Moreover, significant progress has been made in the field of nanomedicine to improve the efficiency of antiglaucoma medications. Nanofabrication systems such as microelectromechanical systems have overcome the limitations of nanodevices and tissue regeneration vesicles for developing glaucoma treatments independent of intraocular pressure (IOP) management based approaches (Cetinel and Montemagno 2016). The first commercial oph-

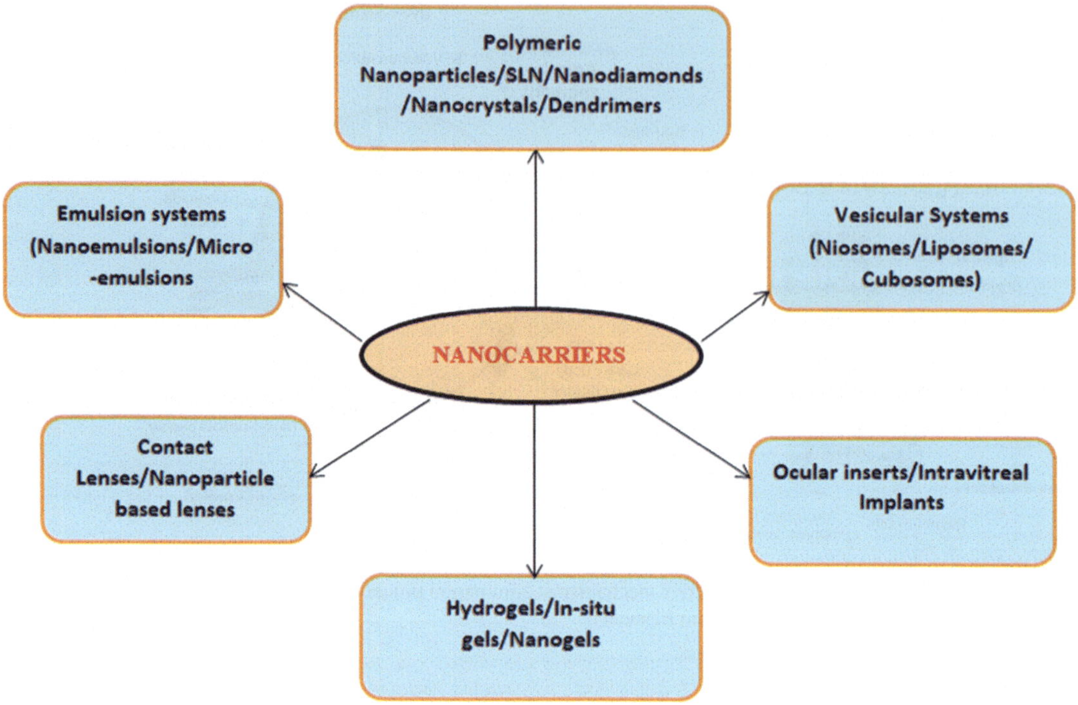

Fig. 11.2 Various novel nanocarriers for ocular drug delivery

thalmic preservative-free anionic nanoemulsion (trade name—Restasis® containing 0.05% cyclosporin A) was developed in early 2000 and approved by US FDA in 2002 for a dry eye condition. Another topical nanoemulsion was marketed as Cyclokat® based on Novasorb® technology by Santen Pharmaceutical Co. Ltd. Further, a drug delivery ophthalmic platform named "*Durasite*" based on biodegradable polymer polycarbophil has also been commercialized for the condition bacterial conjunctivitis (pink eye). Since then numerous nanotechnologies and drug delivery platforms for ocular conditions related to anterior and posterior eye have been successfully marketed.

11.3 Emerging Ocular Manifestations Related to Anterior Segment of the Eye

Disorders of the anterior segment of the eye are the leading causes of ocular morbidity. Such conditions include dry eye conditions, infections, and traumas of various types, inflammatory reactions, hereditary disorders, and cataracts. The conventional drugs and formulations which are fabricated for the major diseases related to anterior chamber (i.e., dry eye, keratitis, conjunctivitis, and cataract) primarily suffer from poor bioavailability because of corneal barrier and precorneal factors. Studies have revealed that conventional systems such as eye drops may cause damage to the corneal surface, film instability, and inflammation (Chung et al. 2016). Figure 11.3 illustrates the major disease burden to both the segments of the eye.

11.4 Emerging Ocular Manifestations Related to the Posterior Segment of the Eye

In contrast to diseases of the anterior eye, diseases related to posterior segment occur most commonly in the retina and choroid.

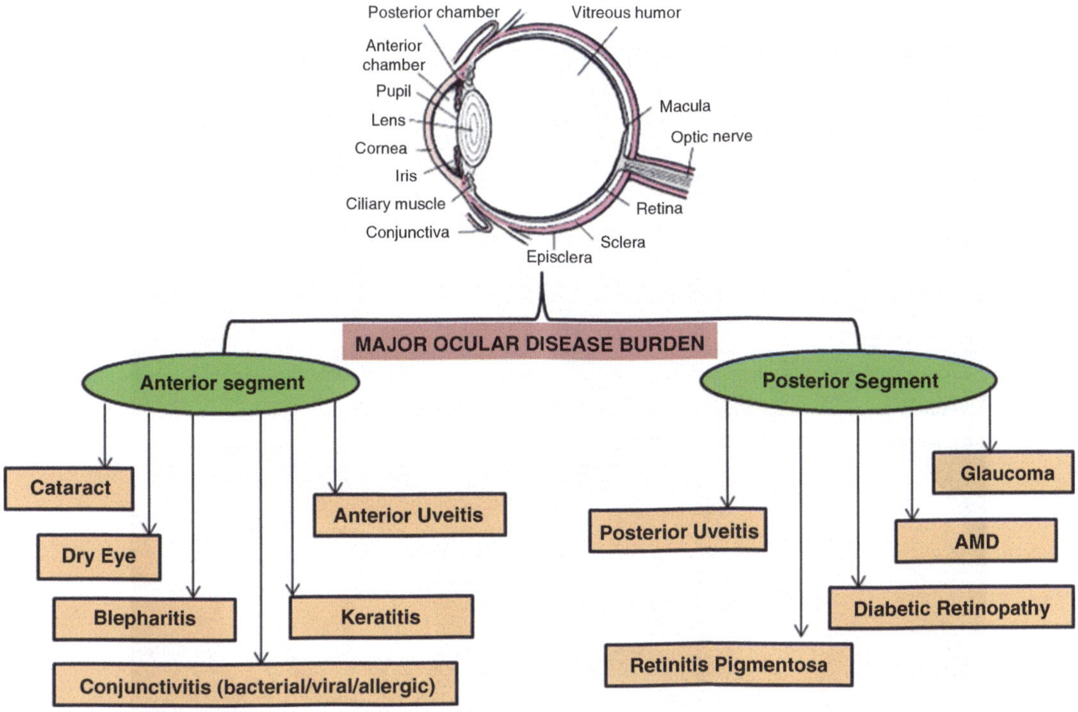

Fig. 11.3 Major disease burden to both segments of the eye

11.4.1 Glaucoma

11.4.1.1 History and Prevalence

The use of the term "glaucoma" (*glaukos* means bluish gray) first featured in Aphorisms of Hippocrates (460–375 BC) primarily due to characteristic color assumed by the anterior segment of the eye and not due to depiction of any disease form. The term was largely misinterpreted with cataract until the characteristic features of the disease appeared in the first English book of ophthalmology by Richard Banister.

As far as prevalence is concerned, glaucoma is the second leading cause of irreversible vision loss worldwide. According to the World Health Organization (WHO) statistics, it is responsible for blindness to >12% of patients (approx. 4.5 million cases) globally. Further, the projections indicate that approximately 79.6 million people will be affected by glaucoma by 2020 (Tham et al. 2014). Some of the potential risk factors which may lead to glaucoma are as follows:

- Age > 40 years
- African, Hispanic, or Asian heritage
- Family history of glaucoma
- Myopic/poor vision
- Diabetes, migraines, high blood pressure, and poor blood circulation
- High eye pressure
- Chronic use of steroids
- Injury/trauma to the eye
- Corneas that are thin in the center
- Thinning of the optic nerve

11.4.1.2 Pathobiogenesis and Mechanism

This multifactorial disorder is primarily a group of optic neuropathies characterized by progressive degeneration of retinal ganglion cells (central nervous system (CNS) neurons having their cell bodies in the inner retina and axons in the optic nerve). The pathological progression of the disease in the inner retina is indicated by degeneration of the optic nerve head termed as "*cup-*

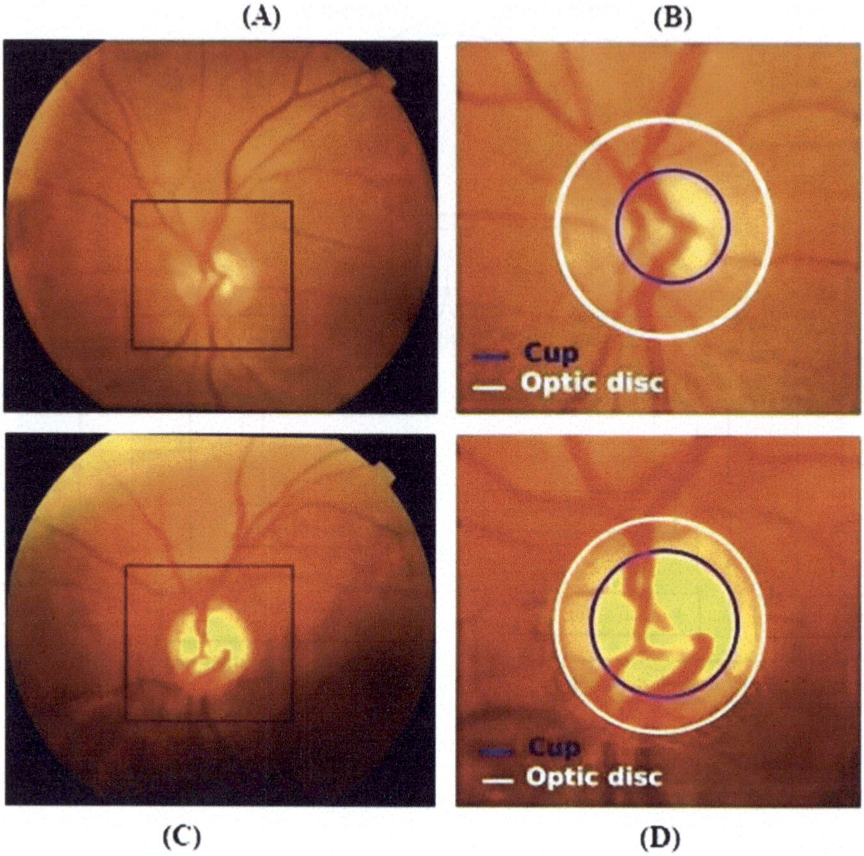

Fig. 11.4 Schematic illustration of regions: (**a**) healthy retina, (**b**) normal optic disc regions of retina, (**c**) glaucomatous retina, and (**d**) optic disc and optic cup regions of retina with neurodegenerative changes associated in glaucoma and relatively high CDR. (Reused in original form with licenced permission from Elsevier)

ping of optic disc" (neuroretinal rim thinning, and sectoral retinal nerve fiber layer thinning) (Chang and Goldberg 2012; Lee et al. 2019). Figure 11.4 depicts the schematic view of healthy state of retina (Fig. 11.4a) along with normal optic cup and disc regions of retina (Fig. 11.4b) in comparison to glaucomatous retina (Fig. 11.4c) along with neurodegenerative disease progression possessing relative high cup/disc ratio (CDR) (Fig. 11.4d). This neurodegenerative progression transpires owing to abnormally high IOP, ocular blood flow, oxidative stress, decreased axoplasmic flow, and genetic predisposition which may be asymptomatic in the earlier stages (a primary reason for the frequently delayed diagnosis) (Weinreb et al. 2014). However, during the late stages of the disease, progressions of neuronal loss include the lateral geniculate nucleus and the visual cortex. Figure 11.5 summarizes the cascade of the events involved in the pathobiogenesis of glaucoma and the management strategies (based on IOP-dependent and non-IOP-dependent approaches) to resolve the ocular condition. The normal range of IOP is 2–22 mm Hg, whereas eye pressure of greater than 22 mm Hg is considered higher than normal. When the IOP is greater than 22 mm Hg without any symptom, the condition is termed as state of ocular hypertension, and the person with high IOP is referred to as "*glaucoma suspect*". This term may also be used in case of suspicious optic nerve or with strong family history of glaucoma.

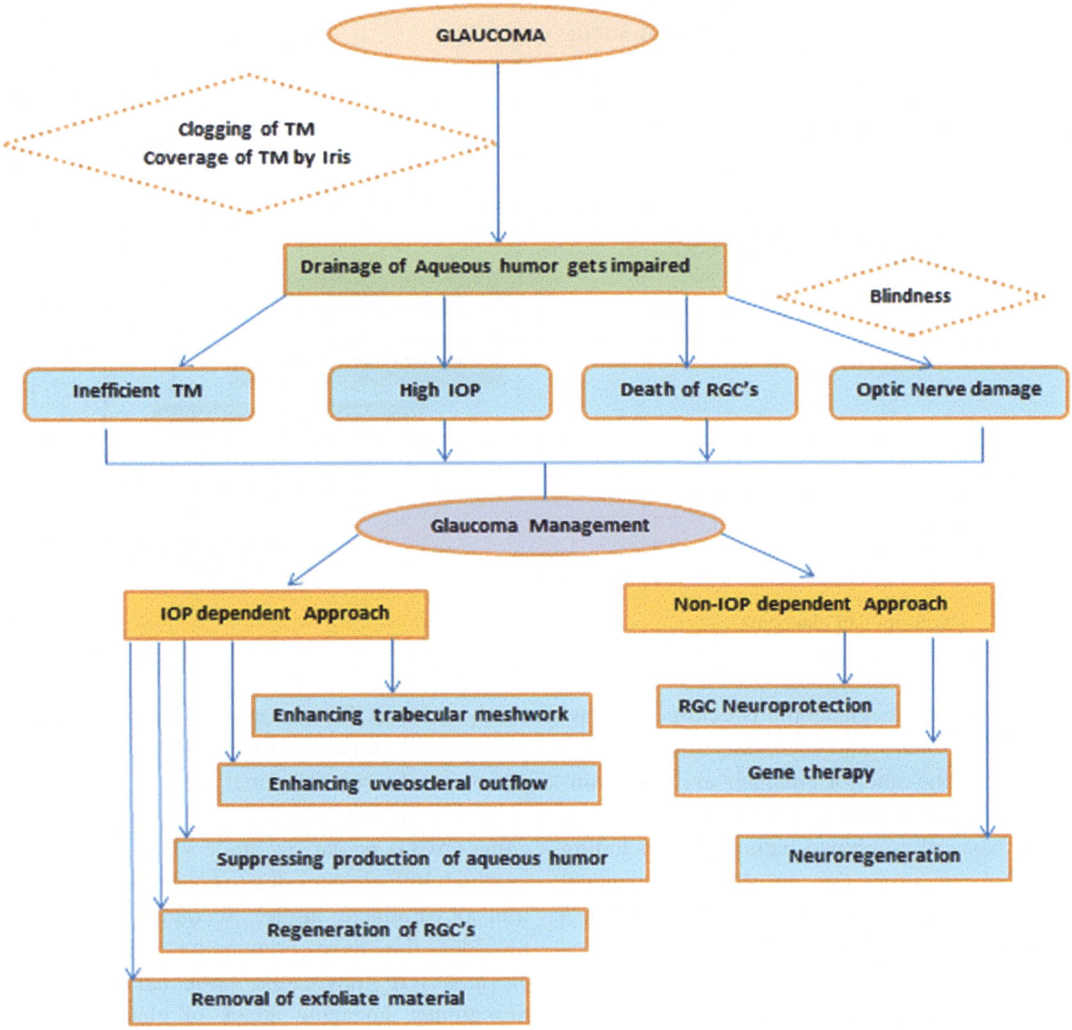

Fig. 11.5 Schematic representation of pathogenesis and management of glaucoma

The vertical cup/disc ratio (CDR) for normal individuals is 0.3 which is used for the assessment of the glaucoma suspect, as cup size is related physiologically to disc size and pathologically to glaucomatous damage. Further, IOP compensation is also highly indispensable for maintaining the physiological homeostasis of the eye. A significant quantitative relationship for IOP determination is

$$IOP = F / C + PV$$

(where F denotes for aqueous fluid formation rate, C is outflow rate, and PV is episcleral venous pressure). Although the elevated IOP is one of the prime causes for glaucoma, however, it is not the only contributory factor for glaucoma. Further, exfoliation syndrome also causes glaucoma due to defects in the microfibrils, which alter the biomechanical properties of surrounding tissue and affect the signaling. The biological mechanism of glaucoma has not been still fully elucidated, and several key factors (such as mechanical compression, ischemia, oxidative stress, neurotrophic growth factor deprivation, intracellular calcium toxicity, activation of autoimmunity, and glutamate neurotoxicity) play a significant role in its progression, which are yet under investigation (Tian et al. 2015).

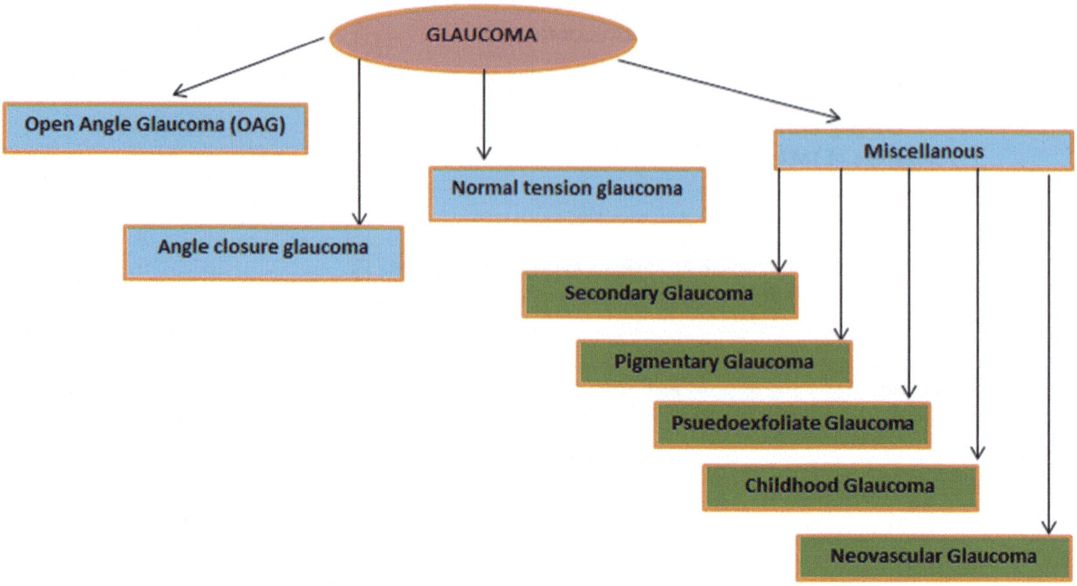

Fig. 11.6 Classification of glaucoma

In the literature, glaucoma is commonly classified into primary and secondary based on the anatomy of the anterior chamber and the drainage pathway (open and narrow angles). However, on the basis of combined pathologies including comorbid conditions (i.e., infection, mechanical injury, or neovascularization that often affect a single eye alone), it may be best classified as shown in Fig. 11.6.

Open-angle glaucoma (OAG) or wide-angle glaucoma (WAG) is the primary form of the disease with 80% rate of incidence and occurs due to inadequate drainage in front of the eye. Figure 11.7 represents the anatomical representation of primary OAG, which is characterized by the abnormal elevated IOP levels transmitted from anterior segment to posterior segment of globe containing retina and optical disc (where retinal ganglion cells (RGCs) and axons reside) (Fig 11.7a). In aqueous outflow pathways, the entrance to the drainage canals remains clear, but congestion occurs inside the drainage canals (the drain space between iris and cornea becomes too narrow), which results in aqueous humor accumulation leading to abnormal IOP (Fig 11.7b). Thus, the occurrence of primary OAG is primarily characterized by elevated IOPs or significantly low IOPs (known as normal-tension glaucoma, which affects 40% of glaucoma patients and results in visual loss).

The secondary type is angle-closure glaucoma (ACG) or narrow-angle glaucoma (NAG) in which IOP elevates due to coverage or congestion of drainage angle. Secondary glaucoma provides the most convincing evidence that elevated IOP may cause optic nerve damage. Sometimes, an acute attack of glaucoma may occur having any of such symptoms such as blurredness, eye pain, headache, nausea, and vomiting.

The causative factors for the congestion of drainage angle could be trauma, certain medications such as corticosteroids, inflammation, tumor, or conditions such as pigment dispersion or pseudo-exfoliation.

11.4.2 Conventional Therapies (IOP-Dependent Approaches)

Among the non-invasive applications, topical administration of eye drops, eye lotions, and solutions is still widely preferred to maintain the aqueous humor production, IOP, facilitate tra-

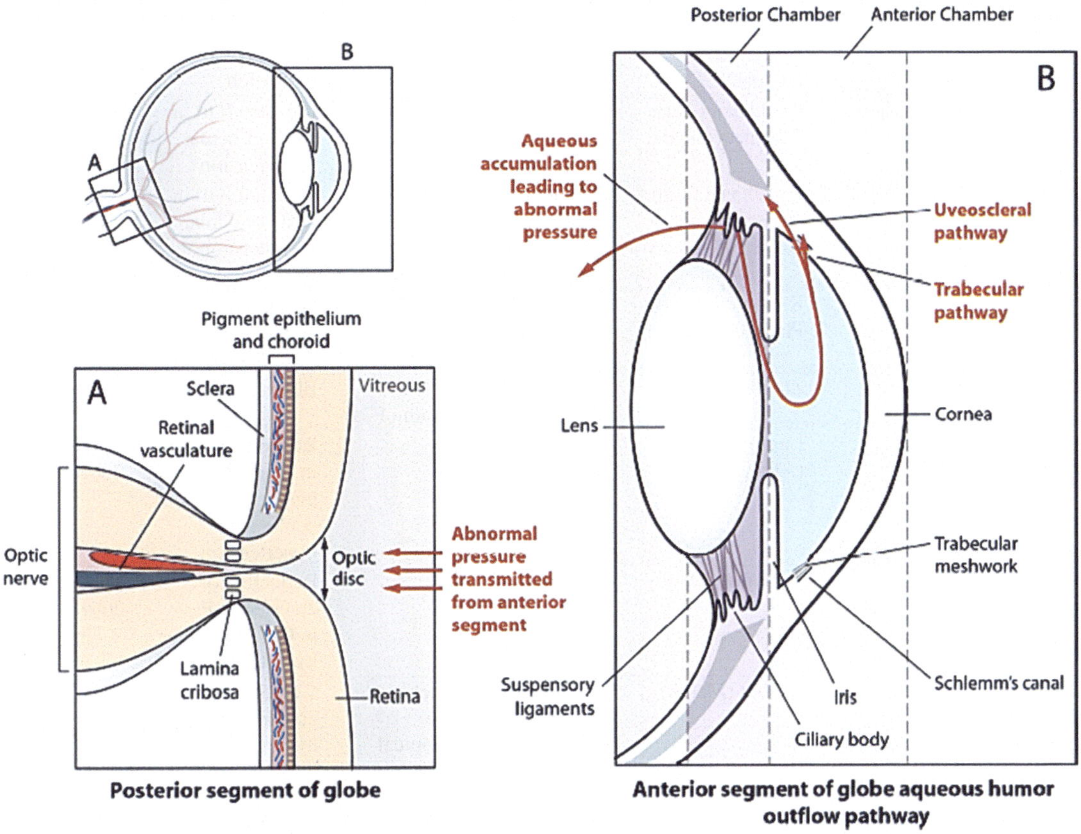

Fig. 11.7 Schematic anatomical representation of primary form of open-angle glaucoma: (**a**) abnormal elevated IOP levels transmitted from anterior segment to posterior segment of globe containing retina and optical disc; (**b**) aqueous outflow pathways from anterior segment. (Reused in original form with licenced permission from Elsevier)

becular meshwork (TM), and enhance uveoscleral outflow. Table 11.1 summarizes the top-listed (based on IOP-dependent approaches involving maintenance of IOP) ocular products approved by US FDA during the last decade in chronological order, which is currently under clinical use for glaucoma treatment.

To date, there are numerous drugs that control IOP, which are most commonly used as a topical solution applied to the eye (eye drops)—a convenient noninvasive method of administration. These topical drugs (which primarily act to decrease the production of aqueous humor and facilitate drainage through the TM, increasing uveoscleral outflow) majorly belong to five categories: β-blockers, carbonic anhydrase inhibitors, prostaglandin analogs, sympathomimetic drugs, and parasympathomimetic drugs as shown in Table 11.2.

In addition, some fixed combination therapies have also been approved by US FDA for effective IOP control when the patient does not respond to one pure form of medication. Some of the fixed combination therapies for glaucoma mainly include prostaglandin analogs/β-blockers, carbonic anhydrase inhibitors/β-blockers, and α2-adrenergic agonists/β-blockers and carbonic anhydrase inhibitors/α2-adrenergic agonists.

Table 11.1 Top-listed US FDA approved products for glaucoma during the last decade in chronological order

Ocular Condition	Formulation	Trade name/ company	Active agent/mechanism of action	Therapeutic indication	Approved year
Glaucoma	Eye solution (drops)	Rocklatan (Aerie Pharmaceuticals)	Netarsudil and latanoprost	Elevated IOP in OAG or ocular hypertension	March 2019
		Vyzulta (Bausch & Lomb)	Latanoprostene (nitric oxide-donating prostaglandin F2-alpha analog)	Elevated IOP in OAG or ocular hypertension	November 2017
		Rhopressa (Aerie Pharmaceuticals)	Netarsudil (Rho kinase inhibitor)	Glaucoma or ocular hypertension	December 2017
		Zioptan (Merck)	Tafluprost (fluorinated analog of prostaglandin F2a)	Elevated IOP	February 2012
		Lumigan (Allergan)	Bimatoprost	Reduction of IOP in open-angle glaucoma or ocular hypertension	March 2001
		Travatan (Alcon)	Travoprost	Reduction of elevated IOP in OAG or ocular hypertension	March 2001
		Cosopt (Merck)	Dorzolamide hydrochloride and timolol maleate (combination of a topical carbonic anhydrase inhibitor + beta-adrenergic receptor blocker)	Glaucoma or ocular hypertension	April 1998
	Ophthalmic suspension or drops	Betaxon (Alcon)	Levobetaxolol hydrochloride (beta-adrenergic antagonist)	Lowering IOP in chronic OAG or ocular hypertension	February 2000
	Ophthalmic solution	Rescula (Ciba Vision)	Unoprostone isopropyl	OAG or ocular hypertension	August 2000
	Ophthalmic Solution	Alphagan (Allergan)	Brimonidine	OAG and ocular hypertension	September 1996

11.4.3 Novel Therapies (Non-IOP-Dependent Approaches)

There is a wide acceptance among the clinicians and technologists that management of glaucoma based on IOP-dependent approaches only is not sufficient enough to provide comprehensive treatment of the disease. Thus, more attention has been focused on non-IOP-based approaches which include neuroprotectives and neurodegenerative procedures to preserve neuronal structure and function. Another view is the combination of IOP (use of IOP-lowering drugs) and non-IOP approaches (neurotrophic factors and antioxidants) simultaneously for effective management of glaucoma (Nafissi and Foldvari 2015).

11.4.3.1 Neurotrophic Factor (NTF)

With the advent of genome engineering and the profound understanding of the mechanism of neurodegenerative disorders related to ocular diseases such as glaucoma, novel gene therapies such as neurotrophic factor (NTF), cell replacement, and therapeutics have shown the potential to become the new ray of hope for the patient's nonresponsive IOP-dependent approaches.

Table 11.2 Classification of commercial proprietary drugs available in the market with historical timeline of treatment options for the management of glaucoma

Class of drugs/methods currently used in glaucoma	Timeline of drugs introduced for IOP reduction in glaucoma
Sympathomimetic drugs—Brimonidine (*Alphagan, Alphagan-p, Bimonidintartrat, Brimoratio, Glaudin*); apraclonidine (*Iopidine*); dipivefrin (*Propine*); epinephrine (*Gluacon, Epifrin*) **Parasympathomimetic drugs—**Pilocarpine (*Pilokarpin, Isopto Carpine, pilocar, Pilopine HS*); echothiophate (*Phospholine Iodide*) **Beta-blockers—**Timolol (*Optimol, Timacar Depot, Timoptol-LA, Timolol, Nyogel L.P., Timogel, Timosan, Aquanil*); levobunolol; carteolol (*Ocupress*); metipranolol (*OptiPranolol*); betatoxol (*Betoptic*); nipradilol **Carbonic anhydrase inhibitors—**Dorzolamide (*Trusopt, Arzolamid, Dorzolamid*); brinzolamide (*Azopt*); acetazolamide (*Diamox*); methazolamide (*Neptazane*) **Prostaglandin analogs—**Tafluprost (*Taflutan, Saflutan, Zioptan*); latanoprost (*Xalatan, Monoprost, Latanoprost*); bimatoprost (*Lumigan*); travoprost (*Travatan*); unoprostone isopropyl (*Rescula*) **Surgery**—Laser trabeculoplasty; iridotomy	Pilocarpine—1875 Epinephrine—1925 Diamox—1956 Timolol—1978 Pilocarpine/timolol—1992 Dorzolamide—1994 Latanoprost and brimonidine—1996 Brinzolamide and dorzolamide/timolol—1998 Bimatoprost—2000 Travoprost and latanoprost/timolol—2001 Brimonidine/timolol—2005 Bimatoprost/timolol and travoprost/timolol—2006 Tafluprost—2008 Brinzolamide/timolol—2009 Monoprost—2013 Brimonidine/brinzolamide and tafluprost/timolol—2014

Recently in August 2018, US FDA has approved an ophthalmic product (trade name–*Oxervate*®, by *Dompe*), a novel recombinant human nerve growth factor (rhNGF; structurally similar to NGF protein synthesized in the body including ocular tissues), for neurotrophic keratitis (which causes corneal scarring and vision loss).

NTF belongs to a group of proteins secreted by the central and peripheral nervous system which are critical for its role in neuroprotection during glaucoma. The various NTF's nerve growth factor (NGF) family members such as glial cell derived neurotrophic factor (GDNF), brain derived neurotrophic factor (BDNF), and cerebral dopamine neurotrophic factor (CDTF) have been the subject of comprehensive investigation and have shown experimentally immense application for the long-term effective management of glaucoma (Kimura et al. 2016).

Many investigators have vowed for the exogenous supplementation of NTF, apoptotic inhibitors, and survival factors for the regeneration of RGC in glaucoma. Targeted gene therapies for the delivery of transgenes employing viral/nonviral vectors encoding NTFs have also been studied (Pietrucha-Dutczak et al. 2018). However, direct targeting of NTFs by living cells and direct replacement of growth/survival factors, apoptosis inhibiting factors manipulated genetically ex vivo would be highly beneficial and facilitate long-term expression for sustained neuroprotection. Some authors have revealed the useful application of stem and progenitor cells expressing and secreting NTFs for neuroprotection and long-term expression in preclinical animal models of glaucoma (Johnson et al. 2011; Chamling et al. 2016).

11.4.3.2 Role of DNA Therapeutics

The management of neurodegenerative disorders such as glaucoma employing DNA vectors owing to their small sizes offers a potential substitute to the conventional plasmids for superior biosafety standards, immune and biocompatibility, and improved gene transfer in rapidly dividing cells and tissues with higher regenerative capacity (Khar et al. 2010). Therefore, the gene therapy for glaucoma requires sustained and stable expression of tightly controlled DNA vectors as most of the DNA vectors become diluted after subsequent mitosis.

11.4.3.3 RGC Survival Therapies

The progression of optic neuropathy in glaucoma is primarily characterized by loss of RGCs and typical visual field defects. Some of the other reasons for RGC death are the reduction in neurotrophic factors owing to local vascular insufficiency at optic nerve head. In some cases, if neuroprotection is overdue because of severe cell loss, RGC replacement therapy could be preferably used in such cases.

With the advent of the concept of neuroprotection, various neuroprotectives have been investigated to minimize the RGC loss and retinal damage. Guo et al. studied the topical application of CoQ10 on RGC apoptosis in vivo in a rat model. It was observed that CoQ10 (0.1%) significantly regressed the staurosporine-induced RGC apoptosis with respect to 0.05% CoQ10. The possible mechanism for this apoptosis inhibition could be potentiated by inhibition of mitochondrial depolarization, cytochrome c release, and caspase-9 activation (Guo and Cordeiro 2008). In addition to RGC survival, the role of CoQ10 has also been implicated in the IOP-lowering treatment in glaucoma. Another significant neuroprotective agent is citicoline, which promulgates the stimulation of phospholipid synthesis and phosphatidylcholine in the inner mitochondrial membranes. Various investigations have embarked on the basis of experimental evidence which confirms the neuroprotective role of citicoline. In an investigation, Matteucci et al. studied the role of citicoline in terms of apoptosis and caspase activation in retinal cultures (extracted from rat embryos) in a concentration-dependent manner. It was observed that citicoline restricted neuronal cell damage both in glutamate-treated and high glucose-treated retinal cultures by decreasing proapoptotic effects and conflicting synapse loss (Matteucci et al. 2014). Few other investigations have also hypothesized the antiapoptotic effect of citicoline in mitochondria-dependent cell death and axon regeneration (Oshitari et al. 2002; Park et al. 2005; Schuettauf et al. 2006; Nucci et al. 2018).

11.4.3.4 Gene Therapy

Gene therapy is also another approach for neuroprotection employed to deliver protective or antiapoptotic genes for regeneration and small interference RNA (siRNA) molecules for silencing inhibitory factors in advanced stages of glaucoma (Martínez et al. 2014). Investigations have been carried out to study axon regeneration (or by blocking axonal growth-inhibitory factors such as oligodendrocyte myelin glycoproteins and myelin-associated glycoproteins) using siRNA protein system (Yang and Schnaar 2008; Schnaar and Lopez 2009).

Few approaches such as cell-based regeneration of TM tissue or whole tissue regeneration have been studied as a part of future treatment strategies. TM stem cells have been investigated in terms of their localization into TM and then further differentiated into functionalized TM cells. The replacement therapy using artificial TM tissues with improved cell attachment has also been studied in cultured human TM cells.

11.4.3.5 Role of Nanomedicine in the Management of Glaucoma

Nanotechnology-based treatments show a great deal of promise in overcoming these complications and form the basis for next-generation glaucoma treatment strategies, with the help of applications such as controlled release, targeted delivery, increased bioavailability, diffusion limitations, and biocompatibility. Although topical application in glaucoma still exhibits significant primary and adjunctive role, however, diverse novel strategies have been devised with the application of nanocarriers. During the last two decades, the prime focus of preclinical investigations involving antiglaucomatic nano-drug delivery approaches (as summarized in Table 11.3) has been to revolutionize the mode of drug administration in ocular tissues by improving the precorneal residence time (e.g., formulating sus-

Table 11.3 Summary of preclinical investigations carried out in the last two decades involving nanotechnological platforms and devices for glaucoma

Nanotechnological platform	Payload	Biomaterial	Clinical stage/Therapeutic indication	Remarks	Reference/Trial no.
Hydrogel	Mitomycin-C	Pluronic F127 loaded thermogel	Preclinical/glaucoma	Hydrogel showed good compatibility and sustained release in intraocular after glaucoma surgery	Xi et al. (2014)
	Timolol maleate (Timoptic-XE®)	Thermogel	Commercially marketed/glaucoma	Topical treatment for glaucoma	Schenker and Silver (2000)
Contact lenses	Brimonidine	(PLGA-PEG-PLGA) copolymer	Preclinical/glaucoma	Sustained drug release; relief in IOP; good biocompatibility to epithelial cells	Sun et al. (2017)
		Propoxylated glyceryl triacrylate nanoparticles in contact lens		In vivo studies (beagle dogs) with hydrogel lenses (incorporated with timolol-PGT nanoparticles) showed sustained release for one month after an initial burst and a reduction in IOP	Jung et al. (2013)
		Vitamin E-coated narafilcon A lenses		In vivo study showed over 4 days of treatment, significant reduction of IOP in dogs	Peng et al. (2012)
		Unmodified commercial vasurfilcon A, etafilcon A, and vifilcon		In vivo study showed no toxicity after 2 weeks, IOP levels decreased to similar to daily eye-drop therapy	Schultz et al. (2009)
		MAA molecularly imprinted pHEMA gels		In vitro study showed enhanced loading and pH-dependent hydrogel swelling for drug release	Alvarez-Lorenzo et al. (2002)
	Timolol and Dorzolamide	Vitamin E-coated senofilcon-A lenses		Treatment with vitamin E lenses demonstrated a prolonged IOP-lowering effect compared to eye drop	Hsu et al. (2015)
	Latanoprost	Senofilcon-A (ACUVUE®)		In vivo studies showed that drug–polymer contact lenses films provided an initial burst in the aqueous humor followed by a steady-state concentration comparable to the concentration of marketed eye drops	Ciolino et al. (2014)
	Acetazolamide and ethoxzolamide	Poly(2-hydroxyethyl methacrylate) (pHEMA)		pHEMA hydrogels loaded contact lens were highly cytocompatible, better drug release and possessed good oxygen permeability	Ribeiro et al. (2011)
	Puerarin	Poly(2-hydroxyethyl methacrylate-co-N vinylpyrrolidone-co-methyl acrylate) (pHEMA-NVP-MA)		Contact lenses extended the mean resident time of puerarin to 77.45 min from 12.88 min of 1% puerarin eye drops and exhibited similar bioavailability with puerarin eye drops in tear fluid	Xu et al. (2010)
Nano-opthalmic injection	Latanoprost	Controlled release patented liposomes (with size of 100 nm) for subconjuctival injection	Phase II/glaucoma	POLAT-001® (controlled release liposmal injection sponsored by Peregrine Ophthalmic Pvt. Ltd., Singapore) compared with latanoprost eye solution for reduction of mean IOP from 28 mm Hg to 15 mm Hg in an open labeled study on 6 patients	NCT02466399

(continued)

Table 11.3 (continued)

Nanotechnological platform	Payload	Biomaterial	Clinical stage/Therapeutic indication	Remarks	Reference/Trial no.
Nanoparticles	Curcumin	Pluronic-F127 stabilized D-α-tocopherol polyethylene glycol 1000 succinate	Preclinical/neuroprotective therapy in glaucoma	Neuroprotection against glutamate and $CoCl_2$ – induced injury in retinal cultures in vitro and significantly preserved RGC density in rodent Models of ocular injury	Davis et al. (2018)
	Brimonidine	Chitosan methylcellulose (gelling agent)	Preclinical/glaucoma	Nanoparticles incorporated gel showed sustained release and sustained IOP reduction (>25 h) compared to eye drops	Ibrahim et al. (2015)
	Dorzolamide HCl	Chitosan and sodium alginate		Nanoparticles showed sustained release and slower corneal permeation compared to commercial eye drops in rabbits	Katiyar et al. (2014)
		Poly (lactide-co-glycolide)		Enhanced corneal permeation w.r.t. Trusopt® and higher drug concentration in aqueous humor with IOP reduction	Warsi et al. (2014)
		6-O-Carboxymethyl chitosan		Showed sustained drug release, and in vivo studies revealed non-irritant particles with prolonged antiglaucoma effect	Shinde et al. (2013)
	Betaxolol HCl	Chitosan		Nanoparticles exhibited sustained release up to 12 h and significant IOP reduction reaching a peak of 9.9 ± 0.5 mmHg, compared to control after 5 h.	Jain et al. (2013)
Cationic solid lipid nanoparticles (SLNs)	Melatonin	Softisan® 100 (solid lipid) stearic acid (lipid modifier)		Showed enhanced ocular retention time, and effective in IOP reduction for 24 h	Kouchak et al. (2016)
Modified SLNs	Methazolamide	GMS (solid lipid) and lecithin		Chitosan modified SLNs exhibited prolonged in vitro release, better corneal permeation and better reduction in IOP than unmodified SLN and marketed eye drops	Yu et al. (2015)
SLNs		GMS (solid lipid) phospholipid-S100		SLNs exhibited sustained release and significant IOP reduction compared to marketed eye drops	Leonardi et al. (2015)
SLN and nanolipid carriers		GMS (solid lipid) Castor oil (liquid lipid)		Both SLNs and NLCs (after autoclaving) were non-irritant to ocular mucosa and exhibited high entrapment compared to non-autoclaved ones	Mehnert and Mäder (2001)
Cationic nanostructured lipid matrix		Compritol® 888 ATO cetostearyl alcohol stearylamine		The optimized formulation showed reduction of IOP by 8.3 mm Hg within 3 h and was maintained for 12 h	Wang et al. (2014)
Microparticles	Dorzolamide	Poly(ethylene glycol)-co-poly (sebacic acid) (PEG3-PSA) polymer	Preclinical/neuroprotective therapy in glaucoma	Dorzolamide-based formulation caused IOP reduction with significant RGC protection	Pitha et al. (2018)

Nanosheets	Latanoprost	Chitosan and sodium alginate	Preclinical/glaucoma	One day application of LP loaded NS (on cornea) significantly reduced IOP in rats (sustained effect for 7 days)	Kashiwagi et al. (2013)
Nanoliposomal carrier		Egg phosphatidylcholine		Sustained release for subconjunctival injection; successful preclinical study on rabbit and monkey	Natarajan et al. (2012) and NCT01987323
Liposomes	Pilocarpine HCl	Dipalmitoyl phosphatidylcholine		Showed reduced IOP in glaucomatous pigmented rabbits	Monem et al. (2000)
Unilamellar liposomes	Diltiazem HCl	Soyaphosphatidyl choline and cholesterol		Vesicles, rigidified using cholesterol showed high entrapment efficiency, prolonged release and high reduction in IOP activity in rabbits w.r.t solution	Mokhtar Ibrahim et al. (2014)
Small unilamellar liposomes	Brimonidine tartrate	Cholesterol DPPC (1,2 dipalmitoyl-sn-glycero-3-phosphocholine)		Liposomes showed prolonged release of drug, and IOP reducing activity in normotensive rabbits was sustained for a longer period of time than drug solution	Prabhu et al. (2010)
Large unilamellar liposomes	Latanoprost	Egg phosphatidylcholine		Exhibited sustained in vitro release for 2 weeks; subconjunctival injection of liposomes maintained a sustained IOP-lowering effect in rabbits w.r.t topical daily administration	Natarajan et al. (2012)
Liposomal gels		Phospholipon® 90G, cholesterol, and Pluronic® F127 (gelling agent)		Liposomes vesicles with enhanced entrapment efficiency were incorporated Pluronic® F127 gels for sustained drug release (~45% in 48 h) and maintained IOP reduction for 72 h w.r.t marketed eye drops	Fathalla et al. (2015)
Liposomes	Brinzolamide	Soybean phosphatidylcholine (S100), cholesterol		Liposomes showed 6.2-fold increase in the corneal permeability and sustained IOP reduction in rabbits compared to commercial suspension	Li et al. (2016)
Nanoliposomes	Dorzolamide HCl	Phospholipon 85G®· cholesterol		Liposomes showed enhanced transcorneal permeation compared to dorzolamide solution and greater IOP reduction compared to marketed eye drops	Kouchak et al. (2016)
Liposome in ion-sensitive in situ gel	Timolol maleate	Soybean phosphatidylcholine, cholesterol, and deacetylated gellan gum (gelling agent)		Liposomes in in situ gel revealed a corneal retention time superior to commercial eye drops and to liposomes and were non-irritant to ocular tissues and showed fast IOP reduction compared to eye drops	Yu et al. (2015)
Nanofiber patch	Timolol maleate Dorzolamide HCl	Polyvinyl alcohol and polycaprolactone		The patch possessed very high mucoadhesive strength and retained for a longer period in the eyes (maintained IOP for 72 h)	Gagandeep et al. (2014)
Nanofilms	Timolol maleate	Chitosan		In vivo study showed IOP reduction same commercial eye drops in rabbits	Fulgêncio Gde et al. (2012)
Nano-ocular inserts	Brimonidine tartrate	HPMC, SA, Na-CMC		Na-CMC inserts showed significant IOP lowering in normotensive rabbits. SA-based inserts showed a stable IOP-lowering effect for 5 h	Labib et al. (2013)
		PVP K-90, HPMC, Carbopol, SA, Chitosan		Ocular inserts showed superior sustained effect w.r.t plain drug solution and exhibited more IOP-lowering effect compared to its non-coated or dual-side-coated counterpart in albino rabbits	Aburahma and Mahmoud (2011)

pensions and ointments, viscous vehicles, bioadhesive vehicles, and in situ gelling systems), sustained corneal permeation (e.g., pro-drugs, penetration enhancers, ion pairs, iontophoresis, and cyclodextrins), improved tissue adherence (e.g., liposomes, emulsions, nanoparticles, and nanocapsules), ocular biocompatibility (e.g., degradable/non-degradable matrices, collagen shields, nanoparticle embedded contact lenses, drug loaded into performed lenses and membrane-controlled devices), and lowering ocular irritation with improved patient compliance (e.g., implantable devices).

11.4.4 Age-Related Macular Degeneration (AMD)

11.4.4.1 Prevalence

Age-related macular degeneration (AMD), or also known as age-related maculopathy, is one of the most prominent and commonest causes of adult blindness in industrialized nations and people age more than 50 years. Globally, AMD ranks third as a cause of blindness after cataract and glaucoma (WHO, 2019). Approximately, 11 million people in the United States have some form of AMD, and these numbers are expected to double to nearly 22 million by 2050. The statistical projections about AMD indicate that the number of people living with macular degeneration is expected to reach 196 million worldwide by 2020 and increase to 288 million by 2040 (Pennington and DeAngelis 2016).

As per the statistics of Macular Society, UK, nearly 600,000 people are affected by vision loss due to some form of AMD, and around 70,000 new cases are being reported annually (with a rate of 200 cases per day). It has been projected that by 2050, the number of AMD patients will be more than double to 1.3 million. In terms of cost, it is estimated that AMD burdens huge health costs to at least £1.6bn a year. Some of the causative factors which may lead to AMD condition are as follows:

- Obese/overweight population (or patients with high cholesterol)
- Smoking; alcohol consumption
- Age (>50 years)
- Arterial hypertension
- Cardiovascular disease or high cholesterol levels
- Light exposure (UV-A or UV-B rays)
- Low dietary intake of antioxidants, zinc
- Family history (siblings with AMD have four times more chances to get AMD than the no relatives with AMD)

11.4.4.2 The Current Line of Treatment Options

Dry AMD

During the initial phase of dry AMD (or atrophic AMD), oral vitamin supplementation (such as lutein, zeaxanthin, lycopene, or tocopherol or centrophenoxine, vitamin C, and beta carotene) and zinc are prescribed in order to ameliorate the lipofuscin accumulation and reduce the symptoms in AMD (Age-Related Eye Disease Study Research Group 2001; Birch and Liang 2007; Khoo et al. 2019). However, patients with advanced dry AMD, also called geographic atrophy (GA), have no effective treatments available to them.

Wet AMD

The pharmacological interventions for wet AMD are based on periocular or intraocular drug administration. These intravitreal injections achieve improved therapeutic concentrations at the target tissues; however, the rapid clearance of these agents is still a big challenge. Moreover, frequent intravitreal injections are not desirable due to the risk of surgery. Although some treatments to slow the progression of AMD are available, there is currently no cure for this irreversible disease. For Wet AMD, intravitreal injection of therapeutic agents (commercially available as *Eylea®, Lucentis®, or Avastin®*) that block vascular endothelial growth factor (VEGF) helps the patient to mitigate the symptoms only for 4–8 weeks; therefore, repeated therapy of these intraocular injections at monthly intervals in patients with wet AMD is required to preserve their vision. Nanotechnology can devise novel

Table 11.4 Top-listed US FDA approved products for AMD during the last decade in chronological order

Ocular condition	Formulation	Trade name/company	Active agent/ mechanism of action	Therapeutic indication	Approved year
Age-related macular degeneration (AMD)	Intravitreal injection	Eylea (Regeneron Pharmaceuticals)	Aflibercept (VEGF inhibitor)	Neovascular type AMD	November 2011
		Lucentis (Genentech)	Ranibizumab	Neovascular (wet) age-related macular degeneration	June 2006
		Macugen (Eyetech Pharmaceuticals)	Pegaptanib (Pfizer)	Wet age-related macular degeneration	December 2004
	Injection or photosensitive therapy/laser (non-thermal) therapy using red light	Visudyne (QLT Phototherapeutics)	Verteporfin	Wet AMD	April 2000
	Injection or photosensitive therapy/laser (non-thermal) therapy using red light	Visudyne (QLT Phototherapeutics)	Verteporfin	Wet AMD	April 2000

approaches to target VEGF and simultaneously can assist in reducing the injection frequency.

Other therapies such as argon laser for the photocoagulation of abnormal vessels, photodynamic therapy with verteporfin, and vitreoretinal surgery are also being employed (Lin et al. 2015). Table 11.4 summarizes the top-listed range of ophthalmic products or devices approved by US FDA for the AMD condition during the last decade.

11.4.4.3 Pathobiogenesis and Mechanism

This multifactorial disease occurs due to environmental as well as genetic factors. It involves damage to the macula (a part of retina) which causes irreversible loss of central field of vision [i.e., sharp/fine details cannot be seen at far and near distance (e.g., inability to read, drive, see color, and recognize face), or "straight head vision loss"]. The exact causes and underlying pathophysiological mechanisms for AMD are yet to be fully understood. Among several forms of AMD, it can be classified primarily into two types: dry AMD (involve 90% of cases and undergoes slow progression) and wet AMD (rarely involves only 10% of the cases and results in severe progression). It has been investigated that wet AMD affects one eye at a time, and it takes nearly more than 5 years of period to develop this condition in another eye in the majority of the wet AMD population (Birch and Liang 2007). The cascade of events and detailed mechanisms of progression of the disease have been elucidated in Fig. 11.8.

Several preclinical investigations have established the efficacy of nutraceuticals and functional foods rich in antioxidants in conjunction with anti-AMD pharmacological treatments. However, a new dimension of the role of gut microbiome in the pathophysiology of AMD has been the focus of scientific attention in recent years (Andriessen et al. 2016). The alteration of gut microbiota has been associated with various intestinal and extraintestinal disorders or inflammatory conditions (inflammatory bowel disease, colon cancer, obesity, and fatty liver disease) causing permeation of endotoxin lipopolysaccharides and pathogen-associated molecular pattern molecules, which ultimately induce low-grade

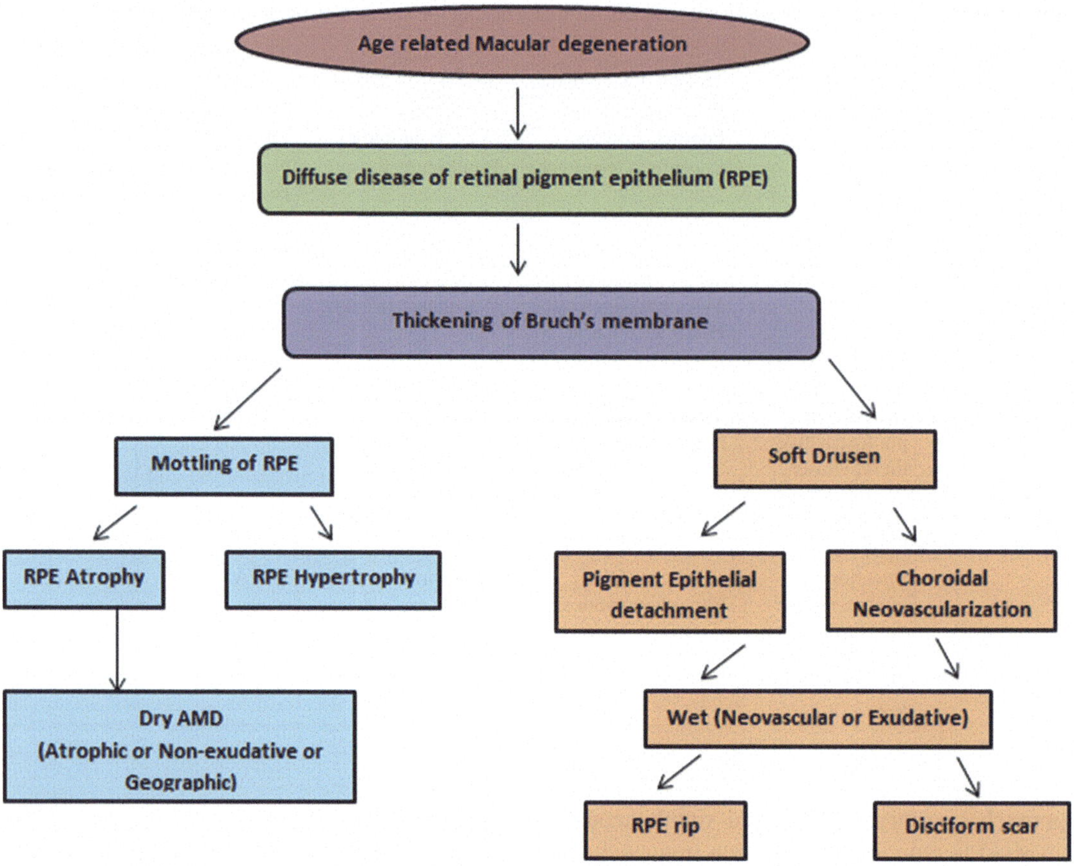

Fig. 11.8 Pathophysiology of various types of AMD

inflammation through pattern recognition receptors. Scientific reports have revealed similar links or concepts of "gut–retina axis" in the pathogenesis of ocular conditions (such as in case of RPE cells in AMD) (Rinninella et al. 2018). Further, some studies have underscored the significant immunomodulatory role of ocular and non-ocular microbiota (low diversity microbiome) and their compositional changes in various ocular and retinal disorders including AMD (Ozkan and Willcox 2019).

11.4.4.4 Dry AMD

The dry AMD (also known as atrophic or non-exudative AMD or geographic atrophy) occurs due to thinning of the macula with an accumulation of yellowish deposit, a protein 'lipofuscin' as tiny clumps within the retinal pigment epithelial (RPE) cells known as '*drusen grow*' which is a non-curable condition. The accumulation of these clumps leads to the gradual death of associated photoreceptors, and then, the patients progressively become blind. It has been found that the disease progression of dry AMD is quite slow with respect to wet AMD. Dry AMD is often difficult to diagnose in early stages. The stages of AMD are characterized by early, intermediate, and late.

The soft *drusen* of particle size <63 μm indicate early-stage characteristics and dry nature of AMD, which are the discreet, round, and slightly elevated clumps capable of causing hyperpigmentation or hypopigmentation within the RPE of the macula and fundus in the eyes. A small number of medium drusen (63–125 μm in size) also lie under the retina. However, the intermediate form of AMD is characterized by at least one large druse (>125 μm). Late form of AMD is quite threatening leading to irreversible vision loss. The overlying RPE indicates thinning, whereas RPE between *drusen* is indicative of thickening (De Jong 2018).

11.4.4.5 Wet AMD

The wet AMD (as known as neovascular or exudative AMD) is the leading cause of central vision loss due to macular edema from vascular hyperpermeability (i.e., leakage of blood and fluid under the macula) and abnormal new blood vessel growth behind the macula (Daruich et al. 2018).

Basically, the movement of the growth of new blood vessels occurs from the side of the retina and tends to grow toward the center. The newly formed blood vessels (which happen to be very fragile and tend to leak easily) initiate from the choriocapillaris (through Bruch's membrane) under or above the retinal pigment epithelium (RPE). Finally, the growth of blood vessels moves toward macula within a span of a few weeks. The abnormal blood vessel growth tends to reoccur even till years. The consequence of this growth is hemorrhage, scar formation, retinal detachment, and irreversible loss of central field of vision with 2 years from the day of its progression in most of the cases (if left untreated).

The pathophysiological mechanism of AMD involves multifactorial pathogenesis. IL-17 pathway has been reported to be involved in the AMD pathogenesis (Parmeggiani et al. 2012; Kauppinen et al. 2016). Further, studies have shown that vascular endothelial growth factor (VEGF), a protein essential in angiogenesis and vascular hyperpermeability, is highly associated with wet AMD (Pechan et al. 2014; Al-Khersan et al. 2019). Some studies have reported the identification of few genetic factors (such as the complement factor H (CFH) Y402H polymorphism) responsible for AMD (Landowski et al. 2019).

Another significant factor that plays a critical role in vascular leakage and neovascularization is the angiopoietin pathway (Ng et al. 2017; Saharinen et al. 2017). Angiopoietin-2 inhibitors such as RG7716 and nesvacumab are under the developmental phase and have been investigated for their potential role (in the angiopoietin pathway) by Genentech and Regeneron Pharmaceuticals, respectively (Hussain and Ciulla 2017). Further, AKB-9778 another molecule under investigation (Aerpio Therapeutics) activates Tie-2 an intermediate found in endothelial cells that plays a key role in the angiopoietin pathway.

Integrins are transmembrane proteins that are involved in regulating cellular adhesion, kinase signaling pathways, endothelial cell migration, apoptosis, VEGF receptor-2 activation, and vascular development, making them potential targets for wet AMD therapy. Two integrin inhibitors, *Volociximab* (Ophthotech) and *Luminate* (Allegro Ophthalmics), have demonstrated good safety in phase I trials.

Moreover, several attempts have been made to identify biomarkers; for instance, carboxyethylpyrrole and C-reactive protein have been found to be associated with the pathogenesis of AMD. Investigators while studying the proteomic characterization of drusen observed that carboxyethylpyrrole adducts were abnormally high in AMD than in normal Bruch's membrane/RPE/choroid tissues. The formation of CEP protein adducts results from docosahexaenoate containing lipids (found in abundance in ocular tissues) which are responsible for free radical-induced oxidative stress in AMD (Crabb et al. 2002). Further, elevated plasma levels of carboxyethylpyrrole adduct and C-reactive protein have been reported in AMD donors as well (Renganathan et al. 2013; Chirco and Potempa 2018).

Diagnostic Tests These techniques are employed to screen and diagnose the condition at various stages, which include the Amsler test, preferential hyperacuity perimetry, shape discrimination hyperacuity, macular mapping test, and noise-field (entoptic) perimetry (Singh et al. 2017).

11.4.4.6 Conversion from Dry to Wet AMD

The ground reality is all patients initiate with the dry form of AMD in their earlier form of disease. At present, there is no diagnostic technique or method available to predict the time and state of the disease when the dry form will get converted to wet AMD. This is primarily due to the uneven pattern of AMD, as sometimes dry AMD results in blindness without undergoing conversion into wet form. As the dry AMD undergoes slow progression, it is highly difficult for the patient and the physician to detect the initiation point and endpoint of the disease. Further, some patients suddenly turn into wet AMD and within a span of years undergo choroidal neovascularization. Therefore, the exact etiology and mechanism of conversion of dry state to wet state of AMD are fully understood; however, investigations have clearly shown that change in the pigmentation within the RPE is the prime causative or risk factor for the conversion of dry AMD into Wet AMD.

11.4.4.7 Role of Nanotechnology in AMD

With the inception of anti-VEGF aptamers in 2004 (Macugen, Pegaptanib Sodium; OSI Pharmaceuticals, NY, USA) and monoclonal antibody in 2006 (Lucentis; Ranibizumab; Genentech, California, USA), the growth of biopharmaceutical drug (protein/peptide-based therapies) market has presented spectacular evolution. It is estimated that global sales of biopharmaceutical drugs for ophthalmic indications may touch $35.7 billion by 2025.

Nanotechnology can provide a possible solution to manage the AMD by prolonged drug delivery, administration of nanoparticle-based enzyme formulation to dissolve and metabolize lipofuscin intracellularly. The nanotechnology-based targeted delivery of anti-VEGF therapies would suppress the growth factor and will assist in the recurrence of choroid neovascularization (Hussain and Ciulla 2017). Table 11.5 represents the various nanotechnological platforms for the management of AMD along with its associated conditions.

11.5 Formulation Issues and Challenges with Anti-VEGF Therapies

The major challenges associated with the intravitreal anti-VEGF therapies are the adverse effects that include infectious and non-infectious endophthalmitis, retinal detachment, and enhanced IOP.

Apart from various significant caveats associated with the intravitreal administration, sterile compounding of intravitreal injections often leads to contamination (as no prefilled syringe packing is available except ranibizumab) and, thus, results in bacterial and fungal endophthalmitis. In addition, variable concentrations of active drug and silicone oil droplets have been reported with repackaged syringes of bevacizumab from the compounding pharmacies. Further, the syringes which are often utilized to administer anti-VEGF agents are not suitably designed for intravitreal administration. Therefore, these syringes tend to release silicone droplets causing "floaters" which ultimately obstruct the patient's vision. Hence, the issues related to sterility, therapeutic efficacy, and validated packaging of the containers are still required to be addressed for better patient compliance.

11.6 Novel Agents and Therapies

Among the novel targets, VEGF is one of the most significant cellular factors determining the growth and proliferation of blood vessels. It has become the major target for wet AMD therapies such as *ranibizumab* (Lucentis®), *bevacizumab* (Avastin®), both of which target VEGF-A; *pegaptanib* (Macugen®), a selective inhibitor of VEGF165; and *aflibercept* (Eylea®), which inhibits VEGF-A, as well as placental growth factor (PGF), has become established treatments for wet AMD. *Brolucizumab*, another anti-VEGF molecule likely to get approved by FDA (Biological Licensing Application accepted in 2019), is in phase III clinical trials and can last as long as 12 weeks between treatments. *Abicipar* is another drug that is injected into the eye to target VEGF. A phase II trial shows that it can last as long as 12 weeks. Therefore, longer acting drugs can be another possibility to enhance patient compliance in wet AMD treatment. Another molecule, OPT-302, targets VEGF forms C and D, which is under phase II trials and injected in combination with a traditional VEGF inhibitor. US FDA has also approved various treatments

Table 11.5 Schematic representation of significant nanotechnological platforms used in the management of AMD and associated pathologies

Platform	Payload	Biomaterial	Function/use/target	Stage	Ref.
Carbon- dots	Hybrid aptamer nanocomposite	Bevacizumab	Hybrids showed no toxicity for both in vitro and in vivo murine animal model, and effectively inhibited VEGF-stimulated angiogenesis in choroidal blood vessels	Preclinical	Shoval et al. (2019)
Nanoparticle	Cerium oxide	Oligochitosan and alginate	The hydrogels showed control release for 2 months and suppressed inflammation response in ARPE-19 cell lines (AMD cellular models)	Preclinical	Wang et al. (2018)
	IgG-Fab antibody	Composite pentablock copolymer (PB-1: PCL-PLA-PEG-PLA-PCL)	Sustained-release nanoformulation was demonstrated as ocular platform with in vitro cell viability in mouse macrophage cell lines	Preclinical	Agrahari et al. (2016)
	Nintedanib	UV-sensitive polymer	Intravitreal administration of UV light-triggered NP release attenuated laser-induced choroidal neovascularization (CNV) in rats	Preclinical	Huu et al. (2015)
	Triamcinolone	Folate-functionalized poly(ethylene glycol)-β-polycaprolactone (PEG-β-PCL)	RPE targeting and Neovascular AMD	Preclinical	Suen and Chau (2013)
	Integrin-binding liner RGD peptide	PLGA	Restored vision function in primate and murine macular degeneration model	Preclinical	Luo et al. 2013
	Bevacizumab	PLGA/PLA	Intravitreal administration showed in a rat model of wet AMD	Preclinical	Li et al. (2012)
	anti-αvβ3 monoclonal antibody, DM101	Gold-perfluorodichlorooctane	Restored visual function in corneal neovascularization	Preclinical	Anderson et al. (2000)

(continued)

Table 11.5 (continued)

Platform	Payload	Biomaterial	Function/use/target	Stage	Ref.
Nanowafer	Axitinib	Four different polymers such as PVA, PVP, HPMC, and CMC were used	Drug loaded nanowafers successfully treated corneal neovascularization in (CNV) in a murine ocular burn model compare commercial eye drop even at a low dose range	Preclinical	Yuan et al. (2015)
Dendrimer	Gene	Hydroxyl-terminated polyamidoamine (PAMAM)	Dendrimer-gene complex showed effective gene transfection in RPE cells	Preclinical	Mastorakos et al. 2015
Liposome	Small interfering RNA (siRNA)	Arg(R)-Gly(G)-Asp(D) motif peptide conjugated to PEGylated liposomes	The peptide modified liposomes targeted RPE cells and enhanced the delivery of siRNA fourfold more than non-modified liposomes	Preclinical	Chen et al., (2011, 2013)
	Visudyne®; Verteporfin	Lactose monohydrate, egg phosphatidylglycerol, dimyristoyl phosphatidylcholine, ascorbyl palmitate, and butylated hydroxytoluene (E321)	Photodynamic therapy with light-activated drug Verteporfin (commercialized by QLT phototherapeutics; 2002)	Phase III	NCT00121407
Verisome	Biodegradable polymeric system	Triamcinolone acetonide	Verisome™ is an injectable, biodegradable, and effective delivery system for sustained intraocular administration	Phase I/II	NCT01175395
Hydrogel	Polycaprolactone dimethacrylate (PCM) and hydroxyethyl methacrylate (HEMA)	Bevacizumab	The delivery platform successfully exhibited sustained release of bevacizumab in suprachoroidal space of SD rats for 4 months	Preclinical	Tyagi et al. (2013)
Micelle	Chitosan nanoparticle coated with cationic lipid	Triamcinolone acetonide	The micellar gel system showed sustained release for one year after intravitreal injection	Preclinical	Jiang et al. (2012)
Micelle	Polyion complex (PIC) micelle	Plasmid DNA	IV injection of polyion complex (PIC) micelle encapsulating plasmid DNA (pDNA) showed significant inhibition in CNV in a mice CNV model	Preclinical	Iriyama et al. (2011)

and therapies for neovascular age-related macular degeneration (AMD) and complications associated with diabetic retinopathy requiring frequent anti-VEGF intravitreal injections.

Anti-VEGF therapies are injected into the vitreous, where they bind to abnormal VEGF proteins and prevent them from stimulating further blood vessel growth and leakage. Therefore, frequent intravitreal injections require technicians to handle the patient and precision-based delivery. However, it becomes burdensome for the patient as well as for the practitioners to provide injection therapy at regular intervals and sometimes involves the risk for surgery.

Nanotechnology has contributed immensely to innovating noninvasive therapeutic platforms or minimally invasive technologies that are under various phases (phase I/II or III) of clinical investigation for the safe and effective administration of anti-VEGF therapies in AMD as displayed in Table 11.6. Most recently, a surgically refillable port delivery system (PDS) which can be refilled (once the delivery system runs out of the drug completely) in the wall of the eye for slow release of drug *Lucentis*® is in phase II trials and is expected to complete in 2019. This novel approach may provide a big relief to wet AMD patients requiring frequent intraocular injections. Sunitinib, another anti-VEGF receptor agent, is in phase II trials and has shown good potential as a sustained-release depot (known as version GB-102) by injecting into the eye as well as for oral administration (known as version X-82). Moreover, some physicians have reported patients becoming nonresponsive or less effective to repeated anti-VEGF injection therapies at some point in time during the therapy. Hence, this prompted the ophthalmic clinicians to look for new targets in wet AMD.

11.6.1 Stem Cell Therapies

Various reports have shown the induction of pluripotent stem cells (iPSCs) which differentiate into photoreceptors and RPE cells and integrate into the host cell structure to significantly improve the retinal function in retinal dystrophic and degenerative rat and mouse models (Kanemura et al. 2014). Further, stem cells are also being injected into the eye in trials for dry AMD. Some studies have revealed that if stem cells are injected precisely within the clinical trials, they can be therapeutically helpful; however, treatments outside clinics with imprecise localization and insertion may result in loss of vision. Some initial studies revealed improvement in the visual activity of patients (in the order of 9–19 letters on visual acuity test) within few months of the subretinal ESC transplantation in the Asian population affected with wet AMD. The study showed the huge potential of stem cells as a regenerative therapy in AMD (Song et al. 2015). Furthermore, in another investigation, subretinal transplantation of iPSC-derived RPE cells was premeditated in advanced wet AMD patients. Although no improvement in the visual acuity was observed, however, no worsening of the condition post one year of transplantation was reported (Mandai et al. 2017). The study yielded no significant outcome in terms of therapeutic efficacy, but still it is a big matter of investigation and debate that why the diseased condition was not progressed. Thus, in the light of above facts, it can be implied that the role of stem cell therapy is still in its nascent stages and more investigations are required to implement this therapy at a specific endpoint of the disease for better results.

11.6.2 Gene Therapies

More attention has been paid to the potential of gene therapy in AMD, the delivery of nucleic acid polymers into host cells to treat retinal diseases in recent times. The gene therapy could be exploited to ameliorate the burden of chronic intravitreal therapy via the expression of anti-VEGF proteins. Phase I investigations have shown the application of adeno-associated virus vector (such as AAV2 and AAV8 encoding genes for anti-angiogenic proteins) delivered RPE derived factor gene in advanced stages of neovascular AMD (Moore et al. 2017). Further, endogenous expression of various VEGF inhibitors (such as soluble fms-like tyrosine kinase-1 and

Table 11.6 List of few ophthalmic devices/delivery systems under clinical investigation for the management of AMD

Drug/dosage form	Therapeutic indication	Stage	Manufacturer/stage of development	Polymeric device/excipient	Reference/trial no.
Intravitreal implant	Dry AMD	Phase II	Allergan Inc.	Intravitreal implant containing brimonidine tartrate	NCT02087085
IVT (Verisome®) of triamcinolone acetonide	AMD	Phase I/II	Verisome™ is an injectable, biodegradable gel for sustained intraocular administration	Biodegradable gel	NCT01175395
Liposomal formulation PDT with light-activated Verteporfin (Visudyne®)	Wet AMD	Phase III	QLT phototherapeutics	Systemic route; composed of lactose monohydrate, egg phosphatidylglycerol, dimyristoyl Phosphatidylcholine, ascorbyl palmitate, and BHT	Visudyne® product information EMA (http://www.ema.europa.eu); NCT00121407
Semipermeable hollow fiber membrane NT-501 implant	AMD	Phase I/II	Renexus & Noah Group	Semipermeable hollow fiber membrane with ciliary neurotrophic factor producing RPE cells	NCT00447954
NT-503 implant	AMD	Phase I/II	Neurotech	Semipermeable hollow fiber membrane with VEGF receptor Fc-fusion protein (VEGFR-Fc)-releasing cells	NCT02228304
Photrex® (liposomal Rostaporfin)	AMD	Phase III	Mitravant Medical Technologies	Liposomal formulation of Rostaporfin for intravitreal injection	NCT00157976
PDDS® Ranibizumab	AMD	Phase II	Genetech, ForSight vision 4 Inc.	Novel refillable system designed to provide release rate of 10 mg/ml for decreasing macular thickness and choroidal neovascular leakage	NCT02510794

iTrack microcatheter (a triamcinolone acetonide-based DDS)	Neovascular AMD	Phase I, II	iScience Interventional; Janssen Research & Development	Injection device for suprachoroidal delivery of TA	NCT01226628
LADDER (long-acting delivery of ranibizumab)	Wet AMD	Phase II	PDS, Genentech	Sustained-release port delivery system for ranibizumab	Campochiaro et al. (2019); and NCT02510794
SalutarisMD treatment	Wet AMD	Phase I	Salutaris Medical Devices, Inc. USA	Using radiation (strontium 90 radioisotope) to cause the AMD lesions to regress	NCT02988895
The IRay™	Wet AMD	Phase II	Oraya therapeutics, USA	Three tightly focused, low-energy beams of X-ray radiation using special contact lens	NCT01016873
The AdaptDx dark adaptometer	Wet AMD	Phase I	Maculogix Inc. PA, USA	A tabletop device (FDA approved, 2008) tests the patients into darkened tunnel and focuses on a red dot, which lights the center of a viewing screen	NCT03225131

sFLT-1) has also been explored for binding and neutralizing VEGF-A. It is a well-documented fact that the success of gene therapy for management of AMD depends on various factors such as selection of therapeutic protein, expression level, associated adverse effects, optimized vector, promoter, and method of transfection.

RGX-314 is an anti-VEGF treatment delivered by AAV-associated gene therapy that has been approved by the FDA for another disease known as *Leber's congenital amaurosis*. This could pave the way to the potential application of gene therapies in diverse retinal conditions of AMD.

11.6.3 Complement-Associated Specific Targeted Therapies

The complement system, an intrinsic component of innate immunity, imparts a significant role in maintaining immune surveillance and homeostasis of ocular microenvironment (Park et al. 2019). The mechanism of complement disease dissemination is yet to be fully understood. However, the targeted modulation of complement specific proteins has emerged as a viable therapeutic approach to mitigate disease progression in AMD. Studies have shown the potential application of complement cascade inhibitors to target the modulation of complement proteins C3, C5, factor B, factor D, and properdin in AMD as listed in Table 11.7.

A phase II trial for new molecule APL-2 in combination with anti-VEGF agent is under investigation for the inhibition of complement factor C3. Avacincaptad pegol (Zimura®) is another drug targeting a different complement protein, C5. The literature studies have revealed dysregulation of gene encoding complement factor H, and patients having a copy of Y402H polymorphism (a tyrosine-to-histidine substitution at amino acid position 402 within the CFH protein) are more susceptible to AMD (approximately fivefold increase in risk). Other factors are B, D, C2, and C3, and I have also been observed to be associated with the risk of AMD. Various other clinical studies of Potentia (C3 inhibitor), ARC1905 (C5 inhibitor), eculizumab (humanized monoclonal antibodies binding C5), Tanox (complement factor D inhibitor), and TA106 (complement factor B inhibitor) are also under investigation to assess the role of complement system in AMD.

11.6.4 Targeting Factors/Pathways—IL-7, Rap1 GTPase

The inflammatory response in macula along with various inflammatory biomarkers such as IL-7, cytokines has been found to be associated with AMD. The members of interleukin family which primarily play a vital role in the pathogenesis of AMD are IL-17A cytokine and IL-17 receptor (R)-C. Therefore, the targeting of IL-17, IL-17R-C, or cells producing IL-17 may mini-

Table 11.7 Some significant clinical trials for various complement-based therapeutics in AMD (credit: https://clinicaltrials.gov)

Agent/therapy	Target	Class	Clinical indication	Phase (P)/trial no.
CLG561 (Novartis)	Properdin	Antibody	AMD	P2 (NCT02515942)
APL-2 (Apellis)	C3	Peptide (PEGylated)	Geographical atrophy	P2 (NCT02503332)
LFG316 (Novartis)	C5	Antibody	AMD	P2 (NCT02763644)
Zimura (Ophthotech)	C5	Aptamer	AMD	P2/3 (NCT02686658)
Lampalizumab (Genentech)	Factor D	Antibody	AMD	P3 (NCT02247531)
IONIS-FB-Lrx	Factor B	Antibody	AMD	P2 (NCT03446144)
AMY-101	C3	Peptide	Complement-mediated diseases	P1 (NCT03316521)

mize the retinal degeneration and could be considered as a potential therapeutic target for AMD.

Rap1 GTPase (small guanosine triphosphatase, GTPase) is involved in regulating both endothelial and epithelial cell junctions (critical factor involving RPE barrier function leading to the development of AMD) (Wittchen et al. 2013). Recently in 2018, Li et al. investigated the functional role and mechanism of Rap 1 in CNV in vivo (laser-induced CNV rat model) (Li et al. 2018). It was observed from the findings that activation of Rap1 using 8CPT-2′-O-Me-cAMP was able to produce a significant reduction in CNV size and VEGF expression.

11.6.5 Miscellaneous Therapies

Several agents such as *Oracea*® (an antibiotic famously known as doxycycline) are under phase II/III investigation for the possible anti-inflammatory effects, which could be beneficial in patients with geographic atrophy (or dry AMD). Antidiabetic drugs like metformin have also been explored for an anti-inflammatory role in AMD. Agents such as lipoic acid are being tested in dry AMD patients for their antioxidant properties. This agent has shown immense application by protecting the retinal degeneration in preclinical models of mice.

11.7 Conclusions and Current Perspectives

The confined position of the eye and the challenging eye conditions make it an excellent target for the development and testing of minimally invasive, safe, and effective nanomedical technologies. Further, the global market has also shown tremendous expansion over the last decade as eye diseases like macular degeneration, glaucoma, and diabetic retinopathy had hugely impacted the health care costs. Recent trends in ocular drug delivery care have demonstrated novel technological platforms based on nanoscale systems that can be rapidly and successfully translated into clinically relevant treatments in the eye. Implantable devices such as nano-ocular pumps are capable of dispensing nanoliter-sized dose delivery for the management of glaucoma and AMD.

Nanotechnological tools have produced tangible solutions by facilitating innovative approaches generated by the clinical knowledge based on pathophysiological mechanisms. For example, nanodevices and nanosystems are capable of determining the physiology of the ocular tissues and cells (IOP or oxygen tension), valves for glaucoma drainage, prosthetics for ion channels (which are sensitive to light and can cure blindness), and tools for surgical intervention based on nanoneedles and nanotweezers.

Further, design of contact lenses with novel applications, integration of gels into drug delivery devices like intraocular pumps, injections, and implants have been devised to reduce the burden of comorbidities caused by emerging ocular conditions such as glaucoma, diabetic retinopathies, and AMD. The current summarization of literature is an attempt to provide a critical appraisal of the clinical aspects with pathophysiological bases while employing nanotechniques and novel drug delivery systems used in the characterization of ophthalmic products along with a thorough insight into the safety and biocompatibility of these systems. Finally, a new dimension has been added in the ocular drug delivery segment with the design of stimuli-responsive gels, molecularly imprinted gels, and 3D printed nanogels/hydrogels; 3D printed devices comprise ophthalmic gels. This novel application of gelling systems would generate huge currents in the treatment and management of ocular drug delivery markets by paving a way forward in the production of artificial corneas, corneal wound healing, and hydrogel-based contact lenses.

In the light of above-discussed summary, it can be remarked that nanotechnology-based treatments offer immense potential and application in overcoming the complications (such as diffusional limitation and ocular barriers) by improving the therapeutics in the field of ocular nanomedicine, nanodevices, and tissue regeneration. It can revolutionize the methodology of ocular drug delivery (such as treatment-based IOP-independent therapies in glaucoma) via targeted or controlled or microelectromechanical approaches.

Conflicts of Interest There are no conflicts of interest to declare.

References

Aburahma MH, Mahmoud AA (2011) Biodegradable ocular inserts for sustained delivery of brimonidine tartarate: preparation and in vitro/in vivo evaluation. AAPS PharmSciTech 12:1335–1347

Age-Related Eye Disease Study Research Group (2001) A randomized, placebo-controlled, clinical trial of high-dose supplementation with vitamins C and E, beta carotene, and zinc for age-related macular degeneration and vision loss. Arch Ophthalmol 119(10):1417–1436

Agrahari V, Agrahari V, Hung WT, Christenson LK, Mitra AK (2016) Composite Nanoformulation therapeutics for long-term ocular delivery of macromolecules. Mol Pharm 13(9):2912–2922

Al-Khersan H, Hussain RM, Ciulla TA, Dugel PU (2019) Innovative therapies for neovascular age-related macular degeneration. Expert Opin Pharmacother 12:1–13

Alvarez-Lorenzo C, Hiratani H, Gómez-Amoza JL, Martínez-Pacheco R, Souto C, Concheiro A (2002) Soft contact lenses capable of sustained delivery of timolol. J Pharm Sci 91:2182–2192

Anderson SA, Rader RK, Westlin WF, Null C, Jackson D, Lanza GM (2000) Magnetic resonance contrast enhancement of neovasculature with $\alpha v\beta 3$-targeted nanoparticles. Magn Reson Med 44:433–439

Andriessen EM, Wilson AM, Mawambo G, Dejda A, Miloudi K, Sennlaub F, Sapieha P (2016) Gut microbiota influences pathological angiogenesis in obesity-driven choroidal neovascularization. EMBO Mol Med 8:1366–1379

Birch DG, Liang FQ (2007) Age-related macular degeneration: a target for nanotechnology derived medicines. Int J Nanomedicine 2(1):65–77

Campochiaro PA, Marcus DM, Awh CC, Regillo C, Adamis AP, Bantseev V, Chiang Y, Ehrlich JS, Erickson S, Hanley WD, Horvath J, Maass KF, Singh N, Tang F, Barteselli G (2019) The port delivery system with Ranibizumab for Neovascular age-related macular degeneration: results from the randomized phase 2 ladder clinical trial. Ophthalmology 126(8):1141–1154

Cetinel S, Montemagno C (2016) Nanotechnology applications for Glaucoma. Asia Pac J Ophthalmol (Phila) 5(1):70–78

Chamling X, Sluch VM, Zack DJ (2016) The potential of human stem cells for the study and treatment of Glaucoma. Invest Ophthalmol Vis Sci 57:ORSFi1–ORSFi6

Chang EE, Goldberg JL (2012) Glaucoma 2.0: neuroprotection, neuroregeneration, neuroenhancement. Ophthalmology 119(5):979–986

Chen CW, Lu DW, Yeh MK, Shiau CY, Chiang CH (2011) Novel RGD-lipid conjugate-modified liposomes for enhancing siRNA delivery in human retinal pigment epithelial cells. Int J Nanomedicine 6:2567–2580

Chen CW, Yeh MK, Shiau CY, Chiang CH, Lu DW (2013) Efficient downregulation of VEGF in retinal pigment epithelial cells by integrin ligand-labeled liposome-mediated siRNA delivery. Int J Nanomedicine 8:2613–2627

Chirco KR, Potempa LA (2018) C - reactive protein as a mediator of complement activation and inflammatory signaling in age-related macular degeneration. Front Immunol 9:539

Chung SH, Lim SA, Tchach H (2016) Efficacy and safety of carbomer-based lipid-containing artificial tear formulations in patients with dry eye syndrome. Cornea 35(2):181–186

Ciolino JB, Stefanescu CF, Ross AE, Salvador-Culla B, Cortez P, Ford EM et al (2014) In vivo performance of a drug-eluting contact lens to treat glaucoma for a month. Biomaterials 35:432–439

Crabb JW, Miyagi M, Gu X, Shadrach K, West KA, Sakaguchi H, Kamei M, Hasan A, Yan L, Rayborn ME, Salomon RG, Hollyfield JG (2002) Drusen proteome analysis: an approach to the etiology of age-related macular degeneration. Proc Natl Acad Sci U S A 99(23):14682–14687

Daruich A, Matet A, Moulin A, Kowalczuk L, Nicolas M, Sellam A, Rothschild PR, Omri S, Gélizé E, Jonet L, Delaunay K, De Kozak Y, Berdugo M, Zhao M, Crisanti P, Behar-Cohen F (2018) Mechanisms of macular edema: beyond the surface. Prog Retin Eye Res 63:20–68

Davis BM, Pahlitzsch M, Guo L, Balendra S, Shah P, Ravindran N, Malaguarnera G, Sisa C, Shamsher E, Hamze H, Noor A, Sornsute A, Somavarapu S, Cordeiro MF (2018) Topical curcumin nanocarriers are neuroprotective in eye disease. Sci Rep 8(1):11066

De Jong PTVM (2018) Elusive drusen and changing terminology of AMD. Eye (Lond) 32(5):904–914

Fathalla D, Soliman GM, Fouad EA (2015) Development and in vitro/in vivo evaluation of liposomal gels for the sustained ocular delivery of latanoprost. J Clin Exp Ophthalmol 6:390

Fulgêncio Gde O, Viana FA, Ribeiro RR, Yoshida MI, Faraco AG, Cunha-Júnior Ada S (2012) New mucoadhesive chitosan film for ophthalmic drug delivery of timolol maleate: in vivo evaluation. J Ocul Pharmacol Ther 28:350–358

Gagandeep, Garg T, Malik B, Rath G, Goyal AK (2014) Development and characterization of nano-fiber patch for the treatment of glaucoma. Eur J Pharm Sci 53:10–16

Guo L, Cordeiro MF (2008) Assessment of neuroprotection in the retina with DARC. Prog Brain Res 173:437–450

Hodges RR, Dartt DA (2013) Tear film mucins: front line defenders of the ocular surface; comparison with airway and gastrointestinal tract mucins. Exp Eye Res 117:62–78

Hsu KH, Carbia BE, Plummer C, Chauhan A (2015) Dual drug delivery from vitamin e loaded contact lenses for glaucoma therapy. Eur J Pharm Biopharm 94:312–321

https://clinicaltrials.gov. Accessed on 30-8-19

https://www.who.int/blindness/causes/priority/en/index7.html. Accessed on 20-7-19

Hussain RM, Ciulla TA (2017) Emerging vascular endothelial growth factor antagonists to treat neovascular age-related macular degeneration. Expert Opin Emerg Drugs 22(3):235–246

Huu VA, Luo J, Zhu J, Zhu J, Patel S, Boone A, Mahmoud E, McFearin C, Olejniczak J, de Gracia Lux C, Lux J, Fomina N, Huynh M, Zhang K, Almutairi A (2015) Light-responsive nanoparticle depot to control release of a small molecule angiogenesis inhibitor in the posterior segment of the eye. J Control Release 200:71–77

Ibrahim MM, Abd-Elgawad AH, Soliman OA, Jablonski MM (2015) Natural bioadhesive biodegradable nanoparticle-based topical ophthalmic formulations for management of Glaucoma. Transl Vis Sci Technol 4:12

Iriyama A, Oba M, Ishii T, Nishiyama N, Kataoka K, Tamaki Y, Yanagi Y (2011) Gene transfer using micellar nanovectors inhibits choroidal neovascularization in vivo. PLoS One 6(12):e28560

Jain K, Kumar RS, Sood S, Dhyanandhan G (2013) Betaxolol hydrochloride loaded chitosan nanoparticles for ocular delivery and their anti-glaucoma efficacy. Curr Drug Deliv 10:493–499

Jiang M, Gan L, Zhu C, Dong Y, Liu J, Gan Y (2012) Cationic core-shell liponanoparticles for ocular gene delivery. Biomaterials 33:7621–7630

Johnson TV, Bull ND, Martin KR (2011) Stem cell therapy for glaucoma: possibilities and practicalities. Expert Rev Ophthalmol 6(2):165–174

Jung HJ, Abou-Jaoude M, Carbia BE, Plummer C, Chauhan A (2013) Glaucoma therapy by extended release of timolol from nanoparticle loaded silicone-hydrogel contact lenses. J Control Release 165:82–89

Kanemura H, Go MJ, Shikamura M, Nishishita N, Sakai N, Kamao H et al (2014) Tumorigenicity studies of induced pluripotent stem cell (iPSC)-derived retinal pigment epithelium (RPE) for the treatment of age-related macular degeneration. PLoS One 9(1):e85336

Kashiwagi K, Ito K, Haniuda H, Ohtsubo S, Takeoka S (2013) Development of latanoprost-loaded biodegradable nanosheet as a new drug delivery system for glaucoma. Invest Ophthalmol Vis Sci 54(8):5629–5637

Katiyar S, Pandit J, Mondal RS, Mishra AK, Chuttani K, Aqil M et al (2014) In situ gelling dorzolamide loaded chitosan nanoparticles for the treatment of glaucoma. Carbohydr Polym 102:117–124

Kauppinen A, Paterno JJ, Blasiak J, Salminen A, Kaarniranta K (2016) Inflammation and its role in age-related macular degeneration. Cell Mol Life Sci 73:1765–1786

Khar RK, Jain GK, Warsi MH, Mallick N, Akhter S, Pathan SA, Ahmad FJ (2010) Nano-vectors for the ocular delivery of nucleic acid-based therapeutics. Indian J Pharm Sci 72(6):675–688

Khoo HE, Ng HS, Yap WS, Goh HJH, Yim HS (2019) Nutrients for prevention of macular degeneration and eye-related diseases. Antioxidants 8(4):pii: E85

Kimura A, Namekata K, Guo X, Harada C, Harada T (2016) Neuroprotection, growth factors and BDNF-TrkB Signalling in retinal degeneration. Int J Mol Sci 17(9):pii: E1584

Kouchak M, Bahmandar R, Bavarsad N (2016) Ocular Dorzolamide nanoliposomes for prolonged IOP reduction: in-vitro and in-vivo evaluation in rabbits. Iran J Pharm Res 15:205–212

Kwatra D, Mitra AK (2013) Drug delivery in ocular diseases: barriers and strategies. World J Pharmacol 2(4):78–83

Labib GS, El-Salamouni NS, El-Gamal SS (2013) Bioadhesive ophthalmic inserts for treatment of Glaucoma: in vitro-in vivo evaluation. Lat Am J Pharm 32:1457–1466

Landowski M, Kelly U, Klingeborn M, Groelle M, Ding JD, Grigsby D, Bowes Rickman C (2019) Human complement factor H Y402H polymorphism causes an age-related macular degeneration phenotype and lipoprotein dysregulation in mice. Proc Natl Acad Sci U S A 116(9):3703–3711

Lee EJ, Han JC, Park DY, Kee C (2019) Difference in topographic pattern of prelaminar and neuroretinal rim thinning between nonarteritic anterior ischemic optic neuropathy and Glaucoma. Invest Ophthalmol Vis Sci 60:2461–2467

Leonardi A, Bucolo C, Drago F, Salomone S, Pignatello R (2015) Cationic solid lipid nanoparticles enhance ocular hypotensive effect of melatonin in rabbit. Int J Pharm 478:180–186

Li F, Hurley B, Liu Y, Leonard B, Griffith M (2012) Controlled release of bevacizumab through nanospheres for extended treatment of age-related macular degeneration. Open Ophthalmol J 6:54–58

Li H, Liu Y, Zhang Y, Fang D, Xu B, Zhang L et al (2016) Liposomes as a novel ocular delivery system for Brinzolamide: in vitro and in vivo studies. AAPS PharmSciTech 17(3):710–717

Li J, Zhang R, Wang C, Wang X, Xu M, Ma J, Shang Q (2018) Activation of the small GTPase Rap1 inhibits choroidal neovascularization by regulating cell junctions and ROS generation in rats. Curr Eye Res 43(7):934–940

Lin TC, Hung KH, Peng CH, Liu JH, Woung LC, Tsai CY, Chen SJ, Chen YT, Hsu CC (2015) Nanotechnology-based drug delivery treatments and specific targeting therapy for age-related macular degeneration. J Chin Med Assoc 78(11):635–641

Luo L, Zhang X, Hirano Y, Tyagi P, Barabas P, Uehara H et al (2013) Targeted intraceptor nanoparticle therapy reduces angiogenesis and fibrosis in primate and murine macular degeneration. ACS Nano 7:3264–3275

Mandai M, Watanabe A, Kurimoto Y, Hirami Y, Morinaga C, Daimon T (2017) Autologous induced stem-cell-derived retinal cells for macular degeneration. N Engl J Med 376(11):1038–1046

Mandal A, Pal D, Agrahari V, Trinh HM, Joseph M, Mitra AK (2018) Ocular delivery of proteins and peptides: challenges and novel formulation approaches. Adv Drug Deliv Rev 126:67–95

Martínez T, González MV, Roeh I, Wright N, Pañeda C, Jiménez AI (2014) In vitro and in vivo efficacy of SYL040012, a novel siRNA compound for treatment of glaucoma. Mol Ther 22(1):81–91

Mastorakos P, Kambhampati SP, Mishra MK, Wu T, Song E, Hanes J et al (2015) Hydroxyl PAMAM dendrimer-based gene vectors for transgene delivery to human retinal pigment epithelial cells. Nanoscale 7:3845–3856

Matteucci A, Varano M, Gaddini L, Mallozzi C, Villa M, Pricci F et al (2014) Neuroprotective effects of citicoline in in vitro models of retinal neurodegeneration. Int J Mol Sci 15:6286–6297

Mehnert W, Mäder K (2001) Solid lipid nanoparticles: production, characterization and applications. Adv Drug Deliv Rev 47:165–196

Mokhtar Ibrahim M, Tawfique SA, Mahdy MM (2014) Liposomal diltiazem HCl as ocular drug delivery system for glaucoma. Drug Dev Ind Pharm 40:765–773

Monem AS, Ali FM, Ismail MW (2000) Prolonged effect of liposomes encapsulating pilocarpine HCl in normal and glaucomatous rabbits. Int J Pharm 198(1):29–38

Moore NA, Bracha P, Hussain RM, Morral N, Ciulla TA (2017) Gene therapy for age-related macular degeneration. Expert Opin Biol Ther 17(10):1235–1244

Nafissi N, Foldvari M (2015) Neuroprotective therapies in glaucoma: II. Genetic nanotechnology tools. Front Neurosci 9:355

Natarajan JV, Ang M, Darwitan A, Chattopadhyay S, Wong TT, Venkatraman SS (2012) Nanomedicine for glaucoma: liposomes provide sustained release of latanoprost in the eye. Int J Nanomedicine 7:123–131

Ng DS, Yip YW, Bakthavatsalam M, Chen LJ, Ng TK, Lai TY, Pang CP, Brelén ME (2017) Elevated angiopoietin 2 in aqueous of patients with neovascular age related macular degeneration correlates with disease severity at presentation. Sci Rep 7:45081

Nucci C, Martucci A, Giannini C, Morrone LA, Bagetta G, Mancino R (2018) Neuroprotective agents in the management of glaucoma. Eye 32:938–945

Oshitari T, Fujimoto N, Adachi-Usami E (2002) Citicoline has a protective effect on damaged retinal ganglion cells in mouse culture retina. Neuroreport 13:2109–2111

Ozkan J, Willcox MD (2019) The ocular microbiome: molecular characterisation of a unique and low microbial environment. Curr Eye Res 44(7):685–694

Park CH, Kim YS, Noh HS, Cheon EW, Yang YA, Yoo JM et al (2005) 2005 neuroprotective effect of citicoline against KA-induced neurotoxicity in the rat retina. Exp Eye Res 81:350–358

Park DH, Connor KM, Lambris JD (2019) The challenges and promise of complement therapeutics for ocular diseases. Front Immunol 10:1007

Parmeggiani F, Romano MR, Costagliola C, Semeraro F, Incorvaia C, D'Angelo S, Perri P, Palma PD, Nadai KD, Sebastiani A (2012) Mechanism of inflammation in age-related macular degeneration. Mediat Inflamm 2012:546786

Pechan P, Wadsworth S, Scaria A (2014) Gene therapies for neovascular age-related macular degeneration. Cold Spring Harb Perspect Med 5(7):a017335

Peng CC, Ben-Shlomo A, MacKay EO, Plummer CE, Chauhan A (2012) Drug delivery by contact lens in spontaneously glaucomatous dogs. Curr Eye Res 37:204–211

Pennington KL, DeAngelis MM (2016) Epidemiology of age-related macular degeneration (AMD): associations with cardiovascular disease phenotypes and lipid factors. Eye Vis (Lond) 3:34

Pietrucha-Dutczak M, Amadio M, Govoni S, Lewin-Kowalik J, Smedowski A (2018) The role of endogenous neuroprotective mechanisms in the prevention of retinal ganglion cells degeneration. Front Neurosci 12:834

Pitha I, Kimball EC, Oglesby EN, Pease ME, Fu J, Schaub J, Kim YC, Hu Q, Hanes J, Quigley HA (2018) Sustained Dorzolamide release prevents axonal and retinal ganglion cell loss in a rat model of IOP-Glaucoma. Transl Vis Sci Technol 7(2):13

Prabhu P, Nitish KR, Koland M, Harish NM, Dhondge G et al (2010) Preparation and evaluation of liposomes of brimonidine tartrate as an ocular drug delivery system. Int J Res Pharm Sci 1:502–508

Renganathan K, Gu J, Rayborn ME, Crabb JS, Salomon RG, Collier RJ, Kapin MA, Romano C, Hollyfield JG, Crabb JW (2013) CEP biomarkers as potential tools for monitoring therapeutics. PLoS One 8(10):e76325

Ribeiro A, Veiga F, Santos D, Torres-Labandeira JJ, Concheiro A, Alvarez-Lorenzo C (2011) Bioinspired imprinted PHEMA-hydrogels for ocular delivery of carbonic anhydrase inhibitor drugs. Biomacromolecules 12:701–709

Rinninella E, Mele MC, Merendino N, Cintoni M, Anselmi G, Caporossi A, Gasbarrini A, Minnella AM (2018) The role of diet, micronutrients and the gut microbiota in age-related macular degeneration: new perspectives from the gut-retina axis. Nutrients 10(11):pii: E1677

Saharinen P, Eklund L, Alitalo K (2017) Therapeutic targeting of the angiopoietin–TIE pathway. Nat Rev Drug Discov 16:635–661

Schenker HI, Silver LH (2000) Long-term intraocular pressure-lowering efficacy and safety of timolol maleate gel-forming solution 0.5% compared with Timoptic XE 0.5% in a 12-month study. Am J Ophthalmol 130(2):145–150

Schnaar RL, Lopez PHH (2009) Myelin-associated glycoprotein and its axonal receptors. J Neurosci Res 87(15):3267–3276

Schuettauf F, Rejdak R, Thaler S, Bolz S, Lehaci C, Mankowska A et al (2006) Citicoline and lithium rescue retinal ganglion cells following partial optic nerve crush in the rat. Exp Eye Res 83:1128–1134

Schultz CL, Poling TR, Mint JO (2009) A medical device/drug delivery system for treatment of glaucoma. Clin Exp Optom 92:343–348

Shinde U, Ahmed MH, Singh K (2013) Development of dorzolamide loaded 6-o-carboxymethyl chitosan nanoparticles for open angle glaucoma. J Drug Deliv 2013:562727

Shoval A, Markus A, Zhou Z, Liu X, Cazelles R, Willner I, Mandel Y (2019) Anti-VEGF-aptamer modified C-Dots-A hybrid nanocomposite for topical treatment of ocular vascular disorders. Small 15:e1902776

Singh N, Srinivasan S, Muralidharan V, Roy R, Jayprakash V, Raman R (2017) Prevention of age-related macular degeneration. Asia Pac J Ophthalmol 6(6):520–526

Song WK, Park K-M, Kim H-J, Lee JH, Choi J, Chong SY (2015) Treatment of macular degeneration using embryonic stem cell-derived retinal pigment epithelium: preliminary results in Asian patients. Stem Cell Rep 4(5):860–872

Sridhar MS (2018) Anatomy of cornea and ocular surface. Indian J Ophthalmol 66(2):190–194

Suen WL, Chau Y (2013) Specific uptake of folate-decorated triamcinolone-encapsulating nanoparticles by retinal pigment epithelium cells enhances and prolongs antiangiogenic activity. J Control Release 167:21–28

Sun J, Lei Y, Dai Z, Liu X, Huang T, Wu J, Xu ZP, Sun X (2017) Sustained release of Brimonidine from a new composite drug delivery system for treatment of Glaucoma. ACS Appl Mater Interfaces 9(9):7990–7999

Tham YC, Li X, Wong TY, Quigley HA, Aung T, Cheng CY (2014) Global prevalence of glaucoma and projections of glaucoma burden through 2040: a systematic review and meta-analysis. Ophthalmology 121(11):2081–2090

Tian K, Shibata-Germanos S, Pahlitzsch M, Cordeiro MF (2015) Current perspective of neuroprotection and glaucoma. Clin Ophthalmol 9:2109–2118

Tyagi P, Barros M, Stansbury JW, Kompella UB (2013) Light-activated, in situ forming gel for sustained suprachoroidal delivery of bevacizumab. Mol Pharm 10:2858–2867

Wang F, Chen L, Zhang D, Jiang S, Shi K, Huang Y et al (2014) Methazolamide-loaded solid lipid nanoparticles modified with low- molecular weight chitosan for the treatment of glaucoma: vitro and vivo study. J Drug Target 22:849–858

Wang K, Mitra RN, Zheng M, Han Z (2018) Nanoceria-loaded injectable hydrogels for potential age-related macular degeneration treatment. J Biomed Mater Res A 106(11):2795–2804

Warsi MH, Anwar M, Garg V, Jain GK, Talegaonkar S, Ahmad FJ et al (2014) Dorzolamide-loaded PLGA/vitamin E TPGS nanoparticles for glaucoma therapy: pharmacoscintigraphy study and evaluation of extended ocular hypotensive effect in rabbits. Colloids Surf B Biointerfaces 122:423–431

Weinreb RN, Aung T, Medeiros FA (2014) The pathophysiology and treatment of Glaucoma. JAMA 311(18):1901–1911

Weng Y, Liu J, Jin S, Guo W, Liang X, Hu Z (2017) Nanotechnology-based strategies for treatment of ocular disease. Acta Pharm Sin B 7(3):281–291

Wittchen ES, Nishimura E, McCloskey M, Wang H, Quilliam LA, Chrzanowska-Wodnicka M, Hartnett ME (2013) Rap1 GTPase activation and barrier enhancement in rpe inhibits choroidal neovascularization in vivo. PLoS One 8(9):e73070

Xi L, Wang T, Zhao F, Zheng Q, Li X, Luo J, Liu J, Quan D, Ge J (2014) Evaluation of an injectable thermosensitive hydrogel as drug delivery implant for ocular glaucoma surgery. PLoS One 9(6):e100632

Xu J, Li X, Sun F (2010) Preparation and evaluation of a contact lens vehicle for puerarin delivery. J Biomater Sci Polym Ed 21:271–288

Yang LJ, Schnaar RL (2008) Axon regeneration inhibitors. Neurol Res 30(10):1047–1052

Yu S, Wang QM, Wang X, Liu D, Zhang W, Ye T et al (2015) Liposome incorporated ion sensitive in situ gels for opthalmic delivery of timolol maleate. Int J Pharm 480:128–136

Yuan X, Marcano DC, Shin CS, Hua X, Isenhart LC, Pflugfelder SC et al (2015) Ocular drug delivery nanowafer with enhanced therapeutic efficacy. ACS Nano 9:1749–1758

Effect of Drugs and Nanoformulation on Ocular Cells in Various Disease States

12

Sanjeev Kumar Paikra, Janmejaya Bag, and Monalisa Mishra

Abstract

Vision is the most principal sensory organ present in every organism. The mechanism of vision lies behind the ocular cells and various nerves associated with it. Thus, impairment of any of them leads to a faulty photoreceptor. The defect in the eye can be treated by various approaches like refractive surgery, wearing lens or glasses, drug therapy, or nanoformulation. Among all therapy, nanoformulation is the new strategy for the treatment of ocular diseases which can easily pass the ocular barrier and the drug can be targeted at its right place. Thus, nanoformulations are used to treat optic neuropathy, choroidal neovascularization, diabetic retinopathy, and intraocular solid tumors. However, with the wide application, the toxicity of nanoformulation is also reported from various parts of the eye like eyelids, lacrimal apparatus, conjunctiva, periorbital tissues, cornea, lens, ciliary body, iris, retina, and optic nerve. The current chapter summarizes the effect of different drugs and nanoformulation on ocular cells. Nanocarrier-based delivery of polynucleotide at ocular tissue has also been discussed briefly in this chapter.

Keywords

Nanoparticles · Ocular cells · Drug delivery · Nanoformulation · Ocular toxicity

Nomenclature

AMD	Age-related macular degeneration
BCRP	Breast cancer resistance protein
ADC	Antibody-drug conjugates
ChE	Cholinesterase
CYP	Cytochrome P450
DR	Diabetic retinopathy
mRNA	Messenger ribonucleic acid
MRP	Multidrug resistance proteins
OATP	Organic anion transporting polypeptide
PP	Protein phosphatase
RGC	Retinal ganglion cells
RB	Retinoblastoma
siRNA	Small interfering ribonucleic acid
VEGF	Vascular endothelial growth factor
mOsm	Milliosmole

S. K. Paikra · J. Bag · M. Mishra (✉)
Neural Developmental Biology Laboratory, Department of Life Science, National Institute of Technology, Rourkela, Odisha, India
e-mail: mishramo@nitrkl.ac.in

S. Talegaonkar, M. Rai (eds.), *Nanoformulations in Human Health*,
https://doi.org/10.1007/978-3-030-41858-8_12

12.1 Introduction

The eye is the most governing receptive organ present in our body for visual perception. Ninety-five percent of the sensory signal to our body comes through the eye. Thus, any defect in the eye affects the quality of life severely. The proper function of the eye depends on the ocular cells (epithelial cells, fibroblasts, keratocytes, and trabecular meshwork cells), transparent tissues, and ocular barriers present within it. However, in a disease condition like glaucoma and eye-related neurodegenerative disorder, the intraocular cells and tissues are altered and lead to improper function of visual perception. With growing age, dry eye condition is observed, which can damage the ocular surface. In the US, more than 4 billion dollars spent per year for the treatment of visual impairment (Frick et al. 2007). In some eye diseases, visual acuity is altered, inflammation is found, and macular degeneration occurs which leads to a progression of vision loss. To target the drug in the right area, it is essential to have a proper method to deliver the drugs. The ocular drug transporters such as MRP1 (Juuti-Uusitalo et al. 2012; Sreekumar et al. 2012), MRP2 (Vadlapatla et al. 2013), MRP5 (Mannermaa et al. 2009), P-gp (Zhang et al. 2012), BCRP (Vadlapatla et al. 2013), and metabolizing enzyme have an inherent contribution to the activity of ocular cells (del Amo et al. 2017). Metabolic enzymes have a role in improving the extent of drug delivery to the different ocular cells (Argikar et al. 2017). These enzymes have a significant function in the metabolism of the drug and other nanoformulation. Ocular epithelial and endothelial cells possess various membrane transporters, which have a significant role to deliver drugs to different target sites (Mitra 2009). The anterior and posterior region of the eye possesses a tight cellular barrier, which regulates the flow of intraocular fluid. Topical application of eye drops is used for the intervention of anterior segment associated eye diseases. However, bioavailability is very less owing to the presence of various ocular barriers. Nanoformulations have the potential to cross the barriers for the efficient delivery of drugs. Thus, different strategies have been adopted for the controlled delivery of the drugs to the target site. Various polymeric nanoparticles have been engineered to load a large amount of drug to increase the controlled release/sustained release of drug for a protracted period of time.

With the advancement in nanotechnology, the ophthalmologist uses an advanced drug delivery system and devices for the long-term release of drug at the target sites (Fig. 12.1). In cataract, dry eye, inflammation, glaucoma, infectious diseases, injuries, or trauma, the anterior segment of the eye is affected. The cornea is the initial barrier to prevent drug to pass through the eye. The drug clearance rate is 15–30 sec in the anterior region of the eye in case of topical application (Shell 1982). Drug applied through the topical route traverses the static barrier (blood-aqueous barrier, corneal epithelium, corneal stroma) and dynamic barrier (flow of conjunctival blood, lymph, and drainage of tear) to reach the eye anterior segment (Ghate and Edelhauser 2006; Gaudana et al. 2010). Such types of barriers control the transportation of drugs and other substances. Corneal epithelial cells possess the tight junction which controls the paracellular transport of drugs. Lipophilic drugs are modulated by the carrier-mediated P-glycoprotein (P-gp) transporters (Dey et al. 2003; Elsinga et al. 2004).

12.2 The General Structure of the Eye, Cells, and Disease Associated with It

The human eye function like a bio-micromachine with complete harmonization and cooperation with various tissues like muscle contraction in the eye and a reflection of light through the pupil. The eye has two segments: (i) anterior segment and (ii) posterior segment (Fig. 12.2). One-third part of the eye is constituted by the anterior segment and the rest by the posterior segment. The anterior segment includes the ciliary body, cornea, tear film, conjunctiva, iris, and aqueous humor. The posterior

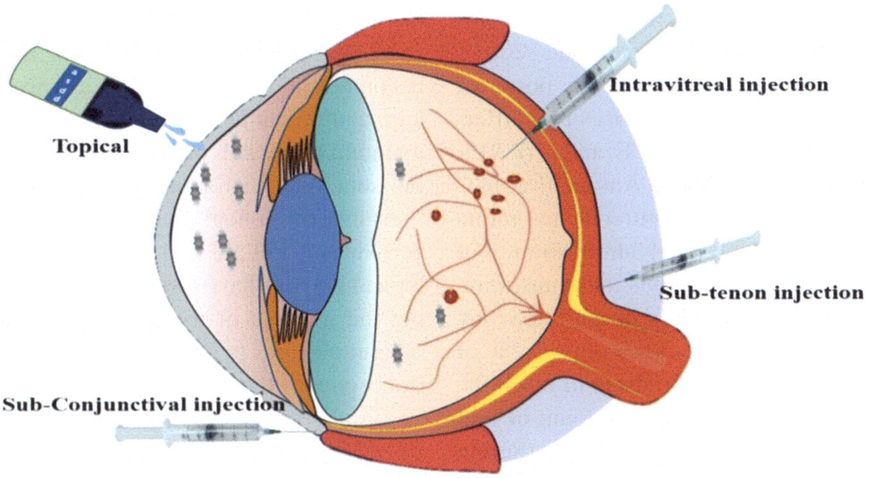

Fig. 12.1 Various modes of administration of drugs for the eye

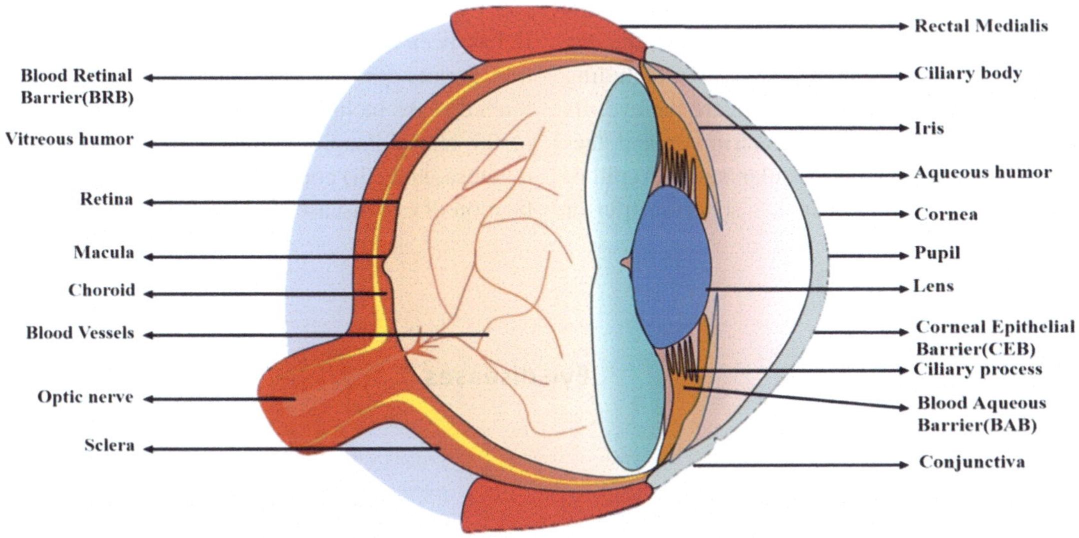

Fig. 12.2 Diagrammatic representation of a human eye depicting various structures

segment includes the retina, Bruch's membrane, sclera, choroid, and vitreous humor (Cholkar et al. 2013). To maintain the electrolytes and fluid homeostasis in the eye, different ocular barriers have played an important role. These barriers include: (a) retinal pigment epithelium (RPE), (b) ciliary body epithelium (CBE), (c) corneal epithelium, (d) iris blood vessel endothelium, and (e) inner barrier of the retina which is composed of retinal capillary endothelial (RCE) cells. Out of these barriers, the blood-ocular barriers consist of two components: (i) blood-aqueous barrier and (ii) blood-retinal barrier. The blood-aqueous barrier has tight junction formed by ciliary epithelial cells and iris vascular endothelium. It is situated in the anterior region of the eye. It prevents the entry of exogenous materials into the posterior segment and helps to maintain the chemical equilibrium of intraocular fluid (Freddo 2001). Blood-retinal barrier is situated at the posterior segment of the eye, and it comprises two different types of cells, i.e., (i) RCE and (ii) RPE (Cunha-Vaz 1997; Runkle and Antonetti 2011).

To deliver the drug at the vitreous and retina region requires the intravitreal administration of drugs because the intravenous administration requires a high dose. Oral dose doesn't have any significant impact since it allows only 1–2% of the total drug present in the plasma to reach the eye posterior segment. A higher amount of oral dose known to have many side effects (Selvin 1983). Lacrimation and tear film formation has a deep impact on the ocular surface including conjunctiva and cornea. It prevents the dryness of the eye by avoiding the attack of external irritants. The eye surface doesn't have any blood vessels on the surface; thus, only tear film helps to supply oxygen and other nutrients to the eye (Craig et al. 2000; Montes-Mico 2007). Including all these, tear film helps to lubricate the eye. Its secretion is controlled by the lacrimal gland, lacrimal sac, orbital gland, ocular surface epithelium, nasolacrimal canal, superior/inferior lacrimal puncta, and superior/inferior lacrimal canal (Rolando and Zierhut 2001). The tear film is composed of nutrient, lipid, electrolytes, protein, and mucin having pH 7.3 to 7.7. It helps to maintain the health of the eye surface by secreting some antimicrobial proteins like lysozyme, lipocalin, immunoglobulin IgA, lactoferrin, and peroxidase (Fullard and Tucker 1994). All biological barriers have a significant role in regulating the traverse of the administered drugs and other molecules to access the anterior and posterior region of the eye.

12.2.1 Various Eye Diseases

The cornea provides physical protection to the inner part of the eye, and thus, it acts as a protective barrier to epithelial cells and inner ocular tissue. Eye diseases are caused by a different reason. It has been noted that a mutation in the drug transporters protein can cause ocular disease. Such disease includes: (i) pinpoint white lesions of the choroid/angioid streaks, (ii) retinitis pigmentosa, and (iii) comet-like streaks. The classification of eye disease is given below.

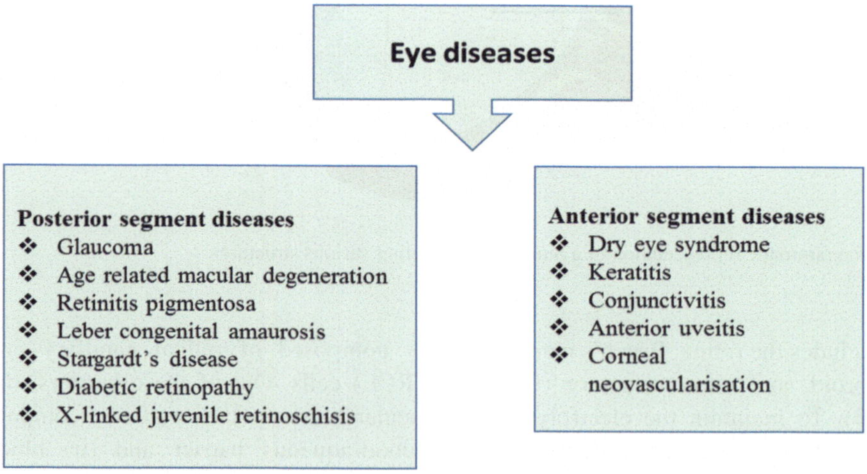

12.2.1.1 Age-Related Macular Degeneration (AMD)

It is one of the preceding causes of blindness. It is caused by the upregulation of vascular endothelial growth factor (VEGF). The macula/macula lutea is the oval-shaped central posterior part of the retina which comprises the photoreceptors and is creditworthy for high-resolution visual acuity. The posterior part of the photoreceptor has the retinal pigment epithelium. Focal dethronement of acellular polymorphous debris near the retinal pigment epithelium causes the formation of drusen, a pale yellowish lesion of 63–124 μm in diameter (Bird et al. 1995). Drusen is the hallmark of AMD and is observed in people over more than 50 years. Damage to the retinal pigment epithelium is observed in severe cases. AMD can be detected by injecting intravenous fluorescein or indocyanine green and taking an angiography to identify the choroidal neovascular lesions. Conventional therapy includes the intravitreal dose of anti-VEGF molecules, dexamethasone, and photodynamic therapy, altogether known as triple therapy for AMD (Yip et al. 2009). A genetic approach for the treatment includes the vector-interceded intravitreal gene transfer of antiangiogenic cytokine and PEDF (pigment epithelium-derived factor). Antiangiogenic cytokine halts the formation of choroidal neovascularization (Campochiaro et al. 2006). Bevasiranib is the small interfering RNA molecule specially designed to silence the VEGF RNA, and it leads to the inhibition of choroidal neovascularization (Chiang and Regillo 2011) in the ocular compartment. Nanoformulation available for the treatment of AMD is aflibercept (AFL), which is encapsulated in the polylactic-co-glycolic acid (PLGA) (Kelly et al. 2018), a nanoparticle synthesized by the double emulsion diffusion method (Kelly et al. 2018). PLGA NPs are used as sustained drug delivery carrier with minimal side effect and low toxicity (Vandervoort and Ludwig 2002; Carroll et al. 2010). The encapsulation efficiency of this nanoparticle is about 75.76% with good drug loading capacity. AFL encapsulated with PLGA NPs inhibits the VEGF and thus protects the eye from degeneration (Kelly et al. 2018). Cytotoxicity study also confirmed that the AFL is nontoxic to ocular cells (Subhani et al. 2016). Nanochitosan peptide also has potential for treatment of AMD. The peptide sequence consists of serine-threonine-tyrosine which acts as a transduction signalling agent between the retinal pigmented cells (Jayaraman et al. 2012). Nanochitosan conjugated with peptide shows the tyrosine kinase activity in the ocular cells (Jayaraman et al. 2012). Chitosan conjugated with peptide acts as an extracellular matrix of ocular cells, which act as a scaffold for the attachment of syndecans, integrins, and glycosylated transmembrane adhesive receptor (Yamagata et al. 2007). It ultimately regulates the antiangiogenic activity in ocular cells (retinal epithelium cells). FDA has already approved three different anti-VEGF agents for treatment of ocular disability or neovascularization: ranibizumab, pegaptanib, and aflibercept (Subhani et al. 2016). The designed material has specificity to target the retinal pigment epithelium for treatment of AMD. Polymeric nanoparticle loaded with doxorubicin also inhibits hypoxia-induced factor-1α (HIF-1α) (Kelly et al. 2019). HIF-1α upregulates the VEGF.

12.2.1.2 Glaucoma

In glaucoma, the permanent vision loss occurs by the degeneration of retinal ganglion cells (RGCs). It is broadly classified as the (i) open-angle glaucoma and (ii) angle-closure glaucoma. RGCs are the part of the central nervous system which has their cell body in the inner part of retina and axon lies in close proximity to the optic nerve (Vrabec and Levin 2007; Gupta and Yucel 2007). At an early stage, the symptoms are not detectable. Although the pathophysiology of glaucoma needs further investigation, it is known that the elevation in intraocular pressure causes the death of RGCs. The imbalance in secretion from the aqueous humor, ciliary body, and its drainage through the uveoscleral outflow and trabecular meshwork disturbs the intraocular pressure. In case of open-angle glaucoma, increment in resistance to aqueous outflow in trabecular meshwork has been observed. In case of angle-closure glaucoma, drainage pathway is occluded by the iris muscles (Quigley 1993; Stone et al. 1997; Kwon et al. 2009). Elevated intraocular pressure causes the increase in mechanical stress at the posterior segment of eye including the lamina cribrosa and its adjacent tissue (Quigley et al. 1981). It results in distortion of lamina cribrosa and subsequently axonal scathe and disruption of axonal transport. Ultrastructural modification in the optic nerve fiber has been observed in a few cases. *Myocilin* (MYOC, GLC1A) (Stone et al. 1997) and *optineurin* (OPTN, GLC1E) (Stone et al. 1997; Rezaie et al. 2002) are the genes responsible for glaucoma. Various strategies adopted to treat glaucoma by reducing intraocular pressure. Several prostaglandin analogues are used to lower intraocular pressure (Stewart et al. 2008). Commercially available nanoformulation for the intervention of glaucoma includes latanoprost, travoprost, bimatoprost, and tafluprost which is available as the cationic oil-in-water-type nanoemulsion (Lallemand et al. 2011; Ako-Adounvo et al. 2014; Bennett 2016). Such type of nanoemulsion is prepared by using the medium-chain triglycerides and benzalkonium chloride (Philips et al. 2012). Oil/water emulsion with neutral zeta potential loaded with prostaglandin analogue is the nanoemulsion used for the glaucoma treatment (Carli et al. 2013). Nanoemulsion prepared with tetrahydrocannabinol-valine-hemisuccinate was tested on rabbit eye (as a model for glaucoma), which reduces the intraocular pressure in the ocular segment (Taskar et al. 2019). It is formulated in the form of lipid-based nanoparticulate carrier which decreases the aqueous humor production and results in a 31% drop in intraocular pressure (Taskar et al. 2019). It permeates the significant amount of drug in ocular tissue with good bioavailability. The current existing treatment strategy for glaucoma includes the prostaglandins analogues, beta-blockers, adrenergic agonists, adenosine receptor agonist, carbonic anhydrase inhibitors, cyclin-dependent kinase inhibitors, and cholinergic agents(Supuran et al. 2019). Carbonic anhydrase inhibitors loaded with nanocarriers diminish the ocular pressure in glaucoma patients by reducing the formation of bicarbonate in aqueous humor region of eye (Supuran et al. 2019). Carbonic anhydrase catalyzes the CO_2 hydration which is required for many physiological processes including homeostasis of bicarbonate ion in aqueous humor and this enzyme is expressed in ocular cells. Mucoadhesive microparticles as a carrier for dorzolamide has specifically enhanced the retention time of drug in ocular site (Fu et al. 2016; Park et al. 2017). Poly(ethylene glycol)-co-poly(sebacic acid)-based nanoformulation shows the long-lasting effect in terms of reduction of intraocular pressure in rabbit eye (Fu et al. 2016). Dorzolamide-loaded nanoliposome is biocompatible and nontoxic, and it can retain its loading capacity as well as physicochemical properties up to several months after its preparation (Kouchak et al. 2018) without causing any harmful effect at ocular site. Dorzolamide-loaded proniosomal gels (Fouda et al. 2018) and acetazolamide-loaded mucoadhesive chitosan-dextran sulfate (Manchanda et al. 2016) were also reported which significantly reduce the intraocular pressure.

12.2.1.3 Cataract

A cataract is an ocular metabolic disorder, wherein the metabolic activity becomes highly saturated and some reactive and toxic metabolites form which can cause tissue damage in the ocular region. A cataract is associated with the cortical, nuclear, and posterior subcapsular region in the eye (Cruickshanks et al. 1992; Delcourt et al. 2000a, b). Univalent reduction of oxygen also leads to metabolic reaction, which causes the generation of reactive oxygen species, i.e., superoxide, hydroxyl, and hydrogen peroxide radical. It is identified by the clouding (opacification) of eye lens with vision impairment (Moreau and King 2012). Lucidity of the eye lens is due to functional lens protein α, β, and γ crystallins (Moreau and King 2012). Lens protein undergoes oxidation and induces the opacification of the lens. Interaction between different proteins (α and γ crystallins) in the eye lens induces the transparency of the lens. The conformational change which occurs due to the oxidation of Cys-131 and Cys-142 (Takemoto 1996) causes oxidative stress. Alteration of osmotic pressure in the ocular region induces the swelling in the eye lens due to increased hydration and decrease in Na + K-ATPase activity. Alteration of osmotic pressure is associated with aging. However, it is also seen in children and neonates after eye injuries, inflammation, or other eye-related complication.

Factors like cigarette smoking, heredity, frequent exposure to UV light, race, nutritional inadequacy, and diabetes cause or worsen the cataract (Khanna et al. 2013). The treatment strategy adopted is the surgical removal of the opaque lens. Nonsurgical therapy includes the multifunctional antioxidant dose which has free radical scavenging and chelation activity. It is also available in the form of nanoformulation (Tzankova et al. 2019). Prodrug of carnosine, N-acetylcarnosine has been developed which controls the lipid peroxidation and ROS generation in the posterior subcapsular region of the eye (Babizhayev et al. 2002). Natural antioxidant molecules prevent the formation of free radicals which can damage the eye lens cells (Moure et al. 2001). These antioxidant molecules are reducing agents such as carotenoids, flavonoids, polyphenols or thiols, vitamins, phenolic acid, and lactoferrins which can terminate the free radical chain reaction (Moure et al. 2001). Topical application of nanoformulation could be adopted as a new strategy for the treatment of cataract (Lee and Robinson 1986). Biodegradable nanoformulation of chitosan which carries the indomethacin and cyclosporine A has the controlled release effect and enhanced drug penetration and absorption from the cornea (Badawi et al. 2008). Few more studies conducted on animal model have suggested that the alginate as a carrier for gatifloxacin (Liu et al. 2006), carboxy methyl cellulose-based nanocarrier for tropicamide (Herrero-Vanrell et al. 2000), polyethylene glycol and poly(ethyl) cyanoacrylate-based carrier for acyclovir (Fresta et al. 2001), and polylactic acid and polyglycolide-based carrier for vancomycin (Gavini et al. 2004) can enhance the macular adhesion and minimize the drug loss from tear. Eudragit-based nanocarrier containing flurbiprofen (Pignatello et al. 2002), pluronic for timolol maleate (El-Kamel 2002), and polyvinyl alcohol as a carrier for ciprofloxacin (Budai et al. 2007) have enhanced the bioavailability of drugs at the ocular site. Some other biodegradable and biocompatible nanocarriers like hydroxypropyl methylcellulose (Liu et al. 2006), hyaluronic acid (Yenice et al. 2008), Carbopol (Aggarwal et al. 2007), and hydroxyethyl methacrylate (Eljarrat-Binstock et al. 2004) are known which enhance the pharmacokinetics and pharmacodynamics property of the encapsulated drugs at the ocular region. Nanoencapsulation of different antioxidant molecules can enhance the bioavailability as well as therapeutic potential of active molecules. Encapsulation of corticosteroid, triamcinolone acetonide, or dexamethasone with a negatively charged polymeric system composed of polycaprolactone and pluronic shell has the potential to minimize the steroid-induced cataract by minimizing the bioavailability of steroid in posterior subcapsular region of the eye (Srinivasarao et al. 2019).

12.2.1.4 Fungal Keratitis

It is characterized by the inflammation of the cornea. The fungus responsible for such infection includes *Candida tropicalis*, *C. albicans*, *C. krusei*, *C. glabrata*, and *C. parapsilosis* (Goldschmidt et al. 2012). In a healthy eye, the fungus cannot access to the cornea. But in an inflamed cornea, fungus and other pathogens can easily enter. In the worst condition, it may cause corneal ulceration and stromal inflammation. The conventional approach of the treatment includes the antifungal eye drops. Natamycin is the FDA-approved drug for fungal keratitis, and its corneal targeted nanoformulation has shown good bioavailability (Chandasana et al. 2014). Nanoparticle synthesized by the nanoprecipitation method has high drug entrapment efficiency (Das et al. 2010). Polycaprolactone NP and polycaprolactone-poly-D-glucosamine nanoparticles carry a positive surface charge which encapsulates natamycin and are effective in low dose as well as in less dosing frequency (Chandasana et al. 2014). Its pharmacokinetics and pharmacodynamics indices have been also compared with marketed preparation which has shown its high therapeutic value. It has high affinity for corneal surface due to positive surface charge of NP. Ocular irritancy test was done in animal model by Draize test (Huhtala et al. 2008) which has shown the positive result. Solid lipid nanoparticle as a carrier for voriconazole is composed of Compritol and palmitic acid with poloxamer and soyalecithin as a surfactant and sodium taurocholate as a co-surfactant which enhance the corneal drug permeation (Kumar and Sinha

2016) and have high bioavailability in aqueous humor region. Amphotericin B-encapsulated lecithin/chitosan nanoparticle for ocular delivery has mucoadhesive property with high precorneal residence time (Chhonker et al. 2015). Chitosan enhances the precorneal residence time through interaction with negatively charged ocular surface which ultimately minimizes the drug loss.

Microemulsion form of voriconazole has been formulated which is efficient for ocular delivery, and it possesses the antifungal activity (Kumar and Sinha 2014). In vitro release studies have confirmed the sustained release of drug at the corneal cells. Poly-(lactide-co-glycolide) nanoparticle loaded with voriconazole improves the agglomeration of drug particles (Peng et al. 2008). These formulations remain stable when dispersed at the site of action. Nanoformulation of voriconazole exhibits threefold higher permeation rate at the cornea in comparison with drug suspension form. Nanostructured dendrimer-based hydrogel is effective in regulating the corneal laceration and promoting wound healing in case of inflammation caused by fungus or any other microorganism (Oelker et al. 2011). Novel therapy employed the use of polymer for encapsulating shRNA which act against VEGF for reducing the corneal neovascularization in vivo (Gonzalez et al. 2013). Many lipid-based nanocarriers also exist which can deliver the antifungal drug with a high propensity to prevent the inflammation and kill fungus.

12.2.1.5 Retinoblastoma (RB)

It is the formation of malignant tumor which affects the retina and it is commonly seen in a child below 5 years of age (Lansingh et al. 2015). It is caused by the mutation in the tumor suppressor gene *rb1* which encode for the retinoblastoma protein and it is responsible for the development of tumor in the ocular region (Van Quill et al. 2005). Formation of a tumor may be unifocal or multifocal. It could be treated by radiotherapy, surgery, systemic chemotherapy, and cryotherapy. Systemic administration of the drug has very low ocular bioavailability due to the blood-retinal barrier. Folate-decorated nanomicelle loaded with curcumin analogue is a novel therapy for targeting retinoblastoma (Alsaab et al. 2017). It targets the folate receptor, and thus, the drug gets internalized by the folate receptor-mediated endocytosis. Carboplatin-containing protein nanoparticles display antiproliferative activity against retinoblastoma (Ahmed et al. 2014). The presence of the charged group in the protein NP supports the easy drug entrapment, and it also supports permeability through the blood-retinal barrier, e.g., doxorubicin. Carboplatin is used as an anticancer drug to treat RB. However, it has several number of side effects such as renal toxicity, neutropenia, thrombocytopenia, and hepatotoxicity (Abramson et al. 1999). The clinical significance of this therapy is also limited to some extent due to its rapid blood clearance, systemic toxicity, and resistance to cancer cells (Chan et al. 1989).

Aptamers are chimerized with drugs or different nanoparticles to target the tumors in case of cancer or retinoblastoma (Subramanian et al. 2015). RNA aptamer conjugated with doxorubicin and encapsulated in nanoparticles can target the retinoblastoma (Subramanian et al. 2018). Folic acid conjugated with silica nanoparticles containing topotecan is also effective against retinoblastoma (Qu et al. 2018). NP surface coated with folic acid enhances the therapeutic efficacy by regulating the sustained release of drug in physiological conditions. It follows the receptor-mediated endocytosis mechanism for internalization of drug molecules. The folic acid receptor is highly expressed in retinoblastoma cells. Thus, NP is fabricated with folic acid to enhance the activity.

12.2.1.6 Conjunctivitis

It is characterized by an inflammatory condition to the conjunctival tissue. It is mostly caused due to the infection in microbes like bacteria (Walker and Claoue 1986; de Kaspar et al. 2005), viruses (Kaufman et al. 1968), and fungi (Wilson et al. 1969; Klotz et al. 2000) and allergens (Ono and Abelson 2005). It is recognized by a red or pink eye appearance, edema with the continuous flow of fluid (ocular discharge) from the eye due to the vasodilation of bulbar and palpebral conjunctiva vessels (Leibowitz 2000). Bacterial conjunctivitis is caused by the *Haemophilus influenzae*, *Neisseria gonorrhoeae*, *Staphylococcus aureus*,

Chlamydia trachomatis, *Streptococcus pneumoniae*, and *Moraxella catarrhalis* (Hovding 2008; Tarabishy and Jeng 2008). Viral conjunctivitis is caused by adenovirus, allergens, pollens, fumes, and dust particles. Antiviral drug acyclovir and ganciclovir are commonly prescribed for the treatment of conjunctivitis. The side effect of acyclovir includes mild stinging, redness in the eye, itching of the eye (allergy), and punctate epithelial erosions. Ganciclovir has side effects which include irritation, redness, rash, and itching in the eye. Dizziness is also reported in severe cases (Smith et al. 1992; Keorochana and Choontanom 2017). Moxifloxacin-loaded gelatin nanoparticle is the novel formulation for the treatment of bacterial conjunctivitis (Mahor et al. 2016). It facilitates the controlled drug release in the corneal region of the eye. It is very effective against *S. aureus* species of bacteria.

12.2.1.7 Diabetic Retinopathy (DR)

It is classified as type I and type II diabetes mellitus. It is evoked due to chronic exposure to high sugar which ultimately causes the thickening of the basement membrane of the retina with progressive damage. Formation of new blood vessels (angiogenesis) and the hypoxic condition also aggravate the DR (Nyengaard et al. 2004; Hammes et al. 2011). Formation of the advanced glycation end product in hypoglycemic condition blocks the blood vessels which ultimately lead to the change in the microvascular structure of eye retinal tissue (Antonetti et al. 2006). Inadequate perfusion in the blood vessels activates the hypoxia-induced factor (HIF-1α) regulated through the PI3K/AKT signalling pathway, which causes the upregulation of VEGF and it led to the unorganized growth of blood vessels. This condition exacerbates the loss of retinal neurons by inducing apoptotic cell death (Ozaki et al. 1999; Cheng et al. 2017).

Vitrectomy is the surgical technique adopted to treat the DR. It involves the complete removal of the vitreous gel and unorganized blood vessels to focus the light on the retina properly (Faulborn et al. 1977; Cairns and Fraco 1988). Corticosteroid is administered through the intravitreal injection to reduce the swelling near the retina (macular region) and to slow down the vision loss (Sarao et al. 2014). Apatinib-loaded nanoparticle are a novel treatment strategy that targets the inhibition of VEGF (Halasz et al. 2019). Antibody-based anti-VEGF agent (ranibizumab and aflibercept) downregulates the expression of VEGF and thus reduces the complication associated with the retina (Fallah et al. 2019). Ranibizumab is a humanized recombinant antibody Fab(48kD) and has an affinity for pan-VEGF-A (Ferrara et al. 2006). Aflibercept (AFL) is also a member of anti-VEGF pharmacotherapy family. Both ranibizumab and AFL have different affinity to bind VEGF-A. Thus, the equilibrium association constant (Kd) is different for both drugs. The binding of AFL to VEGF-A is 100 times faster than ranibizumab. Thus, AFL neutralizes the VEGF-A with high potency (Papadopoulos et al. 2012) and reduces the retina complication (Zehetner et al. 2015).

12.2.1.8 Dry Eye Syndrome

It is a multifactorial ocular disease characterized by pain, inflammation, and ocular discomfort with a change in the composition of the ocular film. The treatment strategy involves the cationic nanoemulsion loaded with the cyclosporine A. Cationic gelatin-based nanoparticles deliver a plasmid encoding for MUC5AC protein which is used for the treatment. MUC5AC is gel-forming mucin released by the goblet cells of the conjunctiva (ocular surface consist of epithelial cells). It plays an important role in the maintenance of homeostasis of lacrimal fluid, and distribution of these components gets altered in dry eye syndrome (Danjo et al. 1998). MUC5AC gelatin NPs are successfully implicated on rabbit conjunctiva for the treatment of dry eye syndrome (Konat Zorzi et al. 2011).

12.3 Advantages of Nanoformulation Over Conventional Therapy

Blood-ocular barrier creates an obstacle in the delivery of drugs at the interior segment of the eye. This problem can be circumvented by nanoformulation-based targeted drug delivery. The biggest challenge in the pharmacotherapy is to achieve the required concentration of drug at the intended site with least toxicity. To tackle this issue potentially active ophthalmic preparation has been employed for the treatment. For ocular delivery of lipophilic drugs, nanoparticles, hydrogel, microparticle, and liposomal formulation have the potency to improve the drug bioavailability (Patravale et al. 2004). The formulation should be done in such a way that it improves the corneal and conjunctival permeability. The biodegradable or bioerodible polymer has a substantial advantage over the non-biodegradable system because the formulation has to be completely absorbed in the system for its easy excretion (Edelman et al. 2019). Drug release at the ocular site largely depends on the association of the drug with the polymeric carrier, and the drug should be completely dispersed within the polymers. Most commonly used polymeric carrier for ocular delivery is poly(alkyl cyanoacrylates) (Obinu et al. 2019), chitosan, poly(lactic acid) (Coolen et al. 2019), poly(acrylic acid) (Bogusz et al. 2019), poly(lactic-co-glycolic acid) (Ma et al. 2019), and Eudragit (Katara et al. 2019).

12.3.1 Advantages of Nanoformulation

(i) Cornea and conjunctival tissue surface have negative charge surface. Thus, cationic colloidal nanoparticles have better penetration through the ocular membrane and barriers. Few nanoparticles like chitosan and Eudragit RL/RS possess the positively charged surface (Bu et al. 2007).

(ii) Drug carrier composed of biodegradable material has no ocular toxicity (Agnihotri and Vavia 2009).

(iii) Polymeric nanoparticles do not have an irritant effect on the cornea, conjunctiva, and iris (Zhou et al. 2013).

(iv) Intravitreal administration of polylactic acid nanosphere loaded with 1% Adriamycin or doxorubicin provides the sustained released delivery of drugs. It follows the first-order kinetics by the efficient release of drug for approximately 2 weeks (Nakhlband and Barar 2011).

(v) Chitosan NP (deacetylated chitin) is a biocompatible and biodegradable polymer that can effectively penetrate the corneal epithelial cells and conjunctiva. It has shown the electrostatic interaction with the negative charge of the mucoadhesive layer (Paolicelli et al. 2009; Basaran and Yazan 2012).

(vi) Lipid-based nanoformulation (containing cationic lipid) has been used for gene delivery at the ocular cells (Liu et al. 2003).

(vii) Dendrimer-based nanoformulation has hydroxyl group, a number of amines, and carboxylate group at its surface which supports the control drug delivery at ocular sites (Kambhampati and Kannan 2013).

(viii) Ocular nanomedicine optimizes the bioavailability of the drugs at the ocular site. For example, the administration of acyclovir-PLA nanosphere in rabbit eye resulted in high drug level at the ocular site with sustained release of drug in comparison to drug formulation without nanocarrier (Giannavola et al. 2003). Nanosuspension shows the higher bioavailability at the ocular site in comparison to the microcrystalline formulation (Kassem et al. 2007).

(ix) Nanoformulation maximizes the drug absorption at ocular sites and increases the drug residence time in the conjunctiva and cornea. It also minimizes the precorneal drug loss (Almeida et al. 2015). The ocular bioavailability of ciprofloxacin hydrochloride can be improved by mucoadhesive chitosan-coated liposomes as a drug carrier which is formulated by thin-film hydration techniques using stearylamine, L-alpha-phosphatidylcholine, cholesterol, and diacetyl phosphate (Abdelbary 2011).

(x) Nanocarrier as a gene delivery approach improves the transport of nucleic acid components across different eye barriers due to its nanometric size (Wadhwa et al. 2009).

(xi) It encourages the intracellular penetration of mRNA, siRNA, or another polynucleotide into the target cells or ocular cells, and it also prevents the degradation of components (Raemdonck et al. 2013).

(xii) Sustained delivery of polynucleotide can also be possible (Saraiva et al. 2017).

12.3.2 Disadvantages of Conventional Dosage Forms

(i) It requires the repetitive administration of the medicaments which cause poor patient compliance (Ako-Adounvo et al. 2014).

(ii) It is difficult to insert the "ocular inserts."

(iii) It is an invasive approach for treatment. So, there is a chance of tissue damage at the ocular site. Sometimes it requires the help of others for instillations or implantation (Agrahari et al. 2016).

12.4 Transportation of Drug and Drug-Metabolizing Enzymes in Different Regions of the Eye

Some of the drug-metabolizing enzymes and drug transporters are endogenously expressed within the ocular cells (Table 12.1). Drugs used for topical application can penetrate the epithelial lining of cornea and conjunctiva. Different drug transporters (peptide and amino acid transporters) are found at this site. Expression of organic anion transporting polypeptide (OATP) is found in rat corneal epithelium (Ito et al. 2003; Gao et al. 2005). This OATP regulates the cellular uptake of neutral and anionic molecules. Organic cation transporters are studied in the rabbit conjunctival epithelium (Ueda et al. 2000). Nucleoside and nucleobase transporters are expressed in the cornea and help in the transport of nucleoside analogues ganciclovir and acyclovir with the involvement of simple passive diffu-

Table 12.1 Distribution of different drug transporters proteins in the human eye

Drug transporters	Site of expression	Substrate molecules	Ref.
L-type amino acid transporters (LAT1)	Cornea	Amino acids	Jain-Vakkalagadda et al. (2003)
Excitatory amino acid carrier (EAAC1)	Pigment retinal epithelium	Glutamate	Maenpaa et al. (2004)
Excitatory amino acid transporters (EAAT4)	Pigment retinal epithelium	Glutamate	(Maenpaa et al. 2004)
Glucose transporters (GLUT1)	Cornea, conjunctiva, retina, iris, ciliary body	Glucose	Bildin et al. (2001)
Monocarboxylate transporters (MCTs)	Pigment retinal epithelium	Monocarboxylate	Philp et al. (2003)
Organic cation transporters 3	Pigment retinal epithelium, conjunctiva	Organic cation	Ueda et al. (2000)
P-glycoprotein	Cornea, conjunctiva, retina, pigment retinal epithelium	Large neutral or cationic compound	Kawazu et al. (1999); Jain-Vakkalagadda et al. (2003); Dey et al. (2004); Pitkanen et al. (2005)
Multidrug resistance protein	Pigment retinal epithelium	Large neutral or anionic molecules, sulfate conjugates, glutathione, glucuronide	Aukunuru et al. (2001)

sion (Majumdar et al. 2003). Expression of different drug transport proteins at the blood-retinal barrier provides us with an opportunity for the successful delivery of the drug to the retina and posterior region of the eye.

Drug-metabolizing enzymes are widely distributed in different regions of the eye. Different isoforms of the CYP family are expressed in different ocular tissues and play a vital role in drug metabolism. It corresponds to the unique function served by the tissue. We put more emphasis on the hydrolytic, oxidative, and conjugating enzymes present in the ocular region. Cytochrome P450 (CYP) enzyme is the heme-containing protein having a preponderant role in the metabolism of commercial drugs and other nanoformulations (Parkinson 1996). The expression level is very high in the liver. The high expression level of CYP1B1 mRNA is found in the nonpigmented epithelium of human eye's ciliary body and in the iris (Coca-Prados and Escribano 2007; Volotinen et al. 2009). CYP catalyzes different chemical reactions such as dehalogenation; N-oxidation; aromatic and side chain hydroxylation; N-hydroxylation; deamination; N-, S-, O-dealkylation; sulfoxidation; and desulfuration (Gilman et al. 2001). The homozygous mutation in CYP1B1 gene that codes for the CYP1B1 is located in chromosome number 2p22-p21, and this is linked to congenital glaucoma (Messina-Baas et al. 2007).

12.4.1 Cytochrome P450 in the Ocular Region

The microsomal electron transport system is first identified in the bovine retinal epithelium (Shichi 1969) to elaborate the CYP distribution in the ocular region. With the advancement of molecular biology, various genes and proteins are identified in the ocular region which supports different functional activity and helps in the drug metabolism. The expression of CYP1A2 and CYP1A1 is identified in the mouse iris and ciliary epithelium by using in situ hybridization and immunohistochemistry. It helps in the metabolism of polyaromatic hydrocarbon compounds (McAvoy et al. 1996). Similarly, CYP2B1/2 is expressed in rat lens (McAvoy et al. 1996). CYP2C is an enzyme that participated in the metabolism of diclofenac and propranolol, and it was identified in the mouse eye (Tsao et al. 2001). This drug-metabolizing enzyme shows the tissue-specific distribution within the eye (Table 12.2). Corneal

Table 12.2 Drug-metabolizing enzyme at the ocular site

Name of the enzyme	Substrate involved	Description	Ref.
Aldehyde oxidase	Brimonidine	Molybdenum-containing enzyme has a role in the nicotine metabolism (Berkman et al. 1995) and synthesis of retinoic acid (Huang et al. 1999). It is expressed in rabbit ocular tissue (Huang et al. 1999). Brimonidine is a selective α2-adrenoceptor agonist used to minimize the intraocular pressure	Acheampong et al. (1995)
Ketone reductase	Levobunolol and ketanserine	It is NADPH dependent and its activity is identified in the epithelium of the cornea, lens, conjunctiva, and iris-ciliary (Lee et al. 1988). Both substrates reduce the intraocular pressure. Its activity is pH dependent within the cornea	Schoenwald and Zhu (2000)
Hydrolytic enzymes like N-acetyl-beta glucosamidase, acid phosphatase, arylsulfatase, esterase (Essner et al. 1978)	Dipivefrin and echothiophate as esterase inhibitors	Esterase like acetylcholinesterase and carboxylesterase is found in the retina and other ocular tissue (Lee et al. 1985; Stampfli and Quon 1995). Esterase enzymes hydrolyze the ester linkage in the xenobiotics	Mindel et al. (1981)
Conjugating enzymes Arylamines acetyltransferase, glutathione-S-transferase	Aminozolamide and paraminobenzoic acid, polyunsaturated fatty acid	It controls ocular hypertension. Glutathione-S-transferase identified in the cornea, retina and iris-ciliary body (Srivastava et al. 1994)	Campbell et al. (1991); Srivastava et al. (1994)

cells contain a number of detoxifying enzymes which provide defense mechanism for the eye.

12.5 Drug-Associated Ocular Toxicity

12.5.1 Methanol-Induced Ocular Toxicity

Methanol has environmental public health concern since it can produce neurotoxic metabolites like formic acid, in the retina, in the CNS, and on the optic nerve. Formic acid causes ocular toxicity in an animal model. It is less toxic at a lower concentration. However, the adverse effect is shown when it is accumulated within the ocular region. Consumption of alcohol, surplus use of perfumes, anti-freezing agent, and inhalation of formaldehyde causes an increase in the level of methanol within the body. Toxic effect of methanol on ocular vision has been tested on animal models such as rat (Andrews et al. 1987; Stanton et al. 1995), mice (Bolon et al. 1993), and rabbit (Hayasaka et al. 2001). Excess of methanol administration causes the optic edema (observed within 48 hours), metabolic acidosis due to formate accumulation in the blood. Methanol undergoes metabolic activity and forms a toxic metabolite formic acid and it causes the ocular toxicity. The serum concentration of methanol exceeding more than 20 mg/dl correlates to ocular toxicity (Martin-Amat et al. 1978). Optical injury can be cured by the elimination of toxic metabolites by hemodialysis or antidote therapy.

12.5.2 Ocular Toxicity Induced by the Fluoroquinolones

Fluoroquinolone classes of drugs are commonly used for the treatment against bacterial infection (Sharma 2011). Fluoroquinolones are 4-oxo-1,4-dihydroquinoline and have antibacterial property. Position of carboxylic acid and ketocarboxyl group in the quinolone ring is responsible for antimicrobial activity. It inhibits the bacterial DNA gyrase (topoisomerase II) which is four subunits bacterial enzyme responsible for DNA supercoiling and replication of DNA in bacteria (Mustaev et al. 2014). Topical and systemic administration of fluoroquinolones can penetrate the ocular tissue to achieve the MIC_{90} value for inhibition of bacteria (von Gunten et al. 1994; Levine et al. 2004). Eye skin is very prone to phototoxicity which can be induced by the fluoroquinolones. Phototoxicity is mainly caused by the halogen group (fluorine or chlorine) present at the eight positions of the quinolones ring identified in lomefloxacin, clinafloxacin, fleroxacin, and sparfloxacin (Domagala 1994; Tripathi et al. 2002; Stahlmann 2002). Ofloxacin has antibacterial tendency, but including that topical application of ofloxacin reduces the number of goblet cells. It also affects the corneal epithelium by forming a white crystalline deposit or precipitate, this event identified due to topical application of ciprofloxacin and norfloxacin. SEM analysis has revealed the polydisperse crystalline needle-like precipitate having length 183 μm due to ciprofloxacin toxicity (Essepian et al. 1995). Low aqueous solubility of the drug facilitates the precipitation at the physiological pH (Cutarelli et al. 1991). Other toxicity caused by this drug may lead to cellular disorganization. Stromal edema induced by the drug is dose-dependent, and it is observed due to topical administration of the drug. Prolonged administration of these drugs may cause the cataract with the opacification of the eye lens. Intravitreal safety of fluoroquinolones needs to be checked in a different age group.

12.5.3 Pesticide Exposure and Ocular Toxicity

Pesticide exposure via inhalation, ingestion, ocular contact, and dermal contact can affect different parts of the body including the eye (Jaga and Dharmani 2006; Damalas and Eleftherohorinos 2011). It shows the dose-dependent response in various parts of the body. It mostly affects the cornea, conjunctiva, eye lens, optic nerve, and retina. Farmers working in the agricultural field are very prone to pesticide exposure. Opticoautonomic peripheral neuropathy has been reported in Japan where the organophosphates (OPs) as pesticide are most commonly used (Ishikawa 1996). Carbamate insecticide has high potency to penetrate the retina via the cornea, aqueous humor, and vitreous humor (Budai et al. 2004). Ocular toxicity caused by pesticide (namely, organophosphate fenthion, malathion, ethylthiometon, ethyl parathion, and fenitrothion) has been studied in different animal species (Dementi 1994). Organophosphate inhibits the activity of cholinesterase (ChE) enzyme in the whole blood, in the red blood cells, and mainly in the serum (Jaga and Dharmani 2003). ChE is also found in the ocular tissue, retina, cornea, choroid, iris, and extraocular muscles with high extent of acetylcholinesterase activity (Dementi 1994). Conjunctiva gets the highest exposure to different pesticides as compared to another part of the eyes, and it reacts to the chemical and causes the inflammation, edema, and congestion (Jaga and Dharmani 2006). Several studies also suggested that the farmers exposed to OP are more prone to change in the structure of retina with damage to macula region which ultimately leads to complete loss of vision in a short span of time and sometimes it has also shown the symptom of age-related macular degeneration (Kirrane et al. 2005).

Exposure to pesticides also impacts the cell cycle, and sometimes it leads to cell death, keratectasia, and corneal neovascularization (Sanyal et al. 2017). Increased rate of apoptosis in the ocular cells has been also identified (Jaga and Dharmani 2006), and sometimes slower cell growth is observed due to organophosphate exposure (Sanyal and Law 2019). Pesticide exposure causes a decrease in the expression of cyclin-D1/CDK4, which disturbs the G1/S phase of the cell cycle in the corneal cells (Sanyal and Law 2019). It also decreases the expression of PCNA which declines the DNA synthesis. It also affects the G2/M phase of the cell cycle. Protein phosphatase (PP) has a paramount role in the cell cycle. Decreased expression of PP1 and PP2A was found with increasing the phosphor-cdc25c (Sanyal and Law 2019). Dephosphorylation of cdc25c at serine residue activates the protein, and it is the hallmark of inhibition of G2/M phase due to pesticide exposure with decreasing PP1, aurora kinase A, and PP2A expression (Sanyal and Law 2019). Chronic exposure of pesticides also induces some cell cycle inhibitors like p21, GSK3β, and p18 which have an adverse effect on corneal epithelial cells.

12.5.4 Ocular Toxicity by Ophthalmic Anesthetics

Cocaine, proparacaine, tetracaine, oxybuprocaine, and lidocaine are the most commonly used ophthalmic anesthetics with some known adverse reactions such as corneal ulceration, corneal perforation, and corneal infiltrates with the least systemic side effect (McGee and Fraunfelder 2007). Ophthalmic anesthetics may also cause refractory corneal lesion and neurotrophic ulcers (McGee and Fraunfelder 2007). It acts by blocking the sodium channels and preventing the conduction of nerve impulses along the axon. It has the potential to inhibit the migration of corneal epithelial cells and causes damage specifically to microvilli (Burns and Gipson 1978). The formation of yellowish-white stromal infiltrate represents the antigen-antibody immune complex formation within the stromal region, and this condition is also observed in herpetic keratitis (Meyers-Elliott et al. 1980).

12.5.5 Ocular Toxicity Associated with Antibody-Drug Conjugates (ADCs)

The eye is susceptible to ADC-induced toxicity due to the presence of a number of cell surface receptors, high blood supply, and high population of rapidly dividing cells (Table 12.3). Similarly, monoclonal antibodies have a diverse effect on various regions of the eye. IMGN242 (huC242-DM4) is the humanized antibody having an affinity for tumor-associated epitope that causes the decrease in visual acuity, keratitis, and corneal deposits (Mita et al. 2007). Mechanism of ocular toxicity is not clearly understood.

Table 12.3 Ocular toxicity associated with administration of antibody-drug conjugates (ADC)

ADC	Indication	Target antigen or linker molecules	Ocular toxicity or symptom	Ref.
Trastuzumab emtansine (T-DM1)	Advanced HER2+ Breast cancer	HER2/DM1/SMCC	Swollen tear duct, conjunctivitis, photophobia	Krop et al. (2010)
Trastuzumab emtansine (T-DM1)	Advanced HER2+ Breast cancer	HER2/DM1/SMCC	Cataract, dry eye, ocular surface disease, punctuate keratitis	Beeram et al. (2012)
SAR3419 (huB4-DM4)	Relapsed/refractory B-cell NHL	CD19/DM4/SPDB	Corneal deposit/microcysts, weekly blurred vision, optic neuropathy	Ribrag et al. (2014)
SGN-CD19A	Relapsed or refractory B-lineage acute leukemia and highly aggressive lymphoma	CD19/MMAF (auristatin)/mc	Superficial microcystic keratopathy, blurred vision, dry eye	Fathi et al. (2014)
Gemtuzumab ozogamicin	Acute myeloid leukemia	CD33/calicheamicin/hydrazine	Ocular bleeding (anatomic location not identified)	Piccaluga et al. (2004)
Lorvotuzumab mertansine (IMGN901)	CD56+ solid tumors	CD56/DM1/SPP	Eye redness	Woll et al. (2010)
IMGN853	Platinum-resistant epithelial ovarian cancer	FRa/DM4/SPDB	Blurred vision, eye pain, keratitis, corneal cyst, punctate keratitis, corneal epithelial microcysts, retinal vein occlusion/vision impairment	Moore et al. (2015)

12.5.6 Ocular Toxicity Associated with Homeostasis Imbalance

Various pharmaceutical preparations cause the toxicity due to poor quality of preservative and vehicle used for the preparation (Table 12.4). For example, excess of benzyl alcohol in ocular preparation causes the injurious effect in the intraocular segment of the eye(Lang et al. 2007). Change in pH and osmolarity of preparation also have a deleterious effect on the retina. Osmolarity higher than 500 mOsm causes the cellular damage in the vitreoretinal interface with disruption of cellular machinery in the eye. Intravitreal injection of dye also induces the drastic change in the osmolarity of the vitreous cavity. Homeostasis of electrolyte balance, pH, and osmolarity is essential for the delicate tissue of the intraocular site. Intravitreal route of administration has been used in high frequency for the treatment of retinal disease which requires a solvent with balanced pH and osmolarity (Brissette et al. 2019).

12.6 Gene Delivery with Nanoformulation at Ocular Site

Newly designed lipid nanoparticles can be employed for the delivery of mRNA to the posterior region of the eye. Lipid nanoparticles enter the cell by using the inducible and constitutive pathway by using the clathrin-mediated endocytosis and micropinocytosis (Diebold and Calonge 2010; Oh and Park 2014). Retinal gene therapy has garnered much attention to the treatment of vision loss (Patel et al. 2019). mRNA therapy has expatiated the ability to attain a high level of gene expression. Gene therapy is cell specific with high expression level at retinal pigmented epithelium. Dysfunctional retinal protein is associated with diabetic retinopathy, glaucoma, and age-related macular degeneration. Gene therapy-based treatment strategy has been adopted in this disorder. The surface of nanoparticles can be fab-

Table 12.4 Ocular toxicity/retinal toxicity associated with current existing drug

A major class of drug	Indication	Toxicity symptom	Ref.
Corticosteroid	Retinal disease, uveitis, glaucoma, cataract	Damage to photoreceptor, endophthalmitis and pseudoendophthalmitis, in around 0.5% of patients (Maia et al. 2007)	Holekamp et al. (2005); Penha et al. (2010)
Antibiotics	Infectious endophthalmitis and uveitis, posterior segment viral uveitis	Intravitreal injection of antibiotics leads to retinal toxicity	Penha et al. (2010)
Aminoglycosides	Amikacin used in treatment of endophthalmitis	Toxicity are seen in the retina, nerve fibre and inner plexiform layer (Hancock et al. 2005)	Penha et al. (2010)
Cephalosporins	Ceftazidime used in the treatment of endophthalmitis	No toxicity at 2.25 mg dose but cause retinal toxicity at high dose (Campochiaro and Green 1992)	Penha et al. (2010)
Vancomycin	Kill gram-positive microorganisms	Postoperative cystoid macular edema (Hegazy et al. 1999)	Penha et al. (2010)
Antifungal agents	Prevent the fungal infection in the eye, intraocular fungal infection	10, 20, 30 to 50 μg doses of amphotericin B cause stronger degrees of retinal toxicity(Khan et al. 2007)	Penha et al. (2010)
Antiviral agents	Cytomegalovirus infection and other viral infection	Ganciclovir in doses >300 μg induces the retinal damage, macular infarction; intravitreal injection of ganciclovir (40 mg/0.1 ml) for CMV retinitis in a subject suffering from AIDS led to irreversible retinal damage resulting in complete visual loss (Saran and Maguire 1994)	Hegazy et al. (1999); Penha et al. (2010)
5-fluorouracil	Inhibits the proliferation and contraction of intraocular fibroblasts	Retinal toxicity caused by 5-FU reported in animal models	Blumenkranz et al. (1984)
Nonsteroidal anti-inflammatory drugs	Cystoid Macular edema	Commercially available NSAIDs ketorolac (3 mg/0.1 ml) is toxic observed in albino rabbit eyes	Komarowska et al. (2009)

ricated with targeting ligand for the cell surface-specific delivery of gene or nucleic acid (Pollinger et al. 2013). These lipid nanoparticles are composed of different cationic or anionic lipid which is assembled in such a way that it can mix with the aqueous solution containing the nucleic acid by using the microfluidic mixing techniques (Belliveau et al. 2012). Ionizable lipid is responsible for electrostatic binding with the nucleic acid and its encapsulation within the nanocarrier. Amphiphilic nature of ionizable lipid is responsible for the binding with mRNA due to the positive charge of this lipid that binds with mRNA and organized itself in the lipid nanoparticles structure. Two regions of this ionizable lipid have a role in endosomal escape and encapsulation efficiency. Lipid nanoparticles possess the ionizable lipid with the low pKa value and having unsaturated hydrocarbon chain showing the reporter gene transfection in the retina after subretinal injection. Unsaturated hydrocarbon supports the membrane destabilization to facilitate the endosomal escape (Heyes et al. 2005).

Gene delivery by using the viral and nonviral vector has great promise for the intervention of ocular diseases. This therapy either depends on gene replacement or gene regulation. To increase the intracellular delivery of mRNA, more than 212 lipid molecules have been screened which modulate the cell signalling events (Patel et al. 2017). Lipid nanoparticles are adopted as the most advanced technique to deliver the siRNA; here also the multiple lipid system encapsulates the SiRNA (Gilleron et al. 2013). Lipid nanoparticles as a carrier have shown the robust mRNA silencing in the human clinical trial (Gilleron et al. 2013). Compact DNA nanoparticles are also used for nonviral gene transfer in ocular cells (Farjo et al. 2006). Hyaluronic acid-chitosan NP has also been used for the ocular gene delivery. It facilitates the delivery of a gene to the cornea and conjunctiva (De la Fuente et al. 2008). This nanoparticle is synthesized by the ionotropic gelation method. The mucoadhesive NP has a high residence time with the ocular surface.

12.7 Conclusion

The current chapter summarizes how different pharmaceuticals product affects the ocular cells. Molecular biology research has already elaborated the genetic basis of the different eye diseases. By keeping this in mind, different nanoformulation has been successfully employed as a carrier for delivery of drug molecules, mRNA, siRNA, and other polynucleotides for the treatment of diseases. This treatment strategy directly impacts the target cells. Several eye diseases linked with eye's posterior and anterior segment can be cured with the nanocarrier based on gene delivery. All ophthalmic preparations are not safe, and many drugs associated with ocular toxicity have been also reported. Thus, utmost care should be taken before administration of the nanoformulations to the patient, and dosage regimen should be fixed for the different age groups.

Acknowledgments SP is thankful to MHRD and JB is thankful to BT/PR21857/NNT/28/1238/2017 for financial support. MM lab is supported by Grant No. BT/PR21857/NNT/28/1238/2017, EMR/2017/003054, Odisha DBT 3325/ST(BIO)-02/2017.

References

Abdelbary G (2011) Ocular ciprofloxacin hydrochloride mucoadhesive chitosan-coated liposomes. Pharm Dev Technol 16(1):44–56

Abramson DH, Frank CM, Dunkel IJ (1999) A phase I/II study of subconjunctival carboplatin for intraocular retinoblastoma. Ophthalmology 106(10):1947–1950

Acheampong AA, Shackleton M, Tang-Liu D (1995) Comparative ocular pharmacokinetics of brimonidine after a single dose application to the eyes of albino and pigmented rabbits. Drug Metab Dispos 23(7):708–712

Aggarwal D, Pal D, Mitra AK, Kaur IP (2007) Study of the extent of ocular absorption of acetazolamide from a developed niosomal formulation, by microdialysis sampling of aqueous humor. Int J Pharm 338(1–2):21–26

Agnihotri SM, Vavia PR (2009) Diclofenac-loaded biopolymeric nanosuspensions for ophthalmic application. Nanomedicine 5(1):90–95

Agrahari V, Agrahari V, Hung W-T, Christenson LK, Mitra AK (2016) Composite nanoformulation therapeutics for long-term ocular delivery of macromolecules. Mol Pharm 13(9):2912–2922

Ahmed F, Ali MJ, Kondapi AK (2014) Carboplatin loaded protein nanoparticles exhibit improve antiproliferative activity in retinoblastoma cells. Int J Biol Macromol 70:572–582

Ako-Adounvo A-M, Nagarwal RC, Oliveira L, Boddu SH, Wang XS, Dey S, Karla PK (2014) Recent patents on ophthalmic nanoformulations and therapeutic implications. Recent Pat Drug Deliv Formul 8(3):193–201

Almeida H, Amaral MH, Lobao P, Frigerio C, Manuel Sousa Lobo J (2015) Nanoparticles in ocular drug delivery systems for topical administration: promises and challenges. Curr Pharm Des 21(36):5212–5224

Alsaab H, Alzhrani R, Kesharwani P, Sau S, Boddu S, Iyer A (2017) Folate decorated nanomicelles loaded with a potent curcumin analogue for targeting retinoblastoma. Pharmaceutics 9(2):15

Andrews L, Clary JJ, Terrill J, Bolte HF (1987) Subchronic inhalation toxicity of methanol. J Toxicol Environ Health 20(1–2):117–124

Antonetti DA, Barber AJ, Bronson SK, Freeman WM, Gardner TW, Jefferson LS, Kester M, Kimball SR, Krady JK, LaNoue KF (2006) Diabetic retinopathy: seeing beyond glucose-induced microvascular disease. Diabetes 55(9):2401–2411

Argikar UA, Dumouchel JL, Kramlinger VM, Cirello AL, Gunduz M, Dunne CE, Sohal B (2017) Do we need to study metabolism and distribution in the eye: why, when, and are we there yet? J Pharm Sci 106(9):2276–2281

Aukunuru JV, Sunkara G, Bandi N, Thoreson WB, Kompella UB (2001) Expression of multidrug resistance-associated protein (MRP) in human retinal pigment epithelial cells and its interaction with BAPSG, a novel aldose reductase inhibitor. Pharm Res 18(5):565–572

Babizhayev MA, Deyev AI, Yermakova VN, Semiletov YA, Davydova NG, Doroshenko VS, Zhukotskii AV, Goldman IM (2002) Efficacy of N-acetylcarnosine in the treatment of cataracts. Drugs R D 3(2):87–103

Badawi AA, El-Laithy HM, El Qidra RK, El Mofty H (2008) Chitosan based nanocarriers for indomethacin ocular delivery. Arch Pharm Res 31(8):1040

Basaran E, Yazan Y (2012) Ocular application of chitosan. Expert Opin Drug Deliv 9(6):701–712

Beeram M, Krop IE, Burris HA, Girish SR, Yu W, Lu MW, Holden SN, Modi S (2012) A phase 1 study of weekly dosing of trastuzumab emtansine (T-DM1) in patients with advanced human epidermal growth factor 2–positive breast cancer. Cancer 118(23):5733–5740

Belliveau NM, Huft J, Lin PJ, Chen S, Leung AK, Leaver TJ, Wild AW, Lee JB, Taylor RJ, Tam YK (2012) Microfluidic synthesis of highly potent limit-size lipid nanoparticles for in vivo delivery of siRNA. Mol Ther Nucleic Acids 1:e37

Bennett L (2016) Drug delivery to specific compartments of the eye. In: Ocular drug delivery: advances, challenges and applications. Springer, USA. pp 37–52

Berkman CE, Park SB, Wrighton SA, Cashman JR (1995) In vitro-in vivo correlations of human (S)-nicotine metabolism. Biochem Pharmacol 50(4):565–570

Bildin VN, Iserovich P, Fischbarg J, Reinach PS (2001) Differential expression of Na: K: 2CI cotransporter, glucose transporter 1, and aquaporin 1 in freshly isolated and cultured bovine corneal tissues. Exp Biol Med 226(10):919–926

Bird A, Bressler NM, Bressler SB, Chisholm I, Coscas G, Davis M, De Jong P, Klaver C, Klein B, Klein R (1995) An international classification and grading system for age-related maculopathy and age-related macular degeneration. Surv Ophthalmol 39(5):367–374

Blumenkranz M, Hernandez E, Ophir A, Norton EW (1984) 5-fluorouracil: new applications in complicated retinal detachment for an established antimetabolite. Ophthalmology 91(2):122–130

Bogusz K, Zuchora M, Sencadas V, Tehei M, Lerch M, Thorpe N, Rosenfeld A, Dou SX, Liu HK, Konstantinov K (2019) Synthesis of methotrexate-loaded tantalum pentoxide–poly (acrylic acid) nanoparticles for controlled drug release applications. J Colloid Interface Sci 538:286–296

Bolon B, Dorman DC, Janszen D, Morgan KT, Welsch F (1993) Phase-specific developmental toxicity in mice following maternal methanol inhalation. Fundam Appl Toxicol 21(4):508–516

Brissette AR, Drinkwater OJ, Bohm KJ, Starr CE (2019) The utility of a normal tear osmolarity test in patients presenting with dry eye disease like symptoms: a prospective analysis. Cont Lens Anterior Eye 42(2):185–189

Bu H-Z, Gukasyan HJ, Goulet L, Lou X-J, Xiang C, Koudriakova T (2007) Ocular disposition, pharmacokinetics, efficacy and safety of nanoparticle-formulated ophthalmic drugs. Curr Drug Metab 8(2):91–107

Budai P, Varnagy L, Fejes S, Somlyay I, Linczmayer K, Pongracz A (2004) Irritative effects of some pesticides and a technical component on tissue structure of the chorioallantoic membrane. Commun Agric Appl Biol Sci 69(4):807–809

Budai L, Hajdu M, Budai M, Grof P, Beni S, Noszal B, Klebovich I, Antal I (2007) Gels and liposomes in optimized ocular drug delivery: studies on ciprofloxacin formulations. Int J Pharm 343(1–2):34–40

Burns RP, Gipson I (1978) Toxic effects of local anesthetics. JAMA 240(4):347–347

Cairns JD, Fraco WGC (1988) Vitrectomy techniques in the treatment of giant retinal tears: a flexible approach. Aust N Z J Ophthalmol 16(3):209–214

Campbell D, Schoenwald R, Duffel M, Barfknecht C (1991) Characterization of arylamine acetyltransferase in the rabbit eye. Invest Ophthalmol Vis Sci 32(8):2190–2200

Campochiaro PA, Green WR (1992) Toxicity of intravitreous ceftazidime in primate retina. Arch Ophthalmol 110(11):1625–1629

Campochiaro PA, Nguyen QD, Shah SM, Klein ML, Holz E, Frank RN, Saperstein DA, Gupta A, Stout JT, Macko J (2006) Adenoviral vector-delivered pigment epithelium-derived factor for neovascular age-related macular degeneration: results of a phase I clinical trial. Hum Gene Ther 17(2):167–176

Carli F, Baronian M, Schmid R, Chiellini E (2013) Ophthalmic oil-in-water emulsions containing prostaglandins. Google Patents

Carroll RT, Bhatia D, Geldenhuys W, Bhatia R, Miladore N, Bishayee A, Sutariya V (2010) Brain-targeted delivery of Tempol-loaded nanoparticles for neurological disorders. J Drug Target 18(9):665–674

Chan H, Canton M, Gallie B (1989) Chemosensitivity and multidrug resistance to antineoplastic drugs in retinoblastoma cell lines. Anticancer Res 9(2):469–474

Chandasana H, Prasad YD, Chhonker YS, Chaitanya TK, Mishra NN, Mitra K, Shukla PK, Bhatta RS (2014) Corneal targeted nanoparticles for sustained natamycin delivery and their PK/PD indices: an approach to reduce dose and dosing frequency. Int J Pharm 477(1–2):317–325

Cheng L, Yu H, Yan N, Lai K, Xiang M (2017) Hypoxia-inducible factor-1α target genes contribute to retinal neuroprotection. Front Cell Neurosci 11:20

Chhonker YS, Prasad YD, Chandasana H, Vishvkarma A, Mitra K, Shukla PK, Bhatta RS (2015) Amphotericin-B entrapped lecithin/chitosan nanoparticles for prolonged ocular application. Int J Biol Macromol 72:1451–1458

Chiang A, Regillo CD (2011) Preferred therapies for neovascular age-related macular degeneration. Curr Opin Ophthalmol 22(3):199–204

Cholkar K, Patel SP, Vadlapudi AD, Mitra AK (2013) Novel strategies for anterior segment ocular drug delivery. J Ocul Pharmacol Ther 29(2):106–123

Coca-Prados M, Escribano J (2007) New perspectives in aqueous humor secretion and in glaucoma: the ciliary body as a multifunctional neuroendocrine gland. Prog Retin Eye Res 26(3):239–262

Coolen A-L, Lacroix C, Mercier-Gouy P, Delaune E, Monge C, Exposito J-Y, Verrier B (2019) Poly (lactic acid) nanoparticles and cell-penetrating peptide potentiate mRNA-based vaccine expression in dendritic cells triggering their activation. Biomaterials 195:23–37

Craig JP, Singh I, Tomlinson A, Morgan PB, Efron N (2000) The role of tear physiology in ocular surface temperature. Eye 14(4):635

Cruickshanks KJ, Klein B, Klein R (1992) Ultraviolet light exposure and lens opacities: the Beaver Dam Eye Study. Am J Public Health 82(12):1658–1662

Cunha-Vaz JG (1997) The blood-ocular barriers: past, present, and future. Doc Ophthalmol 93(1–2):149–157

Cutarelli PE, Lass JH, Lazarus HM, Putman SC, Jacobs MR (1991) Topical fluoroquinolones: antimicrobial activity and in vitro corneal epithelial toxicity. Curr Eye Res 10(6):557–563

Damalas CA, Eleftherohorinos IG (2011) Pesticide exposure, safety issues, and risk assessment indicators. Int J Environ Res Public Health 8(5):1402–1419

Danjo Y, Watanabe H, Tisdale AS, George M, Tsumura T, Abelson MB, Gipson IK (1998) Alteration of mucin in human conjunctival epithelia in dry eye. Invest Ophthalmol Vis Sci 39(13):2602–2609

Das S, Suresh PK, Desmukh R (2010) Design of Eudragit RL 100 nanoparticles by nanoprecipitation method for ocular drug delivery. Nanomedicine 6(2):318–323

de Kaspar HM, Koss MJ, He L, Blumenkranz MS, Ta CN (2005) Antibiotic susceptibility of preoperative normal conjunctival bacteria. Am J Ophthalmol 139(4):730–733

De la Fuente M, Seijo B, Alonso MJ (2008) Novel hyaluronic acid-chitosan nanoparticles for ocular gene therapy. Invest Ophthalmol Vis Sci 49(5):2016–2024

del Amo EM, Rimpela A-K, Heikkinen E, Kari OK, Ramsay E, Lajunen T, Schmitt M, Pelkonen L, Bhattacharya M, Richardson D (2017) Pharmacokinetic aspects of retinal drug delivery. Prog Retin Eye Res 57:134–185

Delcourt C, Carriere I, Ponton-Sanchez A, Lacroux A, Covacho M-J, Papoz L (2000a) Light exposure and the risk of cortical, nuclear, and posterior subcapsular cataracts: the Pathologies Oculaires Liees a l'Age (POLA) study. Arch Ophthalmol 118(3):385–392

Delcourt C, Cristol J-P, Tessier F, Leger CL, Michel F, Papoz L, Group P S (2000b) Risk factors for cortical, nuclear, and posterior subcapsular cataracts: the POLA study. Am J Epidemiol 151(5):497–504

Dementi B (1994) Ocular effects of organophosphates: a historical perspective of Saku disease. J Appl Toxicol 14(2):119–129

Dey S, Patel J, Anand BS, Jain-Vakkalagadda B, Kaliki P, Pal D, Ganapathy V, Mitra AK (2003) Molecular evidence and functional expression of P-glycoprotein (MDR1) in human and rabbit cornea and corneal epithelial cell lines. Invest Ophthalmol Vis Sci 44(7):2909–2918

Dey S, Gunda S, Mitra AK (2004) Pharmacokinetics of erythromycin in rabbit corneas after single-dose infusion: role of P-glycoprotein as a barrier to in vivo ocular drug absorption. J Pharmacol Exp Ther 311(1):246–255

Diebold Y, Calonge M (2010) Applications of nanoparticles in ophthalmology. Prog Retin Eye Res 29(6):596–609

Domagala JM (1994) Structure-activity and structure-side-effect relationships for the quinolone antibacterials. J Antimicrob Chemother 33(4):685–706

Edelman JL, Hughes PM, Malone TC, DeVries GW, Chang-Lin J-E, Shiah J-G, Nivaggioli T, Spada LT, Blanda WM (2019) Biodegradable intravitreal tyrosine kinase implants. Google Patents

Eljarrat-Binstock E, Raiskup F, Stepensky D, Domb AJ, Frucht-Pery J (2004) Delivery of gentamicin to the rabbit eye by drug-loaded hydrogel iontophoresis. Invest Ophthalmol Vis Sci 45(8):2543–2548

El-Kamel A (2002) In vitro and in vivo evaluation of Pluronic F127-based ocular delivery system for timolol maleate. Int J Pharm 241(1):47–55

Elsinga PH, Hendrikse NH, Bart J, Vaalburg W, Waarde AV (2004) PET studies on P-glycoprotein function in the blood-brain barrier: how it affects uptake and binding of drugs within the CNS. Curr Pharm Des 10(13):1493–1503

Essepian JP, Rajpal R, O'Brien TP (1995) Tandem scanning confocal microscopic analysis of ciprofloxacin corneal deposits in vivo. Cornea 14(4):402–407

Essner E, Gorrin GM, Griewski RA (1978) Localization of lysosomal enzymes in retinal pigment epithelium of rats with inherited retinal dystrophy. Invest Ophthalmol Vis Sci 17(3):278–288

Fallah A, Sadeghinia A, Kahroba H, Samadi A, Heidari HR, Bradaran B, Zeinali S, Molavi O (2019) Therapeutic targeting of angiogenesis molecular pathways in angiogenesis-dependent diseases. Biomed Pharmacother 110:775–785

Farjo R, Skaggs J, Quiambao AB, Cooper MJ, Naash MI (2006) Efficient non-viral ocular gene transfer with compacted DNA nanoparticles. PLoS One 1(1):e38

Fathi AT, Chen R, Trippett TM, O'Brien MM, DeAngelo DJ, Shah BD, Cooper TM, Foran JM, Hale GA, Pressey J (2014) Interim analysis of a phase 1 study of the antibody-drug conjugate SGN-CD19A in relapsed or refractory B-lineage acute leukemia and highly aggressive lymphoma. Am Soc Hematology

Faulborn J, Atkinson A, Olivier D (1977) Primary vitrectomy as a preventive surgical procedure in the treatment of severely injured eyes. Br J Ophthalmol 61(3):202–208

Ferrara N, Damico L, Shams N, Lowman H, Kim R (2006) Development of ranibizumab, an anti–vascular endothelial growth factor antigen binding fragment, as therapy for neovascular age-related macular degeneration. Retina 26(8):859–870

Fouda NH, Abdelrehim RT, Hegazy DA, Habib BA (2018) Sustained ocular delivery of Dorzolamide-HCl via proniosomal gel formulation: in-vitro characterization, statistical optimization, and in-vivo pharmacodynamic evaluation in rabbits. Drug Deliv 25(1):1340–1349

Freddo TF (2001) Shifting the paradigm of the blood–aqueous barrier. Exp Eye Res 73(5):581–592
Fresta M, Fontana G, Bucolo C, Cavallaro G, Giammona G, Puglisi G (2001) Ocular tolerability and in vivo bioavailability of poly (ethylene glycol)(PEG)-coated polyethyl-2-cyanoacrylate nanosphere-encapsulated acyclovir. J Pharm Sci 90(3):288–297
Frick KD, Gower EW, Kempen JH, Wolff JL (2007) Economic impact of visual impairment and blindness in the United States. Arch Ophthalmol 125(4):544–550
Fu J, Sun F, Liu W, Liu Y, Gedam M, Hu Q, Fridley C, Quigley HA, Hanes J, Pitha I (2016) Subconjunctival delivery of dorzolamide-loaded poly (ether-anhydride) microparticles produces sustained lowering of intraocular pressure in rabbits. Mol Pharm 13(9):2987–2995
Fullard RJ, Tucker D (1994) Tear protein composition and the effects of stimulus. In: Lacrimal gland, tear film, and dry eye syndromes. Springer, USA. pp 309–314
Gao B, Huber RD, Wenzel A, Vavricka SR, Ismair MG, Remé C, Meier PJ (2005) Localization of organic anion transporting polypeptides in the rat and human ciliary body epithelium. Exp Eye Res 80(1):61–72
Gaudana R, Ananthula HK, Parenky A, Mitra AK (2010) Ocular drug delivery. AAPS J 12(3):348–360
Gavini E, Chetoni P, Cossu M, Alvarez MG, Saettone MF, Giunchedi P (2004) PLGA microspheres for the ocular delivery of a peptide drug, vancomycin using emulsification/spray-drying as the preparation method: in vitro/in vivo studies. Eur J Pharm Biopharm 57(2):207–212
Ghate D, Edelhauser HF (2006) Ocular drug delivery. Expert Opin Drug Deliv 3(2):275–287
Giannavola C, Bucolo C, Maltese A, Paolino D, Vandelli MA, Puglisi G, Lee VH, Fresta M (2003) Influence of preparation conditions on acyclovir-loaded poly-d, l-lactic acid nanospheres and effect of PEG coating on ocular drug bioavailability. Pharm Res 20(4):584–590
Gilleron J, Querbes W, Zeigerer A, Borodovsky A, Marsico G, Schubert U, Manygoats K, Seifert S, Andree C, Stoter M (2013) Image-based analysis of lipid nanoparticle–mediated siRNA delivery, intracellular trafficking and endosomal escape. Nat Biotechnol 31(7):638
Gilman A, Hardman J, Limbird L (2001) Goodman and Gilman's, the pharmacological basis of therapeutics. McGraw-Hill, New York
Goldschmidt P, Degorge S, Sarria PC, Benallaoua D, Semoun O, Borderie V, Laroche L, Chaumeil C (2012) New strategy for rapid diagnosis and characterization of fungal infections: the example of corneal scrapings. PLoS One 7(7):e37660
Gonzalez L, Loza RJ, Han K-Y, Sunoqrot S, Cunningham C, Purta P, Drake J, Jain S, Hong S, Chang J-H (2013) Nanotechnology in corneal neovascularization therapy—a review. J Ocul Pharmacol Ther 29(2):124–134
Gupta N, Yucel YH (2007) Glaucoma as a neurodegenerative disease. Curr Opin Ophthalmol 18(2):110–114
Halasz K, Kelly SJ, Iqbal MT, Pathak Y, Sutariya V (2019) Utilization of Apatinib-loaded nanoparticles for the treatment of ocular neovascularization. Curr Drug Deliv 16(2):153–163
Hammes H-P, Feng Y, Pfister F, Brownlee M (2011) Diabetic retinopathy: targeting vasoregression. Diabetes 60(1):9–16
Hancock HA, Guidry C, Read RW, Ready EL, Kraft TW (2005) Acute aminoglycoside retinal toxicity in vivo and in vitro. Invest Ophthalmol Vis Sci 46(12):4804–4808
Hayasaka Y, Hayasaka S, Nagaki Y (2001) Ocular changes after intravitreal injection of methanol, formaldehyde, or formate in rabbits. Pharmacol Toxicol 89(2):74–78
Hegazy HM, Kivilcim M, Peyman GA, Unal MH, Liang C, Molinari LC, Kazi AA (1999) Evaluation of toxicity of intravitreal ceftazidime, vancomycin, and ganciclovir in a silicone oil-filled eye. Retina (Philadelphia, Pa) 19(6):553–557
Herrero-Vanrell R, Fernandez-Carballido A, Frutos G, Cadorniga R (2000) Enhancement of the mydriatic response to tropicamide by bioadhesive polymers. J Ocul Pharmacol Ther 16(5):419–428
Heyes J, Palmer L, Bremner K, MacLachlan I (2005) Cationic lipid saturation influences intracellular delivery of encapsulated nucleic acids. J Control Release 107(2):276–287
Holekamp NM, Thomas MA, Pearson A (2005) The safety profile of long-term, high-dose intraocular corticosteroid delivery. Am J Ophthalmol 139(3):421–428
Hovding G (2008) Acute bacterial conjunctivitis. Acta Ophthalmol 86(1):5–17
Huang D-Y, Furukawa A, Ichikawa Y (1999) Molecular cloning of retinal oxidase/aldehyde oxidase cDNAs from rabbit and mouse livers and functional expression of recombinant mouse retinal oxidase cDNA inEscherichia coli. Arch Biochem Biophys 364(2):264–272
Huhtala A, Salminen L, Tahti H, Uusitalo H (2008) Corneal models for the toxicity testing of drugs and drug releasing materials. Topics in Multifunctional Biomaterials and Devices, N Ashammakhi (Ed) © 2008, 1(2), pp 1–23
Ishikawa S (1996) Ophthalmopathy due to environmental toxic substances especially intoxication by organophosphorus pesticides. Nippon Ganka Gakkai Zasshi 100(6):417–432
Ito A, Yamaguchi K, Tomita H, Suzuki T, Onogawa T, Sato T, Mizutamari H, Mikkaichi T, Nishio T, Suzuki T (2003) Distribution of rat organic anion transporting polypeptide-E (oatp-E) in the rat eye. Invest Ophthalmol Vis Sci 44(11):4877–4884
Jaga K, Dharmani C (2003) Sources of exposure to and public health implications of organophosphate pesticides. Rev Panam Salud Publica 14:171–185
Jaga K, Dharmani C (2006) Ocular toxicity from pesticide exposure: a recent review. Environ Health Prev Med 11(3):102–107
Jain-Vakkalagadda B, Dey S, Pal D, Mitra AK (2003) Identification and functional characterization of a Na+–independent large neutral amino acid trans-

porter, LAT1, in human and rabbit cornea. Invest Ophthalmol Vis Sci 44(7):2919–2927
Jayaraman MS, Bharali DJ, Sudha T, Mousa SA (2012) Nano chitosan peptide as a potential therapeutic carrier for retinal delivery to treat age-related macular degeneration. Mol Vis 18:2300
Juuti-Uusitalo K, Vaajasaari H, Ryhanen T, Narkilahti S, Suuronen R, Mannermaa E, Kaarniranta K, Skottman H (2012) Efflux protein expression in human stem cell-derived retinal pigment epithelial cells. PLoS One 7(1):e30089
Kambhampati SP, Kannan RM (2013) Dendrimer nanoparticles for ocular drug delivery. J Ocul Pharmacol Ther 29(2):151–165
Kassem M, Rahman AA, Ghorab M, Ahmed M, Khalil R (2007) Nanosuspension as an ophthalmic delivery system for certain glucocorticoid drugs. Int J Pharm 340(1–2):126–133
Katara R, Sachdeva S, Majumdar DK (2019) Design, characterization, and evaluation of aceclofenac-loaded Eudragit RS 100 nanoparticulate system for ocular delivery. Pharm Dev Technol 24(3):368–379
Kaufman H, Brown D, Ellison E (1968) Herpes virus in the lacrimal gland, conjunctiva and cornea of man—a chronic infection. Am J Ophthalmol 65(1):32–35
Kawazu K, Yamada K, Nakamura M, Ota A (1999) Characterization of cyclosporin A transport in cultured rabbit corneal epithelial cells: P-glycoprotein transport activity and binding to cyclophilin. Invest Ophthalmol Vis Sci 40(8):1738–1744
Kelly S, Hirani A, Shahidadpury V, Solanki A, Halasz K, Varghese Gupta S, Madow B, Sutariya V (2018) Aflibercept nanoformulation inhibits VEGF expression in ocular in vitro model: a preliminary report. Biomedicine 6(3):92
Kelly SJ, Halasz K, Smalling R, Sutariya V (2019) Nanodelivery of doxorubicin for age-related macular degeneration. Drug Dev Ind Pharm 45(5):715–723
Keorochana N, Choontanom R (2017) Efficacy and safety of an extemporaneous preparation of 2% ganciclovir eye drops in CMV anterior uveitis. BMJ Open Ophthalmol 2(1):e000061
Khan FA, Slain D, Khakoo RA (2007) Candida endophthalmitis: focus on current and future antifungal treatment options. Pharmacotherapy 27(12):1711–1721
Khanna RC, Murthy GV, Giridhar P, Krishnaiah S, Pant HB, Shantha GPS, Chakrabarti S, Gilbert C, Rao GN (2013) Cataract, visual impairment and long-term mortality in a rural cohort in India: the Andhra Pradesh Eye Disease Study. PLoS One 8(10):e78002
Kirrane EF, Hoppin JA, Kamel F, Umbach DM, Boyes WK, DeRoos AJ, Alavanja M, Sandler DP (2005) Retinal degeneration and other eye disorders in wives of farmer pesticide applicators enrolled in the agricultural health study. Am J Epidemiol 161(11):1020–1029
Klotz SA, Penn CC, Negvesky GJ, Butrus SI (2000) Fungal and parasitic infections of the eye. Clin Microbiol Rev 13(4):662–685
Komarowska I, Heilweil G, Rosenfeld PJ, Perlman I, Loewenstein A (2009) Retinal toxicity of commercially available intravitreal ketorolac in albino rabbits. Retina 29(1):98–105
Konat Zorzi G, Contreras-Ruiz L, Parraga JE, Lopez-Garcia A, Romero Bello R, Diebold Y, Seijo B, Sanchez A (2011) Expression of MUC5AC in ocular surface epithelial cells using cationized gelatin nanoparticles. Mol Pharm 8(5):1783–1788
Kouchak M, Malekahmadi M, Bavarsad N, Saki Malehi A, Andishmand L (2018) Dorzolamide nanoliposome as a long action ophthalmic delivery system in open angle glaucoma and ocular hypertension patients. Drug Dev Ind Pharm 44(8):1239–1242
Krop IE, Beeram M, Modi S, Jones SF, Holden SN, Yu W, Girish S, Tibbitts J, Yi J-H, Sliwkowski MX (2010) Phase I study of trastuzumab-DM1, an HER2 antibody-drug conjugate, given every 3 weeks to patients with HER2-positive metastatic breast cancer. J Clin Oncol 28(16):2698–2704
Kumar R, Sinha V (2014) Preparation and optimization of voriconazole microemulsion for ocular delivery. Colloids Surf B: Biointerfaces 117:82–88
Kumar R, Sinha VR (2016) Solid lipid nanoparticle: an efficient carrier for improved ocular permeation of voriconazole. Drug Dev Ind Pharm 42(12):1956–1967
Kwon YH, Fingert JH, Kuehn MH, Alward WL (2009) Primary open-angle glaucoma. N Engl J Med 360(11):1113–1124
Lallemand F, Phillips B, Garrigue J-S (2011) Cationic oil-in-water emulsions containing prostaglandins and uses thereof. Google Patents
Lang Y, Leibu R, Shoham N, Miller B, Perlman I (2007) Evaluation of intravitreal kenalog toxicity in humans. Ophthalmology 114(4):724–731
Lansingh VC, Eckert KA, Haik BG, Phillipps BX, Bosch-Canto V, Leal-Leal C, Ramirez-Ortiz MA (2015) Retinoblastoma in Mexico: part I. A review of general knowledge of the disease, diagnosis, and management. Boletin Medico del Hospital Infantil de Mexico 72(5):299–306
Lee VH, Robinson JR (1986) Topical ocular drug delivery: recent developments and future challenges. J Ocul Pharmacol Ther 2(1):67–108
Lee VH, Chang S-C, Oshiro CM, Smith RE (1985) Ocular esterase composition in albino and pigmented rabbits: possible implications in ocular prodrug design and evaluation. Curr Eye Res 4(11):1117–1125
Lee V, Chien D, Sasaki H (1988) Ocular ketone reductase distribution and its role in the metabolism of ocularly applied levobunolol in the pigmented rabbit. J Pharmacol Exp Ther 246(3):871–878
Leibowitz HM (2000) The red eye. N Engl J Med 343(5):345–351
Levine JM, Noecker RJ, Lane LC, Herrygers L, Nix D, Snyder RW (2004) Comparative penetration of moxifloxacin and gatifloxacin in rabbit aqueous humor after topical dosing. J Cataract Refract Surg 30(10):2177–2182

Liu D, Ren T, Gao X (2003) Cationic transfection lipids. Curr Med Chem 10(14):1307–1315
Liu Z, Li J, Nie S, Liu H, Ding P, Pan W (2006) Study of an alginate/HPMC-based in situ gelling ophthalmic delivery system for gatifloxacin. Int J Pharm 315(1–2):12–17
Ma K, Liu G-J, Yan L, Wen S, Xu B, Tian W, Goldys EM, Liu G (2019) AIEgen based poly (L-lactic-co-glycolic acid) magnetic nanoparticles to localize cytokine VEGF for early cancer diagnosis and photothermal therapy. Nanomedicine. https://doi.org/10.2217/nnm-2018-0467
Maenpaa H, Gegelashvili G, Tahti H (2004) Expression of glutamate transporter subtypes in cultured retinal pigment epithelial and retinoblastoma cells. Curr Eye Res 28(3):159–165
Mahor A, Prajapati SK, Verma A, Gupta R, Iyer AK, Kesharwani P (2016) Moxifloxacin loaded gelatin nanoparticles for ocular delivery: formulation and in-vitro, in-vivo evaluation. J Colloid Interface Sci 483:132–138
Maia M, Farah ME, Belfort RN, Penha FM, Lima Filho AA, Aggio FB, Belfort R (2007) Effects of intravitreal triamcinolone acetonide injection with and without preservative. Br J Ophthalmol 91(9):1122–1124
Majumdar S, Tirucherai GS, Pal D, Mitra AK (2003) Functional differences in nucleoside and nucleobase transporters expressed on the rabbit corneal epithelial cell line (SIRC) and isolated rabbit cornea. AAPS PharmSci 5(2):72
Manchanda S, Sahoo PK, Majumdar DK (2016) Mucoadhesive chitosan-dextran sulfate nanoparticles of acetazolamide for ocular hypertension. Nanotechnol Rev 5(5):445–453
Mannermaa E, Vellonen K-S, Ryhanen T, Kokkonen K, Ranta V-P, Kaarniranta K, Urtti A (2009) Efflux protein expression in human retinal pigment epithelium cell lines. Pharm Res 26(7):1785–1791
Martin-Amat G, McMartin K, Hayreh S, Hayreh M, Tephly T (1978) Methanol poisoning: ocular toxicity produced by formate. Toxicol Appl Pharmacol 45(1):201–208
McAvoy M, Singh AK, Shichi H (1996) In situ hybridization of Cyp1a1, Cyp1a2 and Ah receptor mRNAs expressed in murine ocular tissues. Exp Eye Res 4(62):449–452
McGee HT, Fraunfelder F (2007) Toxicities of topical ophthalmic anesthetics. Expert Opin Drug Saf 6(6):637–640
Messina-Baas O, Gonzalez-Huerta L, Chima-Galán C, Kofman-Alfaro S, Rivera-Vega M, Babayan-Mena I, Cuevas-Covarrubias S (2007) Molecular analysis of the CYP1B1 gene: identification of novel truncating mutations in patients with primary congenital glaucoma. Ophthalmic Res 39(1):17–23
Meyers-Elliott RH, Pettit TH, Maxwell WA (1980) Viral antigens in the immune ring of herpes simplex stromal keratitis. Arch Ophthalmol 98(5):897–904
Mindel JS, Yablonski ME, Tavitian HO, Podos SM, Orellana J (1981) Dipivefrin and echothiophate: efficacy of combined use in human beings. Arch Ophthalmol 99(9):1583–1586
Mita M, Ricart A, Mita A, Patnaik A, Sarantopoulos J, Sankhala K, Fram R, Qin A, Watermill J, Tolcher A (2007) A phase I study of a CanAg-targeted immunoconjugate, huC242-DM4, in patients with Can Ag-expressing solid tumors. J Clin Oncol 25(18_suppl):3062
Mitra AK (2009) Role of transporters in ocular drug delivery system. Springer 26(5):1192–6. https://doi.org/10.1007/s11095-009-9862-x
Montes-Mico R (2007) Role of the tear film in the optical quality of the human eye. J Cataract Refract Surg 33(9):1631–1635
Moore KN, Martin LP, Seward SM, Bauer TM, O'Malley DM, Perez RP, Oza AM, Jeong W, Kirby MW, Zhou Y (2015) Preliminary single agent activity of IMGN853, a folate receptor alpha (FRα)-targeting antibody-drug conjugate (ADC), in platinum-resistant epithelial ovarian cancer (EOC) patients (pts): phase I trial. American Society of Clinical Oncology
Moreau KL, King JA (2012) Protein misfolding and aggregation in cataract disease and prospects for prevention. Trends Mol Med 18(5):273–282
Moure A, Cruz JM, Franco D, Dominguez JM, Sineiro J, Dominguez H, Nunez MJ, Parajo JC (2001) Natural antioxidants from residual sources. Food Chem 72(2):145–171
Mustaev A, Malik M, Zhao X, Kurepina N, Luan G, Oppegard LM, Hiasa H, Marks KR, Kerns RJ, Berger JM (2014) Fluoroquinolone-gyrase-DNA complexes two modes of drug binding. J Biol Chem 289(18):12300–12312
Nakhlband A, Barar J (2011) Impacts of nanomedicines in ocular pharmacotherapy. Bioimpacts 1(1):7
Nyengaard JR, Ido Y, Kilo C, Williamson JR (2004) Interactions between hyperglycemia and hypoxia: implications for diabetic retinopathy. Diabetes 53(11):2931–2938
Obinu A, Rassu G, Corona P, Maestri M, Riva F, Miele D, Giunchedi P, Gavini E (2019) Poly (ethyl 2-cyanoacrylate) nanoparticles (PECA-NPs) as possible agents in tumor treatment. Colloids Surf B: Biointerfaces 177:520–528
Oelker AM, Berlin JA, Wathier M, Grinstaff MW (2011) Synthesis and characterization of dendron cross-linked PEG hydrogels as corneal adhesives. Biomacromolecules 12(5):1658–1665
Oh N, Park J-H (2014) Endocytosis and exocytosis of nanoparticles in mammalian cells. Int J Nanomedicine 9(Suppl 1):51
Ono SJ, Abelson MB (2005) Allergic conjunctivitis: update on pathophysiology and prospects for future treatment. J Allergy Clin Immunol 115(1):118–122
Ozaki H, Yu A, Della N, Ozaki K, Luna JD, Yamada H, Hackett SF, Okamoto N, Zack DJ, Semenza GL (1999) Hypoxia inducible factor-1alpha is increased in ischemic retina: temporal and spatial correlation with VEGF expression. Invest Ophthalmol Vis Sci 40(1):182–189

Paolicelli P, de la Fuente M, Sanchez A, Seijo B, Alonso MJ (2009) Chitosan nanoparticles for drug delivery to the eye. Expert Opin Drug Deliv 6(3):239–253
Papadopoulos N, Martin J, Ruan Q, Rafique A, Rosconi MP, Shi E, Pyles EA, Yancopoulos GD, Stahl N, Wiegand SJ (2012) Binding and neutralization of vascular endothelial growth factor (VEGF) and related ligands by VEGF trap, ranibizumab and bevacizumab. Angiogenesis 15(2):171–185
Park CG, Kim YK, Kim S-N, Lee SH, Huh BK, Park M-A, Won H, Park KH, Choy YB (2017) Enhanced ocular efficacy of topically-delivered dorzolamide with nanostructured mucoadhesive microparticles. Int J Pharm 522(1–2):66–73
Parkinson A (1996) An overview of current cytochrome P450 technology for assessing the safety and efficacy of new materials. Toxicol Pathol 24(1):45–57
Patel S, Ashwanikumar N, Robinson E, DuRoss A, Sun C, Murphy-Benenato KE, Mihai C, Almarsson O, Sahay G (2017) Boosting intracellular delivery of lipid nanoparticle-encapsulated mRNA. Nano Lett 17(9):5711–5718
Patel S, Ryals RC, Weller KK, Pennesi ME, Sahay G (2019) Lipid nanoparticles for delivery of messenger RNA to the back of the eye. J Control Release 303:91–100
Patravale V, Date AA, Kulkarni R (2004) Nanosuspensions: a promising drug delivery strategy. J Pharm Pharmacol 56(7):827–840
Peng H-S, Liu X-J, Lv G-X, Sun B, Kong Q-F, Zhai D-X, Wang Q, Zhao W, Wang G-Y, Wang D-D (2008) Voriconazole into PLGA nanoparticles: Improving agglomeration and antifungal efficacy. Int J Pharm 352(1–2):29–35
Penha FM, Rodrigues EB, Maia M, Furlani BA, Regatieri C, Melo GB, Magalhaes O Jr, Manzano R, Farah ME (2010) Retinal and ocular toxicity in ocular application of drugs and chemicals–part II: retinal toxicity of current and new drugs. Ophthalmic Res 44(4):205–224
Philips B, Bague S, Rabinovich-Guilatt L, Lambert G (2012) Ophthalmic emulsions containing prostaglandins. Google Patents
Philp NJ, Wang D, Yoon H, Hjelmeland LM (2003) Polarized expression of monocarboxylate transporters in human retinal pigment epithelium and ARPE-19 cells. Invest Ophthalmol Vis Sci 44(4):1716–1721
Piccaluga PP, Martinelli G, Rondoni M, Malagola M, Gaitani S, Visani G, Baccarani M (2004) First experience with gemtuzumab ozogamicin plus cytarabine as continuous infusion for elderly acute myeloid leukaemia patients. Leuk Res 28(9):987–990
Pignatello R, Bucolo C, Spedalieri G, Maltese A, Puglisi G (2002) Flurbiprofen-loaded acrylate polymer nanosuspensions for ophthalmic application. Biomaterials 23(15):3247–3255
Pitkanen L, Ranta V-P, Moilanen H, Urtti A (2005) Permeability of retinal pigment epithelium: effects of permeant molecular weight and lipophilicity. Invest Ophthalmol Vis Sci 46(2):641–646
Pollinger K, Hennig R, Ohlmann A, Fuchshofer R, Wenzel R, Breunig M, Tessmar J, Tamm ER, Goepferich A (2013) Ligand-functionalized nanoparticles target endothelial cells in retinal capillaries after systemic application. Proc Natl Acad Sci 110(15):6115–6120
Qu W, Meng B, Yu Y, Wang S (2018) Folic acid-conjugated mesoporous silica nanoparticles for enhanced therapeutic efficacy of topotecan in retina cancers. Int J Nanomedicine 13:4379
Quigley HA (1993) Open-angle glaucoma. N Engl J Med 328(15):1097–1106
Quigley HA, Addicks EM, Green WR, Maumenee A (1981) Optic nerve damage in human glaucoma: II. The site of injury and susceptibility to damage. Arch Ophthalmol 99(4):635–649
Raemdonck K, Martens TF, Braeckmans K, Demeester J, De Smedt SC (2013) Polysaccharide-based nucleic acid nanoformulations. Adv Drug Deliv Rev 65(9):1123–1147
Rezaie T, Child A, Hitchings R, Brice G, Miller L, Coca-Prados M, Heon E, Krupin T, Ritch R, Kreutzer D (2002) Adult-onset primary open-angle glaucoma caused by mutations in optineurin. Science 295(5557):1077–1079
Ribrag V, Dupuis J, Tilly H, Morschhauser F, Laine F, Houot R, Haioun C, Copie C, Varga A, Lambert J (2014) A dose-escalation study of SAR3419, an anti-CD19 antibody maytansinoid conjugate, administered by intravenous infusion once weekly in patients with relapsed/refractory B-cell non-Hodgkin lymphoma. Clin Cancer Res 20(1):213–220
Rolando M, Zierhut M (2001) The ocular surface and tear film and their dysfunction in dry eye disease. Surv Ophthalmol 45:S203–S210
Runkle EA, Antonetti DA (2011) The blood-retinal barrier: structure and functional significance. In: The blood-brain and other neural barriers. Springer Nature Switzerland AG, pp 133–148
Sanyal S, Law S (2019) Ocular surface and chronic pesticide exposure: evaluating the alterations in corneal cellular turnover concerning cell cycle and apoptosis. Exp Eye Res 178:122–132
Sanyal S, Law A, Law S (2017) Chronic pesticide exposure and consequential keratectasia & corneal neovascularisation. Exp Eye Res 164:1–7
Saraiva SM, Castro-Lopez V, Paneda C, Alonso MJ (2017) Synthetic nanocarriers for the delivery of polynucleotides to the eye. Eur J Pharm Sci 103:5–18
Saran BR, Maguire AM (1994) Retinal toxicity of high dose intravitreal ganciclovir. Retina (Philadelphia, Pa) 14(3):248–252
Sarao V, Veritti D, Boscia F, Lanzetta P (2014) Intravitreal steroids for the treatment of retinal diseases. Sci World J 2014
Schoenwald RD, Zhu J (2000) The ocular pharmacokinetics of ketanserin and its metabolite, ketanserinol, in albino rabbits. J Ocul Pharmacol Ther 16(5):481–495
Selvin BL (1983) Systemic effects of topical ophthalmic medications. South Med J 76(3):349–358

Sharma S (2011) Antibiotic resistance in ocular bacterial pathogens. Indian J Med Microbiol 29(3):218

Shell JW (1982) Pharmacokinetics of topically applied ophthalmic drugs. Surv Ophthalmol 26(4):207–218

Shichi H (1969) Microsomal electron transfer system of bovine retinal pigment epithelium. Exp Eye Res 8(1):60–68

Smith TJ, Pearson PA, Blandford DL, Brown JD, Goins KA, Hollins JL, Schmeisser ET, Glavinos P, Baldwin LB, Ashton P (1992) Intravitreal sustained-release ganciclovir. Arch Ophthalmol 110(2):255–258

Sreekumar PG, Spee C, Ryan SJ, Cole SP, Kannan R, Hinton DR (2012) Mechanism of RPE cell death in α-crystallin deficient mice: a novel and critical role for MRP1-mediated GSH efflux. PLoS One 7(3):e33420

Srinivasarao DA, Reddy SS, Reddy GB, Katti DS (2019) Spatio-temporal control on the delivery of triamcinolone acetonide using polymeric nanoparticles reduces steroid induced cataract. Int J Pharm 568:118474

Srivastava SK, Singhal SS, Bajpai KK, Chaubey M, Ansari NH, Awasthi YC (1994) A group of novel glutathione S-transferase isozymes showing high activity towards 4-hydroxy-2-nonenal are present in bovine ocular tissues. Exp Eye Res 59(2):151–159

Stahlmann R (2002) Clinical toxicological aspects of fluoroquinolones. Toxicol Lett 127(1–3):269–277

Stampfli HF, Quon CY (1995) Polymorphic metabolism of flestolol and other ester containing compounds by a carboxylesterase in New Zealand white rabbit blood and cornea. Res Commun Mol Pathol Pharmacol 88(1):87–97

Stanton ME, Crofton KM, Gray LE, Gordon CJ, Boyes WK, Mole ML, Peele DB, Bushnell PJ (1995) Assessment of offspring development and behavior following gestational exposure to inhaled methanol in the rat. Toxicol Sci 28(1):100–110

Stewart WC, Konstas AG, Nelson LA, Kruft B (2008) Meta-analysis of 24-hour intraocular pressure studies evaluating the efficacy of glaucoma medicines. Ophthalmology 115(7):1117–1122.e1111

Stone EM, Fingert JH, Alward WL, Nguyen TD, Polansky JR, Sunden SL, Nishimura D, Clark AF, Nystuen A, Nichols BE (1997) Identification of a gene that causes primary open angle glaucoma. Science 275(5300):668–670

Subhani S, Vavilala DT, Mukherji M (2016) HIF inhibitors for ischemic retinopathies and cancers: options beyond anti-VEGF therapies. Angiogenesis 19(3):257–273

Subramanian N, Kanwar JR, Kanwar RK, Krishnakumar S (2015) Targeting cancer cells using LNA-modified aptamer-siRNA chimeras. Nucleic Acid Ther 25(6):317–322

Subramanian N, Balachandran A, Subramanian K (2018) Aptamer as therapeutics for cancer with focus on retinoblastoma. In: Gene and cell therapy: biology and applications. Springer Nature Singapore Pvt Ltd. pp 147–194

Supuran CT, Altamimi ASA, Carta F (2019) Carbonic anhydrase inhibition and the management of glaucoma: a literature and patent review 2013–2019. Expert Opin Ther Pat 29(10):781–792

Takemoto LJ (1996) Oxidation of cysteine residues from alpha-A crystallin during cataractogenesis of the human lens. Biochem Biophys Res Commun 223(2):216–220

Tarabishy AB, Jeng BH (2008) Bacterial conjunctivitis: a review for internists. Cleve Clin J Med 75(7):507

Taskar PS, Patil A, Lakhani P, Ashour E, Gul W, ElSohly MA, Murphy B, Majumdar S (2019) Δ9-tetrahydrocannabinol derivative-loaded nanoformulation lowers intraocular pressure in normotensive rabbits. Transl Vis Sci Technol 8(5):15–15

Tripathi A, Chen SI, O'sullivan S (2002) Acute psychosis following the use of topical ciprofloxacin. Arch Ophthalmol 120(5):665–666

Tsao C-C, Coulter SJ, Chien A, Luo G, Clayton NP, Maronpot R, Goldstein JA, Zeldin DC (2001) Identification and localization of five CYP2Cs in murine extrahepatic tissues and their metabolism of arachidonic acid to regio-and stereoselective products. J Pharmacol Exp Ther 299(1):39–47

Tzankova V, Aluani D, Yordanov Y, Kondeva Burdina M, Petrov P, Bankova V, Simeonova R, Vitcheva V, Odjakov F, Apostolov A (2019) Micellar propolis nanoformulation of high antioxidant and hepatoprotective activity. Revista Brasileira de Farmacognosia

Ueda H, Horibe Y, Kim K-J, Lee VH (2000) Functional characterization of organic cation drug transport in the pigmented rabbit conjunctiva. Invest Ophthalmol Vis Sci 41(3):870–876

Vadlapatla RK, Vadlapudi AD, Ponnaluri VC, Pal D, Mukherji M, Mitra AK (2013) Molecular expression and functional activity of efflux and influx transporters in hypoxia induced retinal pigment epithelial cells. Int J Pharm 454(1):444–452

Van Quill KR, Dioguardi PK, Tong CT, Gilbert JA, Aaberg TM Jr, Grossniklaus HE, Edelhauser HF, O'Brien JM (2005) Subconjunctival carboplatin in fibrin sealant in the treatment of transgenic murine retinoblastoma. Ophthalmology 112(6):1151–1158

Vandervoort J, Ludwig A (2002) Biocompatible stabilizers in the preparation of PLGA nanoparticles: a factorial design study. Int J Pharm 238(1–2):77–92

Volotinen M, Maenpaa J, Kankuri E, Oksala O, Pelkonen O, Nakajima M, Yokoi T, Hakkola J (2009) Expression of cytochrome P450 (CYP) enzymes in human non-pigmented ciliary epithelial cells: induction of CYP1B1 expression by TCDD. Invest Ophthalmol Vis Sci 50(7):3099–3105

von Gunten S, Lew D, Vaudaux P, Brazitikos PD, Leuenberger PM, Paccolat F (1994) Aqueous humor penetration of ofloxacin given by various routes. Am J Ophthalmol 117(1):87–89

Vrabec J, Levin L (2007) The neurobiology of cell death in glaucoma. Eye 21(S1):S11

Wadhwa S, Paliwal R, Paliwal SR, Vyas S (2009) Nanocarriers in ocular drug delivery: an update review. Curr Pharm Des 15(23):2724–2750

Walker C, Claoue C (1986) Incidence of conjunctival colonization by bacteria capable of causing postoperative endophthalmitis. J R Soc Med 79(9):520–521
Wilson LA, Ahearn DG, Jones DB, Sexton RR (1969) Fungi from the normal outer eye. Am J Ophthalmol 67(1):52–56
Woll P, O'Brien M, Fossella F, Shah M, Clinch Y, O'Keeffe J, Qin A, O'Leary J, Lorigan P (2010) Phase I study of lorvotuzumab mertansine (IMGN901) in patients with CD56-positive solid tumors. Ann Oncol 21(Suppl. 8)
Yamagata N, Hozumi K, Kikkawa Y, Nomizu M (2007) Peptide Mosaic Chitosan Membranes Promote Diverse Biological Functions. In: 4th International Peptide Symposium in conjunction with the 7th Australian Peptide Conference and the 2nd Asia-Pacific International Peptide Symposium, pp 21–25
Yenice I, Mocan MC, Palaska E, Bochot A, Bilensoy E, Vural I, Irkec M, Hıncal AA (2008) Hyaluronic acid coated poly-ε-caprolactone nanospheres deliver high concentrations of cyclosporine A into the cornea. Exp Eye Res 87(3):162–167
Yip PP, Woo CF, Tang HHY, Ho CK (2009) Triple therapy for neovascular age-related macular degeneration using single-session photodynamic therapy combined with intravitreal bevacizumab and triamcinolone. Br J Ophthalmol 93(6):754–758
Zehetner C, Kralinger MT, Modi YS, Waltl I, Ulmer H, Kirchmair R, Bechrakis NE, Kieselbach GF (2015) Systemic levels of vascular endothelial growth factor before and after intravitreal injection of aflibercept or ranibizumab in patients with age-related macular degeneration: a randomised, prospective trial. Acta Ophthalmol 93(2):e154–e159
Zhang Y, Li C, Sun X, Kuang X, Ruan X (2012) High glucose decreases expression and activity of p-glycoprotein in cultured human retinal pigment epithelium possibly through iNOS induction. PLoS One 7(2):e31631
Zhou H-Y, Hao J-L, Wang S, Zheng Y, Zhang W-S (2013) Nanoparticles in the ocular drug delivery. Int J Ophthalmol 6(3):390

Part IV

Nanoformulations in Topical Diseases

Nanosized Labile and Particulate Ingredients in Topical Formulations: A Strategic Approach Against Photoageing and Photocarcinogenesis

13

Surbhi Dhawan, Pragya Sharma, and Sanju Nanda

Abstract

Skin being the largest and fastest-growing organ of the body acts as a protective coat for the body. It is not only a barrier to environmental insults and pathogenic invasions but is also a site of beauty, a mirror of internal health and a route of drug delivery. The topical problems often lead to cosmetic aberrations, for example, dandruff, baldness, acne, rosacea, urticaria, melasma, and wrinkles. The epidermal and dermal layers are viable layers, and free radicals pose a big threat to their viability. The UV radiations have been infamous for their role in the production of reactive oxygen species (ROS), causing sunburn, tanning, itching, inflammation, hyperpigmentation, etc. Additionally, UVB rays have the power to reach dermal layers and lead to the activation of matrix metalloproteinases (MMPs), disturb the skin structure and cause premature skin ageing. Photoageing has become one of the major cosmetic concerns and designing a broad spectrum photoprotective formulation is the need of the hour. Drugs generally used in treating skin ailments fall in the category of anti-allergic and anti-inflammatory agents, antioxidants, anti-infectives, immunosuppressants and anticancer agents. There is no dearth of therapeutic molecules for dermatological problems but making effective, safe and non-irritant formulations is always a challenge for the cosmetic scientist. Nanotechnology inspired strategies are being used for better product performance and site-specific targeting. Nanosized labile carriers such as liposomes, niosomes, nanoemulsions, nanospheres and nanostructured lipid carriers have been designed in the cosmetic and dermatological product categories with the aim to achieve enhanced skin penetration, controlled and sustained release, better entrapment and better product stability of the drug. Regulations and guidance on the use of nanomaterials and nanocosmetics are being promulgated by regulatory agencies so as to ensure consumer safety and address environmental concerns. This chapter will cover all these aspects and will also update on the manufacturing, testing, packaging and labelling directions for nanomaterials in cosmetics and topical products.

Keywords

Skin disorders · Cosmetics · Photoageing · Photocarcinogenesis · Antioxidants · Sunscreens · Particulate ingredients · Nanobiomaterials · Drug delivery systems · Regulations

S. Dhawan · P. Sharma · S. Nanda (✉)
Department of Pharmaceutical Sciences, Maharshi Dayanand University, Rohtak, Haryana, India

S. Talegaonkar, M. Rai (eds.), *Nanoformulations in Human Health*,
https://doi.org/10.1007/978-3-030-41858-8_13

13.1 Introduction

The skin stands out to be the largest and fastest-growing body organ. It covers a total surface area of around 1.8 m^2 and is highly exposed to the environment. It acts as an interface between body's internal organs and the environment. Therefore, skin serves as the first line of defense for the body. Several tasks are performed by the skin in order to maintain the body's homeostasis. This involves both non-immune and immune functions. Some of the non-immune functions include shielding against physical and biochemical insults, acting as a sensory receptive area, maintaining hydration, allowing synthesis of vitamins and hormones, etc. The skin also has an effectual immune system that provides protection to deeper body tissues. It has a well-coordinated system of epithelial and immune cells. Together they work against trauma, toxins and infections. It tries to maintain self-tolerance, prevent allergy and inhibit autoimmunity (Di Meglio et al. 2011). But apart from this, skin is also a site of beauty, a mirror of internal health that reflects the state of the body and a route for local and systemic drug administration.

Skin is regarded as a multifunctional organ due to its structural organization and composition. The skin is composed of three layers, namely the outermost epidermis, dermis and the innermost hypodermis. The basement membrane separates the epidermis from dermis. The epidermis is further divided into different layers. From the uppermost observable part of the epidermis to the lowermost layer are the stratum corneum (SC), the stratum granulosum, the stratum spinosum and the stratum basale. Epidermal keratinocytes, acidic (due to sweat) and hydrolipidic nature (due to sebum, lipids and antimicrobial peptides) of the skin help to attain its barrier function. The epidermal layer is also composed of melanocytes, Merkel and immune cells (Langerhans cells and T lymphocytes). The dermis makes the thickest layer and is divided into an upper papillary region known as stratum papillare containing thin collagen fibres and lower reticular region known as stratum reticulare containing thick collagen fibers. Dermis has three types of tissues, namely collagen, elastin and reticular fibers spread throughout the dermis. These fibres provide mechanical strength, elasticity and structural framework (Losquadro 2017). Dermis hosts blood vessels as well as many significant immune cells like dermal dendritic cells, αβ T cells, γδ T cells, natural killer cells, B cells, mast cells and macrophages. The hypodermis or subcutaneous fatty tissue acts as a support to the dermis and epidermis layers of the skin. The management of body temperature is one of the key roles played by cutaneous blood vessels.

The skin acts as a port for delivering useful drug molecules to achieve cutaneous, targeted, or systemic effects in the body. The drug's efficacy is highly affected by the way it is administered into the body. The skin constitutes an efficient barrier system due to the 'bricks and mortar' structure of the stratum corneum, where bricks represent corneocytes and mortar represents intercellular lipids (Michaels and Shaw 1975). This structure restricts the passage of harmful xenobiotics as well as most therapeutic compounds into the body. The SC layer (horny layer) is 10–15 cells deep. These are high density and low hydrated cells that are 10–20 μm thick. Hence, it causes difficulty in drug administration through the skin (Ellias 1981). Only a handful of the drugs possess the characteristics (weight less than 500 Da and logP 1–3) that allow them to diffuse passively across the stratum corneum in adequate amount to obtain the therapeutic concentration in the blood. Hence, drug delivery through skin route is a challenging task for the formulators. The process of designing topical or transdermal drug delivery systems involves a detailed knowledge of skin anatomy, the disorder, the area or layer of the skin to be targeted, severity of the disorder, the physicochemical properties of the drug chosen and the drug delivery method.

There are three possible routes by which a drug molecule can penetrate the skin when applied topically (Keleb et al. 2010). It is not necessary that the drug molecule will penetrate through only one of the pathways since the physiochemical properties of the active molecule

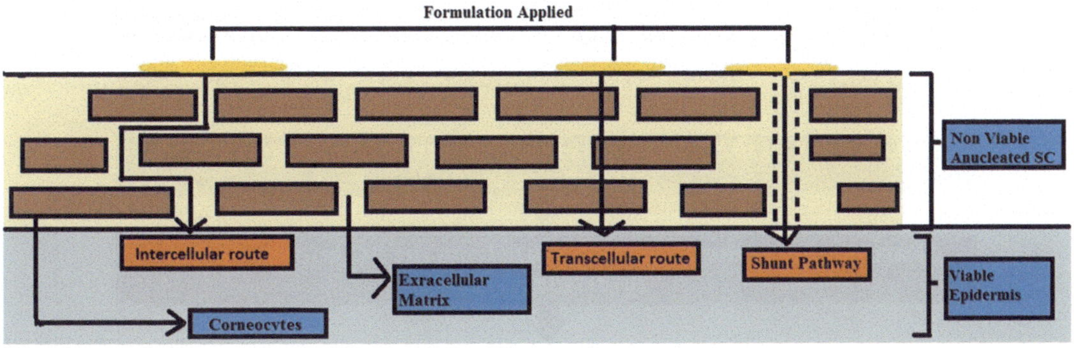

Fig. 13.1 Various penetration routes via skin

determine its permeation pathway. There are several compounds that enter the skin via multiple ways. The various pathways are discussed below with a pictorial representation in Fig. 13.1.

(a) *Shunt pathway (through the appendages)*: Just 0.1% of the skin's total surface area contributes to the skin appendages. Hence, this passage contributes very little in drug permeation when the formulation is applied to the skin. Hair follicles make easy access to the dermal microcirculation as they penetrate through the stratum corneum. Charged molecules and large polar compounds like peptide-based drugs are enabled to permeate through this pathway.
(b) *Transcellular route (via corneocytes)*: This pathway involves the movement of drugs through both the phospholipid membranes and the cytoplasm of the dead keratinocytes that constitute the SC. The drug faces high permeation resistance because it has to repeat these steps multiple times to cross the full width of the SC. Only a few drugs have the desired characteristics to follow this pathway.
(c) *Intercellular route (through matrix layer)*: Though only a small area is occupied by the intercellular lipid, they make the only uninterrupted passage through the SC. This route allows the transportation of both lipidic and polar molecules. The physiochemical characteristics of the active molecule outline the amount and rate of the molecule's diffusion. Drug molecule has to move along the small spaces that exist between the cells thus, the actual path increases 20-fold times than the normal thickness of the SC which is just around 20 μm. This reduces the rate of drug penetration.

Drug permeation from topical or transdermal formulation into the skin follows a series of processes that are depicted in Fig. 13.2. For transdermal drug delivery, it is required that the drug needs to enter the blood circulation after crossing all the three layers of the skin. Whereas for the topical delivery, it is required that drug needs to be retained in the skin layers after crossing the stratum corneum (Wilbur 2017).

13.2 Problems of the Skin and Topical Disorders

There is a pool of skin conditions that affect human beings. The skin disorder can be either temporary or permanent. Some conditions can be cured, and some can only be treated to lessen the symptoms and effects of a disease. The severity and symptoms of the skin conditions may vary depending upon the individual, type and level of disorder and the status of the immune system of the body. These disorders may be painless or

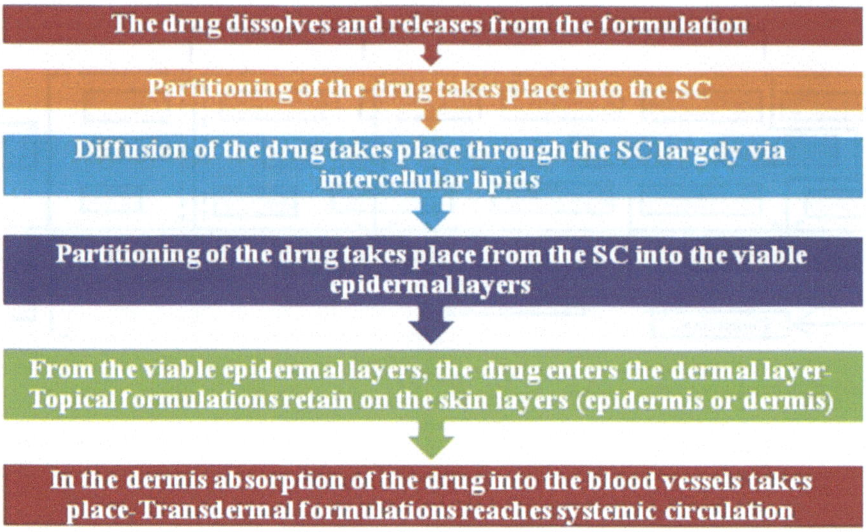

Fig. 13.2 Permeation process for topical/transdermal formulations

painful. The main cause behind them may be known or unknown. Generally, environmental factors, allergens, genetic make-up, irritants, certain diseases and affected immune system lead to skin problems. But overall these skin disorders or conditions affect the patient's mental health. Disorders like psoriasis, eczema and skin cancer possess a significant psychological and social impact on the patients. Patients limit their lives because they feel self-conscious about their symptoms (Tuckman 2016). Some of the common skin disorders are acne (caused by blockage of skin follicles due to the plug formed by oil from glands, bacteria, dead cells, etc.), eczema (leads to itchy, swelled, cracked and scaly skin), alopecia areata (affects hair follicles and makes the hair falls out in small and round patches), psoriasis (caused by overactive immune system), rosacea (long-term disease with reddened skin and pimples usually on the face) and vitiligo (loss of skin color in blotches).

13.2.1 Photoageing

The damaging UV rays affect all the layers of the skin and their effects depend upon the duration and extent of the UV exposure. Excessive sun exposure leads to the penetration of UV rays to the deeper skin layers. The effects of these rays are different in different skin layers. UVA rays penetrate deeper into the dermal layer, while UVB rays penetrate the epidermal layer. These rays increase the prevalence of sunburn, tanning, itching, inflammation, hyperpigmentation, etc. UVA reaches dermal layer and leads to the activation of matrix metalloproteinases (MMPs), elastase, hyaluronidase, etc. that disturb the skin structure and cause premature skin ageing. The harmful UV rays also affect the skin's natural antioxidant defence system and suppress the immune system making it more prone to serious issues. The mechanism involved during photoageing has been illustrated in Fig. 13.3 (Gilchrest 2007).

13.2.2 Photocarcinogenesis

Numerous clinical interpretations and epidemiological data suggest that UV rays are the primary stimuli for human skin cancer formation. Continuous and excess exposure causes skin cells to die, damage or develop cancer in the epidermal layer. Photocarcinogenesis develops in a stepwise manner that involves initiation of the tumor

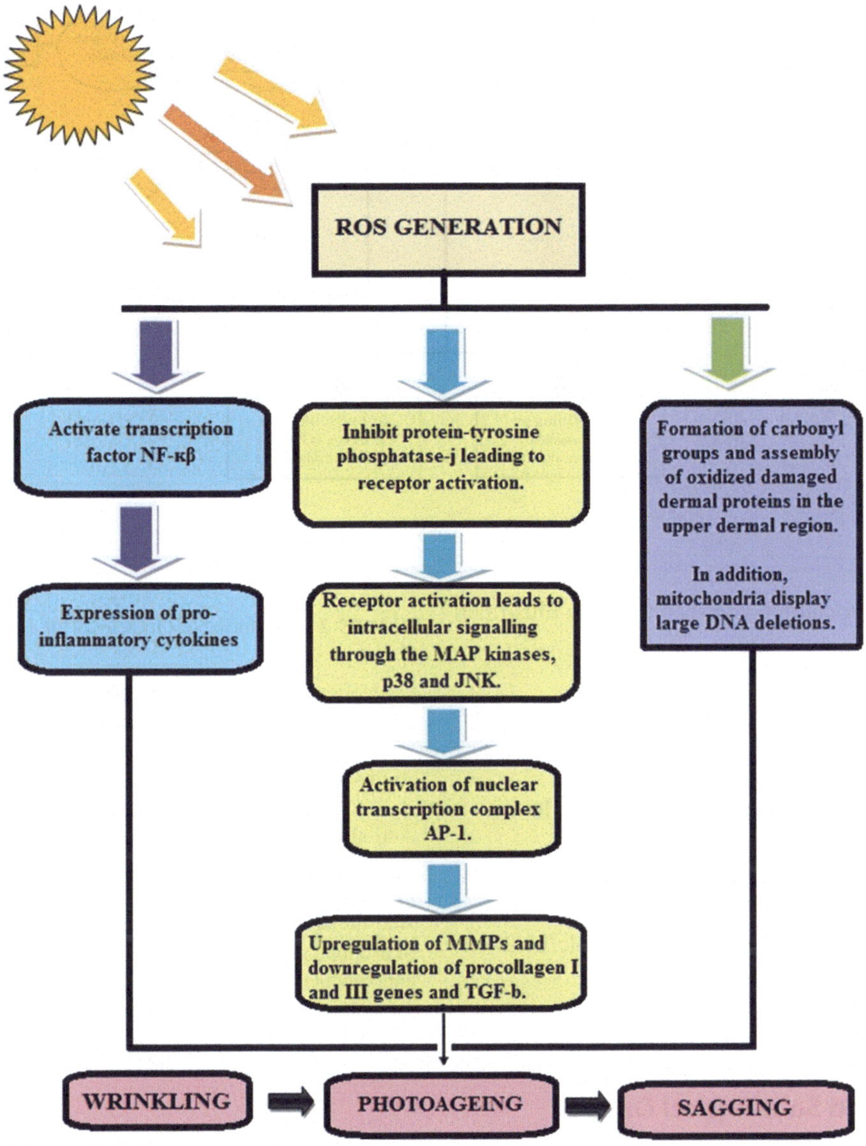

Fig. 13.3 Mechanism involved behind photoageing

growth, its promotion, and further its progression. The pathway involved in the photocarcinogenesis is a complex mixture of several cell-related, biochemical and molecular level changes that are generally related to each other (Bosch et al. 2015). The features observed on a photodamaged skin according to the types of skin are listed down in Table 13.1 and illustrated in Fig. 13.3 (Gilchrest 2007). The incidences that

Table 13.1 Characteristics of the UV damaged skin based on the type of skin

Skin type	Features
Type I and II	Atrophy of the epidermal region of the skin, immune exhaustion, focal hypopigmentation pseudoscars, mutations and dysplasia, lentigo maligna, melanoma and nonmelanoma skin cancer, solar elastosis, small brown spots, naevi
Type III and IV	Skin hyperplasia, tanning, thickening of the epidermis, Lentigines

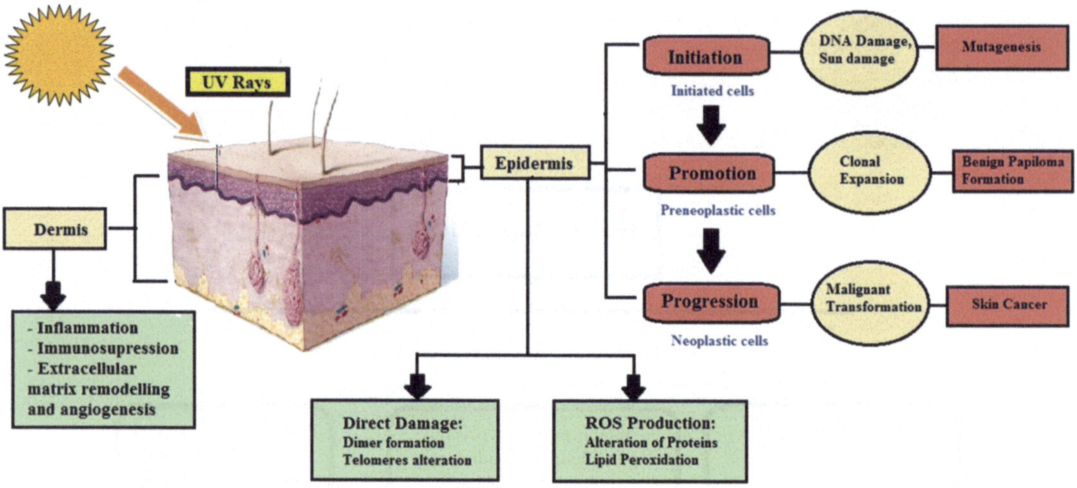

Fig. 13.4 Incidences involved in photocarcinogenesis

lead to photocarcinogenesis have been illustrated in Fig. 13.4.

13.3 Categories of Drugs Generally Used for Dermatological Problems

There are several categories of drugs that are used to treat dermatological disorders. Some of them have been enlisted below in Table 13.2.

Table 13.2 Categories of drugs used for dermatological problems

Categories	Examples
Anti-fungal	Clotrimazole, Econazole, Fluconazole
Antibacterial	Dicloxacillin, Erythromycin and Tetracycline
Anti-allergic	Fexofenadine, Diphenhydramine
Immunosuppressants	Azathioprine, Methotrexate
Anti-tumor	Fluorouracil, Imiquimod
Skin supplements/ antioxidants	Vitamin C, Vitamin B
Steroids	Hydrocortisone, Triamcinolone, Fluocinonide and Clobetasol

13.4 Formulation Design Strategies for Effective and Safe Topical Drug Delivery

There is no dearth of therapeutic molecules for dermatological problems but making effective, safe and non-irritant formulations is always a challenge for the cosmetic scientist. Strategies for designing topical formulation involve consideration of the following points:

A. *Type of skin disorder*:

Human beings get suffered from numerous skin disorders. It is essential to know the severity and symptoms of the disease for which formulation is to be prepared. While formulating, it is necessary to make sure that the formulation is working against the desired symptoms and the disease.

B. *Layer to be targeted*:

Various skin disorders affect different skin layers and definite skin structure. Before designing a topical formulation it is required to have prior knowledge about the affected skin area and accordingly design the strategy to deliver the drug there.

C. *Drug's physical and chemical characteristics*:

The physicochemical properties of the drugs like solubility, partition coefficient, the dissociation constant, hydrogen bonding, ionization, etc. must be known. These properties define the penetration ability of the active moiety through the SC. Considering these properties, the components and the delivery systems for the topical drug delivery need to be decided.

D. *Penetration enhancement of the active moiety through SC*:

The structural make-up and biochemical composition of the SC impart selective permeability to the drug molecule. Hence, it acts as a rate-limiting barrier that prevents penetration of the drug through the skin. Therefore, the rate of penetration and permeation of the active molecule into the dermis depends highly on the rate at which it diffuses across the SC. In order to deliver the drug dermally or transdermally, it becomes highly significant to overcome the SC barrier. A series of passive and active strategies have been introduced to achieve the same.

Passive Strategies:

- *Use of penetration enhancers*: These are also known as absorption promoters or accelerants. They reversibly decrease the SC's barrier resistance by interacting with skin constituents to promote the drug flux. Some of the commonly used penetration enhancers are sulphoxides (e.g. dimethylsulphoxide), azones (e.g. laurocapram), pyrrolidones (e.g. 2-pyrrolidone) alcohols and alkanols (ethanol or decanol), glycols (e.g. propylene glycol), surfactants and terpenes (Williams and Barry 2004).
- *Nanocarriers*: The recent trend in the field of dermatology involves the use of nanocarrier systems that promise better penetration, higher dermal localization of actives into the region concerned, i.e. targeted drug delivery, controlled and sustained release. For example, nanoemulsions (NEs), ethosomes, dendrimers, solid lipid nanoparticles (SLNs), nano-lipid carriers, etc. (Gupta et al. 2012).
- *Prodrugs*: Drugs's physical and chemical characteristics also restrict their entry into and through the skin. It is essential for a drug to get dissolved and pass through several lipidic and aqueous phases that constitute the SC in order to overcome this rate-limiting barrier (SC). Hence, prodrugs are designed with properties like increased lipid and aqueous solubility for better penetration (N'Da 2014).

Active Strategies:

- *Microneedles*: This technique involves the use of needles that are in micrometer range (microneedles) which creates microchannels through the SC. These microchannels cause the topically applied drug to bypass the SC. It is a technique that involves minimal invasiveness and pain as the needles do not enter the papillary dermal region where nerve endings are present (Tanner and Marks 2008).
- *Iontophoresis*: This technique involves the use of electrical potential difference (0.5 mA/cm^2 or less) that is applied externally to improve the passage and rate of drug release (for molecules having poor absorption/permeation property) across the membrane. The effectiveness of this technique depends on multiple factors like polarity, valency and mobility of the active moeity, the electrical cycle and type of drug formulation (Green 1996).
- *Electroporation*: This technique involves the use of high voltage pulses generally given for microseconds or milliseconds to temporary disturb the membrane's lipid bilayer structure. This enhances the skin permeability of drugs. The efficacy is determined by electrical parameters and the drug's physical and chemical characteristics (Denet et al. 2004).
- *Sonophoresis*: This technique also known as phonophoresis, involves the use of ultrasound waves as a means to deliver the active ingredients across the skin. It provides enhanced efficacy of the topical/transdermal formulations and improved users' compliance in therapeutic areas like diabetes, psychiatry and vaccines delivery (Polat et al. 2011).
- *Jet injection*: This technique uses a needleless device to deliver the powders or liquids into the skin at high pace. For example, Vitajet (Bioject), Biojector (Bioject) and Medi-Jector systems are used to inject proteins in the liquid form. The major advantage of this system

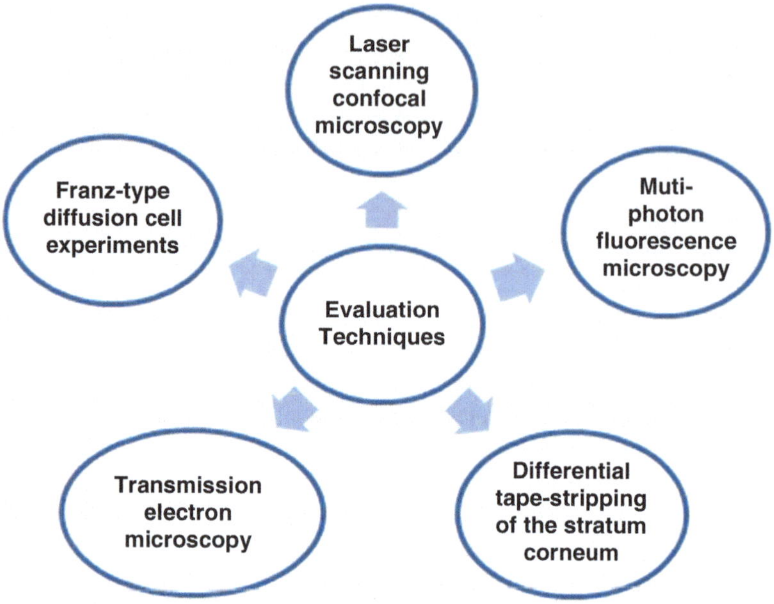

Fig. 13.5 Techniques to evaluate disposition of nanocarrier sytems on and within the skin

is that it provides better patient compliance as it causes less pain than that caused by conventional needles (Benson and Namjoshi 2008).

There are several techniques that are being used to monitor the disposition of nanocarrier system on and within the skin (Fig. 13.5). These techniques provide the estimation of the extent and mechanism involved in the penetration of nanocarriers into the SC (Wu and Guy 2009).

13.5 Nanosized Labile and Particulate Ingredients in Sunscreens, Anti-Photoageing and Anticancer Topical Formulations

A topical delivery system is considered successful if it acts locally and delivers the therapeutic molecule to the affected cells of the skin. Several drawbacks like patient compliance, safety and efficacy issues are faced with conventional systems (Schmid and Korting 1996). The use of nanotechnology-based drug delivery systems promise the required formulation goals and overtake the drawbacks that are experienced with the conventional systems. These nanocarriers make the sunscreens more efficient by enhancing UV protection in them. The minuscule particle size increases the surface area that allows drug to actively move into the skin (Kaul et al. 2018). The recent focus of the formulators is to choose biodegradable excipients for designing nanocarriers for drug delivery. The various merits offered by nanosystems include:

- Sustained and controlled release with localized effect as it creates the reservoirs.
- Precise delivery of potent drugs to the designated site
- Efficient drug targeting and greater drug retention
- The strategy of entrapment of an active molecule prevents their degradation
- Reduction in the adverse effects
- Enhanced skin penetration
- Higher stability
- Offer occlusive properties

Some of the novel nanocarriers used in cosmeceuticals have been discussed below:

13.5.1 Liposomes

These are widely used vesicular nanocarriers. They have a hydrophilic core that is covered by a hydrophobic lipidic bilayer (generally made up of phospholipids). They can entrap both hydrophobic and hydrophilic compounds. These are biocompatible and biodegradable systems that offer improved efficacy, enhanced dermal penetration and reduced toxicity. This system faces some challenges like high production cost, drug leakage, inadequate stability and susceptibility to oxidation and hydrolysis reaction (Tripura and Anushree 2017).

13.5.2 Niosomes

These are also vesicular systems having a bilayer structure that is made up by self-assembly of hydrated nonionic surfactants, with or without incorporation of cholesterol or their lipid. They overcome challenges like instability, expensiveness and susceptibility to oxidation and reduction reactions that were faced in case of liposomes. But niosomes have limited shelf life, require specialized manufacturing equipment and is a time consuming manufacturing process. Improved version of niosomes is known as proniosomes that need to be hydrated right away before use to get aqueous dispersions of niosome (Chandu et al. 2012). They are preferred over niosomes for their better stability and product performance. Coenzyme Q10 proniosomes were formulated and tested on photodamaged skin of mice (Yadav et al. 2015).

13.5.3 Solid Lipid Nanoparticles (SLN)

This system is composed of the oily or lipoidal core that is enclosed by a single-layer shell. They are prepared using lipids that can be biodegraded or using physiological lipids. Hence, surmounts the toxicity issues. Their minuscule size enables better penetration of the actives into the skin. Apart from being a carrier, SLNs also possess UV protective properties that make them act as a physical sunscreen on their own. Therefore, they can be considered as a good choice for sunscreen preparations (Arora and Murthy 2012).

13.5.4 Nanostructured Lipid Carriers (NLCs)

These are second-generation lipidic vesicles designed to surmount the limitations of SLNs. NLC is prepared by blending solid lipids along with liquid lipids leading to amorphous solids in preferable ratio of 70:30 up to 99.9:0.1, being solid at body temperature. They are physically stable, provide extended drug release, higher drug loading and can be easily prepared and scaled up. The use of biodegradable and physiological lipids makes them safer carriers. They provide better UV protection with lesser side effects (Purohit et al. 2016).

13.5.5 Nanoemulsions (NEs)

These are kinetically or thermodynamically stable dispersion systems containing an oily phase, aqueous phase and a combination of surfactant and co-surfactant. NEs are generally transparent or translucent in appearance. They have low viscosity, high absorption rate, interfacial area and solubilization capacity (Ronak and Jay 2012).

13.5.6 Nanospheres

These are core-shell type nanosystems with particle size ranging from 10 to 200 nm in diameter. They can be either crystalline or amorphous systems in which active moiety is enclosed, dissolved, attached, or encapsulated to the polymer matrix. Nanospheres provide protection against chemical and enzymatic degradation of the drug. They can be used to deliver a wide range of actives like poorly soluble and absorbable drugs, labile bioactives, enzymes, genes, etc. (Mamo 2015).

13.5.7 Gold Nanoparticles

These are inert, biocompatible, non-toxic, stable and noncytotoxic particles having size in the range of 5–400 nm. They promise high drug loading and targeted drug release. They are very

Table 13.3 Nanoformulations against photodamage

Nanosized labile system	Purpose	Active ingredients	References
Nanoemulsion	Anti-Photoageing	*Centella asiatica* extract	Lala and Patel (2019)
Solid-in-oil nanodispersion	Anti-Photoageing	Competitive inhibitor peptide of Human Neutrophil Elastase with hyaluronic acid	Madalena et al. (2015)
Nanosuspension	Against Oxidative stress	Resveratrol	Kobierski et al. (2009)
Lipid nanocarriers	Sunscreen	Rice bran and raspberry seed oil	Niculae et al. (2014)
Lipid nanoparticles	Cutaneous alteration-Skin hydration & elasticity	Rosemary Essential Oil	Montenegro et al. (2017)
Nanocapsule	Against UVB distress	Curcumin	Suwannateep et al. (2012)
Nanoemulsion	Sunscreen	Pomegranate	Baccarin et al. (2015)
Niosomes	Antioxidant	Resveratrol, Curcumin	Tavano et al. (2014)
Ultra-small lipid nanoparticles	Antioxidant	Q10 Enzyme	Lohani et al. (2014)
Nanoemulsion	Photoprotection	Pomegranate Seed Oil	Dhawan and Nanda (2019)
Nanoparticles	Sunscreen	Titanium Dioxide	Lin and Lin (2011)
Encapsulation into lipid nanostructures	Photoprotection	Benzimidazole derivatives	Manescu et al. (2015)
Bioadhesive nanoparticles	Sunblock-UV protection	Padimate O	Deng et al. (2015)
Nanoparticles	Sunscreen	Cerium Dioxide	Herrling et al. (2013)
Nanoemulsion	Against UVA radiation	Propolis and lycopene extract	Butnariu and Giuchici (2011)
Nanoparticles	Sunscreen	TiO_2 and	Hosseinzadeh et al. (2017)
Nanoparticles	Suncreen	TiO_2 and ZnO	Smijs and Pavel (2011)
Nanostructured lipid carriers	Sunscreen/skin cancer	Rutin	Kamel and Mostafa (2015)
Nanoparticles	Sunscreen-Safety Confirms	Zinc Oxide	Zvyagin et al. (2008)
Poly(lactic-co-glycolic acid) Nanoparticles	Squamous cell carcinoma	5-aminolevulinic acid	Shi et al. (2013)
Nanoemulsion	Skin carcinoma	Betulin	Dehelean et al. (2013)
Chitosan nanogel	Skin cancer	Bleomycin	Sahu et al. (2017)
Calcium carbonate-polydopamine Nanoparticle	Skin Phototoxicity and tumor	Chlorin e6	Dong et al. (2018)
Nanoparticle	Skin photodamage.	5-aminolevulinic acid	Passos et al. (2013)
Biodegradable liposome gold nanoparticles	Skin cancer	Curcumin	Singh et al. (2018)
Chitin nanogels	Skin cancer	5-fluorouracil	Sabitha et al. (2013)
Chitin	Skin melanoma	(−)-epigallocatechin-3-gallate	Siddiqui et al. (2014)
Gold nanoparticles	Skin cancer	Fluorouracil	Safwat et al. (2018)
Nanostructured systems-Co-encapsulated	Skin carcinoma	Imiquimod and copaiba oil	Venturini et al. (2015)
Pegylated ethosomal nanoencapsule	Melanoma	Paclitaxel	Eskolaky et al. (2015)
Carboxymethyl cellulose/casein nanogels	Skin cancer	Curcumin and folic acid	Alamelu et al. (2017)
Lecithin–chitosan nanoparticle	Antioxidant, delay UV-mediated oxidant	Quercetin	Tan et al. (2011)

(continued)

Table 13.3 (continued)

Nanosized labile system	Purpose	Active ingredients	References
Chitosan nanoparticle	Anti-wrinkle, Acne	Retinol	Kim et al. (2006)
Poly(ε-caprolactone) nanoparticles	Sunscreen	Octyl methoxycinnamate	Alvarez-Roman et al. (2001)
PLGA nanoparticles	Melanoma	Coumarin	Bhattacharyya et al. (2011)
Chitosan nanoparticles	Melanoma	EGCG	Siddiqui et al. (2014)
Silver nanoparticles	Skin cancer	Naphthoquinone-Plumbagin	Duraipandy et al. (2014)
Solid lipid nanoparticles	Skin carcinoma	5-Fluorouracil	Khallaf et al. (2016)
Nanospheres	Skin cancer metastasis	Doxorubicin	Minotti et al. (2004)
Nanoparticle	Skin melanoma	Dacarbazine	Hafeez and Kazmi (2017)
Proniosome	Photoageing	Coenzyme Q10	Yadav et al. (2015)
Lipid-core nanocapsules	Antioxidant, anti-inflammatory, Anticarcinogenic	Curcumin, Resveratrol	Friedrich et al. (2015)
Solid lipid nanosystems	Delayed UV mediated DNA damage & necrosis	Quercetin	Bose et al. (2013)
Nanostructured lipid carrier and Nanoemulsion	Antioxidant, Protect the drug from UV degradation	Tocopherol	Abla and Banga (2014)

stable both in liquid and in dry forms. These nanoparticles improve blood circulation, skin elasticity and firmness, provide anti-inflammatory and antiseptic properties and are widely used in anti-ageing skin care formulations (Thakor et al. 2011).

Tables 13.3, 13.4, and 13.5 enlists some of the photoprotective and anticancer nanoformulations, patents and marketed formulations, respectively.

13.6 Regulatory Requirements of Manufacturing, Testing and Labelling

Nanotechnology is incorporated in cosmetics with a thought that the small particles are easily absorbed into the skin and repair the damage more competently (Lohani et al. 2014). Every system in this universe possesses some negative aspects along with its benefits.

13.6.1 Risk Factors

Vast development and usage of nanomaterials expose a large number of workforces and consumers to nanomaterials. The human exposure to nanoparticles is through inhalation, ingestion and dermal routes (Lohani et al. 2014). In spite of the versatile nature of the nanoparticles, the lack of inclusive scientific data showed some risk factors. There are four areas in general that come under risk factors (Picecchi 2018), i.e.

- The general toxicity of nanomaterials
- The accumulation of nanomaterials within the biological systems
- The non-biodegradability of nanomaterials
- The transboundary harm caused by nanomaterials

It has been established by several studies that nanoparticles due to its small size merely reach to the systemic circulation (and then to organs), where it shows some toxicity. Sometimes the

Table 13.4 Patents on Antiaging and Anticancer Topical Nanoformulations

Patents	Nanoformulation	Active agent	Asignee/Inventor	Purpose	References
CA2894370A1	Nanoparticles	Metadichol	NanorRx Inc.	Various skin disorders	Raghavan (2014)
WO2008057562A1	Nanoparticles	Paclitaxel and albumin with Bevacizumab	Abraxis Bioscience, Llc	Cancer including Skin	Desai and Shiong (2007)
US9757453B2	Nanoparticles	Anti-CD20 antibodies, albumin and Paclitaxel	Mayo Foundation for Medical Education and Research	Skin cancer	Markovic and Navela (2017)
US20100179103A1	Solid lipid nanoparticle	Curcumin	Ketan Desai	Skin tumor	Desai (2009)
US20110262499A1	Nanoemulsion	Lemon juice/rose water	Sunev Pharma Solution Ltd	Skin disorders and ageing	Chaudhary and Naithani (2009)
US20040208902A1	Controlled-release nanodiffusion delivery by Zeolites	Zeolites	Shyam Gupta	Anti-ageing, antioxidant, skin whitening, acne, rosacea sunscreens, etc.	Gupta (2003)
WO2019046978A1	Nanoemulsions and nanocapsules	Carotenoids- curcumin and astaxanthin	Felipe Andres OyarzunAmpuero	Photoprotection	Ampuero et al. (2017)
EP3340962A1	Nanocrystals complex	ZnO or Avobenzone	Indian Institute of Tech Bombay	Sunscreen-UVA	Adersh and Kulkarni (2016)
201711030008A	Nanoformulation	Pomegranate Seed Oil		Photoprotection	Dhawan and Nanda (2017)
201711030132A	Nanoformulation	Rosehip Seed Oil		Photoprotection	Kayath and Nanda (2017)
US 20130022655A1	Nanocomposites	Metal oxide	BASF SE	UV protection	Sachweh et al. (2013)
US 20090220556A1	Nanodiamond	ZnO and TiO_2	International Technology Center	UV protection	Shenderova and Grichko (2009)

Table 13.5 Marketed nanoformulations (Duarah et al. 2016; Sharma and Sharma 2012)

Nanoformulation	Trade name	Company/Manufacturer	Active agent	Purpose
Nanosomes	Revitalift Double Lifting	L'Oreal	Pro-Tensium, Pro-Retinol A	Anti-wrinkle
Nanocrystals	Renergie Microlift	Lancome	Black tea ferment, tetrapeptide-9	Anti-ageing
Fullerene C-60	Zelens Fullerene C-60 Night Cream	Zelens	Fullerenes C60	Anti-ageing
Liposomes	Royal Jelly Lift Concentrate	Jafra Cosmetics	Cellspan Complex with Royal jelly	Anti-wrinkle
Nanoparticles	NanoSun™	Micronisers Pty Ltd	Zinc oxide	Sunscreen
Nano-UV filters	Dior Snow Pure UV Base SPF 50	Dior	Titanium dioxide, Octinoxate, Oxybenzone	Sunscreen
Nanosphere	Nanosphere Plus	Derma Swiss	Hydrolyzed Collagen, Elastin, Allantoin, Hyaluronic Acid, Alpha-Lipoic acid, Apple, Rose	Anti-ageing
Nanoparticles	TEGO® Sun TS plus	Degussa	Titanium dioxide	Sunscreen
Liposomes	Rovisome ACE Plus	Rovi Cosmetics International GmbH	Ascorbyl palmitate, Tocopherol, retinol	Sun protection, Anti-ageing
Nanotopes	Tinoderm E	Ciba Specialty Chemicals	Vitamin E	Photoageing
Liposomes	Ageless Facelift cream	I-Wen Naturals	Coenzyme Q10, Niacinamide	Anti-ageing, whitening, Antioxidant
Micro-encapsulated	Ultimate Anti-Ageing Cream	Promise Cosmeceuticals	Vitamin C	Anti-ageing
Nanoemulsion	Nano-Lipobelle H-EQ10 cream	Mibelle Biochemistry, Switzerland	Coenzyme Q10, Vitamin E acetate	Anti-ageing, anti-inflammatory
Nanoparticles	Revitalift	L'Oreal	Pro-Retinol A	Anti-ageing
Nanoemulsion	Nano-Lipobelle H-AECL	Mibelle Biochemistry, Switzerland	Vitamins A. E, C & borage oil	Anti-wrinkle
Nanocapsules	Lancome Soleil Soft-Touch Anti-Wrinkle Sun Cream SPF 15	L'Oreal	Vit E, Panthenol	Anti-wrinkle, Sunscreen
Fullerenes	Sircuit Addict Firming Antioxidant Serum	Sircuit Skin Cosmeceuticals Inc.	Green tea extract, Grape seed extract, Vitamin E	Anti-ageing, Rejuvenating
Liposomes	DOXIL	TTY Biopharm Company Limited	Doxorubicin hydrochloride	Skin cancer
Nanostructured lipid carriers	Cutanova Nano Repair Q10 Cream	Dr.Rimpler GmbH	CoenzymeQ10	Anti-ageing
Nanostructured lipid carriers	Nanolipid Restore CLR	CLR Chemisches Laboratorium, Dr. Kurt Richter GmbH	Black current seed oil	Revitalising, anti-ageing
Liposomes	Capture	Dior		Anti-ageing
Nanocapsules	Soleil Instant Cooling Sun Spritz SPF 15	Lancome	Vitamin	Sun protection spray

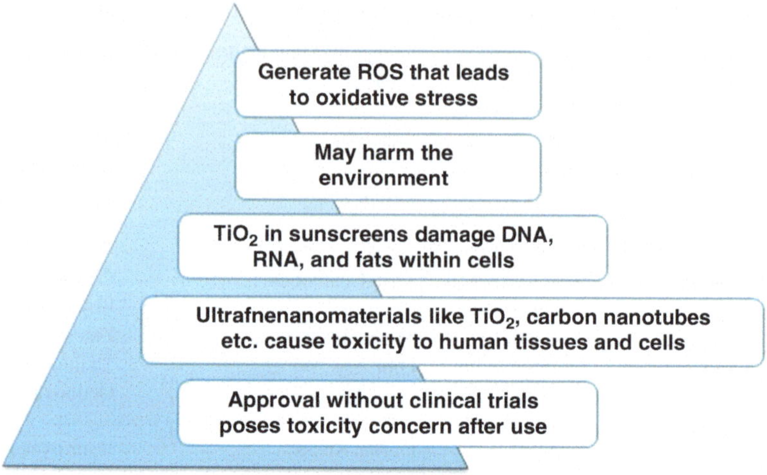

Fig. 13.6 Negative aspects of nanomaterials

nanosized particles produce free radicals and hence toxic to cells. A toxicity study of titanium dioxide (TiO_2) nanoparticles revealed the transfer of particles to the progeny that caused brain damage and reduced sperm count in male children when it was subcutaneously administered to pregnant mice (Lohani et al. 2014).

With the emergence of nanotechnology, the concerns of materials and products having the potential for adverse biological and environmental effects are also intensifying. Nanotechnology imparts environmental problems as well as human health problems. The issues on humans regarding nanoformulations are carcinogenesis, respirational effects, toxicity, life expectancy, etc. The limitations of nanocosmeceuticals in general are depicted in Fig. 13.6. Hence, a need arises to establish some stringent regulations on nanocosmeceuticals.

13.6.2 Safety Assessment

The parameters which are related to the manufacturing of nanoproducts should be reviewed during their life cycle. Life-cycle assessment (LCA) is a means for the quantification of the environmental bearings of a nanoproduct. It can identify or measure all sources of nano-waste from upstream processes (like manufacturing of compounds, equipment, etc.) to the downstream processes (nano-waste capture, recycling, treatment and disposal) (Charitidis et al. 2014).

The safety assessment of nanomaterials used in cosmetic products must consider the following factors: (US FDA, Regulations 2014)

- The physicochemical properties
- Accumulation of nanomaterials and their size distribution
- Possible routes of nanoparticles exposure
- Dosimetry for toxicological interpretation
- Skin diffusion
- Toxicological data on nanomaterial ingredients, potential inhalation, irritation (skin and eye) and mutagenicity/genotoxicity studies
- Impurities etc.

13.6.3 Regulations Governing Manufacturing and Usage of Nanoformulations

At first, the agencies of the world did not realize that the nanomaterials and their traditional forms would be completely different in their properties. The Royal Society of Sciences, UK treated nanomaterials as new entities for the first time (Nanda et al. 2016). In the competitive commercialization of nanotechnology-based products including cosmetics, there is a need to clarify or to reduce the risks involved in the nanoformulations. The concern regarding safety of nanomaterials became the initial step for regulatory bodies to provide guidelines all over the world by means of ethical, legal and regulatory bodies (Declaration, Canadian Environmental Law Association 2007). The basic regulatory approaches towards risk management are as follows:

- Precautionary basis
- Compulsory nano-specific regulations
- Health and safety of the community and workforces
- Environmental safety
- Transparency
- Public contribution
- Insertion of wider impacts
- Manufacturer responsibility

From the production of the material to its packaging and shipping the health, safety and environmental risks are of great concern that require an action. Internationally, the community should have an undivided regulatory system between regions because of the universal nature of the risks of nanomaterials. The regulations in one region will eventually affect the entire environment (Picecchi 2018). Therefore, Governments around the world create regulations and standards for research and the use of nanomaterials, while the most of the nations are currently deficient in specific legislation on nanomaterials. The Food and Drug Administration (FDA) and European Medicines Agency (EMEA) have the leading nanotechnology regulations followed by Health Canada (Canada), Therapeutic Goods Administration (TGA) and the Australia's *National Industrial Chemicals Notification and Assessment Scheme* (NICNAS) (Nanda et al. 2016).

13.6.3.1 US Regulations

The United States has a federal system of regulation. In 2000, the US FDA took up the US National Nanotechnology Initiative (NNI). The first Nano Initiative Task Force was set up by FDA in 2006, to develop safe, efficient and innovative FDA regulated nanomaterial-based products. After the Task Force endorsement in 2007, the US FDA provided a drafted document in 2012 under the title of "Guidance for Industry: Safety of Nanomaterials in Cosmetic Products" and this draft was open for public commenting from June 2014. The FDA initiates the development of new methods to successfully evaluate the toxicity of the nanomaterial in cosmetics when the traditional testing methods are not suitable. It provides a general criterion for the evaluation of nanomaterials in cosmetics either adulterated or misbranded. The nanotechnology also needs modification in nomenclature and dose metrics of the compounds (Nanda et al. 2016).

In June 2014, FDA issued guidance for industry titled "Considering Whether an FDA-Regulated Product Involves the Application of Nanotechnology." This draft provides direction to industry and other investors in order to identify the safety issues of nanomaterials in cosmetic products and helps in designing their evaluation parameters. These guidelines considered the information (like recent advances, publications, etc.) provided by the cosmetic industry to the International Cooperation on Cosmetics Regulations (ICCR) and relevant reports of Organization for Economic Co-operation and Development (OECD) on "Manufactured Nanomaterials," the Scientific Committee on Consumer Safety (SCCS) on "Safety Assessment of Nanomaterials in Cosmetics," relevant ICCR reports on the "Currently Available Methods for Characterization of Nanomaterials," and the "Principles of Cosmetic Product Safety Assessment"(US FDA, Regulations 2014).

The US government entities: the US Environmental Protection Agency (EPA) and the US FDA are involved in signifying the nanoscale materials. EPA is involved in the identification of the health and environmental risks of nanomaterials with a drafted document (that includes the source of nanomaterial; how it transfers to the environment and their associated problems to human, animal or plant), while FDA regulates nanoproducts, not the materials (Kelley 2009). The EPA can follow the regulatory measures set up by the Toxic Substances Control Act (TSCA). Under the TSCA Sect. 13.4, the EPA can regulate any chemical compound if it involved some health or environmental risk. Also, the TSCA Sect. 13.5 gives power to the EPA to screen new chemical products before they enter in the market. US regulatory approach for nanomaterials is generally market-oriented (Picecchi 2018).

According to FDA, medical products are under regulation of the Centre for Drug

Evaluation and Research (CDER), Centre for Devices and Radiological Health (CDRH) and Office of Combination Products (OCP). The task force has also collaborated with bodies like Food Drug and Cosmetic Act (FDCA), Toxic Substance Control Act (TSCA), Occupational Safety and Health Act (OSHA), National Environmental Policy Act (NEPA), United States Department of Agriculture (USDA), National Institute of Nutrition (NIN), etc. (Dhawan et al. 2018).

In 2015, EPA proposed new rules according to TSCA section 8(a) to involve reporting and record keeping information on those chemical substances which are manufactured or processed as nanoscale materials. This proposed rule would notify EPA about production volume, methods of manufacture and processing, exposure and release information and available health and safety data (Regulations of Nanomaterials in USA 2016).

13.6.3.2 EU Regulations

The European Union (EU) is a cosmopolitan body. In contrast to US, the European Union (EU) follows a more precautionary approach, which permits the regulation of certain constituents without inclusive and conclusive scientific data regarding their potential risks. Due to its precautionary approach, the EU has some nano-specific regulations (Breggin et al. 2009). The EU cosmetics regulations cover the use of nanomaterials in cosmetics and provide a meaning to nanomaterials, their usage, labelling and safety evaluation. The toxicological profile of the nanomaterial of the EU Cosmetic regulation includes percutaneous absorption, toxicokinetics, skin sensitization, mutagenicity, repeated dose toxicity, carcinogenicity and photo-induced toxicity. The Scientific Committee on Consumer Safety (SCCS) and the Scientific Committee on Emerging and Newly Identified Health Risks (SCENIHR) regulate the environmental and health-related risks associated with nanomaterials. The SCENIHR is related with the suitability of prevailing risk valuation practices or methodologies, while the SCCS is related to the safety of nanomaterials in cosmetic products and issued an opinion on the safety of nanomaterials especially in cosmetic products in 2007. In Europe only the validated methods are accepted for assessment of cosmetic ingredients. As there is ban on testing of cosmetic ingredients on animals, the alternative methods for toxicological threat identification are in silico modelling approaches. The objective of these approaches is to reduce, refine or replace the use of animals. The methods involved in such approaches are established at the European Centre for the Validation of Alternative Methods (ECVAM) and are considered by Expert Scientific Advisory Committee (ESAC) (SCCS opinion guidelines 2012).

The SCENIHR advises the European Commission about the emerging and newly acknowledged health risks (Picecchi 2018). The main implementation of EU involves regulations, directions, decisions, communications and recommendations. The EU has specific regulatory agencies. The EU bodies that regulate manufactured nanomaterials are: the European Chemicals Agency (ECHA), the EMEA and the European Agency for Safety and Health at Work (EU-OSHA).

The ECHA regulates the Registration, Evaluation, Authorization and Restriction of Chemical Substances (REACH) and Classification, Labelling and Packaging (CLP) regulations. The EMEA is involved in the scientific assessment of therapeutic products which are marketed across the EU and helps in the development of nanotherapeutic products and discover probable scientific solutions. The European Environment Agency (EEA) and the EU-OSHA coordinate, and monitor national and European regulations in their respective areas (Breggin et al. 2009). The latest nanomaterial regulations in EU update the use of nano register in the EU member states.

13.6.3.3 Indian Regulations

The document titled 'Guidelines for evaluation of nanopharmaceuticals in India' under the headship of Dr. (Prof.) Y. K. Gupta is drafted jointly by All India Institute of Medical Sciences (AIIMS), Translational Health Science and Technology Institute (THSTI), Department of Biotechnology (DBT) and Indian Society of Nanomedicine (ISNM). Recently, these guidelines were again revised and drafted jointly by the Indian Society of Nanomedicines (ISNM) and Department of Biotechnology (DBT) and are published by Central Drug Standard Control Organization (CDSCO) in 2019. Obligatorily, it is required to formulate a comprehensive guideline to create a transparent and consistent regulation regarding quality, safety and efficacy of nanopharmaceuticals for its therapeutic use within the country. The guidelines apply for nanoproducts as well as for new nanomaterials. These guidelines also boost the commercialization of nanotechnology-based innovation with high benefits and low-risk ratio. The safety studies in India for nanomaterials are in accordance with the general guidelines specified in Schedule Y of Drugs and Cosmetics Rules, 1945, the principles of ICH guidelines or OECD guidelines.

The basis of safety and efficacy evaluation for a specific nanopharmaceutical should be 'case by case approach' and it depends on various factors like physicochemical and biological nature, nanocarrier used, the regulatory status in other countries, etc. (CDSCO guidelines 2019).

13.6.3.4 Conventions, Councils and Organizations Regarding Nanotechnology

Apart from the regulations, there are some conventions like the Basel Convention which mainly deals with the transboundary movements of harmful wastes and their disposal. While the international trade of certain hazardous chemicals is under Rotterdam convention (or PIC convention). Likewise, Stockholm convention or persistent organic pollutants (POPs) was implemented in 2001 that deal with the protection of human health and the environment from persistent biological pollutants (Picecchi 2018). Many organizations have their own standards and guidelines for the development and handling of nanomaterials because in some areas the government regulations do not give clarity. International Council on Nanotechnology (ICON) is a governing organization devoted to the safe, responsible and beneficial development of nanotechnology (Kelley 2009).

The first Intergovernmental Forum on Chemical Safety (IFCS) discussed nanomaterials on a global level afterward, limitless international bodies have set up the committees and have initiated reports to measure the risks of nanomaterials. For example, the Strategic Approach to International Chemicals Management (SAICM) deals with the management of chemicals with the promotion of international research and cooperation in the field of nanomaterials. Similarly, standardization governing bodies such as the International Organization for Standardization (ISO) or the European Committee for Standardization (CEN) have presented several documents for the standardization and classification of nanomaterials and nanotechnology. Most importantly, the World Health Organization (WHO), the United Nations Educational Scientific and Cultural Organization (UNESCO), the Food and Agriculture Organization of the United Nations (FAO) and the OECD are all involved in collecting information regarding nanomaterials (Picecchi 2018).

The OECD and the ISO are the most important international entities for regulatory cooperation and information sharing. OECD plays a key role in identifying potential contests posed by nanomaterials to the environment. The Cosmetic Toiletry and Fragrance Association (CTFA) and OECD provided the guidelines for toxicity testing on the basis of toxicological profile of the component and their routes of exposure. Animals are banned for toxicity testing of new chemicals; therefore, the two leading bodies, i.e. European Centre for the Validation of Alternative Methods (ECVAM) and the Interagency Coordinating Committee on the Validation of Alternative Methods (ICCVAM), are referred for the alternative testing methods. The reconstructed human skins such as EPISkin™ and EPIDerm™ are used for skin irritation and corrosion testing (Nanda et al. 2016).

The countries that don't have their own nano regulations must adopt the other country's regulations with the concern of the International Conference on Harmonisation (ICH guidelines). ICH is the treaty or convention signed by many countries in order to fill the regional gaps in the regulations.

13.6.4 Labelling Regulations of Nanoformulations

Presently, there is no generic labelling prerequisite for manufactured nanoparticles (MNPs) as well as for the products containing manufactured nanoparticles (PCMNPs) used by both providers and consumers (BSi, Guidance 2007). The EU or US law provides some nano-specific regulatory guidelines on labelling of nanoformulations. In FDA, the Federal Food, Drug and Cosmetic Act (FFDCA) and the Fair Packaging and Labeling Act (FPLA) regulate cosmetic labelling. The FFDCA has the judicial power to remove adulterated or misbranded products. The labelling requirement of the FDA emphasis the addition or the avoidance of the material's information or misleading information, respectively, but FDA lacks the authority to inspect the records. On the other hand, the EU provides the framework for the regulation of labelling and packaging of the product. It allows the manufacturer to carry out risk assessment regarding the product in relation with the Skinny Client Control Protocol (SCCP) or SANCO's. Hence, both FDA and EU labelling guidelines are the prime tools for regulating nanocosmetic market (Falkner et al. 2009). The listing and labelling are used to address probable adverse effects of nanomaterials over the human health or the environment. The regulations on the format and content of labels for MNPs and PCMNPs are given by Publicly Available Specification (PAS). The PAS also provides guidance on the use of the term "nano" in product labelling. The labelling guidelines are used for the following:

- To promote a uniform approach towards labelling.
- To ensure that consumers of MNPs and PCMNPs can correctly identify the contents for making decisions of their selection, procurement, distribution, handling, use and disposal.
- To establish the use of the term 'nano' in labels etc.

It is essential to mention the term "nano" on product's label if it contains nanosized components or if it depicts a nanoenabled effect. Labelling is recommended for formulated nanoparticles and for products containing formulated nanoparticles except when the product or a complex system could not release nano-component. Additionally, with the identified risks, it is suggested that the labels for nanoformulations should provide required information for user or for specialized persons (BSi, Guidance 2007).

The compliance of the product with specific standards includes the list of ingredients, technical description, directions for their use, cleaning, storage, disposal, name, address and contact details of the manufacturer, etc. This should be directed in instructions or on permanently attached labels of the product itself (Amoabediny et al. 2009).

13.7 Conclusion

The skin itself, in the process of being a protective barrier, suffers from many environmental insults. The UV radiations have been established as a skin carcinogen. The damaging UV rays affect all the layers of the skin and their effects depend upon the duration and extent of UV exposure. UV rays increase the prevalence of sunburn, tanning, itching, inflammation, hyperpigmentation, etc. Consequently causing skin cells to die, damage, develop cancer in the epidermal layer or cause photoageing. The skin has been used as a site for drug administration to avail both topical and systemic effects. Designing a topical formulation against photoageing and photocarcinogenesis requires consideration of several factors like physicochemical properties of drug, targeted layer, symptoms to be addressed, pattern of drug release such as controlled or fast release. The major challenges faced while formulating these topical preparations involve overcoming the stratum corneum barrier, safety and efficacy issues. Several techniques have been employed to overcome the barrier. One such highly recommended strategy is the use of nanocarrier systems for delivering useful and effective drug molecules. These nanosystems provide better product performance, site-specific targeting, enhanced skin penetration, controlled and sustained release, better entrapment and better stability of the drug. Apart from having benefits, these nanosystems also create some risks for human health and environment. Hence, stringent regulations and guidelines on the manufacture, labelling and ethical use of nanomaterials and nanocosmetics are being promulgated by regulatory agencies so as to ensure consumer safety without imbalancing the ecosystem of the planet.

References

Abla MJ, Banga AK (2014) Formulation of tocopherol nanocarriers and *in vitro* delivery into human skin. Int J Cosmet Sci 36(3):239–246

Adersh A, Kulkarni RA (2016) Enhanced photostability, extended range UVA filtering and camouflaging potential of avobenzone-defect rich ZnO nanocrystals complex. European Patent Office EP3340962A1, 29 July 2016

Alamelu PP, Raj R, Vasudevan V, Raj V (2017) Curcumin-loaded layer-by-layer folic acid and casein coated carboxymethyl cellulose/ casein nanogels for treatment of skin cancer. Arab J Chem. https://doi.org/10.1016/j.arabjc.2017.07.010

Alvarez-Roman R, Barre G, Guy RH, Fessi H (2001) Biodegradable polymer nanocapsules containing a sunscreen agent: preparation and photoprotection. Eur J Pharm Biopharm 52:191–195

Amoabediny G, Naderi A, Malakootikhah J, Koohi MK (2009) Guidelines for safe handling, use and disposal of nanoparticles. J Phys Conf Ser 170, 012037

Ampuero OAF, Valenzuela MJ, Silva SM, Rivera G, Villoslada M, Alarcon A, Flores F, Gallegos T (2017). Method for obtaining nanostructures with carotenoids and nanostructures obtained. WIPO (PCT) WO2019046978A1, 5 Sept 2017

Arora SA, Murthy RSR (2012) Latest technology advances in cosmaceuticals. Int J Pharm Sci Drug Res 4(3):168–182

Baccarin T, Mitjans M, Ramos D, Lemos-Senna E, Vinardell MP (2015) Photoprotection by *Punica granatum* seed oil nanoemulsion entrapping polyphenol-rich ethyl acetate fraction against UVB-induced DNA damage in human keratinocyte (HaCaT) cell line. J Photochem Photobiol B Biol 153:127–136

Benson HA, Namjoshi S (2008) Proteins and peptides: strategies for delivery to and across the skin. J Pharm Sci 97:3591–3610

Bhattacharyya SS, Paul S, De A, Das D, Samadder A, Boujedaini N, Khuda-Bukhsh AR (2011) Poly(lactide-co-glycolide) acid nanoencapsulation of a synthetic coumarin: cytotoxicity and bio-distribution in mice, in cancer cell line and interaction with calf thymus DNA as target. Toxicol Appl Pharmacol 253(3):270–281

Bosch R, Philips N, Suárez-Pérez JA, Juarranz A, Devmurari A, Chalensouk-Khaosaat J, González S (2015) Mechanisms of photoaging and cutaneous photocarcinogenesis, and photoprotective strategies with phytochemicals. Antioxidants 4:248–268

Bose S, Du Y, Takhistov P, Michniak-Kohn B (2013) Formulation optimization and topical delivery of quercetin from solid lipid based nanosystems. Int J Pharm 441:56–66

Breggin L, Falkner R, Jaspers N, Pendergrass J, Porter R (2009) Project on Securing the promise of nanotechnologies- towards transatlantic regulatory cooperation. Royal Institute of International Affairs, ISBN 978 1 86203 218 7. http://www.lse.ac.uk/nanoregulation

British Standard Institution (BSi) (2007) Guidance on the labelling of manufactured nanoparticles and products containing manufactured nanoparticles. Available at, https://nanotech.law.asu.edu/Documents/2011/06/PAS130_567_5096.pdf

Butnariu VM, Giuchici VC (2011) The use of some nanoemulsions based on aqueous propolis and lycopene extract in the skin's protective mechanisms against UVA radiation. J Nanobiotechnol 9:3

Central Drugs Standard Control Organization (CDSCO) (2019) Guidelines for evaluation of nanopharmaceuticals in India. Available on web. https://cdsco.gov.in/opencms/resources/UploadCDSCOWeb/2018/UploadPublic_NoticesFiles/newdrunoti7march.pdf

Charitidis C, Georgiou P, Koklioti M, Trompeta A, Markakis V (2014) Manufacturing nanomaterials: from research to industry. Manufacturing Rev 1, 11

Chandu VP, Arunachalam A, Jeganath S, Yamini K, Tharangini K (2012) Niosomes: a novel drug delivery system. Int J Novel Trends Pharm Sci 2(1):2277–2782

Chaudhary M, Naithani V (2009) Topical herbal formulation for treatment of acne and skin disorders. United States US20110262499A1, 30 Dec 2009

Declaration (2007) Principles for the Oversight of Nanotechnologies and Nanomaterials. In: Canadian Environmental Law Association. Retrieved from http://www.cela.ca/publications/principles-oversight-nanotechnologies-and-nanomaterials

Dehelean CA, Feflea S, Gheorgheosu D, Ganta S, Cimpean AM, Muntean D, Amiji MM (2013) Anti-angiogenic and anti-cancer evaluation of betulinnanoemulsion in chicken chorioallantoic membrane and skin carcinoma in Balb/c mice. J Biomed Nanotechnol 9(4):577–589

Denet AR, Vanbever R, Preat V (2004) Skin electroporation for transdermal and topical delivery. Adv Drug Deliv Rev 56:659–674

Deng Y, Ediriwickrema A, Yang F, Lewis J, Girardi M, Saltzman MW (2015) A sunblock based on bioadhesive nanoparticles. Nat Mater 14(12):1278–1285

Desai K (2009) Curcumin cyclodextrin combination for preventing or treating various diseases. United States US20100179103A1, 22 June 2009

Desai PN, Shiong SP (2007). Nanoparticles of paclitaxel and albumin in combination with bevacizumab against cancer. WIPO (PCT) WO2008057562A1, 6 Nov 2007

Dhawan S, Nanda S (2017) A nanoformulation of pomegranate seed oil and uses thereof. Indian Patent office, Application No.201711030008 A, 8 Sept 2017

Dhawan S, Nanda S (2019) *In vitro* estimation of photoprotective potential of pomegranate seed oil and development of a nanoformulation. Curr Nutr Food Sci 15(1):87–102

Dhawan S, Hooda P, Nanda S (2018) Herbal nano formulations- patent and regulatory overview. Appl Clin Res Clin Trials Regul Aff 5:1–22

Di Meglio P, Perera GK, Nestle FO (2011) The multitasking organ: recent insights into skin immune function. Immunity 23:857–869

Dong Z, Feng L, Hao Y, Chen M, Gao M, Chao Y, Zhao H, Zhu W, Liu J, Liang C, Zhang Q, Liu Z (2018) Synthesis of hollow biomineralized CaCO3–polydopamine nanoparticles for multimodal imaging-guided cancer photodynamic therapy with reduced skin photosensitivity. J Am Chem Soc 140:2165–2178

Duarah S, Pujari K, Durai DR, Narayanan BVH (2016) Nanotechnology-based cosmeceuticals: a review. Int J Appl Pharm 8(1):8–12

Duraipandy N, Lakra R, Kunnavakkam VS, Samanta D, Sai P, Kiran MS (2014) Caging of plumbagin on silver nanoparticles imparts selectivity and sensitivity to plumbagin for targeted cancer cell apoptosis. Metallomics 6(11):2025–2033

Ellias PM (1981) Epidermal lipids, membranes, and keratinization. Int J Dermatol 20:1–19

Eskolaky EB, Ardjmand M, Akbarzadeh A (2015) Evaluation of anti-cancer properties of pegylated ethosomal paclitaxel on human melanoma cell line SKMEL- 3. Trop J Pharm Res 14(8):1421

Falkner R, Breggin L, Jaspers N, Pendergrass J, Porter R (2009) Consumer labelling of nanomaterials in the EU and US: convergence or divergence? Chatham House, London, UK, EERG BP 2009/03

FDA (U.S. Food Drug Administration) (2014) Guidance for industry safety of nanomaterials in cosmetic products. U.S. Department of Health and Human Services Food and Drug Administration Center for Food Safety and Applied Nutrition

Friedrich RB, Kann B, Coradini K, Offerhaus HL, Beck RC, Windbergs M (2015) Skin penetration behavior of lipid-core nanocapsules for simultaneous delivery of resveratrol and curcumin. Eur J Pharm Sci 78:204–213

Gilchrest BA (2007) Photoageing: mechanism, prevention and therapy. Br J Dermatol 157(5):874–87

Green PG (1996) Iontophoretic delivery of peptide drugs. J Control Release 41(1–2):33–48

Gupta S (2003) Controlled-release nano-diffusion delivery systems for cosmetic and pharmaceutical compositions. United States US20040208902A1, 18 Apr 2003

Gupta M, Agrawal U, Vyas SP (2012) Nanocarrier-based topical drug delivery for the treatment of skin diseases. Expert Opin Drug Deliv 9(7):783–804

Hafeez A, Kazmi I (2017) Dacarbazine nanoparticle topical delivery system for the treatment of melanoma. Sci Rep 7:16517

Herrling T, Seifert M, Jung K (2013) Cerium dioxide: future UV-filter in sunscreen? SOFW J 139(5):10–14

Hosseinzadeh S, Baharifar H, Amani A (2017) Efficacy of a model nano-TiO2 sunscreen preparation as a function of ingredients concentration and ultrasonication treatment. Pharm Sci 23:129–135

Kamel R, Mostafa MD (2015) Rutin nanostructured lipid cosmeceutical preparation with sun protective potential. J Photochem Photobiol B Biol 153:59–66

Kaul S, Gulati N, Verma D, Mukherjee S, Nagaich U (2018) Role of nanotechnology in cosmeceuticals: a review of recent advances. J Pharm 2018:1–19

Kayath H, Nanda S (2017) A nanoformulation of rosehip seed oil and uses thereof. Indian patent office, application no. 201711030132 A, 8 Sept 2017

Keleb E, Sharma RK, Mosa EB, Aljahwi AZ (2010) Transdermal drug delivery system- design and evaluation. Int J Adv Pharm Sci 1:201–211

Kelley B (2009) Small concerns: nanotech regulations and risk management. In: SPIE Newsroom Retrieved from http://spie.org/newsroom/120109-nanoarticle?SSO=1

Khallaf AR, Salem FH, Abdelbary A (2016) 5-Fluorouracil shell-enriched solid lipid nanoparticles (SLN) for effective skin carcinoma treatment. Drug Deliv 23(9):3452–3460

Kim DG, Jeong YI, Choi C, Roh SH, Kang SK, Jang MK, Nah JW (2006) Retinol-encapsulated low molecular water-soluble chitosan nanoparticles. Int J Pharm 319:130–138

Kobierski S, Ofori-Kwakye K, Muller RH, Keck CM (2009) Resveratrol nanosuspensions for dermal application-production, characterization, and physical stability. Pharmazie 64(11):741–747

Lala RR, Patel HP (2019) Nanoemulsion for improved permeability of *Centellaasiatica* extract: formulation, ex-vivo and in-vivo evaluation. Int J Pharm Sci Res 10(4):1711–1718

Lin CC, Lin WJ (2011) Sun protection factor analysis of sunscreens containing titanium dioxide nanoparticles. J Food Drug Anal 19(1):1–8

Lohani A, Verma A, Joshi H, Yadav N, Karki N (2014) Nanotechnology-based cosmeceuticals. ISRN Derm 2014:843687

Losquadro WD (2017) Anatomy of the skin and the pathogenesis of nonmelanoma skin cancer. Facial Plast Surg Clin North Am 25(3):283–289

Madalena M, Nuno AG, Ana CC, Carla S, Teresa M, Andreia GC, Cavaco-Paulo A (2015) Assessment of a protease inhibitor peptide for anti-ageing. Protein Pept Lett, Bentham Science Publishers 22(11):1041–1049

Mamo B (2015) Literature review on biodegradable nanospheres for oral and targeted drug delivery. Asian J Biomed Pharm Sci 5(51):1–12

Manescu GI, Badea G, Iscrulescu L, Iovu M, Balaci T (2015) Incorporation of new benzimidazole compounds into lipid nanostructures in order to obtain photoprotective formulations. Farmacia 63(4):518–525

Markovic NS, Nevala KW (2017) Nanoparticle complexes of anti-CD20 antibodies, albumin and paclitaxel. United States US9757453B2, 5 July 2017

Michaels AS, Shaw JE (1975) Drug permeation through human skin: theory and *in vitro* experimental measurement. Am Inst Chem Eng J 21:985–996

Minotti GP, Menna ES, Cairo G, Gianni L (2004) Anthracyclines: molecular advances and pharmacological developments in antitumor activity and cardiotoxicity. Pharmacology 56:185–229

Montenegro L, Pasquinucci L, Zappala A, Chiechio S, Turnaturi R, Parenti C (2017) Rosemary essential oil-loaded lipid nanoparticles: *in vivo* topical activity from gel vehicles. Pharmaceutics 9:1–48

N'Da DD (2014) Prodrug strategies for enhancing the percutaneous absorption of drugs. Molecules (Basel, Switzerland) 19(12):20780–20807

Nanda S, Nanda A, Lohan S, Kaur R, Singh B (2016) Nanocosmetics: performance enhancement and safety assurance. In: Nanobiomaterials in galenic formulations and cosmetics, p 47–67. https://doi.org/10.1016/B978-0-323-42868-2.00003-6

Niculae G, Lacatusu I, Badea N, Stan R, Vasile BS, Meghea A (2014) Rice bran and raspberry seed oil-based nanocarriers with self-antioxidative properties as safe photoprotective formulations. Photochem Photobiol Sci 13(4):703–716

Passos KS, de Souza ENP, Soares KPP, Eid RMD, Primo LP, Tedesco CA, Lacava GMZ, Morais CP (2013) Quantitative approach to skin field cancerization using a nanoencapsulated photodynamic therapy agent: a pilot study. Clin Cosmet Investig Dermatol 6, 51–59

Picecchi D (2018) Tiny Things with a Huge Impact: The International Regulation of Nanomaterials, *Mich. J. Envtl. & Admin. L.*,*7*, 447

Polat BE, Hart DP, Langer R, Blankschtein D (2011) Ultrasound-mediated transdermal drug delivery: mechanisms, scope, and emerging trends. J Control Release 152(3):330–348

Purohit DK, Nandgude TD, Poddar SS (2016) Nano-lipid carriers for topical application: current scenario. Asian J Pharm 9(5):544–553

Raghavan PR (2014) Metadichol.rtm. liquid and gel nanoparticle formulations. Canada Patent CA2894370A1, 3 Nov 2014

Regulations of Nanomaterials in USA (2016) Chem Safety Pro. Available on web. https://www.chemsafetypro.com/Topics/USA/Regulations_of_Nanomaterials_in_USA.html

Ronak PP, Jay RJ (2012) An overview on nanoemulsion: a novel approach. Int J Pharm Sci Res 3(12):4640–4650

Sabitha M, Rejinold SN, Nair A, Lakshmanan KV, Nair VS, Jayakumar R (2013) Development and evaluation of 5-fluorouracil loaded chitin nanogels for treatment of skin cancer. Carbohydr Polym 91(1):48–57

Sachweh B, Koban W, Wohlleben W, Peukert W, Taylor RK, Distaso M (2013) Metal oxide nanocomposites for UV protection. US Patent Office US20130022655A1, Jan 2013

Safwat AM, Soliman MG, Sayed D, Attia AM (2018) Fluorouracil-loaded gold nanoparticles for the treatment of skin cancer: development, *in vitro* characterization, and *in vivo* evaluation in a mouse skin cancer xenograft model. Mol Pharm 15:2194–2205

Sahu P, Kashaw KS, Kushwah V, Sau S, Jain S, Iyer KA (2017) pH responsive biodegradable nanogels for sustained release of bleomycin. Bioorg Med Chem 25(17):4595–4613

Schmid MH, Korting HC (1996) Therapeutic progress with topical liposome drugs for skin disease. Adv Drug Deliv Rev 18:335–342

Scientific Committee on Consumer Safety (SCCS) (2012) In: Opinion on guidance on the safety assessment of nanomaterials in cosmetics. SCCS/1484/12. Available on web. http://ec.europa.eu/health/scientific_committees/consumer_safety/index_en.htm

Sharma B, Sharma A (2012) Future prospect of nanotechnology in development of anti-ageing formulations. Int J Pharm Pharm Sci 4(3):57–66

Shenderova OA, Grichko V (2009) Nanodiamond UV protectant formulations. US Patent Office US20090220556A1, 3 Sept 2009

Shi L, Wang X, Zhao F, Luan H, Tu Q, Huang Z, Huang Z, Wang H, Wang H (2013) *In vitro* evaluation of 5-amino levulinic acid (ALA) loaded PLGA nanoparticles. Int J Nanomedicine 8:2669–2676

Siddiqui IA, Bharali DJ, Nihal M, Adhami VM, Khan N, Chamcheu JC, Khan MI, Shabana S, Mousa SA, Mukhta H (2014) Excellent anti-proliferative and pro-apoptotic effects of (−)-epigallocatechin-3-gallate encapsulated in chitosan nanoparticles on human melanoma cell growth both *in vitro* and *in vivo*. Nanomedicine 10(8):1619–1626

Singh PS, Alvi BS, Pemmaraju BD, Singh DA, Manda VS, Srivastava R, Rengan AK (2018) NIR triggered liposome gold nanoparticles entrapping curcumin as in situ adjuvant for photothermal treatment of skin cancer. Int J Biol Macromol 110:375–382

Smijs GT, Pavel S (2011) Titanium dioxide and zinc oxide nanoparticles in sunscreens: focus on their safety and effectiveness. Nanotechnol Sci Appl 4:95–112

Suwannateep N, Wanichwecharungruang S, Haag SF, Devahastin S, Groth N, Fluhr JW, Lademann J, Meinke MC (2012) Encapsulated curcumin results in prolonged curcumin activity *in vitro* and radical scavenging activity ex vivo on skin after UVB-irradiation. Eur J Pharm Biopharm 82(3):485–490

Tan Q, Liu W, Guo C, Zhai G (2011) Preparation and evaluation of quercetin-loaded lecithin-chitosan nanoparticles for topical delivery. Int J Nanomedicine 6:1621–1630

Tanner T, Marks R (2008) Delivering drugs by the transdermal route: review and comment. Skin Res Technol 14:249–260

Tavano L, Muzzalupo R, Picci N, Cindio B (2014) Co-encapsulation of lipophilic antioxidants into niosomal carriers: percutaneous permeation studies for cosmeceutical applications. Colloids Surf B Biointerfaces 114:144–149

Thakor AS, Jokerst J, Zavaleta C, Massoud TF, Gambhir SS (2011) Gold nanoparticles: a revival in precious metal administration to patients. Nano Lett 11(10):4029–4036

Tripura P, Anushree H (2017) Anushree novel delivery systems: current trend in cosmetic industry. Eur J Pharm Med Res 4(8):617–627

Tuckman A (2016) The potential psychological impact of skin conditions. Dermatol Ther 7(Suppl 1): S53–S57

Venturini GC, Bruinsmann AF, Contri VR, Fonseca NF, Frank AL, D'Amore MC, Raffin RP, Buffon A, Pohlmann AR, Guterres SS (2015) Co-encapsulation of imiquimod and copaiba oil in novel nanostructured systems: promising formulations against skin carcinoma. Eur J Pharm Sci 79:36–43

Wilbur RL (2017) The difference between topical and transdermal medications. Gensco Pharma. Available on web. https://genscopharma.com/difference-topical-transdermal-medications/. Cited 24 May 2019

Williams AC, Barry BW (2004) Penetration enhancers. Adv Drug Deliv Rev 56:603–618

Wu X, Guy RH (2009) Applications of nanoparticles in topical drug delivery and in cosmetics. J Drug Delivery Sci Technol 19(6):371–384

Yadav NK, Nanda S, Sharma G, Katare OP (2015) Systematically optimized Coenzyme Q10 – loaded novel proniosomal formulations for treatment of photo-induced aging in mice: characterization, biocompatibility studies, biochemical estimations and antiaging evaluation. J Drug Target 24(3):257–271

Zvyagin AV, Zhao X, Gierden A, Sanchez W, Ross JA, Roberts MS (2008) Imaging of zinc oxide nanoparticle penetration in human skin *in vitro* and *in vivo*. J Biomed Opt 13(6):064031–064039

Nanoethosomes for Topical Fungal Therapeutics

14

Kamla Pathak

Abstract

Topical treatment of fungal infections results in efficacious treatment as the drug is intended to target the site of infection; systemic side effects are minimized and patient compliance improves significantly. The conventional topical antifungal formulations offer restricted drug delivery across the skin resulting in inefficient therapeutics and non-targeted distribution of drugs leading to systemic side effects. Topical drug delivery needs to accomplish two aspects: overcome the stratum corneum barrier and deposit the drug in the targeted skin layers to limit percutaneous absorption for fungicidal/fungistatic activity. To achieve this, various nanocarriers have been developed and nanoethosomes hold promise. The ethanolic vesicular nanosized system (classical ethosomes) has evolved as variants in the form of binary ethosomes, composite ethosomes, transethosomes, and polymeric ethosomes. The chapter provides an insight into the occurrence and therapy approaches of fungal infection, usefulness of topical therapy, nanoethosomes and its variants, and their applications in the delivery of antifungal agents.

K. Pathak (✉)
Pharmacy College Saifai, Uttar Pradesh
University of Medical Sciences, Etawah, India

Keywords

Fungal therapeutics · Nanoethosomes · Ethosomal variants

14.1 Introduction

Fungal diseases are caused by a wide variety of fungi and are a growing threat to human health. While healthy people rarely suffer from potentially serious fungal infections, individuals with weakened immune systems like cancer patients, HIV/AIDS patients, organ and stem cell transplant patients, and hospitalized patients are predominantly vulnerable to fungal infection that may be fatal. Fungi are ubiquitous, and among the many different species of fungi, only few are pathogenic. Table 14.1 is a cross-sectional summary of common and rare fungal diseases, the causative fungi, prevalence, and epidemiology. The data has been collected from www.cdc.gov/fungal accessed on 29 April 2019.

The skin fungal infections are caused by (i) dermatophytes that manifest as tinea cruris, tinea corporis, tinea manuum, tinea faciei, tinea capitis, tinea pedis, and tinea barbae; (ii) yeasts, manifesting clinically as candida intertrigo and pityriasis versicolor; and (iii) molds, manifesting as tinea nigra and nail plate infections in humans. The infections of keratinized tissues (skin, hair, and nails) are caused by dermatophytes. Three

S. Talegaonkar, M. Rai (eds.), *Nanoformulations in Human Health*,
https://doi.org/10.1007/978-3-030-41858-8_14

Table 14.1 A compilation of fungal infections, the causative fungi, and epidemiological data

Pathology	Causative fungi	Epidemiological data
Aspergillosis	*Aspergillus*	Occurs in people with lung diseases or weakened immune systems
Candidiasis	*Candida*	Can occur in the mouth, throat, vagina, or bloodstream
Coccidioidomycosis (valley fever)	*Coccidioides*	Prevalent in southwestern USA and parts of Mexico and Central and South America
C. gattii infection	*Cryptococcus gattii*	Prevalent in tropical and subtropical areas of the world, the US Pacific Northwest and British Columbia
Fungal nail infections (onychomycosis)	*Trichophyton rubrum, Candida parapsilosis, C. guilliermondii, C. albicans*	Prevalent worldwide
Mucormycosis	*Mucormycetes*	Rare infection that affects people with weakened immune system
Pneumocystis pneumonia	*Pneumocystis jirovecii*	Prevalent worldwide
Sporotrichosis	Sporothrix schenckii	Omnipresent, cutaneous skin infection is a common form
Blastomycosis	*Blastomyces*	US and Canadian soil
Candida auris infection	*Candida auris*	Multidrug-resistant fungus found in health-care settings
C. neoformans infection	*Cryptococcus neoformans*	Infects the brain, causing meningitis in people with weakened immune system
Fungal eye infection	*Candida* sp.	Rare infection that develops after an eye injury or surgery
Histoplasmosis	*Histoplasma*	Associated with bird and bat droppings
Mycetoma		Caused by bat/fungi in rural regions of Africa, Latin America, and Asia
Ringworm (dermatophytosis)	*Tinea pedis*	Prevalent worldwide
Talaromycosis	*Talaromyces marneffei*	Affects people with weakened immune system, prevalent in Southeast Asia, Southern China, and Eastern India

genera of dermatophytes, namely, *Trichophyton, Epidermophyton, and Microsporum*, are significant, clinically. It is important to identify the causative fungal organism in order to select an appropriate topical antifungal agent. For the majority of the tinea infections other than tinea unguium and tinea capitis, topical antifungals may be a good choice. However, for effective therapy of tinea capitis, an oral antifungal is the therapy of choice. Likewise, oral antifungals are necessary especially if onychomycosis manifests itself as moderate to severe. Furthermore, when the tinea infection involves a large human area in an immunocompromised host (cancer/HIV-infected or AIDS patient) or if infection becomes recurrent with clinically poor response to the established topical agents, then therapy by oral antifungals may be desirable (Gupta et al. 1998).

Fungal infections of skin are categorized into superficial (limited to outermost skin layers), cutaneous, and subcutaneous (Fig. 14.1 corresponding to the depth of invaded tissue (Bseiso et al. 2015)). Superficial infection causes an increase in pH of the skin, redness, inflammation, and scaling at the infection site, thereby disrupting the barrier offered by skin (Hawkins and Smidt 2014). Cutaneous fungal infection is the infection of epidermal layer and is termed as dermatomycoses and may also include fungal infection of nails and hairs. This type of infection may trigger cellular immune response manifesting pathological variations in the patients (Watanabe

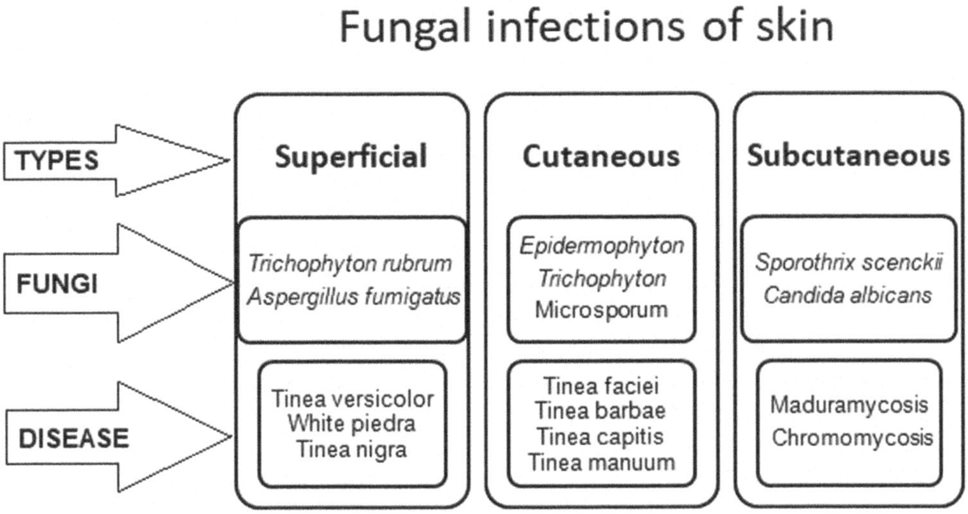

Fig. 14.1 Diagrammatic representation of fungal infections of skin

2008). The fungal infection by *Sporothrix schenckii* and *Candida albicans* of the dermis results in subcutaneous fungal infection (Elgart 2014). The infection is manifested as ulcerated/infiltrated nodular lesions at the site of infection (Patel et al. 2011).

14.2 Antifungal Agents

The antifungal agents (also known as antimycotic agents) are therapeutic agents intended to fungal infections with minimal toxicity to the host. The mechanisms by which these drugs act are (a) inhibition of fungal membrane and/or cell wall synthesis, (b) structural alterations of fungal membranes, (c) destructive effects on microtubules, and (d) inhibition of nucleic acid synthesis. Based on these mechanisms, the antifungal agents may be classified into four classes, and alarmingly, fungal strains resistant to these drugs are emerging.

Depending on the mode of use, the antifungal agents can be classified as systemic and topical, although the classification has diffused boundaries as many antifungals may be administered either ways. The systemic antifungals include polyenes (e.g., candicidin, amphotericin B), imidazoles (e.g., clotrimazole, econazole) and triazoles (e.g., posaconazole, fluconazole), griseofulvin, flucytosine, and ciclopirox. The newer systemic antifungals are terbinafine (synthetic allylamine) and caspofungin (echinocandins). The systemic antifungals manifest numerous side effects like altered estrogen levels and hepatic damage; some antifungals have the potential to cause allergic reactions in patients (Kyriakidis and Tragiannidis 2017). The azole antifungals are known to cause anaphylaxis, and toxicity to mammalian cells has been reported with amphotericin B.

Topical antifungals, on the other hand, have negligible/low systemic toxicity due to poor absorption across the skin. Other advantages include low incidence of drug interactions, economical, ease of use, and additional benefit of anti-inflammatory activity of topical antifungals including azoles and allylamines (Poojary 2017). Clinically, antifungal agents are applied topically on the skin, inserted into vagina, or are allowed to dissolve/disperse in the oral cavity. The topical antifungals include imidazoles (terconazole, econazole, omoconazole, etc.), polyenes (amphotericin and nystatin), tolnaftate, butenafine, terbinafine, haloprogin, naftifine, potassium iodide, and undecylenic acid. The topical antifungal agents may be classified into specific and nonspecific agents. The specific agents are the polyenes, azoles, allylamines, ciclopirox, butenafine, and amorolfine. Many of these antifungals have a wide spectrum of activity and are effective against both dermatophytes and yeasts. The topical antifungal agents are effective against most forms of tinea pedis (Greywal and Friedlander 2018). Some traditional agents without specific antimicrobial function are still used in clinical practice, including Whitfield's ointment, KOH preparation, and Castellani's paint (Weinstein and Berman 2002). The efficacy of these preparations has not been well defined/ quantified. Nevertheless, a research report claims development of ethosomal gel of clove oil for candidiasis. Shetty et al. (2019) formulated ethosomes of clove oil using varying concentrations of soya phosphatidylcholine and ethanol and later incorporated the vesicles into Carbopol 974 base to form ethosomal gel. The optimized formulation was nonirritant and was more effective against *C. albicans* than pure clove oil.

The topical antifungals are cream, gel, nail lacquer, nail solution, powder, or spray, for clinical use. Although these conventional formulations find wide usage in clinical practice, they have issues related to therapeutic efficacy, stability, and safety (Goldstein et al. 2000). This has propagated researchers across the globe to develop efficacious drug delivery systems (Kumar et al. 2014a, b). Various approaches developed for topical delivery of antifungal agents include nanoparticles (polymeric and lipidic), vesicles (liposomes, niosomes, ethosomes, transfersomes, and invasomes), microemulsions, and microspheres. These formulations exhibit controlled or sustained release, minimize side effects, enhance permeability, and minimized dosing frequency.

The most significant aspect is to improve penetration of the drug into the deeper layers of the skin to treat invasive fungal infections (Kumar et al. 2014a, b). The transdermal route of delivery has also been proved to be useful in providing noninvasive treatment of fungal infections using the skin as a route for the delivery of systemically acting drugs. Systemic antifungal drugs are used only for the treatment of fungal infections like onychomycosis, tinea capitis, systemic candidiasis, and invasive fungal infections (Zhang et al. 2007). Numerous drugs have been reported to be delivered via this route to overcome the drawbacks of oral and parenteral routes. However, the topical administration is preferred for the treatment of skin infections because it favours ease of administration, localization of high drug concentration at the site of action, and minimization of systemic drug levels and consequently the systemic adverse effects (Akhtar and Pathak 2012a, b).

14.2.1 Topical Delivery of Antifungals

In order to maintain desired therapeutic concentration, permeation across the skin is a prerequisite step. Physicochemical properties of drug and development of an effective carrier system play pivotal roles in topical delivery. The key to efficient topical delivery is to prevent or reduce diffusion of drug into the systemic circulation and target the drug to specific skin layer (Hamishehkar et al. 2013). The conventional dosage forms such as gels, lotions, creams, and ointments appear to fail in achieving the optimum concentration at the desired site of action. The failures may be attributed to physiological and structural features of the skin (presence of lipids, cellular structure in the cornified layers of intrafollicular epidermis, presence of ceramides, free fatty acids, and cholesterol), drug-related properties, and formulation constraints (Garg et al. 2010). The conventional dosage forms are also inefficient in shielding the normal tissues leading to certain adverse effects, viz., dermal atrophy related to corticosteroids. Additionally, the drug is also required to be protected from metabolic milieu of the skin to avoid its metabolic degradation. The presence of inactive metabolites might reduce drug action, require repeated application, and cumulative accumulation of harmful metabolites may accentuate adverse effects. Thus a specific system is required to target the drug in the most appropriate manner using novel drug delivery systems (Kaur and Kakkar 2010).

In the therapy of cutaneous and subcutaneous infections, the first-line treatment includes the use of amphotericin B, clotrimazole, econazole nitrate, and fluconazole. Amphotericin B is water-insoluble drug and azole antifungals are highly lipophilic in nature (with few exceptions like fluconazole). These can readily partition into the lipophilic intracellular space in the stratum corneum layer (Kyle and Dahl 2004). On the other hand, poor penetration of hydrophilic antifungals via conventional formulations reduces their effectiveness against pathogenic skin fungi (Akhtar et al. 2017). In case of amphotericin B and fluconazole, unwanted systemic absorption is observed. The conventional topical formulations available till date generally lead to local reactions such as burning sensation, irritation, stinging, erythema, pruritic rash, and tenderness in patients leading to noncompliance by the patient, and hence mycological eradication may not be achieved. Pharmaceutical issues like chemical instability or physical instability of creams and limited penetration of drugs via gel/ointment/cream are major limitations (Higa et al. 2013). The latter hampers the deep-seated fungal infection therapeutics.

14.2.1.1 Novel Approaches to Topical Therapy

The poor penetration of antifungal agents into the distinct skin layers results in strenuous topical fungal therapeutics. To overcome the dermatopharmacotherapy issues, a selective delivery system that could enhance penetration of the active moiety into the desired skin layers, localize the drug at the site of action, and minimize percutaneous absorption is desirable (Kircik 2016). In comparison to conventional dosage forms, the nanocarriers can effectively transport the drug topically (Güngör et al. 2013). The fact that clinical efficacy of antifungal agents depends on the therapeutic concentration achieved at the site of action that in turn is dependent on the molecular mass, residence time, and penetration ability of the agent; physicochemical considerations are of great importance. For example, a molecular weight of more than 500 Da results in poor drug penetration across the skin. Thus, enclosing the drug in a suitable carrier system may enhance its efficacy (Kaur and Kakkar 2010). New formulation approaches like nanoparticulate drug carriers such as solid lipid nanoparticles, polymeric nanoparticles, and nanostructured lipid carries have been extensively researched (Devi et al. 2011). Vesicular systems, namely, transfersomes, ethosomes, and invasomes, have also been investigated to ensure effective dermatopharmacotherapy (Kumar et al. 2014a, b).

14.2.1.2 Vesicular Carriers

Vesicles are water-filled colloidal carriers capable of entrapping both hydrophilic and lipophilic drugs. The carrier wall is composed of amphiphilic molecules, lipids, or surfactants in a bilayer conformation that undergo transformation to form unilamellar or multilamellar concentric bilayers in aqueous milieu. The hydrophilic drug is entrapped in the aqueous milieu, whereas the lipophilic drug interacts with lipid bilayer (Pirvu et al. 2010). Of lately, extensive research has been carried on vesicles for dermal delivery and transdermal delivery. In early research stages, these carriers were developed to systemically deliver the drugs. Later, these systems showed potential for localized effect on the skin, and today, these are the most versatile systems for overcoming the penetration barrier across the skin (Arora et al. 2012). In various pathological and cosmetic ailments related to skin, drug delivery to the several layers of the skin is a must. While the ailments (like acne, alopecia, dermatitis, psoriasis) are not life-threatening but may significantly alter the appearance. The infectious diseases include herpes simplex, scabies, and fungal infections. Certain skin pathologies can be cancerous in nature, viz., basal cell carcinoma and squamous cell carcinoma. Chemotherapy and radiation lower the white blood cell count, and the patient becomes susceptible to mild to life-threatening fungal infections (Crawford et al. 2004).

Vesicular carrier systems offer a plethora of benefits like penetration enhancement of drugs across the stratum corneum, control over drug release rate from the formulation, localization of drug, and optimization of targeted dermal drug delivery (Verma and Pathak 2012).

Various approaches to overcome the barrier offered by stratum corneum have been put forward by the researchers. Primarily, the application area can be increased; the secondary approach is to enhance skin permeability; and thirdly, pursuing activation of concentration-independent diffusion-driving forces (Banga 2011). While the second approach uses penetration enhancers, the third method makes use of iontophoresis, jet devices, and vesicular systems. The elastically deformable vesicles can enclose both hydrophilic and lipophilic drugs, increase the half-life of drugs by prolonging the duration in systemic circulation due to encapsulation, target organs for drug delivery, biodegradability, and lack of toxicity. The use of vesicles has been purported for treating deep-seated fungal infections. Decades of research on liposomes has deduced that these vesicles have limited permeability across the skin and remain localized in the upper layers of the stratum corneum (Verma and Pathak 2010). Thus, they are inefficient in treating deep-seated fungal infections. Hence, for topical delivery of soft lipoidal biocarriers, transfersomes, ethosomes, and invasomes have been specifically recognized as efficient skin delivery systems. The term soft lipid carriers defines them relevantly as these carriers are malleable phospholipid vesicular carriers, flexible enough to adjust their shape to the pore size of the skin, and can work either as a carrier or as a penetration enhancer. As a carrier system, they enable the transportation of large molecular weight drugs, across the skin or into the systemic circulation. While as penetration enhancers, they cause perturbation of stratum corneum organization, thus improving the transport rate of low molecular weight drugs (Sharma et al. 2013).

14.2.1.3 Ethosomes

Ethosomes are soft, malleable lipid based vesicular systems composed of phospholipids, ethanol, and water for enhanced delivery of actives. Their ability to penetrate intact through the human skin is correlatable to their high elastic nature. The size of ethosomes may vary from tens of nanometers to micrometers for effective drug delivery. The use of high ethanol concentration in ethosomes makes them unique. Ethanol in the vesicles causes disorganization of skin lipid bilayer thereby improving the vesicle's ability to penetrate the stratum corneum. Additionally, high ethanol concentration leads to formation of less tightly packed vesicular layer in comparison to conventional phospholipid vesicles but has equivalent stability, allows malleability and improves drug distribution in the stratum corneum. The synergistic effect of the phospholipids and ethanol in the vesicular formulations is responsible for deeper penetration and distribution of drug in the deep skin layers (Pathak 2014).

As a novel vesicular carrier, ethosomes have several advantages in comparison to other carriers. These benefits include predominantly uniform and penetration of drug into the skin for effective dermal delivery as well as for transdermal delivery. The system is useful for delivery of small and large molecules (peptides, protein molecules) in the form of gel or cream. It presents a noninvasive system that has been explored commercially for pharmaceutical, cosmetic, and veterinary use (Gangwar et al. 2010). Though acclaimed as an effective dermal carrier, the system presents drug-related constraints. The system is appropriate for delivery of potent drugs (daily dose of 10 mg or less) but is not suited for the drugs that require high systemic blood levels. The drug to be loaded must have optimum solubility both in the lipophilic and hydrophilic arenas of the vesicle in order to effectively target the dermal layers. The molecular size should be optimum for efficient percutaneous delivery. From a commercial viewpoint, the constraints may be exhibited as a limited percentage yield and high production cost (Kumar et al. 2012).

14.3 Formulation Considerations

Phospholipids, the main component, are the vesicles-forming ingredient which helps in the formation of vesicle bilayer. Examples are egg phosphatidylcholine, soya phosphatidylcholine, etc. Polyols (e.g., propylene glycol) are employed as a penetration enhancer, and cholesterol provides stability to the vesicle. Ethanol acts as solvent and skin penetrant and imparts negative charge to the vesicle surface which retards vesicle aggregation (Lopez-Pinto et al. 2005). Due to small size, the nanoethosomes readily penetrate through the intercellular space to reach deeper skin layers (Pandey et al. 2015).

14.3.1 Mechanism of Penetration

The penetration of drug via ethosomal system across the stratum corneum occurs by two mechanisms involving two effects, namely, ethanol effect and ethosomes effect. The first effect is related to the role of ethanol in enhancing penetration across the skin. It penetrates into the intercellular lipids, enhances the cell membrane lipid fluidity, and reduces the density of lipid layer of cell membrane. The fluidizing effect of ethanol causes disorganization of the skin lipid bilayer, and this leads to easy penetration of soft vesicles through it. On the contrary, ethosomal effect is dependent on the effect exerted by ethanol resulting in improved penetration of ethosomes in the skin, where ethosomes fuse with skin lipids and release the drug into deeper skin layers. The permeation enhancement via ethosomes is significantly higher than the effect of topical application of ethanol alone, signifying a combinatorial effect exerted by vesicles, ethanol, and skin lipids. The ethanol enhances the solubility of the drug, disturbs the stratum corneum lipid bilayer organization, and thus increases the lipid fluidity. The interaction between phospholipids and stratum corneum lipids is reported to improve the skin permeability. Ethanol being a volatile constituent may cause extraction of some lipid fractions of stratum corneum, with the consequence of enhanced drug flux when used for prolonged duration (Verma and Pathak 2010).

14.4 Ethosomes for Antifungals

Numerous studies have been conducted by various researchers across the globe to evaluate the potential of ethosomes in treating fungal infections of skin. An antifungal agent that exhibits severe systemic side effects can be employed for topical treatment of fungal infections if it possesses excellent antifungal activity. An efficient carrier system might be plausible solution; ethosomes hold considerable promise. The ethanolic vesicles tend to become leaky due to presence of ethanol hence researchers across the globe are finding ways to stabilize these vesicular systems. A simple approach would be to partly replace ethanol with glycols to get stable binary ethosomes. Another approach would be to incorporate beta-cyclodextrin in the vesicular system to get composite ethosomes. These and other variants have been detailed below.

14.4.1 Classical Ethosomes

Classical ethosomes can be interpreted as modified classical liposomes and are reported superior over classical liposomes because they are smaller in size and have negative zeta potential and greater entrapment efficiency. Furthermore, classical ethosomes show superior skin permeation and stability than classical liposomes (Sarwa et al. 2013; Touitou et al. 2000; Jain et al. 2015). Verma and Pathak (2012) formulated optimized ethanolic nanovesicles of econazole nitrate as Carbopol 934 NF gels with varied permeation enhancers and compared it with liposomal and hydroethanolic gels. The ethosomal gel demonstrated a flux rate of 0.46 ± 0.22 μg/cm^2 hr$^{1/2}$ and exhibited a controlled release of econazole nitrate for 12 h across rat skin. The total drug diffused from ethosomes was approximately two times higher than either liposomal or hydroethanolic gel(s). Confocal laser scanning microscopy proved drug permeation to the stratum basale (Fig. 14.2). The results conformed superiority of ethosomes over liposomes.

The drugs with molecular weight in the range of 130–24 kDa can be readily entrapped in classical ethosomes (Mishra et al. 2010). While a wide variety of antifungals have been entrapped in classical ethosomes, interestingly, numerous research reports on nanoethosomal delivery of fluconazole are cited in the literature. Fluconazole is a proven imidazole derivative with broad antifungal spectrum. Usually well tolerated, it can be safely used for treatment of cutaneous or systemic fungal

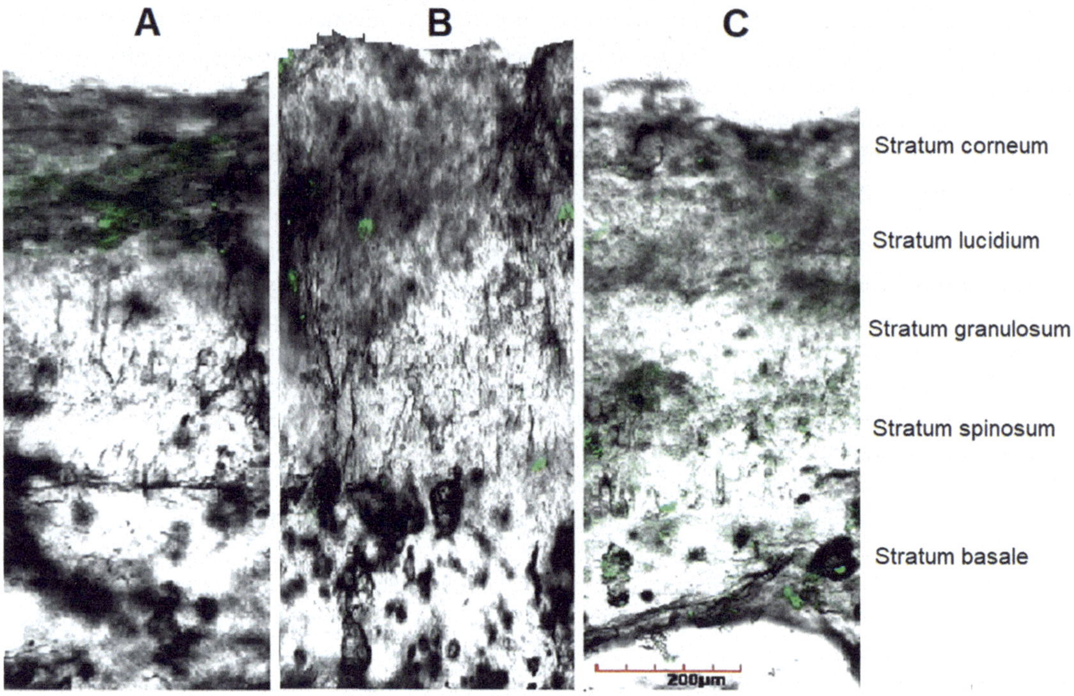

Fig. 14.2 Confocal laser scanning micrographs of econazole nitrate ethosomes deep up to stratum basale (**c**) in comparison to less permeation for liposomal gel (**b**) and plain gel (**a**) of the drug (Verma and Pathak 2012)

Table 14.2 Ethosomal research reports on fluconazole

Description of vesicle	Size and EE	Remarks on efficacy	Reference
Multilamellar spherical vesicles with a smooth surface	144 ± 6.8 nm 82.68%	The developed novel delivery system demonstrated enhanced antifungal activity compared to liposomal formulation, marketed formulation, and hydroethanolic solution of the drug; mean % reduction in dimension of candidiasis lesion	Bhalaria et al. (2009)
Unilamellar vesicles with smooth surface	5–200 nm 90%	Not reported	Indora and Kaushik (2015)
Multilamellar vesicles	3.057–5.449 μm 76%	Not reported	Chandran et al. (2012)
Lamellarity not reported	794.2–5425 μm 85%	Not reported	Yassin and Sayed (2018)
Lamellarity not reported	3.46–5.98 μm 70%	Not reported	Dhurve and Mishra (2019)

infections. However, anaphylactic reactions and cardiorespiratory toxicity in many cases have led to premature termination of therapy. Therefore, attempts have been made to formulate efficacious dermal therapy of fluconazole. Table 14.2 compiles a significant cross section of ethosomal formulations reported for fluconazole. The data clearly shows that only two research reports claim development of nanosized ethosomes and only one research report proved efficacy of the developed formulation against candidiasis.

Another imidazole derivative, ketoconazole is widely used for topical treatment of *C. albicans* infection. The ethosomes of ketoconazole developed by hot-process method were incorporated into water-miscible cream base and assessed for in vitro release profile and stability. The uniform vesicles had average diameter of 4.154 μm at 30% ethanol concentration. Both the ethosomes and cream were stable, and the latter was efficient in drug delivery across the cellophane membrane than the non-ethosomal ketoconazole cream. The authors reiterated the cream's capability for treating topical fungal infections effectively. A cream containing ethosomal vesicles implicated clear edge over non-ethosomal creams, since more than 50% of the incorporated drug was unreleased from the latter, confirming the importance of drug encapsulation in ethosomal vesicle (Chandran et al. 2011).

In an attempt to achieve skin targeting of ketoconazole, Guo et al. (2015) formulated lipidic vesicular systems, namely, classical liposomes, deformable liposomes, ethosomes, and ethanolic deformable liposomes. Sodium dodecyl sulfate was used as edge activator for deformable lipidic vesicles in a concentration of 0.08% w/v. The spherical lipid vesicles with a low polydispersity index (<0.3) were of <160 nm. The ethanolic deformable liposomes demonstrated superior in vitro and in vivo skin deposition that was confirmed by confocal laser scanning microscopy. In vivo pharmacodynamic studies showed enhanced antifungal activity against *Candida albicans* with minimum lag time. The authors purported enhanced skin targeting and micro drug-deposition of the antifungal via nanoethosomes for local therapy. Marto et al. (2016) aimed to prepare a topical ethosomal system of griseofulvin that could exhibit targeted permeation and penetration. The ethanolic vesicles (mean size = 130 nm) were composed of soya phosphatidylcholine, ethanol, and water. The permeation and penetration assays revealed that griseofulvin-loaded ethosomes presented adequate profile to be used as a topical formulation since significant drug retention in the stratum corneum was achieved by the vesicular gel. Furthermore, in vitro cell viability tests on HaCaT cells confirmed that the formulation was devoid of cytotoxicity at concentrations below 50 μg/mL. The diffusion test across rat skin signified the therapeutic potential of the optimized formulation to effectively target skin dermatophytes.

A plethora of research reports on classical ethosomes/nanoethosomes can be found in literature. A cross section of these is presented in Table 14.3.

14.4.2 Binary Ethosomes

Binary ethosomes developed by Zhou et al. (2010) were made using propylene glycol and isopropyl alcohol (Dave et al. 2010; Li et al. 2012; Shen et al. 2014). Propylene glycol has stabilizing effect in formulations by preventing aggregation of vesicles. Binary ethosomes have an intact spherical shape (Fig. 14.3), have the ability to penetrate into deep skin layers, and are more stable than classical ethosomes (Yan et al. 2010).

In a research report, the skin permeability of terbinafine hydrochloride was compared via ethosomes, binary ethosomes, and transfersomes. The topical dose of the drug was applied, and the skin deposition of the applied dose of the drug from ethosomes, binary ethosomes, and transfersomes was found to be 3.34-, 9.88-, and 2.52-fold, respectively, higher than from control (non-vesicular formulation). The penetration depth and fluorescence intensity of the marker (Rhodamine B) from binary ethosomes was much higher than ethosomes and transfersomes as revealed by CLSM experiments (Zhang et al. 2012). Another research report on binary ethosomes of terbinafine hydrochloride by Shruti et al. (2018) claims development and antifungal evaluation of ethosomal gel for onychomycosis. The researchers optimized binary ethosomes in the size range of 200–320 nm with an entrapment efficiency of 70–92%. The hydro-alcoholic binary (ethanol/propylene glycol 7:3 by volume) phase vesicular formulation exhibited faster release and enhanced flux across rat skin. Its gel formulation, however, exhibited lower antifungal activity than the ethosomal formulation against *Candida albicans* which the authors attributed to the gelling effect in agar gel diffusion studies.

Table 14.3 A cross section of research reports on classical ethosomes/nanoethosomes of antifungals

Drug	Indication	Highlight of the study	Reference
Amphotericin B	Dermal fungal infection	Enhanced penetration/negligible irritation scores	Higa et al. (2013)
Clotrimazole	Candidiasis	Growth inhibition of *Candida albicans*	Maheshwari et al. (2012)
	Topical skin infection	Enhanced delivery of drug and localization at the targeted site	Charyulu et al. (2009)
	Ringworm	60–70% improvement in the skin lesions	Goti and Patel (2007)
Ciclopirox olamine	Dermal fungal infection	Targeted delivery to dermis, formulation safe, and nonirritant	Girhepunje et al. (2010)
Fluconazole	Candidiasis	50–75% reduction lesion dimensions	Bhalaria et al. (2009)
Miconazole nitrate	Topical skin infections	Enhanced permeation and localized action of drug	Dubey et al. (2007)
Terbinafine HCl	Deep skin infection Superficial *Candida* infection	Better skin permeability Vesicles containing 4% limonene showed high drug deposition in the skin (53%) and high local accumulation efficiency (35.3%). Low fungal burden was produced with chitosan gel. 86% clinical cure rate within 7 days of treatment as compared to 20% for market product (Lamisil® cream)	Singh et al. (2010) AbdelSamie et al. (2016)
Voriconazole	Antifungal efficacy and improved skin delivery	Twice as effective as DMSO solution against *Aspergillus flavus*. Higher ex vivo drug permeability through rat abdominal skin, and skin deposition was higher for the ethosomes compared with the drug hydroalcoholic solution	Faisal et al. (2018)

14.4.3 Composite Ethosomes

Composite ethosomes incorporate additives that can stabilize the leaky nature of the ethosomes and are added during the preparation of ethosomes. Composite ethosomes can improve drug delivery and at the same time reduce the amount of ethanol so as to reduce the risk of adverse effects associated with the higher concentration of ethanol used in ethosomes. Akhtar and Pathak in 2012 reported composite ethosomes of clotrimazole wherein the researchers experimented the incorporation of Cavamax W7 (β-CD) in ethosomes in a concentration of 0.5%w/v. The research proposed that the molecules of Cavamax W7 imparted rigidity to the vesicle wall by intercalating with the lipid bilayer or the molecules of Cavamax may be positioned at the interface of the lipid bilayer and the hydro-ethanolic core. The hydrophilic exterior and hydrophobic interior of the phospholipid bilayer presumably defined the orientation of Cavamax W7 molecules, both in the lipid bilayer and the interface. The size of composite ethosomes was narrower than classical ethosomes due to partial replacement of phospholipid(s) by Cavamax W7 that resulted in an inward bending of the phospholipid layer and consequently smaller vesicles (Fig. 14.4).

Vesicle size plays an important role in topical drug delivery. Vesicle size less than 300 nm is considered to be efficient in localizing the drug deep into the skin, but a vesicle size of less than 200 nm is considered optimum for drug delivery to the skin (Verma and Pathak 2012). Antifungal activity was titrated for control gel, classical ethosomal gel, and composite ethosomal gel against *C. albicans* and *A. niger*. The antifungal activity was higher for *C. albicans* as compared to *A. niger*. High drug-loaded composite ethosomal gel facilitated higher drug diffusion across the fungal cell membrane, exerting better antifungal activity than ethosomal gel. In vivo CLSM study confirmed uniform permeation of composite ethosomes deep into the epidermis signifying

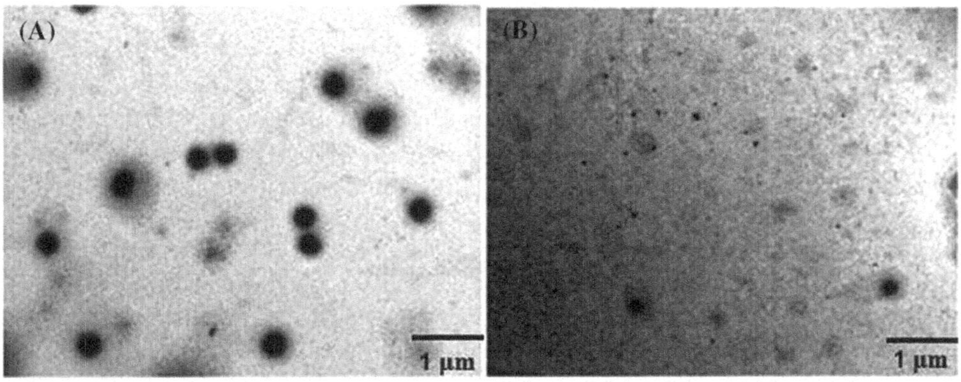

Fig. 14.3 (**a**, **b**) Transmission electron micrographs of binary ethosomes of triamcinolone acetonide in comparison to classical ethosomes (Akhtar et al. 2017)

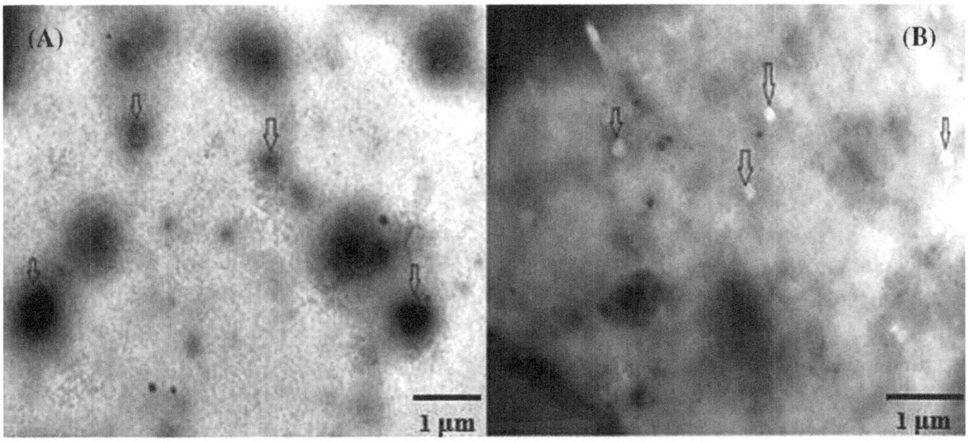

Fig. 14.4 (**a**, **b**) Transmission electron micrographs of non-drug-loaded composite ethosomes in comparison to classical ethosomes

superior ethosomal system for topical drug delivery.

14.4.4 Transethosomes

In addition to the components of classical ethosomes, this system consists of a penetration enhancer or an edge activator (surfactant) in its formulation. The novel vesicle combines the benefits of classical ethosomes and transfersomes to produce transethosomes. Transethosomes first reported by Song et al. in 2012 are composed of phospholipid, ethanol, water, and edge activator (surfactants) or permeation enhancer (oleic acid). The research evaluated the in vivo skin deposition of the drug from voriconazole-loaded transethosomes in mice. The vesicular system showed enhanced in vivo skin deposition (approximately two times) of voriconazole in the dermis and epidermis layers in comparison to conventional liposomes, deformable liposomes, ethosomes, and polyethylene glycol drug solution. Many reports can be found in literature citing superior properties of transethosomes over classical ethosomes (Limsuwan and Amnuaikit 2012; Ascenso et al. 2015) attributable to the intriguing formulation components.

Various penetration enhancers and edge activators have been explored to produce ethosomal systems with superior features. Transethosomes can entrap drugs ranging from low molecular weight to high molecular weight (130 Da to 325 kDa) and can be used for either topical or systemic delivery (Ainbinder and Touitou 2011). As the bioactive agent is encapsulated within the vesicle, the drug is released gradually and in a controlled manner. Transethosomes are biodegradable and biocompatible and present high entrapment efficiency (Honeywell-Nguyen and Bouwstra 2003; Trotta et al. 2004).

14.4.5 Polymeric Ethosomes

Polymeric ethosomes are an ethosomal variant first reported by Liang et al. (2012). These ethosomes are capable of simultaneously encapsulating both the hydrophobic and hydrophilic drug. A study undertaken by Rasheed et al. (2018) focused on the development of oxiconazole-loaded ethosomal gel using hydroxypropyl methylcellulose (HPMC K4M), chitosan, Carbopol 934, and sodium alginate. The in vitro diffusion studies concluded that the gel made with Carbopol 934 exhibited best control on release rate of oxiconazole that was governed by non-Fickian diffusion. The researchers did not use phospholipids in the ethosomal formulation. Table 14.4 depicts typical comparative features of classical ethosomes, binary ethosomes, composite ethosomes, transethosomes, and polymeric ethosomes.

14.5 Ethosomal Dosage Forms

The nanoethosomal suspension containing high concentration of alcohol(s) is incorporated in a suitable vehicle for effective dermal/transdermal delivery. The vehicle minimizes the evaporation of ethanol, prolongs contact time with the skin, enhances the therapeutic efficacy of the entrapped antifungal drug, improves the shelf life of the product, and facilitates patient compliance. Nanoethosomal suspensions have been incorporated in various vehicles to produce ethosomal gels, transdermal patches, and creams. Gels being the most popular dosage forms are formulated using various grades of hydroxypropyl methylcellulose and Carbopol. The advantages offered by these gelling agents include compatibility with ethosomal systems and requisite spreadability and bioadhesivity. The research reports detailing the types of polymers used in the preparation of ethosomal gels and their concentrations are listed in Table 14.5.

The formulation and assessment of ethosomal patches is more complicated than ethosomal gels. However, the patches offer application of ethosomes under occlusive conditions, which has potential to enhance permeation across the skin. None have been reported for antifungal drugs. Likewise ethosomal creams have not been reported for antifungal agents. The literature reports only two studies on formulation of ethosomal creams, both based on incorporation of *Curcuma longa* extract-loaded ethosomal systems in a cream base (Kaur and Saraf 2011; Jeswani and Saraf 2014) for photoprotection and antiaging effect. Based on the reported studies, the ethosomal systems as gels, patches, and creams are patient-friendly dosage forms that have the potential to improve skin permeation of the drug. While gels are the most suited for the pharmaceutical formulations, ethosomal creams are the preferred choice for cosmetic preparations. In this context, only two patents on antifungal drugs using nanoethosomes are documented in literature (Table 14.6).

14.6 Stability

Stability of the vesicular structure and size distribution of drug-loaded ethosomes in their initial suspension form and as dosage form (gels, patches, or creams) have been reported by many researchers. Though the results are promising (Guo et al. 2015; Celia et al. 2009), real-time studies are required to evaluate both the physical and chemical stability of ethosomal systems and their dosage forms. Aggregation of vesicles is a serious physical instability.

Table 14.4 Comparative features of classical ethosomes and its variants

Parameter	Classical ethosomes	Binary ethosomes	Composite ethosomes	Transethosomes	Polymeric ethosomes
Composition	PhospholipidsEthanolStabilizerCharge inducerWaterDrug/agent	PhospholipidsEthanolPropylene glycol or other alcoholCharge inducerWaterDrug/agent	Phospholipidsβ-CD EthanolStabilizerCharge inducerWaterDrug/agent	PhospholipidsEthanolEdge activator (surfactant) or penetration enhancerCharge inducerWaterDrug/agent	Polymer Polyethylene glycolsEthanolStabilizerCharge inducerWaterDrug/agent
Morphology	Spherical	Spherical	Spherical	Regular or irregular spherical shape	Spherical
Size	Smaller than the classical liposomes	≤classical ethosomes	≤classical ethosomes	Size based on type and concentration of edge activator used	Size dependent on type of polymer
Zeta potential	Negatively charged	Negatively charged	Negatively charged	Positively or negatively charged	Positively or negatively charged
Entrapment efficiency	Higher than classical liposomes	Typically higher than classical ethosomes	Typically higher than classical ethosomes	Typically higher than classical ethosomes	Typically higher than classical ethosomes
Skin permeation	Typically higher than classical liposomes	Typically equal to or higher than classical ethosomes	Typically equal to or higher than classical ethosomes	Typically higher than classical ethosomes	Typically equal to or higher than classical ethosomes
Stability	Stable than classical liposomes	Stable than classical ethosomes	Stable than classical ethosomes	No particular trend determined	No particular trend

Table 14.5 Summarized list of the gelling agents used for nanoethosomal formulations

Drug	Gelling agent	Concentration (%w/w)	Reference
Econazole nitrate	Carbopol 934	1.0	Verma and Pathak (2012)
Ketoconazole	Carbopol 934	2.0	Ashoniya and Meenakshi (2011)
Clotrimazole	Carbopol 934LR	1.0	Akhtar and Pathak (Akhtar and Pathak 2012a, b)
Griseofulvin	Carbopol 980 NF	0.5	Aggarwal and Goindi (2013)
Fluconazole	Hydroxypropyl methyl cellulose K4M	2.0	Bhalaria et al. (2009)
Oxiconazole	Carbopol 934	2.0	Rasheed et al. (2018)

Table 14.6 Ethosomal patents on antifungal agents

Title of patent	Patent no. and inventors	Brief description
Ethosomes preparation of antimycotics pharmaceutical and method for preparing the same	CN101273971 A Liu Liping, Li Yimin, Shen Ming Jiang Hu, Yang Jin	The invention discloses an ethosomal preparation containing 1–8% phospholipid, 20–45% ethanol, and 40.9–78.9% of water; loaded with anti-fungal drug
Clotrimazole ethosomes for preventing and curing weaning rabbit dermatomycosis and preparation method thereof	CN104873465 A Liu Man, Mou Liming Yong	The invention describes the composition and method of preparation of clotrimazole ethosomes constituting 3% of lecithin and 1% of clotrimazole by weight

14.7 Conclusion

Since the invention of ethosomes, these nanosystems have proven their ability to effectively deliver therapeutic agents of varied physicochemical properties across the skin for both local and systemic use. Continual research inputs have led to the introduction of variants with improved properties and performance. However, the variants need to be extensively explored for the development of nanosystems of the established antifungals. Furthermore, the development of patient-friendly dosage forms is important to achieve better therapeutic results. Investigations are desirable to focus on enhancing the stability of the ethosomal system and addressing safety issues. Though the nanocarrier has positioned itself commercially, intensive in vivo studies and clinical trials reflecting the safety potential of ethosomal systems in dermal and transdermal delivery of antifungals are required.

References

AbdelSamie SM, Kamel AO, Sammour OA, Ibrahim SM (2016) Terbinafine hydrochloride nanovesicular gel: in vitro characterization, *ex vivo* permeation and clinical investigation. Eur J Pharm Sci 88:91–100

Aggarwal N, Goindi S (2013) Dermatopharmacokinetic and pharmacodynamic evaluation of ethosomes of griseofulvin designed for dermal delivery. J Nanopart Res 15:1–15

Ainbinder D, Touitou E (2011) A new approach for skin tumor treatment: from delivery system characterization to in vivo evaluation. Drug Deliv Transl Res 1:53–65

Akhtar N, Pathak K (2012a) Preclinical and clinical aspects of antimicrobial drugs delivered through ethosomal vesicles. Anti-infect Agents 10:15–25

Akhtar N, Pathak K (2012b) Cavamax W7 composite ethosomal gel of clotrimazole for improved topical delivery: development and comparison with ethosomal gel. AAPS PharmSci Tech 13:344–355

Akhtar N, Verma A, Pathak K (2017) Feasibility of binary composition in development of nanoethosomal glycolic vesicles of triamcinolone acetonide using Box-Behnken design: in vitro and ex vivo characterization. Artificial Cells Nanomed Biotechnol 45:1123–1131

Arora S, Lamba HS, Tiwari R (2012) Dermal delivery of drugs using different vesicular carriers: a comparative review. Asian J Pharm 6:237–244

Ascenso A, Raposo S, Batista C, Cardoso P, Mendes T, Praça FG, Bentley MV, Simões S (2015) Development, characterization, and skin delivery studies of related ultradeformable vesicles: transfersomes, ethosomes, and transethosomes. Int J Nanomedicine 10:5837–5851

Ashoniya S, Meenakshi C (2011) Ethosomes as vesicular carrier for enhanced transdermal delivery of ketoconazole – formulation and evaluation. J Pharm Cosmetol 1(3):1–14

Banga AK (2011) Transdermal and intradermal delivery of therapeutic agents: application of physical technologies. CRC Press, Boca Raton

Bhalaria M, Naik S, Misra A (2009) Ethosomes: a novel delivery system for antifungals drugs in the treatment of topical fungal diseases. Indian J Exp Biol 47:369–375

Bseiso EA, Nasr M, Sammour O, El A, Gawad NA (2015) Recent advances in topical formulation carriers of antifungal agents. Indian J Dermatol Venereol Leprol 81:457–463

Celia C, Trapasso E, Cosco D, Paolino D, Fresta M (2009) Turbiscan lab expert analysis of the stability of ethosomes and ultradeformable liposomes containing a bilayer fluidizing agent. Colloids Surf B Biointerfaces 72:155–160

Chandran S, Shirwaikar A, Devi SA, Dominic A (2011) Development and evaluation of ethosomal formulation containing ketoconazole. Asian J Biochem Pharm Res 4:303–309

Chandran S, Shriwaikar A, Kuriakose MR, Sabna NS (2012) Development and evaluation of ethosomes for transdermal delivery of fluconazole. J Chem Biol Phys Sci 2:254–260

Charyulu RN, Harish NM, Sudhakar CK and Udupa G (2009) Formulation and evaluation of clotrimazole ethosomes for topical delivery, November: 7–12

Crawford J, Dale DC, Lyman GH (2004) Chemotherapy induced nutropenia. Cancer 100:228–237

Dave V, Kumar D, Lewis S, Paliwal S (2010) Ethosome for enhanced transdermal drug delivery of aceclofenac. Int J Drug Deliv 2:81–92

Devi M, Kumar MS, Mahadevan N (2011) Amphotericin-B loaded vesicular systems for the treatment of topical fungal infection. Int J Recent Adv Pharm Res 4:37–46

Dhurve R, Mishra A (2019) Formulation and evaluation of ethosomal gel of fluconazole for topical drug delivery. Int J Cur Trends Drug Develop Indust Pharm 3:9–13

Dubey V, Mishra D, Jain NK and Nahar M (2007) Miconazole loaded ethosomes for effective management of topical fungal infection, AAPS Ann Meeting Exposition, December: 9–15

Elgart GW (2014) Subcutaneous (deep) fungal infections. Semin Cutan Med Surg 33:146–150

Faisal W, Soliman GM, Hamdan AM (2018) Enhanced skin deposition and delivery of voriconazole using ethosomal preparations. J Liposome Res 28:14–21

Gangwar S, Singh S, Garg G (2010) Ethosomes: a novel tool for drug delivery through the skin. J Pharm Res 3:688–691

Garg BJ, Saraswat A, Bhatia A, Katare OP (2010) Topical treatment in vitiligo and the potential uses of new drug delivery systems. Indian J Dermatol Venereol Leprol 76:231–238

Girhepunje K, Pal R, Gevaria H, Behera A (2010) Ethosomes: a novel vesicular carrier for enhanced dermal delivery of ciclopirox olamine. Pharm Lett 2:360–367

Goldstein A, Smith K, Ives T (2000) Mycotic infections: effective management of conditions involving the skin, hair, and nails. Geriatrics 55:40–52

Goti A and Patel V (2007) Ethosomally entrapped clotrimazole: a view to improve therapeutic response of antifungal drug, AAPS National Biotechnology Conference, June 23–28

Greywal T, Friedlander SF (2018) Dermatophytes and other superficial fungi. In: Principles and practice of pediatric infectious diseases, 5th edn

Güngör S, Erdal MS, Aksu B (2013) New formulation strategies in topical antifungal therapy. J Cosm Dermatol Sci Appl 3:56–65

Guo F, Wang J, Ma M, Tan F, Li N (2015) Skin targeted lipid vesicles as novel nanocarrier of ketoconazole: characterization, in vitro and in vivo evaluation. J Mater Sci Mater Med 26:175

Gupta AK, Einarson TR, Summerbell RC, Shear NH (1998) An overview of topical antifungal therapy in dermatomycoses: a North American perspective. Drugs 55:645–674

Hamishehkar H, Rahimpour Y, Kouhsoltani M (2013) Niosomes as a propitious carrier for topical drug delivery. Expert Opin Drug Deliv 10:261–272

Hawkins DM, Smidt AC (2014) Superficial fungal infections in children. Pediatr Clin North Am 61:443–455

Higa LH, Schilrreff P, Perez AP, Morilla MJ, Romero EL (2013) The intervention of nano-technology against epithelial fungal diseases. J Biomater Tissue Eng 3:1–19

Honeywell-Nguyen PL, Bouwstra JA (2003) The in vitro transport of pergolide from surfactant based elastic vesicles through human skin: a suggested mechanism of action. J Control Release 86:145–156

Indora N, Kaushik D (2015) Design, development and evaluation of ethosomal gel of fluconazole for topical fungal infection. Int J Eng Sci Invent Res Develop 1:280–306

Jain S, Patel N, Madan P, Lin S (2015) Quality by design approach for formulation, evaluation and statistical optimization of diclofenac-loaded ethosomes via transdermal route. Pharm Dev Technol 20:473–489

Jeswani G, Saraf S (2014) Topical delivery of *Curcuma longa* extract loaded nanosized ethosomes to combat facial wrinkles. J Pharm Drug Deliv Res 3:1000118

Kaur IP, Kakkar S (2010) Topical delivery of antifungal agents. Expert Opin Drug Deliv 7:1303–1327

Kaur CD, Saraf S (2011) Topical vesicular formulations of *Curcuma longa* extract on recuperating the ultraviolet radiation-damaged skin. J Cosmet Dermatol 10:260–265

Kircik LH (2016) Advancements in topical antifungal vehicles. J Drugs Dermatol 15(2 Suppl):s44–s48

Kumar A, Pathak K, Bali V (2012) Ultra-adaptable nanovesicular systems: a carrier for systemic delivery of therapeutic agents. Drug Discov Today 17:1233–1241

Kumar JR, Muralidharan S, Parasuraman S (2014a) Antifungal agents: new approach for novel delivery system. J Pharm Sc Res 6:229–235

Kumar L, Verma S, Bhardwaj A, Vaidya S, Vaidya B (2014b) Eradication of superficial fungal infections by conventional and novel approaches: a comprehensive review. Artifl Cells Nanomed Biotechnol 42:32–46

Kyle AA, Dahl MV (2004) Topical therapy for fungal infections. Am J Clin Dermatol 5:443–451

Kyriakidis I, Tragiannidis A, Munchen S, Groll AH (2017) Clinical hepatotoxicity associated with antifungal agents. Expert Opin Drug Safety 16:149–165

Li G, Fan Y, Fan C, Li X, Wang X, Li M, Liu Y (2012) Tacrolimus-loaded ethosomes: physicochemical characterization and in vivo evaluation. Eur J Pharm Biopharm 82:49–57

Liang XF, Jing-Ying HU, Fu-Hua C, Zong-Hai LI, Jin C (2012) Characterization of chitosan polymeric ethosomes capable of encapsulating hydrophobic an hydrophilic drugs prepared by a microemulsion method. Acta Physico Chimica Sinica 28:879–902

Limsuwan T, Amnuaikit T (2012) Development of ethosomes containing mycophenolic acid. Procedia Chem 4:328–335

Lopez-Pinto JM, Gonzalez-Rodriguez ML, Rabasco AM (2005) Effect of cholesterol and ethanol on dermal delivery from DPPC liposomes. Int J Pharm 298:1–12

Maheshwari RGS, Tekade RK, Sharma PA, Darwhekar G, Tyagi A, Patel RP, Jain DK (2012) Ethosomes and ultradeformable liposomes for transdermal delivery of clotrimazole: a comparative assessment. Saudi Pharm J 20:161–170

Marto J, Vitor C, Guerreiro A, Severino C, Eleutério C, Ascenso A, Simões S (2016) Ethosomes for enhanced skin delivery of griseofulvin. Colloids Surf B Biointerfaces 146:616–623

Mishra D, Mishra PK, Dabadghao S, Dubey V, Nahar M, Jain NK (2010) Comparative evaluation of hepatitis B surface antigen-loaded elastic liposomes and ethosomes for human dendritic cell uptake and immune response. Nanomedicine 6:110–118

Pandey V, Golhani D, Shukla R (2015) Ethosomes: versatile vesicular carriers for efficient transdermal delivery of therapeutic agents. Drug Deliv 22:988–1002

Patel U, Chu J, Patel R, Meehan S (2011) Subcutaneous dermataceous fungal infection. Dermatol Online J 17:19–35

Pathak K (2014) Ethosomes for optimized skin delivery. In: Drug nanocarriers, pp 176–202

Pirvu CD, Hlevca C, Ortan A, Prisada R (2010) Elastic vesicles as drugs carriers through the skin. Farmacia 58:128–135

Poojary SA (2017) Topical antifungals: a review and their role in current management of dermatophytoses. Clin Dermatol Rev:S124–S129

Rasheed SH, Mogili RK, Chandrasekhar KB (2018) Design and evaluation of Oxiconazole based ethosome for novel drug delivery to the skin. Int J Res Pharm Sci 9:572–579

Sarwa KK, Suresh PK, Rudrapal M, Verma VK (2013) Penetration of tamoxifen citrate loaded ethosomes and liposomes across human skin: a comparative study with confocal laser scanning microscopy. Curr Drug Deliv 11:332–337

Sharma M, Yusuf M, Sharma V, Pathak K (2013) Lipoidal soft hybrid biocarriers in pharmacotherapeutics: retrospection through patents. Pharm Pat Anal 2:539–569

Shen LN, Zhang YT, Wang Q, Xu L, Feng NP (2014) Enhanced in vitro and in vivo skin deposition of apigenin delivered using ethosomes. Int J Pharm 460:280–288

Shetty S, Jose J, Kumar L, Charyulu RN (2019) Novel ethosomal gel of clove oil for the treatment of cutaneous candidiasis. J Cosmet Dermatol 18:862–869

Shruthi K, Narender D, Arjun N, Kishan V (2018) Development and antimicrobial evaluation of binary topical ethosomal gel of terbinafine hydrochloride for the treatment of onchomycosis. Int J Pharm Sci Nanotechnol 11:3998–4005

Singh A, Rathore P, Shukla M, Nayak S (2010) Comparative studies on skin permeation of miconazole using different novel carriers. Int J Pharm Sci Res 1:61–66

Song CK, Balakrishnan P, Shim C-K, Chung S-K, Chong S, Kim D-D (2012) A novel vesicular carrier, transethosome, for enhanced skin delivery of voriconazole: characterization and *in vitro/in vivo* evaluation. Colloids Surf B Biointerfaces 92:299–304

Touitou E, Dayan N, Bergelson L, Godin B, Eliaz M (2000) Ethosomes-novel vesicular carriers for enhanced delivery: characterization and skin penetration properties. J Control Release 65:403–418

Trotta M, Peira E, Carlotti ME, Gallarate M (2004) Deformable liposomes for dermal administration of methotrexate. Int J Pharm 270:119–125

Verma P, Pathak K (2010) Therapeutic and cosmeceutical potential of ethosomes: an overview. J Adv Pharm Technol Res 1:274–282

Verma P, Pathak K (2012) Nanosized ethanolic vesicles loaded with econazole nitrate for the treatment of deep skin infections through topical gel formulation. Nanomed Nano-technol Biol 8:489–496

Watanabe S (2008) Dermatomycosis–classification, etiology, pathogenesis, and treatment. Nihon Rinsho 66:2285–2289

Weinstein A, Berman B (2002) Topical treatment of common superficial tinea infections. Am Fam Physician 65:2095–2103

Yan Z, Yu HW, Guo QZ, Xin AW (2010) Synergistic penetration of ethosomes and lipophilic prodrug on the transdermal delivery of acyclovir. Arch Pharm Res 33:567–574

Yassin GE, Sayed MH (2018) Statistical optimization of fluconazole – loaded vesicular systems for the treatment of skin fungal infection. Int J Pharm Sci Sci Res 4:10–23

Zhang AY, Camp WL, Elewski BE (2007) Advances in topical and systemic antifungals. Dermatol Clin 25:165–183

Zhang JP, Wei YH, Zhou Y (2012) Ethosomes, binary ethosomes and transfersomes of terbinafine hydrochloride: a comparative study. Arch Pharm Res 35:109–117

Zhou Y, Wei Y, Liu H, Zhang G, Wu X (2010) Preparation and in vitro evaluation of ethosomal total alkaloids of *Sophora alopecuroides* loaded by a transmembrane pH-gradient method. AAPS PharmSciTech 11:1350–1358

15 Nanostructure Drug Delivery System: An Inimitable Approach for Candidiasis Therapy

Radhika Sharma, Shivani Sharma, and Vikas Rana

Abstract

Candidiasis is among the most frequent healthcare-associated infections and leads to significant morbidity and mortality because of late diagnosis and delayed treatment. Candidiasis is a major problem for immunocompromised individuals and patients in intensive care units. Candidiasis is a fungal infection associated with yeast that belongs to *Candida* genus. There are over 20 species of *Candida* yeasts that can cause infection in humans, the most common of which are *C. albicans* and *C. glabrata*. Candidiasis is majorly categorized into superficial (oral, dermal, and vaginal) and systemic candidiasis, called as invasive candidiasis. Despite the availability of several antifungal agents, their therapeutic outcome is less than optimal due to limitations related to drug physicochemical properties like aqueous solubility, toxicity, and resistance. Nanostructure drug delivery system holds great promise to overcome these limitations due to its ability to enhance drug aqueous solubility, bioavailability, and target-specific delivery. Therefore, nanoscale strategy could be an excellent option to improve the clinical efficacy of antifungal drugs and patient acceptability. This book chapter encompasses the nanostructure-based drug delivery systems that have been exploited for the delivery of antifungal drugs with desirable benefits. It also touches upon the mechanism of azole resistance in candidiasis therapy and the role of nanostructure-based drug delivery systems to reverse this resistance.

Keywords

Nanotechnology · Nanoformulations · Candidiasis · Antifungals · Drug delivery · Resistance · Pathophysiology

15.1 Introduction

The past two decades has perceived an increase in the prevalence of fungal infections, especially in case of immunocompromised or hospitalized patients. The possible causes are disruption of mucosal and/or cutaneous barrier, metabolic dysfunction, and age (Horn et al. 2007; Pfaller and Diekema 2007; Pfaller and Diekema 2010). Extensive use of broad-spectrum antibiotics, chemotherapies, and transplantation also proliferates the risk of opportunistic fungal infections (Sawant and Khan 2017). In addition, around 20–25% of the human population suffer from

R. Sharma · S. Sharma · V. Rana (✉)
Pharmaceutics Division, Department of Pharmaceutical Sciences and Drug Research, Punjabi University, Patiala, Punjab, India
e-mail: vikas@pbi.ac.in

S. Talegaonkar, M. Rai (eds.), *Nanoformulations in Human Health*,
https://doi.org/10.1007/978-3-030-41858-8_15

superficial fungal infections (Ameen 2010). On the other hand, invasive fungal infections such as disseminated candidiasis are progressively becoming a significant cause of morbidity and mortality particularly in patients having acquired immune deficiency syndrome (AIDS), hematologic malignancies, severe aplastic anemia, and myelodysplasia, immunocompromised patients, organ transplant recipients, premature neonates, and the elderly (Vallabhaneni et al. 2016). *Candida* fungus has been found to be the major cause of opportunistic mycoses worldwide. Due to diseases like AIDS or other immunocompromised diseases, the prevention and treatment of candidiasis become a challenge.

C. albicans is responsible for two major types of fungal infections that include superficial (oral, cutaneous, and vaginal) and systemic infections (invasive candidiasis) (Pfaller et al. 2006). Around 75% of human population have *C. albicans* and other *Candida* species in their oral cavity up to a lesser extent. However, in the case of immunocompromised patients, the risk of "oral candidiasis" is often higher (Mayer et al. 2013). Vulvovaginal candidiasis (VVC) is a type of superficial infection affecting approximately 75% of women at least once in their lifetime, while 40–50% experience at least one additional episode of infection and a small percentage of women (5–8%) experiences at least four recurrent VVC per year. Invasive candidiasis, a cluster of various infectious syndromes like disseminated candidiasis, candidemia, endocarditis, endophthalmitis, and meningitis, responsible for infections in the bloodstream, leads to morbidity and mortality in infants (Tripathi et al. 2012). The virulence of *C. albicans* is related to its ability of morphological transitions between yeast and hyphal form, biofilm formation, gene expression, adhesion and invasion on the cell surface, phenotypic switching, hydrolytic enzymes secretion, and adaptability to environmental pH change, stress response, and metabolic flexibility (Nicholls et al. 2011). *C. albicans* is a polymorphic fungus and can either grow as parallel-walled true hyphae at high pH (>7) or ovoid-shaped budding yeast at low pH (<6); however, both forms are important for its pathogenicity (Berman and Sudbery 2002; Sawant and Khan 2017). Another important factor that determines the virulence of *C. albicans* is the ability to form biofilm on the abiotic or biotic surfaces like catheter, dentures, and mucosal surface. Mature biofilm possesses a complex organization comprising expression of drug efflux pumps and metabolic plasticity that are responsible for resistance to antifungal agents (Finkel and Mitchell 2011; Fanning and Mitchell 2012).

Due to major research advances in the development of new antifungal agents, the newer generation has been introduced with improved therapeutic outcomes (Nett and Andes 2016). Thus, after a time span of more than 20 years, the first-generation azole drugs, including fluconazole and itraconazole, were introduced in the 1990s. This was followed by the introduction of second-generation azole drugs, including voriconazole, posaconazole, isavuconazole, and echinocandins (anidulafungin, caspofungin, and micafungin), in the 2000s (Nett and Andes 2016). Further, many of these newly developed antifungal drugs have limited therapeutic efficacy due to their spectrum of activity, physicochemical and biopharmaceutical properties, pharmacokinetics, drug-drug interactions, and pharmacodynamic properties (Lewis 2011).

Several antifungal drugs are hydrophobic which limits water solubility that leads to poor oral bioavailability and limited formulation approaches (Lewis 2011). For example, many commonly used azole antifungal drugs, such as clotrimazole, itraconazole, miconazole, econazole, oxiconazole, tioconazole, voriconazole, and sertaconazole, are hydrophobic and have poor aqueous solubility (Gupta and Cooper 2008; Zhang et al. 2010). On the other hand, drug-drug interactions and toxicity of systemic antifungal agents are major obstacles leading to limited clinical benefits (Ashley et al. 2006). Amphotericin B is the well-known example of antifungal drug toxicity; its administration leads to dose-limited toxicities, particularly nephrotoxicity. In addition, AmB amplifies the nephrotoxicity of many other drugs, such as cyclosporine and aminoglycosides (Churchill and Seely 1977). Despite the availability of several conventional dosage forms for antifungal drugs including tablets, creams, IV infusions, etc., there is a strong need to develop innovative drug delivery systems to overcome limitations. Rationally designed drug delivery systems have the ability to improve drug performance and overcome many of these limitations. Lipid-based formulations of amphotericin B (AmB), such as liposomal AmB, AmB lipid complex, and AmB colloidal dispersion, exhibited a great reduction in AmB nephrotoxicity while maintaining its broad-spectrum antifungal activity (Arikan and Rex 2001). These encouraging results inspired the development of various new drug delivery systems to improve the safety profile of antifungal agents while enhancing their efficacy. Among new delivery systems, nano-based drug delivery systems have emerged as an innovative and promising platform able to minimize undesirable drug side effects while maintaining or enhancing its therapeutic efficacy (Zhang et al. 2010; Zazo et al. 2016). Nano-based drug delivery systems have various attractive features which include sustained drug release, enhanced drug stability, targeting to infected tissue, reduction of off-target side effects, prolongation of residence time in the blood, improved drug efficacy, and enhanced penetration through skin (Fig. 15.1) (Mbah et al. 2014; Chang et al. 2015; Soliman 2017). Amphotericin B is the only antifungal drug marketed in nanoformulations. Careful literature review shows only a limited number of review articles covering nanoscale antifungal drug carriers.

Thus, the authors have made an attempt to provide an in-depth account on various classes of candidiasis, their pathophysiology, and their therapeutic management. This book chapter also highlights the emergence of resistance to available antifungal drugs and their possible mechanisms. This chapter also describes the recent advances in the nano-based drug delivery systems of antifungal agents to overcome the deficiencies of conventional drug delivery systems and enhancement in the overall efficacy of these drugs. Challenges facing this field and impeding clinical translation of some promising nanoformulations are discussed.

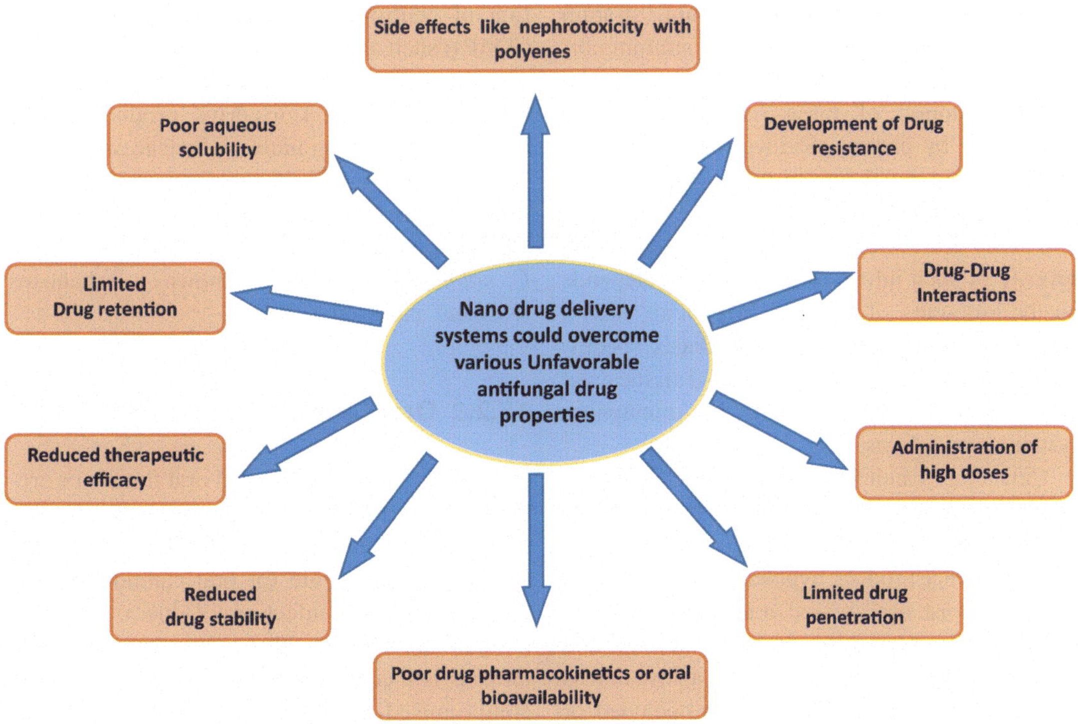

Fig. 15.1 Unpropitious antifungal drug properties that can be overcome through nano-drug delivery systems

15.2 Pathophysiology of Candidiasis

The planning of appropriate treatment of *Candida* infections requires knowledge of local epidemiology of infections, since type and severity of candidiasis are closely related to *Candida* species present at the site of infection. Based on the site of infection, candidiasis can be classified into four types (Table 15.1).

15.2.1 Cutaneous Candidiasis

The intact skin and various appendages act as an integumentary system that protects the body from outer damage. Moreover, this bio-barrier is open to the exchange of heat and air as well as the permeable to materials with low molecular weight (less than 500 Da). The skin is composed of multiple layers of different cells and tissues that are connected to the body via the connective tissues. The epidermis and dermis are the two main layers found in the skin. Further, the epidermis involves different layers of cells performing diverse functions. These layers from deep to superficial are stratum germinativum, stratum spinosum, stratum granulosum, and stratum corneum. The dermis consists of the connective tissues. Disruption of these barriers either by accident or by pathogenic invasion causes skin infection. Among them, an attack by dermatophytes especially *C. albicans* causes severe infection in the skin called cutaneous candidiasis. The severity of such infections significantly depends on the immunity of patients. In patients with a weakened immune system, candidiasis specifically superficial can spread to deeper tissues and may invade the blood causing life-threatening systemic candidiasis.

Cutaneous candidiasis is the most common type of candida infection that arises from candida blastospores which invade epithelial tissue, colonize, and hence produce hyphae. It usually occurs in warm, moist, and creased areas of the skin and is characterized by redness, rashes, itching, and discomfort. Host resistance to yeast invasion is reduced at epidermal sites that are occluded or macerated and is also decreased in patients whose cellular immunity is impaired. This allows commensal yeasts to penetrate the corneal layer. Penetration beyond the horny layer is normally not seen even in patients with defective T-lymphocyte responses. Epidermal and external epithelial surfaces are normally defended against microbial invasion by a range of factors, two of which stand out as particularly significant anti-*Candida* defenses, T-lymphocyte immune responses and epidermal proliferation, as the evidence for the importance of cellular immunity in defense against *Candida* infections comes from the simple observation that in persons with definable T-cell defects and in patients with low CD4 cell counts resulting from HIV infection, chronic cutaneous and mucosal candida infections frequently occur (Odds 1994). The skin has a layered innate immune system. *C. albicans* directly activates cutaneous sensory nerves to induce the release of calcitonin gene-related peptide (CGRP). CGRP acts on CD301b + dermal dendritic cells (dDC), which subsequently release IL-23. IL-23 acts on dermal γδ T cells to drive IL-17 production in the skin, leading to anti-*C. albicans* resistance through the presumed activation of neutrophils and antimicrobial peptides (AMPs) such as β-defensin. In addition, melanocytes in the basal epidermis can also recognize *C. albicans* via TLR-4 to drive production and release of melanin granules, which are antimicrobial in nature. Finally, Langerhans cells (LC) of the epidermis can suppress liver-derived CD49a + natural killer (NK) cells in response to *C. albicans* through unknown mechanisms (Kashem and Kaplan 2016).

15.2.2 Oral Candidiasis

Oral candidiasis is also called oral thrush, or oropharyngeal candidiasis. It is a mycotic infection affecting the oral mucosa. *Candida*, yeast-like fungus, is responsible for oral candidiasis, i.e., the opportunistic infection of the oral cavity (Akpan and Morgan 2002). Oropharyngeal candidiasis is a common manifestation in immunocompromised patients, in elderly individuals

Table 15.1 Causes and symptoms of various types of candidiasis

Category	Causes	Symptoms	Image
Cutaneous candidiasis			
Candidal folliculitis	Penetration of fungus in hair follicle due to bad hygiene or immunosuppression	Pus-filled pimple-like bumps around the hair follicle, itching, tenderness, hair fall, permanent baldness	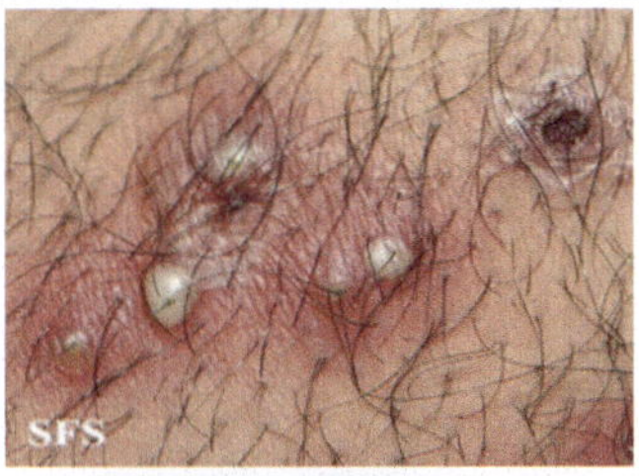
Candidal intertrigo	Friction between folds, heat, humidity, and obesity	Redness, burning, and excessive itching in skin folds most commonly under breast, between fingers, and armpits	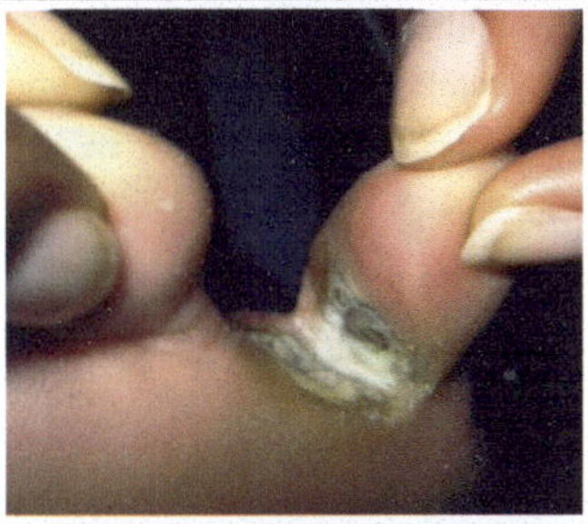
Candidal paronychia	Wet feet and hand for excessive time	Redness of skin around the nail, tenderness of nail, and pus-filled blisters	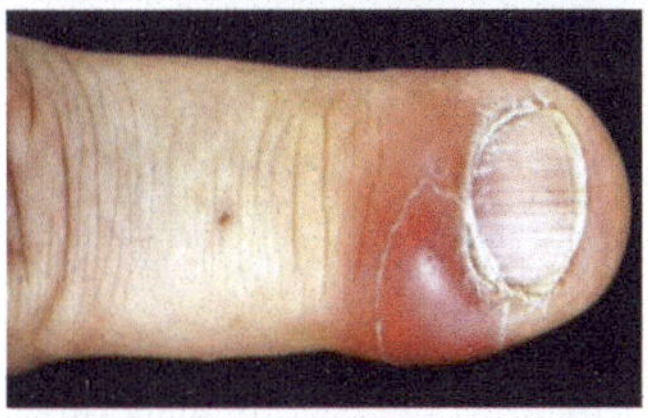
Diaper candidiasis	Poor hygiene	Pimple, blisters, ulcers, and pus sores in diaper area	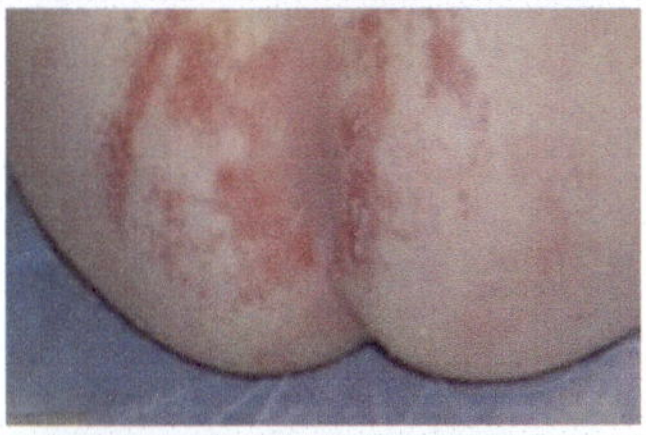
Congenital cutaneous candidiasis	Due to intrauterine candidal infection	Respiratory distress, skin eruptions, presence of macules and papules at birth on head, face, neck, and trunk	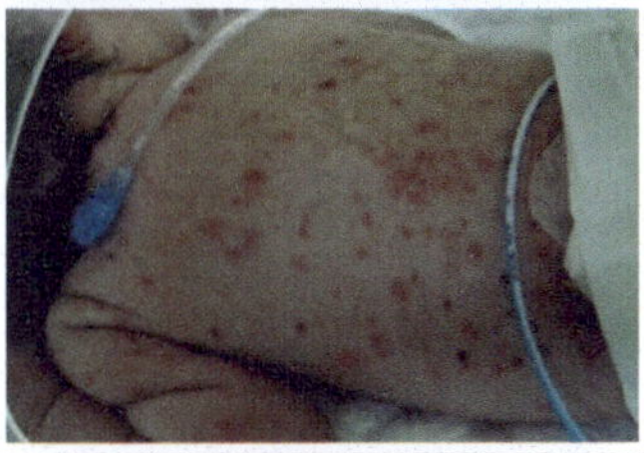
Perianal candidiasis	Poor hygiene and excessive contact with water for longer time	Itching, lesions, and ulcerative appearance in the genitals and area around anal orifice	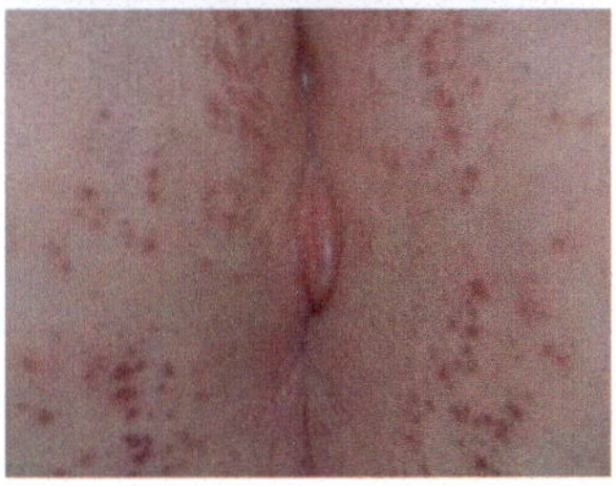

(continued)

Table 15.1 (continued)

Category	Causes	Symptoms	Image
Chronic mucocutaneous candidiasis	Hereditary immunodeficiency disorder caused due to malfunctioning of T-lymphocytes	Persistent infection on skin, nails, and other parts	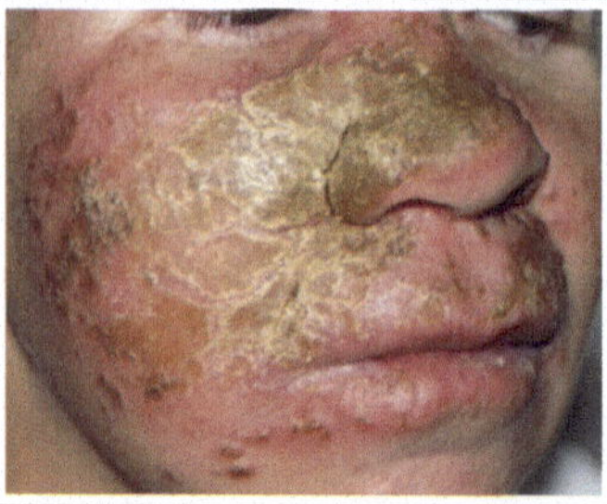
Oral candidiasis			
Pseudomembranous candidiasis	Intake of topical corticosteroid and immunosuppression	Creamy white lesions on the oral mucosa	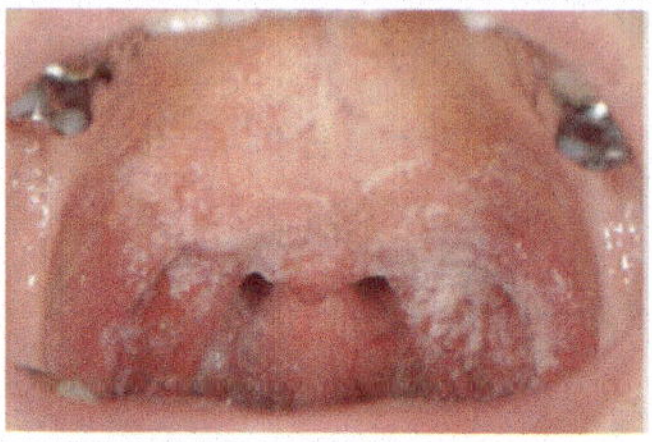
Erythematous candidiasis	Immunosuppression	Red raw-looking lesions, loss of lingual papillae	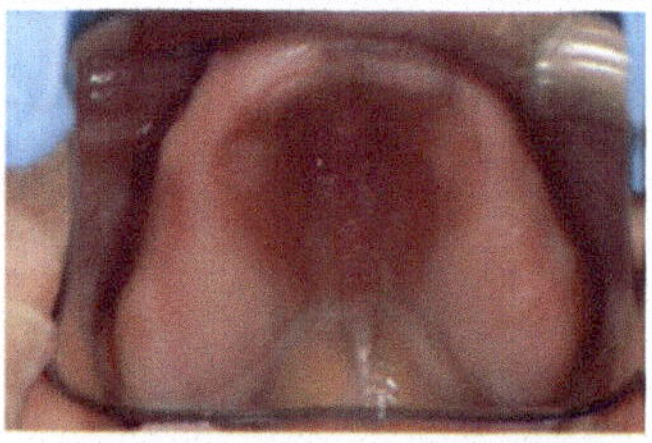
Hyperplastic	Immunosuppression	Rough and nodular lesions resembling white plaque	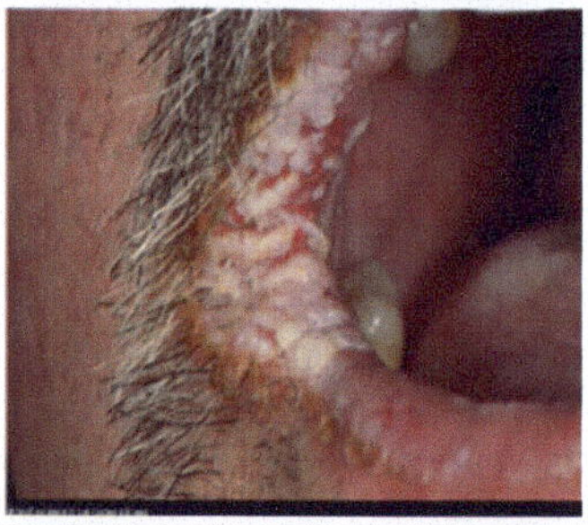
Denture-related stomatitis	Uncleansed dentures, bearing of dentures constantly for long time	Mild inflammation and redness beneath the denture	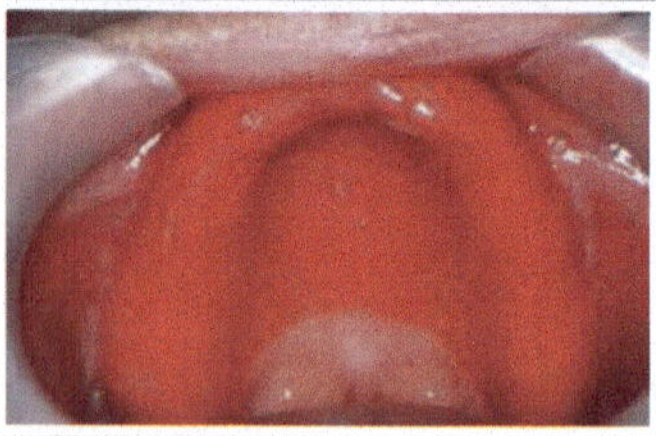

(continued)

Table 15.1 (continued)

Category	Causes	Symptoms	Image
Angular cheilitis	In patients with existing forms of intraoral candidiasis and high candida load	Inflammation and lesions at the angels of mouth	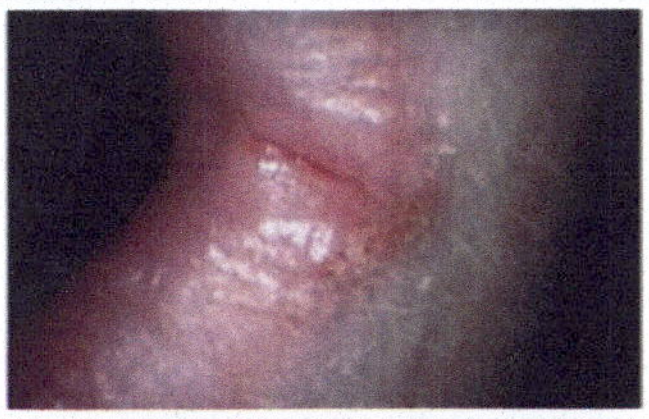
Median rhomboid glossitis	Due to steroid inhalers or in tobacco smokers	Diamond-shaped lesion on the posterior midline on the dorsum of the tongue	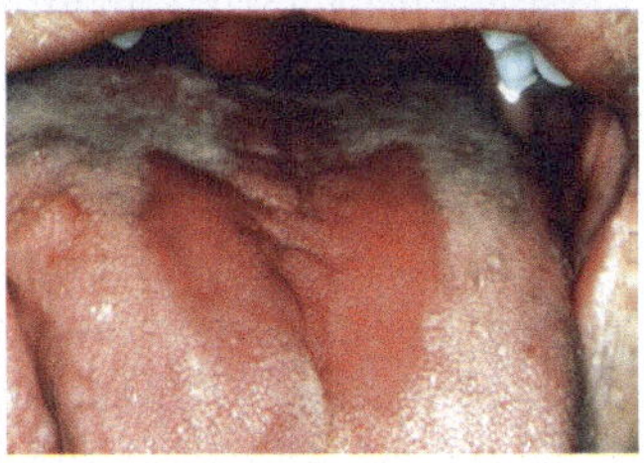

undergoing immunosuppressive therapy for cancer or organ transplantation, and in those exposed to broad-spectrum antibiotics. Most notably, oropharyngeal candidiasis is a major problem in individuals infected with HIV (Clark-Ordóñez et al. 2017). These individuals may suffer from painful, recurrent oral candidiasis which may be complicated by esophageal candidiasis. The latter may rarely lead to gastrointestinal bleeding, perforation, or disseminated candidiasis (Hoepelman and Dupont 1996).

The risk of developing oral and esophageal candidal infection is more with changes in oral flora, in patients with hyposalivation, diabetes mellitus, immunodeficient (AIDS patients), prolonged use of antibiotics or immunosuppressive drugs, denture wearers, poor oral hygiene, heavy smoking, malabsorption, infancy and old age, dysplasia and atopy and xerostomia (Takakura et al. 2003; Mobeen 2014). Clinically, oral candidiasis is diagnosed as white patches that appear as discrete lesions on the buccal mucosa, throat, tongue, and gum linings which emerge as convergent pseudomembranous resembling milk curds. These symptoms can be seen in people undergoing chemotherapy for cancer, people taking immunosuppressive drugs to protect transplanted organs, or people with HIV infection. Most types of oral candidiasis are painless, but a burning sensation may occur in some cases. A burning sensation is more likely with erythematous candidiasis, while hyperplastic candidiasis is normally asymptomatic. Acute atrophic candidiasis may feel like the mouth has been scalded with a hot liquid. Another symptom is a metallic, acidic, salty, or bitter taste in the mouth. The pseudomembranous type rarely causes any symptoms apart from possibly some discomfort or bad taste due to the presence of the membranes (Bruch and Treister 2010). Occasionally, there can be difficulty in swallowing which indicates that candidiasis involves the oropharynx or the esophagus, as well as the mouth. The trachea and the larynx may also be involved where there is oral candidiasis, and this may cause hoarseness of the voice.

15.2.3 Vulvovaginal Candidiasis (VVC)

VVC affects about three-quarters of women with at least one episode of VVC during their reproductive age and during pregnancy (especially during the second and third trimesters) and approximately half of the women population from two or more episodes (Aguin and Sobel 2015). The causative agent is predominantly *C. albicans* followed by *C. glabrata* (Sobel et al. 2004; Achkar and Fries 2010). The most common symptoms of VVC are burning pain and pruritus of the vulva with discomfort that can lead to dysuria and dyspareunia in more severe cases. Clinical signs of VVC are edema and erythema of the vulva and the vagina accompanied by an abnormal vaginal discharge that may be watery, cheese-like, or minimal (Dovnik et al. 2015). VVC is divided into two categories: uncomplicated cases characterized by infrequent episodes of mild infections caused by *C. albicans* in speciously healthy women and complicated cases characterized by a severe infection caused by non-*C. albicans* species during pregnancy or associated medical conditions like immunosuppression or diabetes (Sawant and Khan 2017). Pathophysiology of vulvovaginal candidiasis is mediated by a number of virulence factors that involve five steps.

15.2.3.1 Adhesion

Adhesion of *Candida* to host surfaces is the primary step for initial colonization of human tissues, contribution to the perseverance of the fungus within the host and is essential in the establishing fungal infection. Therefore, adhesion of candida species to vaginal epithelial cells is the principal event in VVC (Silva et al. 2012).

15.2.3.2 Biofilm Formation

Biofilms are structured groups of microorganisms that are irreversibly attached to a surface, with a high degree of organization and a self-produced extracellular matrix (Douglas 2003). Biofilms are the most prevalent growth form of microorganisms in nature, with up to 80% of all microorganisms, in the environment, existing in biofilm organization. Over 65% of all human infections are due to microbial biofilms (Donlan 2002). *Candida* species can form biofilms on vaginal epithelium and have a high capacity to produce biofilms on IUDs promoting VVC (Harriott et al. 2010).

15.2.3.3 Extracellular Hydrolytic Enzyme Production

Several hydrolytic enzymes secreted by *Candida* species play an important role in adhesion, tissue penetration, invasion, and destruction of host epithelial tissue (Schaller et al. 2005). The enzymes most frequently concerned in *Candida* pathogenicity are aspartyl proteinases, but lipases, phospholipases, and hemolysins are also involved in *Candida* virulence (Silva et al. 2012).

15.2.3.4 Hyphae Formation

Hyphae formation is a reversible morphological rotation between unicellular yeast cells and filamentous phase. This is an important virulence factor of some *Candida* species (Silva et al. 2012). Filamentous or hyphae forms give more mechanical strength, enhancing colonization, and they are believed to play an important role in invasion of host tissues (Kumamoto and Vinces 2005; Silva et al. 2012).

15.2.4 Invasive Candidiasis

Invasive candidiasis comprises various types of appalling invasive disorders like disseminated candidiasis, candidemia, endocarditis, endophthalmitis, and meningitis (Pappas 2006). Candidemia is the fourth most common bloodstream infection that affects more than 250,000 individuals worldwide every year and is responsible for more than 50,000 deaths (Kullberg and Arendrup 2015). Recently, additional species of *Candida* like *C. auris*, *C. glabrata, and C. parapsilosis* have also emerged as causative agents alongside *C. albicans* (Wisplinghoff et al. 2004). The major predisposing factors that contribute toward pathogenicity of invasive candidiasis involves increased fungal burden due to inconsistent use of broad-spectrum antibiotics, use of intravascular devices, recent surgery and trauma, and immune dysfunction like chemotherapy-induced neutropenia or corticosteroid therapy (Blumberg et al. 2001; Wisplinghoff et al. 2004). *Candida* species adheres to gastrointestinal, vaginal, and oral epithelial cells, platelet fibrin clots, acrylic and plastic materials like IUDs, etc., lymphocytes, and it forms biofilm with unique phenotypic and genotypic characteristics that are resistant to currently used antifungal drugs (Pittet et al. 1994; Shin et al. 2002). The general risk factors for invasive candidiasis in adults can be categorized into two types:

(i) Intrinsic: colonization with *Candida* spp., diabetes mellitus, gastrointestinal perforation, increased age, pancreatitis, sepsis, and severity of illness
(ii) Iatrogenic: any type of dialysis (especially hemodialysis), broad-spectrum antibiotics, central venous catheter, corticosteroids and other immunosuppressants, gastrointestinal surgery or other major surgery, left ventricular assist device, long-term stay in hospital or intensive care unit, mechanical ventilation, solid organ transplant, stem cell transplant, and total parenteral nutrition.
(iii) Additionally, children and neonates are predisposed to premature birth and congenital defects (Sonnex and Lefort 1999; Sawant and Khan 2017; Soliman 2017).

15.3 Therapeutic Management of Candidiasis

Therapeutic management of candidiasis is usually based upon the anatomic location of the infection, immune status of the patient, risk factors for patients with infection, species responsible, and lastly the susceptibility of the candida species toward the antifungal drug. Antifungal agents are classified into polyenes, azoles, allylamines, or derivatives, and echinocandins, and their targets, mechanistic pathway, and side effects are depicted in Table 15.2.

15.3.1 Polyenes

Polyenes include the drugs amphotericin B and nystatin, and their mode of action is through direct binding to the sterol ergosterol found within fungal cell membranes. Polyene binding to ergosterol induces leakage of cytoplasmic contents leading to fungal cell death (D Sanglard 2002). The equivalent mammalian sterol is cholesterol, which has a lower binding affinity for polyenes, and this makes host cells less susceptible to their toxic effects. Nevertheless, at higher therapeutic concentrations, polyenes do exhibit a degree of toxicity in humans (Williams et al. 2011). Polyenes are frequently used in the treatment of chronic erythematous candidiasis. Oral suspension of amphotericin B (10 mg; four times a day) may be employed in treating refractory oral candidiasis frequently seen in HIV-infected and AIDS patients. Moreover, IV infusion of amphotericin B is used to treat esophageal candidiasis (0.25 mg/kg/day), and nystatin is available as pastilles (10 mg/day) and oral suspension (40 mg/day).

15.3.2 Azoles

The azole antifungals are fungistatic rather than fungicidal. The mechanism of action is by inhibiting the enzyme lanosterol demethylase that is a cytochrome P-450 3-A-dependent enzyme involved in the synthesis of ergosterol. Subsequent depletion of ergosterol in the fungal cell results in inhibition of fungal growth and impairment of membrane permeability (Andes 2003).

Itraconazole and fluconazole are first-generation azoles to be used in the treatment of candidiasis. These are also administered orally because of their easy absorption through the GI tract (Andes 2003). Miconazole is used as a topical preparation in the treatment of angular cheilitis, a type of oral candidiasis. Also, there are various dosage forms of clotrimazole like creams, gels, troches, and mouth paint available for the treatment of oral thrush (Samaranayake et al. 2009; Niimi et al. 2010). Intravaginal creams, suppositories, and vaginal tablets are commonly used to treat VVC and are preferred due to their limited systemic absorption, rapid symptomatic relief, and minimum side effects (Faro 1996; Magliani et al. 2002). Ketoconazole is not administered in immunosuppressed patients or patients with chronic, recurrent, and persistent infection due to side effects like nausea, vomiting, abdominal pain, hepatotoxicity, and inhibition of androgen biosynthesis (Hay

Table 15.2 Classification of antifungal drugs and their mechanistic pathways

S. no.	Antifungal agent	Site of action	Target	Side effects
Polyenes				
1.	Amphotericin B	Fungal cell membrane	Binds irreversibly to ergosterol in cell membrane, resulting in disruption of membrane integrity and ultimately cell death	Nephrotoxicity, renal insufficiency, hypokalemia, hypomagnesemia, polyuria
2.	Nystatin			Itching, mouth and hand swelling, chest tightness, diarrhea, nausea, mild stomach upset
Azoles				
3.	Miconazole	Inhibition of cytochrome P450 and thus ergosterol production inhibition and inhibition of conversion of lanosterol to ergosterol	Cytochrome P450, Gene: cytochrome 51, inhibition of lanosterol 14-alpha demethylase	Oral: vomiting, diarrhea, nausea Topical: itching, mild burning, and stinging sensations
4.	Clotrimazole			Topical: irritation, burning sensation, and contact dermatitis Oral: nausea, vomiting, bad or unusual taste in mouth
5.	Itraconazole			Oral: chest pain, coughing of blood, dark urine or pale stools, numbness, rapid weight gain, hypokalemia on prolonged treatment
6.	Ketoconazole			Oral: GIT disturbances including nausea, vomiting, abdominal pain, liver problems, abnormal heart rhythm, headache, dizziness, fainting Topical: irritation and burning sensation, skin rashes, acne
7.	Fluconazole			Oral: abdominal pain, diarrhea, nausea, vomiting, headache, hepatic toxicity, loss of appetite Topical: blisters, skin rashes, and rare exfoliative cutaneous reactions, such as toxic epidermal necrolysis
8.	Voriconazole			Blurred vision, headache, nausea, dizziness
9.	Econazole			Topical: irritation, burning sensation, and contact dermatitis
Echinocandins				
10.	Caspofungin	Cell wall formation inhibition	Inhibit enzyme (1 → 3)-β-D-glucan synthase thereby disturbing the integrity of the fungal cell wall	Vomiting, diarrhea, mild skin rash, dizziness, headache
11.	Micafungin			Mild nausea, vomiting, diarrhea, headache
12.	Anidulafungin			Nausea, vomiting, diarrhea
Allylamine derivative				
13.	Terbinafine	Cell membrane formation	Inhibition of squalene epoxidase enzyme and thus blocking the ergosterol synthesis	Nausea, upset stomach, rash, headache, change in taste

(continued)

Table 15.2 (continued)

S. no.	Antifungal agent	Site of action	Target	Side effects
14.	Amorolfine	Ergosterol depletion in cell membrane	Inhibit Delta 14 sterol reductase and cholesterol delta isomerase	Nail discoloration, broken or brittle nails, itching, or irritating skin
15.	Butenafine hydrochloride	Ergosterol biosynthesis	Block squalene epoxidation	Irritation, redness, burning, worsening of skin condition
16.	Naftifine	Blocking sterol biosynthesis	Inhibition of squalene 2,3-epoxidase enzyme	Headache, dizziness, redness, dry skin, itching

Source: Gupta et al. (2017); Nigam (2015)

1993). However, in VVC ketoconazole is prescribed for a shorter duration of time, thus having less probability to develop side effects (Faro 1996). Fluconazole, an orally administered antifungal agent, is frequently used because it is active against *C. albicans*, *C. parapsilosis*, *C. glabrata, and C. tropicalis* (Hay 1993; Maiolo et al. 2014).

When patients do not have any response to topical antifungals or there is no patient compliance or there are cases of relapses after topical treatment, then opt for systemic antifungals. Nowadays, there are increasing cases of resistance to antifungal agents, and this is of much more concern in the case of immunocompromised patients. People like newborns and immune-deficient individuals are more prone to the candida infection and thus are given broad-spectrum antibiotics. OTC antifungal dosage forms such as creams and gels can be used for local treatment of candidiasis, whereas for preventing the spread of the disease to deeper vital organs, effective treatment by candidiasis antifungal chemotherapy is preferred. Use of probiotics and development of novel vaccines are an advanced approach for the prevention of the infection (Hani et al. 2015).

15.3.3 Echinocandins

Echinocandins are a family of semisynthetic lipopeptides with a highly selective target, the biosynthesis of 1,3-ß-D-glucan of the fungal wall, by blocking the activity of the enzyme ß-glucan synthetase, with fungicidal effect against *Candida* and few toxic effects for human eukaryotic cells. Its use is exclusively intravenous (Quindós et al. 2019). The first licensed echinocandin product is caspofungin acetate (Cancidas; Merck); subsequent members of the class likely to be licensed include micafungin (Fujisawa) and anidulafungin (Versicor). The initial licensure of caspofungin, however, is for the treatment of patients with invasive aspergillosis refractory to amphotericin B (in its various formulations) and/or itraconazole (Denning 2002). Among the advantages of echinocandins for the treatment of severe and recalcitrant oral candidiasis are their anti-biofilm activities and their prolonged post-antifungal effect. They can be first-choice drugs for the treatment of severe candidiasis in patients with immunodeficiency, the seriously ill, and those with a high probability of drug interactions. They are category C drugs in pregnancy and should be avoided if there is another therapeutic alternative, as during breastfeeding (Quindós et al. 2019).

Appropriate and timely antifungal treatment is necessary as a delay in the treatment is associated with an increased rate of morbidity and mortality. Various systemic antifungal agents available for the treatment of invasive candidiasis include polyenes, azoles, echinocandins, and flucytosine. Azoles are inactive against biofilm, while echinocandins show variable efficacy. The antifungal agents commonly used in candidiasis treatment are mentioned in Table 15.3 along with their available dosage forms.

Table 15.3 Antifungal drugs currently used in therapeutic management of candidiasis

Affected areas	Class of drug	Generic name	Brand name	Dose	Available dosage form
		Oral thrush			
Tongue, buccal mucosa, palate, corners of the mouth, beneath a denture, on gums	Azole	Miconazole	Oravig®	50 mg/day for 14 days	Buccal tablet
			Loramyc®	50 mg/day	Mucoadhesive buccal tablet
			Daktarin	20 mg/kg/day	Oral gel
			Miconazex	50 mg/day for 14 days	Gel
		Clotrimazole	Mycelex troche	1 troche 5 times a day for 14 days	Troche
		Fluconazole	Diflucan	20 mg on day 1 and then 100 mg PO for 2 weeks	Oral suspension
Vaginal candidiasis					
Vagina and vulva	Azole	Miconazole nitrate	Monistat	1200 mg suppository for 1 day	Suppository
			Gyno Daktarin	200 mg capsule; insert one capsule twice a day	Vaginal capsule
			Femizol-M	20 milligrams (for seven nights)	Vaginal cream (2%)
			Miconazex	Apply 5 g intravaginally for 10–14 days	Cream (2%)
			Miconazex	100 mg once daily for 7–14 days	Pessary
		Fluconazole	Diflucan	150 mg/day	Tablet
		Clotrimazole	Cancap-VT	100 mg/day	Tablet
			Candid tab	100/day	Tablet
			Canesten	100 mg/day	Tablet
			Gynostatum	100 mg to 500 mg for 6 days	Tablet
			Surfaz-VT	100 mg to 500 mg for 6 days	Tablet
		Butoconazole	Vaginal cream Antican	20 mg for 7 days 600 mg/day	Cream Tablet

(continued)

Table 15.3 (continued)

Affected areas	Class of drug	Generic name	Brand name	Dose	Available dosage form
Cutaneous candidiasis					
On the whole outer layer of the body	Azole	Miconazole nitrate (2%)	Decocort	100 mg every night for 7–14 days	Pessary
			Decocort	5 g every night for 7–14 days (twice daily)	Cream
			3M™Cavilon™	Apply once every 24 h	Cream
			Miconazex	Apply a thin layer over the affected area for 2–6 weeks and continue for a week after symptoms disappear	Cream
			Monistat-Derm	Apply twice a day for 2 weeks	Cream (2%)
			Aloe Vesta	Twice daily for 2–4 weeks	Cream
			Zimycan	Apply for 2 weeks twice a day	Paste
		Clotrimazole	Lotrimin AF®	Apply twice daily for 4 weeks	Foot cream
			Canesten	Apply two to three times daily	Cream
			Mycelex −7	Apply twice a day	Cream
		Ketoconazole	Nizoral-AD	To be used four times a week	Shampoo
			Xolegel	Apply for 2 weeks over the affected area	Gel
	Polyene	Nystatin	Mycostatin	1 gm applied two to four times a day	Powder and cream
			Nyamyc	Apply four times a day	Gel
Gastrointestinal tract candidiasis					
GIT tract	Polyene	Nystatin	Mycostatin Pastilles	One to two tablets three times daily	Tablets
			Nilstat	Four times a day	Troches, oral suspension
			Mycostatin	Two of them four or five times a day	Pastilles
Esophageal candidiasis					
Mouth extended to the whole esophagus	Azole	Miconazole	Miconazex	Apply one to two times daily over the affected area and continue for a week after lesions disappear	Cream
		Fluconazole	Diflucan	150 mg for 14 days	Tablet
		Itraconazole	Sporanox	100–200 mg per day for 2 weeks	Capsule

(continued)

Table 15.3 (continued)

Affected areas	Class of drug	Generic name	Brand name	Dose	Available dosage form
		Voriconazole	Vfend	200 mg PO q12hr	Lyophilized powder for solution of IV infusion
	Echinocandins	Micafungin	Mycamine	150 mg/day IV infusion for 10–30 days	IV injection
		Anidulafungin	Eraxis	200 mg injection first day followed by 100 mg injections for 14 days	IV injection
		Caspofungin	Cancidas	50 mg IV infused over 1 h, continue for 7–14 days	IV injection
	Polyenes	Amphotericin B	Amphocin	0.25 mg/kg/day	IV injection
			Fungizone	1.5 mg/kg/day	IV injection
Nail candidiasis					
Nail late, nail fold	Azole	Itraconazole	Onmel	200 mg/12 h for 1 week	Liquid
		Miconazole	Miranel AF	Apply thin layer over the affected area for 2–4 weeks	Liquid

15.3.4 Challenges and Issues in Therapeutic Management of Candidiasis

15.3.4.1 Pharmacokinetic Issues

The absorption or metabolism of an antifungal drug readily gets affected by any change in pH of the stomach. The absorption of fluconazole is not affected by drugs that increase gastric pH (Brüggemann et al. 2009). The absorption of itraconazole capsules is pH-dependent requiring an acidic environment. Administration of a drug which tends to lower the pH of the stomach has a deleterious impact on the absorption of itraconazole (Smith and Andes 2008), and thus, administration of any antacid or anticholinergic drug should be done after 2 h of administration of antifungals (Caterina et al. 2013). The absorption of voriconazole is not markedly influenced by antacids or proton pump inhibitors, although the mean C_{max} and AUC values of voriconazole are increased by 15% and 41% when coadministered with omeprazole, because of the inhibition of plasma clearance of voriconazole. C_{max} and AUC values of posaconazole were both reduced by 39% when coadministered with cimetidine (400 mg twice daily), possibly as a result of decreased gastric acid production. Not only the gastric pH but also the integrity of the gastrointestinal tract may be important factors for the absorption of antifungal drugs. Posaconazole absorption appeared to be reduced in patients with grade 1 or grade 2 mucositis, compared with patients without mucositis (AUC for 400 mg of posaconazole twice daily). The mean bioavailability of itraconazole oral solution under steady-state conditions was 43% higher for those who fasted than for those who did not. Single and multiple oral doses of voriconazole with food lowered the bioavailability by 22% and delayed absorption, compared with single and multiple oral doses of voriconazole without food. Administration of voriconazole with a high-fat meal reduced the mean C_{max} and AUC by 34% and 24%, respectively. For this reason, oral administration is recommended either 1 h before or 1 h after meals. The mean AUC and C_{max} values increased by 400% when posaconazole was administered with a high-fat meal, compared with when it was administered under fasting conditions (Brüggemann et al. 2009).

15.3.4.2 Pharmacodynamic Issues

Various kinds of pharmacodynamic issues of antifungal drugs come up along with therapeutic effects shown by these drugs. Itraconazole is available in different dosage forms, and the side effect is also dosage form-dependent. Gastrointestinal disturbances, pruritus, dizziness, and headache are associated with its capsule form, and oral form is associated with increased levels of aminotransferases. Intravenous administration of itraconazole is associated with injection site reaction and headache (Willems et al. 2001). Fluconazole is associated with nausea, vomiting, skin rash, and abdominal pain. The side effects noted with voriconazole are mild to moderate to well tolerated. Reversible disturbances include blurred vision, bright spot, altered color discrimination, mild skin rashes, facial erythema, and cheilitis. Posaconazole is associated with gastrointestinal tract disturbances, abdominal disturbances, and nausea (Schiller and Fung 2007).

15.4 Antifungal Resistance in Candidiasis: Definition, Mechanism, and Epidemiology

Antifungal resistance can be well-defined as clinical resistance or microbiologic, or as a composite of both. When the concentration of antifungal agent is higher than the range seen in wild type strain to inhibit the growth of infecting pathogen or organism, then the condition is said to be microbiologic resistance. Clinical resistance is said to occur in a situation in which the infecting organism is inhibited by a concentration of an antifungal agent that is associated with a high likelihood of therapeutic failure. In other words, the pathogen is inhibited by an antimicrobial concentration that is higher than could be safely achieved with normal dosing. By the composite definition, resistance is present when isolates are not inhibited by the usually achievable concentrations of the agent with normal dosage schedules and/or when they demonstrate MICs that fall in the range where specific microbial resistance mechanisms are likely, and where clinical efficacy against the isolate has not been reliably shown in treatment studies (Pfaller 2012).

Dermatophytosis is frequently associated with relapses following the termination of antifungal therapy. Until the late 1990s, clinical resistance to antifungal agents was rare, with only isolated cases in patients with chronic mucocutaneous candidiasis (Lupetti et al. 2002; Stephenson 1997). During the last 5 years, the prevalence of fungal infections as well as resistant infections has increased, and this may be due to irregular or inadequate use of antifungal drugs or increased frequency of immunodeficiency conditions (Stephenson 1997; White et al. 1998). In recent years, the use and over-the-counter sale of antifungal drugs and antibiotics have increased, which may be a major cause of prevalence of clinical resistance to these drugs. Drug resistance in azole, especially against fungi, is becoming more prevalent clinically. Minimum inhibitory concentration (MIC) is the main parameter to quantify antifungal drug resistance in which fungal growth is measured in the presence of antifungal drug concentration over a definite time period (Nigam 2015). The minimum drug concentration that results in a substantial reduction of growth (usually either 50% or 90% reduction) is called the MIC; however, it does not always predict the clinical outcome of antifungal therapy (Sanglard and Odds 2002). In 1997, the NCCLS proposed a standardized technique that can be used to determine the level of resistance of the yeast strain (Hudson 2001).

15.4.1 Drug Resistance Biochemical and Molecular Mechanisms

The main molecular and biochemical mechanisms that contribute to antifungal resistance include reduction in uptake of the drug, an active efflux of the cell, alteration in the interaction of the drug to the target site or other enzymes involved in the same enzymatic process by point mutations, overexpression of the target molecule, overproduction or mutation of the target enzyme, amplification and gene conversion (recombination), and increased cellular efflux (Sanglard 2002; Martinez-Rossi et al. 2008) (Fig. 15.2).

Ergosterol is the principal component of the fungal cell membrane and responsible for membrane fluidity and therefore membrane integrity in fungal cells. Azole uptake by fungal cells may be decreased by alterations in the sterol and/or the phospholipid composition of the fungal cell membrane and membrane fluidity. Similarly, reduced intracellular accumulation of the drug may occur due to increased active transport of the drug out of the cell. Azoles, polyenes, allylamine, and thiocarbamates owe their antifungal activities to inhibition of synthesis of or direct interaction with ergosterol (Revie et al. 2018).

Resistant strains either exhibit a modification in the quality or quantity of target enzyme, reduced access to the target, or a combination of these mechanisms. Various mechanisms by which microbial cells might develop resistance include (Ghannoum and Rice 1999) (i) the target enzyme is overproduced, so that the drug does not inhibit the biochemical reaction completely; (ii) the drug target is altered so that the drug cannot bind to the target; (iii) the drug is pumped out by an efflux pump; (iv) the entry of the drug is prevented at the cell membrane/cell wall level; (v) the cell has a bypass pathway that compensates for the loss-of-function inhibition due to the drug activity; (vi) some fungal enzymes that convert an inactive drug to its active form are inhibited; and (vii) the cell secretes some enzymes to the extracellular medium, which degrade the drug.

Several studies observed an alteration in the quantity or quality of 14α-demethylase in the expression of resistance to azole antifungal agents (Martinez-Rossi et al. 2018). A role of upregulation of the ERG11 gene, which encodes the major target enzyme of the azoles lanosterol 14α-demethylase, has been observed in azole-resistant *C. albicans and C. glabrata* isolates (Henry et al. 2000; Chau et al. 2004). On the other hand, *C. albicans* may possess one or more additional genes encoding ATP-binding cassette MDR-like proteins that are distinct from CDR1,

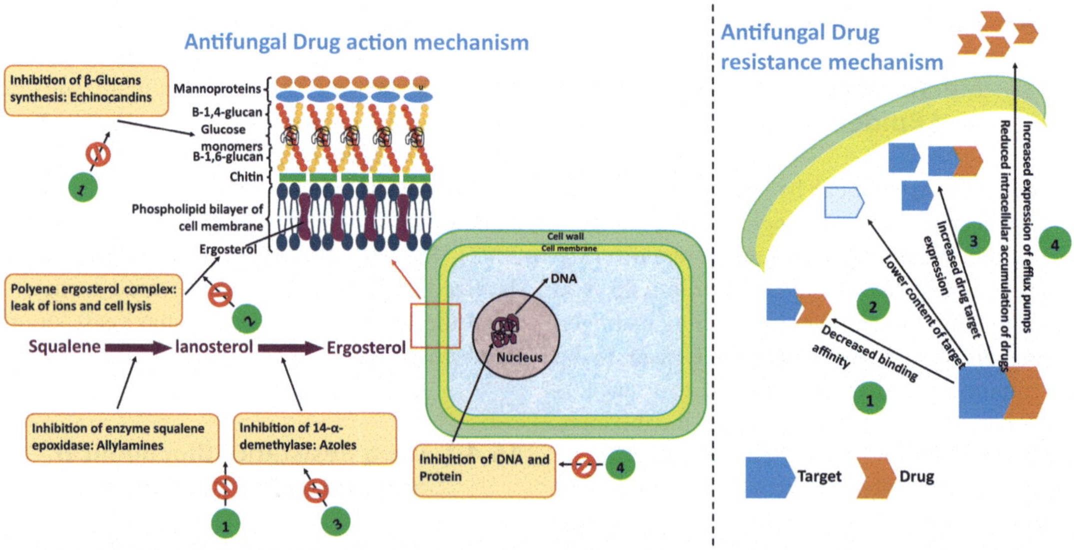

Fig. 15.2 Antifungal drug actions and resistance mechanisms in *Candida* species. (1) Alteration in the structures of enzymes or other proteins due to mutations and drugs cannot bind to it. (2) The drug target content is less; drug cannot bind to it efficiently. (3) Drug targets such as enzymes are overproduced, and drugs cannot inhibit the enzymatic reactions. (4) Drugs are pumped out by efflux pump, and there is less accumulation of drug on the target site

which could participate in the development of azole resistance (Walsh et al. 1997). Considerable evidence implicating drug efflux as an important mechanism of resistance to azole antifungals is forthcoming recently. Studies indicate that fungi possess at least two efflux systems: (i) proteins belonging to the major facilitator superfamily and (ii) ATP-binding cassette superfamily of proteins (Martinez-Rossi et al. 2008; Revie et al. 2018).

Another emerging source of antifungal resistance is the occurrence of a biofilm, the extracellular matrices produced by microbes themselves which serve to help organisms attach to living or nonviable surfaces (Minnebruggen et al. 2010). It is estimated that about 65% of all human microbial infections involve biofilms, and the majority of invasive diseases produced by *C. albicans* are associated with biofilm growth (Donlan and Costerton 2002). It has been demonstrated that drug efflux pumps play a role in the drug resistance of early biofilms. In contrast, resistance of mature biofilms does not rely on the known antifungal efflux pumps (Sanguinetti et al. 2005). It has been hypothesized that a change in membrane sterol composition during biofilm formation might explain resistance to amphotericin B and the azoles (Mateus et al. 2004).

Resistance to polyene antifungal drugs is rare, which is mostly confined to the less common species of *Candida*, such as *C. lusitaniae*, *C. glabrata, and C. guilliermondii* (Martins and Rex 1996). Fryberg suggested that development of resistance occurs by selection of naturally occurring resistant cells, present in small numbers in the population (Fryberg et al. 1974). These naturally resistant cells produce modified sterols that bind nystatin with lower affinity. Athar and Winner, however, have suggested that resistance results from mutation rather than selection (Athar and Winner 1971). Hamilton-Miller (1973) proposed a "biochemical" hypothesis that resistance arises due to alterations, either qualitative or quantitative, in the sterol content of the fungi cells. According to this biochemical hypothesis, resistant cells with altered sterol content should bind smaller amounts of polyene than do susceptible cells. This decreased binding of polyenes in *C. albicans* mutants could be attributed to (Ghannoum and Rice 1999) (i) a decrease in the total ergosterol content of the cell, without concomitant changes in sterol composition; (ii) replacement of some or all of the polyene-binding sterols by ones which bind polyene less well; or (iii) masking or reorientation of existing ergosterol, so that binding with polyenes is sterically or thermodynamically less favored.

15.5 Nano-drug Delivery Approaches for Candidiasis

15.5.1 Lipid-Based Nano-drug Delivery System

15.5.1.1 Liposomes

A liposome is a spherical vesicle having at least one lipid layer. Liposomes are more often composed of phospholipid, especially phosphatidylcholine. The major types of liposomes are the multilamellar vesicle (MLV, 500–5000 nm), the small unilamellar vesicle (SUV, ~100 nm), and large unilamellar vesicle (LUV, 200–800 nm). The structure of liposomes allows them to act as effective delivery systems for both hydrophilic and hydrophobic drugs (Eloy et al. 2014). The amphotericin B (Fungizone, AmB) has long been recognized as a powerful fungicidal and leishmanicidal drug. AmB deoxycholate which is the conventional and most effective form of amphotericin B but have some adverse effect like nephrotoxicity. Therefore, analogues of AmB like liposomal AmB (AmBisome), AmB lipid complex (Abelcet), AmB colloidal dispersion (Amphocil), and intralipid AmB were prepared (Vyas and Gupta 2006). A study shows that the fluconazole-loaded liposomal gel accumulated in various regions of skin or in various strata of skin following topical application. The study signified the localized effect of drug due to sustained release (Gupta et al. 2010). Terbinafine HCl-loaded liposomes dispersed in gum karaya gel had been evaluated for ex vivo drug retention in rat skin. Developed liposomes showed approximately 70% entrapment of terbinafine HCl and prolonged retention of drug in rat skin compared to plain gum karaya gel containing free terbinafine HCl up to 24 h (Sudhakar et al. 2014). For transdermal delivery, Elmoslemany et al. (2012) developed a comparative assessment between propylene glycol liposomes and conventional liposomes loaded with miconazole nitrate. Minimum inhibitory concentration value of 1.46 μg/ml against *C. albicans* showed by propylene glycol liposomes which was low compared to the MIC value of conventional liposomes (2.93 μg/ml). In human skin, propylene glycol liposomes also showed high skin retention and skin permeation of miconazole nitrate compared to conventional liposomes and miconazole nitrate suspension. Two different phospholipids, namely, phosphatidylcholine saturated 97.3% content and phosphatidylcholine unsaturated 98.0% content for topical delivery of miconazole nitrate are used for evaluation of liposomes performed by Agarwal and Katare (2002) which shows high stability and good colloidal characteristics. However, phosphatidylcholine-based liposomes showed higher skin retention of miconazole nitrate than phosphatidylcholine in in vitro mouse skin.

15.5.1.2 Ethosomes

Ethosomes are nanocarrier systems having high ethanol content, phospholipids, and water in them. Ethosomes may contain 2–5% content of phospholipids and 20–40% concentration of ethanol. Enhancement of ethosomes colloidal stability is due to negative surface charge on it. Bhalaria et al. (2009) investigated fluconazole-loaded ethosomes for treatment of cutaneous candidiasis in eight patients for a period of 1 month. Ethosomal gel containing fluconazole showed a 50–70% reduction in skin lesions in patients as compared to liposomes (30–60%) and commercial fluconazole cream (25–30%). Later on, for the treatment of deep fungal infection, econazole nitrate-loaded ethosomes were compared with liposomes loaded with the same in gel form. Ethosomal gel showed twofold higher diffusion of the drug in the albino rat skin compared to liposomal gel after 12 h of application. Results of confocal laser scanning microscopy studies revealed accumulation of econazole nitrate-loaded ethosomes in the stratum basale layer of animal skin (Verma and Pathak 2012). Furthermore, Faisal et al. (2018) prepared voriconazole-loaded ethosomes for effective skin deposition in skin. Ex vivo drug permeation of developed ethosomal formulation in the rat abdominal skin showed sixfold more permeation compared to hydroethanolic solution of voriconazole. If ethanol concentration is more than 30% in ethosomes, it causes excessive release of entrapped material and irritation of skin. Therefore, Akhtar and Pathak (2012) developed Cavamax W7 composite ethosomes to overcome the problem associated with high ethanol concentration. Cavamax W7 is a permeation enhancer for synergistic effect on ethanol's skin penetration power. Developed Cavamax W7 composite ethosomes showed high stability and ex vivo skin permeation and antifungal activity against *C. albicans* and *Aspergillus niger* compared to conventional ethosomes.

15.5.1.3 Transethosomes

To encompass the advantages of transfersomes and ethosomes, there is a new vesicular nanocarrier system named as transethosomes. They include penetration enhancer or an edge activator, and additionally, their composition is exactly similar to ethosomes. For in vivo skin deposition of drug in mice, Song et al. (2012) evaluated voriconazole-loaded transethosomes and showed increased in vivo skin deposition of voriconazole in the dermis and epidermis area compared to other nanocarriers like deformable liposomes, conventional liposomes, ethosomes, and polyethylene glycol drug solution.

15.5.1.4 Solid Lipid Nanoparticles (SLNs) and Nanostructured Lipid Carriers (NLCs)

Solid lipid nanoparticles (SLNs) originate as a new class of colloidal drug carriers at the beginning of the 1990s. SLNs show a wide drug delivery approach in the area of pharmaceutics, clinical medicine, and research. SLNs are colloidal carriers developed in the last decade as an alternative system to the existing traditional carriers (emulsion, liposomes, and polymeric nanoparticles). They are a new generation of submicron (52–100 nm)-sized lipid emulsions where the liquid lipid (oil) has been substituted by a solid lipid (Mukherjee et al. 2009).

The topical delivery of miconazole as SLNs was prepared by Bhalekar et al. (2009). Miconazole-loaded SLNs showed good stability for 1 month. The evaluation studies by using ex vivo cadaver skin and Franz diffusion cell were done and showed significantly enhanced delivery of miconazole to the targeted area by increasing accumulative uptake of miconazole in skin over marketed gel, used as a reference. Tape-stripping experiments concluded that there is a tenfold greater retention with miconazole-loaded SLNs bearing hydrogel as compared to miconazole suspension and miconazole hydrogel.

Fluconazole-loaded SLNs were prepared by ultrasonication techniques which show better effect on fluconazole-resistant strains of various candida species (Kelidari et al. 2017). The spherical-shaped fluconazole SLNs present mean diameter, potential, and entrapment efficiency of 84.8 nm, −25 mV, and 89.6%, respectively. After 30 min, release rate of drug showed initial burst release followed by 24 h sustained release. Fluconazole-resistant strains of *C. albicans*, *C. parapsilosis, and C. glabrata* showed MIC_{50} as 2, 1, and 2 g/ml, respectively.

Butani et al. (2016) improved the topical delivery of amphotericin B via SLNs by using a novel solvent diffusion method. Different SLN formulations were evaluated for particle size, potential, drug entrapment, in vitro antifungal activity, ex vivo permeation, and skin irritation. Different SLN formulations of amphotericin B were prepared, but the best was SLN5 characterized by drug/lipid ratio 1:10 and Pluronic F-127 0.25% as surfactant. These particles showed an average size of 111.1 ± 2.2 nm, zeta potential of −23.98 ± 1.36 mV, and 93.8% of drug entrapment.

Itraconazole-loaded SLNs for ocular delivery were developed by Mohanty et al. (2015). SLNs were prepared by using polyvinyl alcohol as an emulsifier with stearic and palmitic acids, obtained by the melt emulsion sonication and low-temperature solidification method and determine its drug loading, entrapment efficiency, and zeta potential. The mean particle size of SLNs prepared with stearic acid was between 139–199 nm while mean particle size of SLNs prepared with palmitic acid was in the range of 126–160 nm. Stearic acid SLNs have more entrapment efficacy than palmitic SLNs. Franz diffusion cell and excised goat corneas are used for the evaluation of corneal permeability. SA-SLNs show higher itraconazole permeation than palmitic SLNs. Antimicrobial efficacy of these formulations is shown by clear zone of inhibition against *Aspergillus flavus*.

To prolong the action of nystatin, Khalil et al. (2013) developed SLNs of nystatin. In the data from in vitro release study, it has been shown that the rate of drug could be influenced by the concentration of nystatin, type and concentration of surfactant, etc. Due to drug-enriched shell model, nystatin was released more quickly when used in lower concentration. According to drug-enriched shell model of drug incorporation, there is formation of solid lipid core when the recrystallization temperature of the lipid is reached. A year later, Samein (2014) formulated SLNs of nystatin as gel and studied effect of nystatin on skin. Nystatin SLNs had good physical stability after 1-month storage; the SLN dispersion at various temperature parameters showed little difference in particle size and entrapment efficiency. There was no change in clarity, and phase separation was observed. When nystatin SLN gel is compared with the marketed gel, there is sustained release of drug in the case of SLN gel. The primary skin irritation test on rabbit skin was conducted in accordance with guidelines of the Consumer Product Safety Commission, and the primary irritation index was calculated to be 0.00. Centrifugation at 3000 rpm for 30 min showed no precipitation, and the nystatin SLNs had good physical stability.

Kumar and Sinha (2016) fabricated and evaluated the solid lipid nanoparticles (SLNs) for improved ocular delivery of voriconazole. Compritol and palmitic acid were selected as lipid carriers based on drug solubility and partitioning behavior. Poloxamer and soy lecithin were the choice for surfactant, while sodium taurocholate was used as a cosurfactant. The in vitro release study of SLNs exhibited a sustained-release property of the drug. The ex vivo studies displayed enhanced corneal drug permeation from SLNs in comparison to the drug suspension. Further, the corneal hydration studies, histopathology, and Hen's Egg Test-Chorioallantoic Membrane assay confirmed the non-irritancy of the nanoformulation. The in vivo study confirmed the higher availability of voriconazole from SLNs in aqueous humor with minimal nasolacrimal drainage in contrast to the drug suspension.

Most of the azoles specifically fluconazole become resistant to *Candida* species. To overcome resistance, Moazeni et al. (2016) prepared solid lipid nanoparticles as a novel antifungal drug delivery system. The fluconazole SLNs presented a spherical shape with a mean diameter, zeta potential, and entrapment efficiency of 84.8 nm, −25 mV, and 89.6%, respectively. The drug release from fluconazole SLNs exhibited burst-release behavior at the initial stage (the first 30 min) followed by a sustained release over 24 h. Fluconazole-resistant yeast strains behaved as susceptible strains after treatment with fluconazole SLNs (≤8 μg/ml). The MIC_{50} drug concentrations were 2 μg/ml, 1 μg/ml, and 2 μg/ml for fluconazole-resistant strains of *C. albicans*, *C. parapsilosis, and C. glabrata*, respectively.

NLC-based hydrogel containing miconazole was prepared and characterized. NLC dispersion shows particles in nanometer range (~200 nm) with low polydispersity index (<0.3), good physical stability, and high encapsulation efficiency (>87%). Encapsulation improved antifungal activity of miconazole against *C. albicans* (Mendes et al. 2013).

Kelidari et al. (2017) made an attempt to improve the yeast delivery of fluconazole with nanostructured lipid carrier system. The fluconazole-loaded nanostructured lipid carriers presented a spherical shape with a mean diameter, zeta potential, and entrapment efficiency of 126.4 ± 15.2 nm, 35.1 ± 3.0 mV, and 93.6 ± 3.5%, respectively. The drug release from fluconazole-loaded nanostructured lipid carriers exhibited burst-release behavior at the initial stage followed by sustained release over 24 h. Using a new formulation of fluconazole led to a significant decrease in MICs for all *Candida* groups ($P < 0.05$). Furthermore, *C. albicans* isolates showed more susceptibility to fluconazole-loaded nanostructured lipid carriers than *C. glabrata* and *C. parapsilosis* ($P < 0.05$). The MIC50 drug concentration was obtained as 0.0625, 0.031, and 0.25 mg/ml for fluconazole-resistant strains of *C. albicans, C. glabrata, and C. parapsilosis*, respectively.

15.5.1.5 Lipid Nanoparticles

15.5.2 Non-phospholipid-Based Vesicular Nanocarriers

15.5.2.1 Niosomes

Niosomes are bilayered vesicular systems which are made up of single alkyl chain nonionic surfactants. Handjani Vila et al. gave the first description of niosomes in 1979. Structurally, hydrophilic tail endorsed inside the bilayer while they have a hydrophilic head of surfactant oriented toward the exterior and interior of bilayer. Therefore, niosomes are capable of encapsulating either hydrophilic or lipophilic drug. To enhance the rigidity of bilayer and reduction of premature drug leakage, cholesterol is also added in the production of niosomes (Sawant and Khan 2017). Alomrani et al. (2014) prepared niosomes loaded with itraconazole (ITZ) for transdermal delivery using different nonionic surfactants. A comparison was done using Span surfactants (Span 60, Span 80, and Span 85), Tween surfactants (Tween 60, Tween 80, and Tween 85), and Brij 35. Niosomes prepared from Tween 85 showed more skin permeation as compared to Span 85 niosomes and Brij 35 niosomes.

15.5.2.2 Spanlastics

Spanlastics are novel vesicular carriers which are also known as "Modified niosomes" as they contain edge activator in niosomal composition. They contain Spans, edge activators like Tweens, and many others. For ocular drug delivery, Kakkar and Kaur (2011) first developed spanlastics loaded with ketoconazole using Span 60 as surfactant and Tween 80 as an edge activator. Terbinafine hydrochloride-loaded spanlastics were developed for the treatment of nail fungal infection, namely, onychomycosis. In this study, Span 60 and Span 65 as surfactants while Tween 80 and sodium deoxycholate as edge activators were used. Spanlastics that have Span 65 as surfactant and sodium deoxycholate as edge activator showed maximum drug entrapment, smaller size, and good colloidal properties. Confocal laser scanning microscopy revealed efficient ex vivo nail permeation of optimized spanlastic formulation (Elsherif et al. 2017).

15.5.3 Polymeric Nano-drug Delivery Systems

15.5.3.1 Polymeric Micelles

Polymeric micelles are self-assembled nanoscopic core-shell structures formed by amphiphilic copolymer inside water above their critical micellar concentration which are able to hold hydrophobic drugs inside the core of micelles and hydrophilic molecules in the outer shell of polymeric micelles. The size of polymeric micelles is usually <100 nm (Biswas et al. 2016). Poly(ethylene glycol) (PEG) is the most commonly used polymer as a hydrophilic micelle corona due to its hydrophilicity and biocompatibility (Suk et al. 2016). Polymeric micelles were also able to achieve high drug concentration in tumor and inflammatory tissues by virtue of their small size, leaky tumor vasculature, and lack of lymphatic drainage through the enhanced permeability and retention effect (Maeda 2015). In the context of antifungal drug delivery, one of the earlier attempts to enhance antifungal drug efficacy was using poly(ethylene oxide)-block-poly(b-benzyl-L-aspartate) copolymers as delivery vehicles for AmB (Yu et al. 1998). In order to target AmB to the brain, it was incorporated into angiopep-2-modified PE-PEG-based micelles, and drug accumulation in the brain was evaluated (Shao et al. 2010). Angiopep-2 is a ligand of low-density lipoprotein receptor-related protein in the blood-brain barrier (BBB). It exhibits higher transcytosis capacity and parenchymal accumulation, and thus, it might facilitate drug targeting to the brain. AmB-incorporated angiopep-2-modified micelles had higher penetration across BBB compared with unmodified micelles and Fungizone1, in vitro and in vivo. When tested in an immunosuppressive murine model with *Cryptococcus neoformans* meningoencephalitis, the micelles had higher AmB level in the brain, significantly reduced the brain fungal burden, and prolonged the median survival time (Shao et al. 2012).

Tonglairoum et al. (2017) developed clotrimazole (CZ)-loaded N-naphthyl-N,O-succinyl chitosan (NSCS) micelles as an alternative for oral candidiasis treatment. The micelles ranged in size from 120 nm to 173 nm. The micelles prepared via the O/W emulsion method offered the highest percentage of entrapment efficiency and loading capacity. The CZ was released from the CZ-loaded micelles at a much faster rate compared to CZ powder. The CZ-loaded NSCS micelles can significantly hinder the growth of *Candida* cells after contact. These CZ-loaded NSCS micelles offer great antifungal activity and might be further developed to be a promising candidate for oral candidiasis treatment.

Ketoconazole is a broad-spectrum imidazole antifungal drug. For the treatment of superficial fungal infections with ketoconazole, it should permeate to deep skin layers. In order to develop a topical formulation of ketoconazole for improving its skin deposition and water solubility, ketoconazole-loaded methoxy poly(ethylene glycol)-b-poly(δ-valerolactone) micelles were developed through the thin-film hydration method. The drug-loaded micelles were obtained with an encapsulation efficiency of 86.39% and a particle diameter of about 12 nm. The micelles made ketoconazole aqueous solubility increase to 86-fold higher than crude one. Ketoconazole-loaded micelles showed no skin permeation of ketoconazole, obviously enhanced skin deposition, and demonstrated similar antifungal activity as compared with marketed ketoconazole cream. Fluorescein-loaded micelles displayed higher skin deposition than fluorescein water solution. These results demonstrate that the

MPEG-PVL micelle is a potential delivery system for ketoconazole in the field of skin delivery (Deng et al. 2017).

Introduction of linolenic acid (LNA) and methoxy poly(ethylene glycol) (MPEG) to the backbone of oligochitosan (CS) afforded LNA-modified MPEG-CS conjugate (MPEG-CS-LNA). Amphotericin B-loaded MPEG-CS-LNA micelles (AmB-M) were prepared via dialysis method with 82.27 ± 1.96% of drug encapsulation efficiency and 10.52 ± 0.22% of drug loading capacity. The AmB-M enhanced AmB's water solubility to 1.64 mg/mL, being 1640-fold higher than native AmB. The AmB-M obviously reduced hemolytic effect and renal toxicity of AmB when compared to marketed AmB injection (AmB-I). Its antifungal activity against *C. albicans* was equivalent to AmB-I although AmB's release from AmB-M was significantly retarded. According to fluorescence microscopy test, the unchanged activity should be attributed to enhanced fungal cellular uptake of AmB-M caused by combined inducement of LNA and CS. The pharmacokinetic studies demonstrated that AmB-M also improved the pharmacokinetic parameters of AmB with AmB-I as control. Conclusively, developed LNA-modified MPEG-CS micellar system could be a viable alternative to the current toxic commercial AmB-I as a highly efficacious drug delivery system (Song et al. 2019).

Kareem et al. (2019) made an attempt to enhance therapeutic efficacy of clotrimazole by delivery through poly(ethylene oxide)-block-poly(ε-caprolactone) copolymer-based micelles. Clotrimazole loaded in micelles was investigated for its antifungal activity through an in vitro assay and scanning electron microscopy. The antifungal activity of drug increased significantly by delivering through polymeric micelles.

15.5.3.2 Polymeric Nanoparticles

Polymeric nanoparticles are synthesized from synthetic polymers like polyacrylamide, polyacrylate, poly(L-lactide), and polyurethane. Among natural polymers, chitosan is the most widely used polymer. In addition to chitosan, many others such as gelatin and sodium alginate overcome some toxicological problems with the synthetic polymers. They are further classified into biodegradable and nonbiodegradable. Polymeric nanoparticles can be prepared from either preformed polymers or polymerization reactions from monomers. The methods of preparing polymeric nanoparticles include solvent evaporation, salting-out, dialysis, and supercritical fluid technology (Sawant and Khan 2017).

Sinha et al. (2013) prepared poly-lactide-co-glycolide nanoparticles (PLGA-NPs) containing voriconazole by multiple emulsification technique. Higher porosity was achieved in the presence of an effervescent mixture that resulted in improved pulmonary drug delivery. The average size of PLGA-NPs was found to be 207–605 nm with a 20% drug release in initial 2 h followed by a sustained release for 15 days. Porous nanoparticles with lower mass median aerodynamic diameter showed better pulmonary deposition and prolonged residence in the lungs (Sinha et al. 2013).

Localized acidity due to fungal metabolism and host immune response often leads to loss of amphotericin B activity in a pH-dependent manner. To overcome this limitation, Tang et al. (2015) designed pH-responsive and surface charge-switching PLGA-b-poly(L-histidine)-b-poly(ethylene glycol) (PLGA-PLH-PEG) nanoparticles incorporating AmB. To further enhance drug antifungal efficacy, AmB-encapsulated PLGA-PLH-PEG NPs were modified with anti-*C. albicans* antibody (CDA) (CDA-AmB-NPs). The results showed that the CDA-AmB-NPs switched their surface charge from negative to positive upon decreasing the pH from 7.35 to 6.8. CDA-AmB-NPs induced nearly complete apoptosis and necrosis in *C. albicans* cells at pH 6.8 due to targetability and higher drug release under acidic conditions. Same formulation induced 60% apoptosis and 30% necrosis at pH 7.34 confirming the efficiency of these nanocarriers as pH-sensitive systems. CDA-AmB-NPs had significantly lower hemolytic activity against red blood cells and lower in vitro toxicity against the immortalized human renal tubular epithelial cell line, as well as lower in vivo nephrotoxicity. Further, in vivo studies showed that CDA-AmB-NPs effectively eliminated fungi in the kidney, liver, and spleen compared with free AmB.

Modi et al. (2013) prepared chitosan mucoadhesive nanoparticles of ketoconazole to improve its bioavailability using ionic gelation method. The nanoparticles had 69.16 ± 5.91% mucin binding efficiency, particle size of 382.6 ± 2.38 nm, and entrapment efficiency of 59.84 ± 1.088%. The results of ex vivo diffusion study showed drug diffusion even after 5 h as compared to conventional solution proving that it can be a very efficient carrier for delivery of ketoconazole in its absorption window.

Current therapies are insufficient to prevent recurrent fungal infection especially in the lower part of the lung. A careful and systematic understanding of the properties of nanoparticles plays a significant role in the design, development, optimization, and in vivo performances of the nanoparticles. Thus, Das et al. (2015) prepared PLGA nanoparticles containing antifungal drug voriconazole. The nanoparticles and the free drug were radiolabeled with technetium-99m with 90% labeling efficiency, and the radiolabeled particles were administered to investigate the effect on their blood clearance, biodistribution, and in vivo gamma imaging. In vivo deposition of the drug in the lobes of the lung was studied by LC-MS/MS study. The particles were found to be spherical and had an average hydrodynamic diameter of 300 nm with a smooth surface. The radiolabeled particles and the free drug were found to accumulate in various major organs. Drug accumulation was more pronounced in the lung in case of administration of the nanoparticles than that of the free drug. The free drug was found to be excreted more rapidly than the nanoparticles containing drug following inhalation route as assessed by gamma scintigraphy study. Thus, the study reveals that pulmonary administration of nanoparticles containing voriconazole could be a better therapeutic choice even as compared to the IV route of administration of the free drug and/or the drug-loaded nanoparticles.

Paul et al. (2018) developed chitosan-coated polylactic-co-glycolic acid nanoparticles of voriconazole to increase residence time and provide sustained drug release locally to treat the recurrent lung-fungal infection. Gamma scintigraphic images showed that Tc-99m-labeled chitosan-coated polylactic-co-glycolic acid voriconazole nanoparticles had better pulmonary retention for a longer period than that of the noncoated formulation. Drastic improvement in the pharmacokinetic profile of chitosan-coated polylactic-co-glycolic acid voriconazole nanoparticles than noncoated formulation was observed.

15.5.4 Nanocrystals

Drug nanocrystals are nanoparticles possessing crystalline character in the nano-size range with a unique composition of 100% drug without the presence of any polymeric carrier. Dispersion of nanocrystals in liquid leads to formation of nanosuspension, which needs to be stabilized by addition of surfactant or polymeric stabilizer. Nanocrystals offer numerous advantages such as increased dissolution rate due to decrease in size leading to an increase in saturation solubility further aiding the dissolution rate of nanocrystals. They are prepared by precipitation, milling, and homogenization methods (Müller and Junghanns 2006).

Sarnes et al. (2014) prepared itraconazole nanocrystals by using rapid wet milling technique for dissolution enhancement and transformed them into solid dosage form by freeze-drying and granulating techniques. The three formulations, i.e., nanocrystal suspension, freeze-dried nanoparticles, and granulated nanoparticles, were subjected to in vitro and in vivo studies along with commercial itraconazole suspension. Their results indicated that the enhanced in vitro dissolution did not translate to superior in vivo drug absorption.

Pyo et al. (2017) prepared miconazole nitrate nanocrystals by using wet bead milling technique for enhanced antifungal efficacy and deep penetration of miconazole nitrate into skin. The nanocrystals were incorporated into a hydroxypropyl cellulose gel base. These nanocrystal formulations were closely or similarly effective as the microsuspensions and the market products containing the synergistic chlorhexidine digluconate, showing the potential of the nanosuspension formulation. Nanosuspension performance was even further increased when chlorhexidine digluconate was added. Ex vivo skin penetration studies on porcine ears revealed distinctly less remaining miconazole nitrate on the skin surface for nanocrystals (e.g., 76–86%) compared to market products (e.g., 94%). Also, penetration was increased, e.g., in skin depth of 5–10 μm, from <1.0/1.7% to, e.g., 3.3–6.2% for nanocrystals.

15.5.5 Colloidal Carriers

15.5.5.1 Microemulsions and Nanoemulsions

Microemulsions are clear, transparent, thermodynamically stable dispersions of two immiscible liquids stabilized by addition of suitable surfactant and cosurfactant with droplet size usually in the range of 10–100 nm. They offer advantages of ease of preparation with no energy required, are thermodynamically stable, and are suitable for both hydrophilic and lipophilic drugs (Singh et al. 2014). However, nanoemulsions are isotropic mixture of oil and water along with suitable stabilizing surfactant, cosurfactant, and cosolvents and with droplet diameters ranging from 10 to 500 nm (Mundada et al. 2016). Nanoemulsion has good kinetic stability and requires external forces for its preparation. Formulation scientists explored that both MEs and NEs have potential as an attractive option for enhancing cutaneous drug delivery of both hydrophilic and lipophilic drugs compared with conventional vehicles. The ease of simplicity and lower cost make it an attractive approach. Several reports investigated to confirm its potential suitability as dermal and transdermal administration of a wide variety of drug molecules. They increased the dermal drug permeation rate and retention in the skin (Gupta et al. 2017; Heuschkel et al. 2008). Microemulsions and nanoemulsions could also allow targeted topical antifungal drug delivery to maximize local drug effects and avoid systemic toxicity, such as nephrotoxicity (Hussain et al. 2016).

Ofokansi et al. (2013) prepared poloxamer-stabilized miconazole nitrate-loaded topical microemulsion to improve its water solubility and bioavailability. The results indicated that lower content of surfactant and cosurfactant formed water in oil (w/o) while higher quantities formed oil in water (o/w) microemulsions. Poloxamer 407 reduced the interfacial tension between oil and water and solubilized the drug. An increase in in vivo inhibition of *C. albicans* was observed in case of poloxamer-stabilized microemulsion which was 22.87 ± 0.91 mm as compared to commercial miconazole powder (Fungusol ®) 10.91 ± 0.38 mm and non-stabilized microemulsions. It may be due to the increased permeation of miconazole through the fungal cell wall. This study proved that microemulsion is an effective strategy to increase the bioavailability of the poorly absorbed drug.

Fluconazole microemulsion with globule size of 24 nm was prepared for vaginal drug delivery. The drug loaded microemulsion was incorporated into carbopol gel. This microemulsion-based gel showed a faster onset of action and significantly higher in vitro bioadhesion with a retention time of 45 ± 3.0 min and antifungal activity 5.5 ± 0.1 mm than Candid V® gel which had a retention time of 24 ± 1.5 min and antifungal activity 3.0 ± 0.15 mm (Bachhav and Patravale 2009).

Tonglairoum et al. (2015) fabricated a novel scaffold of clotrimazole microemulsion containing nanofibers using an electrospinning process for oral candidiasis applications. The extent of drug release from the fiber mats at 4 h was approximately 64.81–74.15%. The release kinetics appeared to follow Higuchi's model. In comparison with clotrimazole lozenges (10 mg), the nanofiber mats exhibited more rapid killing activity. Moreover, the nanofiber mats demonstrated desirable mucoadhesive properties and were safe for 2 h. Therefore, the nanofiber mats have the potential to be promising candidates for oral candidiasis applications

Nystatin nanoemulsion was prepared and tested as a potential treatment for oral and skin candidosis (Campos et al. 2012; Fernández-Campos et al. 2013). Nystatin nanoemulsion had a minimum inhibitory concentration against *C. albicans* and *Saccharomyces cerevisiae* that was twofold lower than that of the free drug confirming the enhanced drug antifungal efficacy. Systemic administration of nystatin results in serious toxicity. Ex vivo permeability studies through oral porcine mucosa were therefore conducted to confirm the safety of nystatin nanoemulsion. Negligible drug permeation through the mucosa was observed confirming the safety of this delivery system. Drug retention studies in oral porcine mucosa showed that about 50% of the applied drug dose was retained in the tissue after 6 h. This was about 310 times higher than the drug minimal inhibitory concentration value against *C. albicans* confirming the efficacy of this treatment (Campos et al. 2012).

Nanoemulsion of amphotericin B was prepared by Sosa et al. (2017) for the treatment of skin candidiasis and aspergillosis. From the antifungal efficacy and skin tolerability studies, it showed that AmB nanoemulsion showed a MIC of 0.13 μg/mL which was also below the other reported values. No theoretical systemic absorption was expected to occur because no AmB was detected in the receptor chamber from the ex vivo permeation study. Nevertheless, the amount of AmB retained after 36 h application was 17.76 μg/g/cm^2.

Similarly, clotrimazole nanoemulsion was formulated and tested for the topical treatment of candidiasis. Nanoemulsion provided a sustained release of clotrimazole according to the first-order model. Similar skin permeation properties were observed between clotrimazole NE and commercial reference. However, significant higher clotrimazole amounts retained in mucosae when compared with references. Antifungal efficacies against *Candida albicans* were also higher than commercial references, and the in vivo tolerance study confirmed the suitability for topical application, making clotrimazole NE a great tool for clinical investigation of topical candidiasis treatments (Soriano-Ruiz et al. 2019).

Some essential oils also exhibit antifungal activity against candida species. Thus attempts had been made to incorporate herbal oils into nanoemulsion formulation. Quatrin et al. (2017) prepared nanoemulsion of *Eucalyptus globulus* oil and verify its antifungal activity against *Candida* spp. The antimicrobial activity of the nanoemulsion was determined from the macrodilution tests and the cell viability curve, where the minimum fungicidal concentration of 0.7 mg/mL for *C. albicans* and 1.4 mg/mL for *C. tropicalis* and *C. glabrata* were obtained.

Ramteke et al. (2019) evaluated antifungal activity of blended cinnamon oil and usnic acid nanoemulsion using candidiasis model. The maximum zone of inhibition was 1.19 cm for nanoemulsion (10 mg/mL), which was near to the fluconazole (1 mg/mL), i.e., 1.82 cm. The MIC of nanoemulsion for *C. albicans* was 60 μg/mL, which was more than cinnamon oil and usnic acid solution. In vivo study of nanoemulsion in cutaneous candidiasis model showed significant antifungal activity. The log colony-forming unit per infected site of nanoemulsion was 1.36 in comparison to the untreated control group (3.91)

15.6 Formulations for Candidiasis Therapy: FDA Approved and in Recent Clinical Trials

Unique properties of nanoformulations make them available to deliver antifungal drugs to the desired site of action, thus enhancing the therapeutic efficacy and reducing the risk of side effects. However, despite considerable amounts of described nanotechnology-based formulations, only a limited number of them were introduced into clinical trials. Recently, the interest of the researchers has focused on the employment of already used, FDA-approved nanodrugs as the adjuvants in combinatory therapy. Table 15.4 shows the list of new formulations for candidiasis therapy which are approved by FDA or under clinical trials.

Table 15.4 Antifungal drug-based drug delivery systems in clinical trials/FDA approved for candidiasis

Delivery system	Trade name	Active molecule	Indication	Phase of development	Administration route	Sponsor
Probiotic vaginal gel	–	Lactobacillus	Vulvovaginal candidiasis	–	Vaginal	University Hospital, Antwerp
Vaginal ovule	Gynomax® XL	Gynomax	Trichomonal vaginitis, bacterial vaginosis, candidal vulvovaginitis, and mixed vaginal infections	Phase IV	Vaginal	Exeltis, Turkey
Capsule	VT-1161	–	Recurrent vulvovaginal candidiasis	Phase III	Oral	Mycovia Pharmaceuticals Inc.
Nanoparticle in denture base material	–	Titanium dioxide	Denture stomatitis	–	–	Cairo University
Dietary supplement (Oil)	–	Medium-chain triglyceride (MCT) oil	Colonization of preterm infants with *Candida*	Phase I	Oral	Joseph Bliss
Solution	APX001	Fosmanogepix	Candidemia including suspected or confirmed antifungal-resistant candidemia in non-neutropenic patients	Phase II	Oral	Amplyx Pharmaceuticals
Rinse solution	CelAgace™ OraRinse	Silver citrate complex and acemannan	Oral candidiasis	Phases I–II	Oral	CelaCare Technologies, Inc.
Lipid crystal nanoparticle	MAT2203	Amphotericin B	Mucocutaneous candidiasis	Phase II	Oral	Matinas BioPharma Nanotechnologies, Inc.
–	SCY-078	Ibrexafungerp	Invasive candidemia caused by *Candida auris*	Phase III	Oral	Scynexis, Inc.
–	MK 0991	Caspofungin acetate	Esophageal candidiasis	Phase III	IV	Merck Sharp and Dohme corp
–	FK 463	Micafungin	Candidemia	Phase III	IV	Astellas Pharma Inc
Liposomes	AmBisome	Amphotericin B	Invasive Candidiasis	FDA approved	IV infusion	Gilead Sciences
Liposomal lipid complex	Abelcet	Amphotericin B	Invasive Candidiasis	FDA approved	IV infusion	Sigma-Tau
Cream	–	Cumin seed extract	*Candidal vulvovaginitis*	Phases II–III	Vaginal	Assiut University, Egypt

Data recovered from US National Institute of Health website (http://clinicaltrials.gov/) in June 2019

15.7 Challenges of Nano-Based Drug Delivery Systems for Antifungal Agents

The literature reported the success story of nanotechnology in drug delivery systems. In addition, the potential of different nanoformulations to act as efficient delivery systems for antifungal drugs is evident. However, despite several decades of research, patents into this field, and hundreds of published papers, amphotericin is the only antifungal drug that is commercially available in nano-based formulations. This lagging might be due to several reasons; most prominent is industry-related, and others are inherent problems related to nanoformulations and problems related to preclinical studies and clinical trials. Another challenge of research and development (R&D) of nanoformulations for drug delivery is large-scale production. There is always a need to scale up laboratory or pilot technologies for eventual commercialization. A number of nano-drug delivery technologies may not be scalable due to the method and process of production and the high cost of materials employed. This is partially due to the fact that most of the research studies in nano-drug delivery are carried out by researchers in academia with a lack of real support from pharmaceutical industries (Rana and Sharma 2019; Zazo et al. 2016). Therefore, for these technologies to get to the market, there has to be increased partnership with the pharmaceutical companies. Unfortunately, a number of the major pharmaceutical industries are yet to consider nanotechnology as one of their priorities due to lack of regulatory guidelines, lack of standardized methods for nanoformulation synthesis, and challenges of scaling up. Furthermore, a limited number of newly developed nano-based formulations fulfill the important prerequisites of biocompatibility and/or biodegradability. Many promising nanoformulations have some degrees of cytotoxicity and/or immunogenicity, and the effects of their chronic use on the human body are not certain (Lewinski et al. 2008; Sainz et al. 2015). So, these are factors which delay the translation of nano-based drug delivery systems from the lab to the market.

15.8 Conclusion and Future Outlooks

Fungal diseases are becoming a global public health problem especially fungal infections that are resistant to commonly used antifungal drugs and cause significant morbidity and mortality. Although fungal infections can affect anyone, however, they pose a severe risk to people with weakened immune systems (cancer or HIV/AIDS patients). In recent time, some types of *Candida* species are becoming resistant to first-line and second-line antifungal medications, namely, fluconazole and echinocandins (anidulafungin, caspofungin, and micafungin). While there are several antifungal drugs available in market for therapeutic management, their clinical benefits are limited due to high toxicity and their unfavorable physicochemical and biopharmaceutical properties. There is a need to develop newer drug delivery systems over conventional ones to overcome these limitations and improve the clinical efficacy of antifungal drugs. Nano-drug delivery systems like nanoparticles, liposomes, SLNs, NLCs, and microemulsions and nanoemulsions offer advantages like enhanced aqueous solubility, enhanced stability, targeting to infected areas, and reduction in dose, dosing frequency, and side effects. The translation of nano-based drug delivery systems to clinic is an uphill task due to difficulties in their scale-up and commercialization. However, liposomal amphotericin B (AmBisome) is the only antifungal nanoformulation that made it to clinical trials and has been successfully commercialized, whose technology can be used as a platform for translation of other novel antifungals delivery systems to the clinical setting. Additionally, the newer antifungal agents like echinocandins can be designed into novel drug delivery systems for enhancing their clinical effectiveness in the treatment of invasive candidiasis and counteracting the emerging antifungal drug resistance especially for treating infections of *Candida*. Therefore, research in the field of antifungal drug delivery should focus on overcoming the challenges that hinder clinical translation of nano-based drug delivery systems.

References

Achkar JM, Fries BC (2010) Candida infections of the genitourinary tract. Clin Microbiol Rev 23(2):253–273. https://doi.org/10.1128/CMR.00076-09

Agarwal R, Katare O (2002) Miconazole nitrate–loaded topical liposomes. Pharm Tech 26:48–60

Aguin T, Sobel J (2015) Vulvovaginal candidiasis in pregnancy. Curr Infect Dis Rep 17(6):30. https://doi.org/10.1007/s11908-015-0462-

Akhtar N, Pathak K (2012) Cavamax w7 composite ethosomal gel of clotrimazole for improved topical delivery: development and comparison with ethosomal gel. AAPS PharmSciTech 13(1):344–355. https://doi.org/10.1208/s12249-012-9754-y

Akpan A, Morgan R (2002) Oral candidiasis. Postgrad Med J 78(922):455–459. https://doi.org/10.1136/pmj.78.922.455

Alomrani AH, Shazly GA, Amara AA, Badran MM (2014) Itraconazole-hydroxypropyl-β-cyclodextrin loaded deformable liposomes: *in vitro* skin penetration studies and antifungal efficacy using Candida albicans as model. Colloids Surf B Biointerfaces *121*:74–81. https://doi.org/10.1016/j.colsurfb.2014.05.30

Andes D (2003) *In vivo* pharmacodynamics of antifungal drugs in treatment of candidiasis. Antimicrob Agents Chemother 47(4):1179–1186. https://doi.org/10.1128/AAC.47.4.1179-1186.2003

Arikan S, Rex JH (2001) Lipid-based antifungal agents current status. Curr Pharm Des 7(5):393–415. https://doi.org/10.2174/1381612013398031

Ashley ESD, Lewis R, Lewis JS, Martin C, Andes D (2006) Pharmacology of systemic antifungal agents. Clin Infect Dis *43*(Supplement_1):S28–S39. https://doi.org/10.1086/504492

Athar MA, Winner H (1971) The development of resistance by Candida species to polyene antibiotics *in vitro*. J Med Microbiol 4(4):505–517. https://doi.org/10.1099/00222615-4-4-505

Ameen M (2010) Epidemiology of superficial fungal infections. Clin Dermatol 28(2):197–201. https://doi.org/10.1016/j.clindermatol.2009.12.005

Bachhav YG, Patravale VB (2009) Microemulsion based vaginal gel of fluconazole: formulation, *in vitro* and *in vivo* evaluation. Int J Pharm *365*(1-2):175–179. https://doi.org/10.1016/j.ijpharm.2008.08.021

Berman J, Sudbery PE (2002) Candida albicans: a molecular revolution built on lessons from budding yeast. Nat Rev Genet 3(12):918. https://doi.org/10.1038/nrg948

Bhalaria M, Naik S, Misra A (2009) Ethosomes: a novel delivery system for antifungal drugs in the treatment of topical fungal diseases. Indian J Exp Biol 47:368–375

Bhalekar MR, Pokharkar V, Madgulkar A, Patil N, Patil N (2009) Preparation and evaluation of miconazole nitrate-loaded solid lipid nanoparticles for topical delivery. AAPS PharmSciTech 10(1):289–296. https://doi.org/10.1208/s12249-009-9199-0

Biswas S, Kumari P, Lakhani PM, Ghosh B (2016) Recent advances in polymeric micelles for anti-cancer drug delivery. Eur J Pharm Sci *83*:184–202. https://doi.org/10.1016/j,ejps.2015.12.031

Blumberg HM, Jarvis WR, Soucie JM, Edwards JE, Patterson JE, Pfaller MA et al (2001) Risk factors for candidal bloodstream infections in surgical intensive care unit patients: the NEMIS prospective multicenter study. Clin Infect Dis 33(2):177–186. https://doi.org/10.1086/321811

Bruch JM, Treister NS (2010) Clinical oral medicine and pathology. Springer, Cham. https://doi.org/10.1007/978-3-319-29767-5

Brüggemann RJ, Alffenaar J-WC, Blijlevens NM, Billaud EM, Kosterink JG, Verweij PE et al (2009) Clinical relevance of the pharmacokinetic interactions of azole antifungal drugs with other coadministered agents. Clin Infect Dis 48(10):1441–1458. https://doi.org/10.1086/598327

Butani D, Yewale C, Misra A (2016) Topical Amphotericin B solid lipid nanoparticles: design and development. Colloids Surf B: Biointerfaces 139:17–24. https://doi.org/10.1016/j.colsurfb.2015.07.032

Campos FF, Campmany ACC, Delgado GR, Serrano OL, Naveros BC (2012) Development and characterization of a novel nystatin-loaded nanoemulsion for the buccal treatment of candidosis: ultrastructural effects and release studies. J Pharm Sci 101(10):3739–3752. https://doi.org/10.1002/jps.23249

Caterina P, Antonello DP, Chiara C, Giacomo L, Antonio S, Luca G (2013) Pharmacokinetic drug-drug interaction and their implication in clinical management. J Res Med Sci 18(7):600–609

Chang EH, Harford JB, Eaton MA, Boisseau PM, Dube A, Hayeshi R et al (2015) Nanomedicine: past, present and future–a global perspective. Biochem Biophys Res Commun 468(3):511–517. https://doi.org/10.1016/j.bbrc.2015.10.136

Chau AS, Mendrick CA, Sabatelli FJ, Loebenberg D, McNicholas PM (2004) Application of real-time quantitative PCR to molecular analysis of Candida albicans strains exhibiting reduced susceptibility to azoles. Antimicrob Agents Chemother 48(6):2124–2131. https://doi.org/10.1128/AAC.48.6.2124-2131.2004

Churchill D, Seely J (1977) Nephrotoxicity associated with combined gentamicin–amphotericin B therapy. Nephron 19(3):176–181. https://doi.org/10.1159/000180883

Clark-Ordóñez I, Callejas-Negrete OA, Aréchiga-Carvajal ET, Mouriño-Pérez RR (2017) Candida species diversity and antifungal susceptibility patterns in oral samples of HIV/AIDS patients in Baja California, Mexico. Med Mycol 55(3):285–294. https://doi.org/10.1093/mmy/myw069

Das PJ, Paul P, Mukherjee B, Mazumder B, Mondal L, Baishya R, Debnath MC, Dey KS (2015) Pulmonary delivery of voriconazole loaded nanoparticles providing a prolonged drug level in lungs: a promise for treating fungal infection. Mol Pharm 12(8):2651–2664. https://doi.org/10.1021/acs.molpharmaceut.5b00064

Deng P, Teng F, Zhou F, Song Z, Meng N, Feng R (2017) Methoxy poly (ethylene glycol)-b-poly (δ-valerolactone) copolymeric micelles for improved skin delivery of ketoconazole. J Biomater Sci Polym Ed 28(1):63–78. https://doi.org/10.1080/09205063.2016.1244371

Denning DW (2002) Echinocandins: a new class of antifungal. J Antimicrob Chemother 49(6):889–891. https://doi.org/10.1093/jac/dkf045

Donlan RM (2002) Biofilms: microbial life on surfaces. Emerg Infect Dis 8(9):881. https://doi.org/10.3201/eid0809.020063

Donlan RM, Costerton JW (2002) Biofilms: survival mechanisms of clinically relevant microorganisms. Clin Microbiol Rev 15(2):167–193. https://doi.org/10.1128/CMR.15.2.167-193.2002

Douglas LJ (2003) Candida biofilms and their role in infection. Trends Microbiol 11(1):30–36. https://doi.org/10.1016/S0966-842X(02)00002-1

Dovnik A, Golle A, Novak D, Arko D, Takač I (2015) Treatment of vulvovaginal candidiasis: a review of the literature. *Acta Dermatovenerol Alp Pannonica Adriat 24*(1):5–7. https://doi.org/10.15570/actaapa.2015.2

Elmoslemany RM, Abdallah OY, El-Khordagui LK, Khalafallah NM (2012) Propylene glycol liposomes as a topical delivery system for miconazole nitrate: comparison with conventional liposomes. AAPS PharmSciTech 13(2):723–731. https://doi.org/10.1208/s12249-012-9783-6

Eloy JO, de Souza MC, Petrilli R, Barcellos JPA, Lee RJ, Marchetti JM (2014) Liposomes as carriers of hydrophilic small molecule drugs: strategies to enhance encapsulation and delivery. Colloids Surf B: Biointerfaces 123:345–363. https://doi.org/10.1016/j.colsurfb.2014.09.029

Elsherif NI, Shamma RN, Abdelbary G (2017) Terbinafine hydrochloride trans-ungual delivery via nanovesicular systems: *in vitro* characterization and *ex vivo* evaluation. AAPS PharmSciTech 18(2):551–562. https://doi.org/10.1208/s12249-016-0528-9

Faisal W, Soliman GM, Hamdan AM (2018) Enhanced skin deposition and delivery of voriconazole using ethosomal preparations. J Liposome Res 28(1):14–21. https://doi.org/10.1080/08982104.2016.1239636

Fanning S, Mitchell AP (2012) Fungal biofilms. PLoS Pathog 8(4):e1002585. https://doi.org/10.1371/journal.ppat.1002585

Faro S (1996) New treatments for vulvovaginal candidiasis. Infect Dis Obstet Gynecol 4(4):247–254. https://doi.org/10.1371/journal'ppat.1002585

Fernández-Campos F, Clares Naveros B, López Serrano O, Alonso Merino C, Calpena Campmany A (2013) Evaluation of novel nystatin nanoemulsion for skin candidosis infections. Mycoses 56(1):70–81. https://doi.org/10.1111/j.1439-0507.2012.02202.X

Finkel JS, Mitchell AP (2011) Genetic control of Candida albicans biofilm development. Nat Rev Microbiol 9(2):109. https://doi.org/10.1038/nrmicro2475

Fryberg M, Oehlschlager A, Unrau A (1974) Sterol biosynthesis in antibiotic-resistant yeast: nystatin. Arch Biochem Biophys 160(1):83–89. https://doi.org/10.1016/S0003-9861(74)80011-1

Ghannoum MA, Rice LB (1999) Antifungal agents: mode of action, mechanisms of resistance, and correlation of these mechanisms with bacterial resistance. Clin Microbiol Rev 12(4):501–517. https://doi.org/10.1128/CMR.12.4.501

Gupta AK, Cooper EA (2008) Update in antifungal therapy of dermatophytosis. Mycopathologia 166(5–6):353–367. https://doi.org/10.1007/s11046-008-9109-0

Gupta M, Goyal AK, Paliwal SR, Paliwal R, Mishra N, Vaidya B et al (2010) Development and characterization of effective topical liposomal system for localized treatment of cutaneous candidiasis. J Liposome Res 20(4):341–350. https://doi.org/10.3109/08982101003596125

Gupta M, Sharma V, Chauhan NS (2017) Promising novel nanopharmaceuticals for improving topical antifungal drug delivery. In: Nano-and microscale drug delivery systems. Elsevier, Amsterdam, pp 197–228. https://doi.org/10.1016/B978-0-323-52727-9.00011-X

Hamilton-Miller J (1973) Chemistry and biology of the polyene macrolide antibiotics. Bacteriol Rev 37(2):166

Hani U, Shivakumar HG, Vaghela R, Osmani AM, Shrivastava A (2015) Candidiasis: a fungal infection-current challenges and progress in prevention and treatment. Infect Disord Drug Targets (Formerly Current Drug Targets-Infectious Disorders) 15(1):42–52

Harriott M, Lilly E, Rodriguez T, Fidel P Jr, Noverr M (2010) Candida albicans forms biofilms on the vaginal mucosa. Microbiology 156(Pt 12):3635. https://doi.org/10.1099/mic.0.039354-0

Hay RJ (1993) Risk/benefit ratio of modern antifungal therapy: focus on hepatic reactions. J Am Acad Dermatol 29(1):S50–S54. https://doi.org/10.1016/S0190-9622(08)81838-5

Henry KW, Nickels JT, Edlind TD (2000) Upregulation of ERG genes in Candida species by azoles and other sterol biosynthesis inhibitors. Antimicrob Agents Chemother 44(10):2693–2700. https://doi.org/10.1128/AAC.44.10.2693-2700.2000

Heuschkel S, Goebel A, Neubert RH (2008) Microemulsions—modern colloidal carrier for dermal and transdermal drug delivery. J Pharm Sci 97(2):603–631. https://doi.org/10.1002/jps.20995

Hoepelman I, Dupont B (1996) Oral candidiasis: the clinical challenge of resistance and management. Int J Antimicrob Agents 6(3):155–159. https://doi.org/10.1016/0924-8579(95)00050-X

Horn DL, Fishman JA, Steinbach WJ, Anaissie EJ, Marr KA, Olyaei AJ et al (2007) Presentation of the PATH Alliance® registry for prospective data collection and analysis of the epidemiology, therapy, and outcomes of invasive fungal infections. Diagn Microbiol Infect Dis 59(4):407–414. https://doi.org/10.1016/j.diagmicrobio.2007.06.008

Hudson MM (2001) Antifungal resistance and over-the-counter availability in the UK: a current perspective. J Antimicrob Chemother 48(3):345–350. https://doi.org/10.1093/jac/48.3.345
Hussain A, Samad A, Singh S, Ahsan M, Haque M, Faruk A, Ahmed F (2016) Nanoemulsion gel-based topical delivery of an antifungal drug: *in vitro* activity and *in vivo* evaluation. Drug Deliv 23(2):642–657. https://doi.org/10.3109/10717544.2014.933284
Kakkar S, Kaur IP (2011) Spanlastics—A novel nanovesicular carrier system for ocular delivery. Int J Pharm 413(1–2):202–210. https://doi.org/10.1016/j.ijpharm.2011.04.027
Kareem F, Bhayo AM, Imran M, Shah MR, Khan KM, Malik MI (2019) Enhanced therapeutic efficacy of clotrimazole by delivery through poly (ethylene oxide)-block-poly (ε-caprolactone) copolymer-based micelles. J Appl Polym Sci:47769. https://doi.org/10.1002/app.47769
Kelidari HR, Moazeni M, Babaei R, Saeedi M, Akbari J, Parkoohi PI et al (2017) Improved yeast delivery of fluconazole with a nanostructured lipid carrier system. Biomed Pharmacother 89:83–88. https://doi.org/10.1016/j.biopha.2017.02.008
Khalil R, Kassem M, Elbary AA, El Ridi M, AbouSamra M (2013) Preparation and characterization of nystatin-loaded solid lipid nanoparticles for topical delivery. Int J Pharm Sci Res *4*(6):2292–2300. https://doi.org/10.13040/IJPSR.0975-8232.4(6).2292-00
Kullberg BJ, Arendrup MC (2015) Invasive candidiasis. N Engl J Med 373(15):1445–1456. https://doi.org/10.1056/NEJMra1315399
Kumamoto CA, Vinces MD (2005) Contributions of hyphae and hypha-co-regulated genes to Candida albicans virulence. Cell Microbiol 7(11):1546–1554. https://doi.org/10.1111/j.1462-5822.2005.00616.x
Kumar R, Sinha VR (2016) Solid lipid nanoparticle: an efficient carrier for improved ocular permeation of voriconazole. Drug Dev Ind Pharm 42(12):1956–1967. https://doi.org/10.1080/03639045.2016.1185437
Kashem SW, Kaplan DH (2016) Skin Immunity to Candida albicans. Trends Immunol 37(7):440–450. https://doi.org/10.1016/j.it.2016.04.007
Lewinski N, Colvin V, Drezek R (2008) Cytotoxicity of nanoparticles. Small 4(1):26–49. https://doi.org/10.1002/smll.200700595
Lewis RE (2011) Current concepts in antifungal pharmacology. Paper presented at the Mayo Clinic Proceedings. https://doi.org/10.4065/mcp.2011.0247
Lupetti A, Danesi R, Campa M, Del Tacca M, Kelly S (2002) Molecular basis of resistance to azole antifungals. Trends Mol Med 8(2):76–81. https://doi.org/10.1016/S1471-4914(02)02280-3
Maeda H (2015) Toward a full understanding of the EPR effect in primary and metastatic tumors as well as issues related to its heterogeneity. Adv Drug Deliv Rev 91:3–6. https://doi.org/10.1016/j.addr.2015.01.002
Magliani W, Conti S, Salati A, Arseni S, Frazzi R, Ravanetti L, Polonelli L (2002) New strategies for treatment of Candida vaginal infections. Revista iberoamericana de micologia 19(3):144–148
Maiolo EM, Tafin UF, Borens O, Trampuz A (2014) Activities of fluconazole, caspofungin, anidulafungin, and amphotericin B on planktonic and biofilm Candida species determined by microcalorimetry. Antimicrob Agents Chemother 58(5):2709–2717. https://doi.org/10.1128/AAC.00057-14
Martinez-Rossi NM, Peres NT, Rossi A (2008) Antifungal resistance mechanisms in dermatophytes. Mycopathologia 166(5–6):369. https://doi.org/10.1007/s11046-008-9110-7
Martinez-Rossi NM, Bitencourt TA, Peres NTDA, Lang EA, Gomes EV, Quaresemin NR et al (2018) Dermatophyte resistance to antifungal drugs: mechanisms and prospectus. Front Microbiol 9:1108. https://doi.org/10.3389/fmicb.2018.01108
Martins M, Rex J (1996) Resistance to antifungal agents in the critical care setting: problems and perspectives. New horizons (Baltimore, Md.) *4*(3):338–344
Mateus C, Crow SA, Ahearn DG (2004) Adherence of Candida albicans to silicone induces immediate enhanced tolerance to fluconazole. Antimicrob Agents Chemother 48(9):3358–3366. https://doi.org/10.1128/AAC.48.9.3358-3366.2004
Mayer FL, Wilson D, Hube B (2013) Candida albicans pathogenicity mechanisms. Virulence 4(2):119–128. https://doi.org/10.4161/viru.22913
Mbah CC, Builders PF, Attama AA (2014) Nanovesicular carriers as alternative drug delivery systems: ethosomes in focus. Expert Opin Drug Deliv 11(1):45–59. https://doi.org/10.1517/17425247.2013.860130
Mendes A, Silva A, Catita J, Cerqueira F, Gabriel C, Lopes C (2013) Miconazole-loaded nanostructured lipid carriers (NLC) for local delivery to the oral mucosa: improving antifungal activity. Colloids Surf B: Biointerfaces 111:755–763. https://doi.org/10.1016/j.colsurfb.2013.05.041
Minnebruggen GV, François I, Cammue B, Thevissen K, Vroome V, Borgers M, Shroot B (2010) A general overview on past, present and future antimycotics. Open Mycol J 4(1):22. https://doi.org/10.2174/1874437001004010022
Moazeni M, Kelidari HR, Saeedi M, Morteza-Semnani K, Nabili M, Gohar AA et al (2016) Time to overcome fluconazole resistant Candida isolates: solid lipid nanoparticles as a novel antifungal drug delivery system. Colloids Surf B: Biointerfaces 142:400–407. https://doi.org/10.1016/j.colsurfb.2016.03.013
Mobeen N (2014) Oral candidiasis-A short review. Int J Curr Res Rev 6(9):89
Modi J, Joshi G, Sawant K (2013) Chitosan based mucoadhesive nanoparticles of ketoconazole for bioavailability enhancement: formulation, optimization, *in vitro* and *ex vivo* evaluation. Drug Dev Ind Pharm 39(4):540–547. https://doi.org/10.3109/03639045.2012.666978
Mohanty B, Majumdar DK, Mishra SK, Panda AK, Patnaik S (2015) Development and characterization of itraconazole-loaded solid lipid nanoparticles for

ocular delivery. Pharm Dev Technol 20(4):458–464. https://doi.org/10.3109/10837450.2014.882935

Mukherjee S, Ray S, Thakur R (2009) Solid lipid nanoparticles: a modern formulation approach in drug delivery system. Indian J Pharm Sci 71(4):349. https://doi.org/10.4103/0250-474X.57282

Müller RH, Junghanns J (2006) Drug nanocrystals/nanosuspensions for the delivery of poorly soluble drugs. Nanopart Drug Carriers 1:307–328

Mundada V, Patel M, Sawant K (2016) Submicron emulsions and their applications in oral delivery. Crit Rev Ther Drug Carrier Syst 33(3). https://doi.org/10.1615/CritRevTherDrugCarrierSyst.2016017218

Nett JE, Andes DR (2016) Antifungal agents: spectrum of activity, pharmacology, and clinical indications. Infect Dis Clin 30(1):51–83. https://doi.org/10.1016/j.idc.2015.10.012

Nicholls S, MacCallum DM, Kaffarnik FA, Selway L, Peck SC, Brown AJ (2011) Activation of the heat shock transcription factor Hsf1 is essential for the full virulence of the fungal pathogen Candida albicans. Fungal Genet Biol 48(3):297–305. https://doi.org/10.1016/j.fgb.2010.08.010

Nigam PK (2015) Antifungal drugs and resistance: current concepts. Our Dermatol Online 6(2):212. https://doi.org/10.7241/ourd.20152.58

Niimi M, Firth NA, Cannon RD (2010) Antifungal drug resistance of oral fungi. Odontology 98(1):15–25. https://doi.org/10.1007/s10266-009-0118-3

Ofokansi KC, Kenechukwu FC, Isah A (2013) Poloxamer-stabilized topical miconazole nitrate-loaded microemulsion: formulation design and characterization. J Dispers Sci Technol 34(11):1563–1574. https://doi.org/10.1080/01932691.2012.752713

Odds FC (1994) Pathogenesis of Candida infections. J Am Acad Dermatol 31(3):S2–S5. https://doi.org/10.1016/S0190-9622(08)81257-1

Pappas PG (2006) Invasive candidiasis. Infect Dis Clin 20(3):485–506. https://doi.org/10.1016/j.idc.2006.07.004

Paul P, Sengupta S, Mukherjee B, Shaw TK, Gaonkar RH, Debnath MC (2018) Chitosan-coated nanoparticles enhanced lung pharmacokinetic profile of voriconazole upon pulmonary delivery in mice. Nanomedicine 13(5):501–520. https://doi.org/10.2217/nnm-2017-0291

Pfaller MA (2012) Antifungal drug resistance: mechanisms, epidemiology, and consequences for treatment. Am J Med 125(1):S3–S13. https://doi.org/10.1016/j.amjmed.2011.11.001

Pfaller M, Diekema D (2007) Epidemiology of invasive candidiasis: a persistent public health problem. Clin Microbiol Rev 20(1):133–163. https://doi.org/10.1128/CMR.00029-06

Pfaller MA, Diekema DJ (2010) Epidemiology of invasive mycoses in North America. Crit Rev Microbiol 36(1):1–53. https://doi.org/10.3109/10408410903241444

Pfaller MA, Pappas PG, Wingard JR (2006) Invasive fungal pathogens: current epidemiological trends. Clin Infect Dis *43*(Supplement_1):S3–S14. https://doi.org/10.1086/504490

Pittet D, Monod M, Suter PM, Frenk E, Auckenthaler R (1994) Candida colonization and subsequent infections in critically ill surgical patients. Ann Surg 220(6):751

Pyo SM, Hespeler D, Keck CM, Müller RH (2017) Dermal miconazole nitrate nanocrystals–formulation development, increased antifungal efficacy & skin penetration. Int J Pharm 531(1):350–359. https://doi.org/10.1016/j.ijpharm.2017.08.108

Quatrin PM, Verdi CM, de Souza ME, de Godoi SN, Klein B, Gundel A et al (2017) Antimicrobial and antibiofilm activities of nanoemulsions containing Eucalyptus globulus oil against Pseudomonas aeruginosa and Candida spp. Microb Pathog 112:230–242. https://doi.org/10.1016/j.micpath.2017.09.062

Quindós G, Gil-Alonso S, Marcos-Arias C, Sevillano E, Mateo E, Jauregizar N, Eraso E (2019) Therapeutic tools for oral candidiasis: current and new antifungal drugs. *Medicina oral, patologia oral y cirugia bucal 24*(2):e172. https://doi.org/10.4317/medoral.22978

Ramteke P, Pandey AC, Pandey H (2019) Evaluation of antifungal activity of blended cinnamon oil and usnic acid nanoemulsion using candidiasis and dermatophytosis models. Biocatal Agric Biotechnol 18:101062. https://doi.org/10.1016/j.bcab.2019.101062

Rana V, Sharma R (2019) Recent advances in development of nano drug delivery. In: Applications of targeted nano drugs and delivery systems. Elsevier, p. 93–131. https://doi.org/10.1016/B978-0-12-814029-1.00005-3

Revie NM, Iyer KR, Robbins N, Cowen LE (2018) Antifungal drug resistance: evolution, mechanisms and impact. Curr Opin Microbiol 45:70–76. https://doi.org/10.1016/j.mib.2018.02.005

Sainz V, Conniot J, Matos AI, Peres C, Zupanŏiŏ E, Moura L et al (2015) Regulatory aspects on nanomedicines. Biochem Biophys Res Commun 468(3):504–510. https://doi.org/10.1016/j.bbrc.2015.08.023

Samaranayake LP, Keung Leung W, Jin L (2009) Oral mucosal fungal infections. Periodontol 49(1):39–59. https://doi.org/10.1111/j.1600-0757.2008.00291.x

Samein LH (2014) Preparation and evaluation of nystatin-loaded solid-lipid-nanoparticles for topical delivery. Asian J Pharm Res 4(1):44–51

Sanglard D (2002) Current understanding of the modes of action of and resistance mechanisms to conventional and emerging antifungal agents for treatment of Candida infections. In: Candida and candidiasis. ASM Press, Washington, DC, pp 349–383

Sanglard D, Odds FC (2002) Resistance of Candida species to antifungal agents: molecular mechanisms and clinical consequences. Lancet Infect Dis 2(2):73–85. https://doi.org/10.1016/S1473-3099(02)00181-0

Sanguinetti M, Posteraro B, Fiori B, Ranno S, Torelli R, Fadda G (2005) Mechanisms of azole resistance in clinical isolates of Candida glabrata collected during a hospital survey of antifungal resistance. Antimicrob

Agents Chemother 49(2):668–679. https://doi.org/10.1128/AAC.49.2.668-679.2005

Sarnes A, Kovalainen M, Häkkinen MR, Laaksonen T, Laru J, Kiesvaara J et al (2014) Nanocrystal-based per-oral itraconazole delivery: superior *in vitro* dissolution enhancement versus Sporanox® is not realized in *in vivo* drug absorption. J Control Release 180:109–116. https://doi.org/10.1016/j.jconrel.2014.02.016

Sawant B, Khan T (2017) Recent advances in delivery of antifungal agents for therapeutic management of candidiasis. Biomed Pharmacother 96:1478–1490. https://doi.org/10.1016/j.biopha.2017.11.127

Schaller M, Borelli C, Korting HC, Hube B (2005) Hydrolytic enzymes as virulence factors of Candida albicans. Mycoses 48(6):365–377. https://doi.org/10.1111/j.1439-0507.2005.01165.x

Schiller DS, Fung HB (2007) Posaconazole: an extended-spectrum triazole antifungal agent. Clin Ther 29(9):1862–1886. https://doi.org/10.1016/j.clinthera.2007.09.015

Shao K, Huang R, Li J, Han L, Ye L, Lou J, Jiang C (2010) Angiopep-2 modified PE-PEG based polymeric micelles for amphotericin B delivery targeted to the brain. J Control Release 147(1):118–126. https://doi.org/10.1016/j.jconrel.2010.06.018

Shao K, Wu J, Chen Z, Huang S, Li J, Ye L et al (2012) A brain-vectored angiopep-2 based polymeric micelles for the treatment of intracranial fungal infection. Biomaterials 33(28):6898–6907. https://doi.org/10.1016/j.biomaterials.2012.06.050

Shin JH, Kee SJ, Shin MG, Kim SH, Shin DH, Lee SK et al (2002) Biofilm production by isolates of Candida species recovered from nonneutropenic patients: comparison of bloodstream isolates with isolates from other sources. J Clin Microbiol 40(4):1244–1248. https://doi.org/10.1128/JCM.40.4.1244-1248.2002

Silva S, Negri M, Henriques M, Oliveira R, Williams DW, Azeredo J (2012) Candida glabrata, Candida parapsilosis and Candida tropicalis: biology, epidemiology, pathogenicity and antifungal resistance. FEMS Microbiol Rev 36(2):288–305. https://doi.org/10.1111/j.1574-6976.2011.00278.x

Singh PK, Iqubal MK, Shukla VK, Shuaib M (2014) Microemulsions: current trends in novel drug delivery systems. J Pharm Chem Biol Sci 1(1):39–51

Sinha B, Mukherjee B, Pattnaik G (2013) Poly-lactide-co-glycolide nanoparticles containing voriconazole for pulmonary delivery: *in vitro* and *in vivo* study. Nanomedicine 9(1):94–104. https://doi.org/10.1016/j.nano.2012.04.005

Smith J, Andes D (2008) Therapeutic drug monitoring of antifungals: pharmacokinetic and pharmacodynamic considerations. Ther Drug Monit 30(2):167–172. https://doi.org/10.1097/FTD.0b013e318167d0e0

Sobel JD, Wiesenfeld HC, Martens M, Danna P, Hooton TM, Rompalo A et al (2004) Maintenance fluconazole therapy for recurrent vulvovaginal candidiasis. N Engl J Med 351(9):876–883. https://doi.org/10.1056/NEJMoa033114

Soliman GM (2017) Nanoparticles as safe and effective delivery systems of antifungal agents: achievements and challenges. Int J Pharm 523(1):15–32. https://doi.org/10.1016/j.ijpharm.2017.03.019

Song CK, Balakrishnan P, Shim C-K, Chung S-J, Chong S, Kim D-D (2012) A novel vesicular carrier, transethosome, for enhanced skin delivery of voriconazole: characterization and *in vitro*/*in vivo* evaluation. Colloids Surf B: Biointerfaces 92:299–304. https://doi.org/10.1016/j.colsurfb.2011.12.004

Song Z, Wen Y, Deng P, Teng F, Zhou F, Xu H et al (2019) Linolenic acid-modified methoxy poly (ethylene glycol)-oligochitosan conjugate micelles for encapsulation of amphotericin B. Carbohydr Polym 205:571–580. https://doi.org/10.1016/j.carbpol.2018.10.086

Sonnex C, Lefort W (1999) Microscopic features of vaginal candidiasis and their relation to symptomatology. Sex Transm Infect 75(6):417–419. https://doi.org/10.1136/sti.75.6.417

Soriano-Ruiz JL, Calpena-Capmany AC, Cañadas-Enrich C, Bozal-de Febrer N, Suñer-Carbó J, Souto EB, Clares-Naveros B (2019) Biopharmaceutical profile of a clotrimazole nanoemulsion: evaluation on skin and mucosae as anticandidal agent. Int J Pharm 554:105–115. https://doi.org/10.1016/j.ijpharm.2018.11.002

Sosa L, Clares B, Alvarado HL, Bozal N, Domenech O, Calpena AC (2017) Amphotericin B releasing topical nanoemulsion for the treatment of candidiasis and aspergillosis. Nanomedicine 13(7):2303–2312. https://doi.org/10.1016/j.nano.2017.06.021

Stephenson J (1997) Investigators seeking new ways to stem rising tide of resistant fungi. JAMA 277(1):5–6. https://doi.org/10.1001/jama.1997.03540250013006

Sudhakar B, Ravi Varma J, Ramana Murthy K (2014) Formulation, characterization and *ex vivo* studies of terbinafine HCl liposomes for cutaneous delivery. Curr Drug Deliv 11(4):521–530. https://doi.org/10.2174/1567201810666140109113830

Suk JS, Xu Q, Kim N, Hanes J, Ensign LM (2016) PEGylation as a strategy for improving nanoparticle-based drug and gene delivery. Adv Drug Deliv Rev 99:28–51. https://doi.org/10.1016/j.addr.2015.09.012

Takakura N, Sato Y, Ishibashi H, Oshima H, Uchida K, Yamaguchi H, Abe S (2003) A novel murine model of oral candidiasis with local symptoms characteristic of oral thrush. Microbiol Immunol 47(5):321–326. https://doi.org/10.1111/j.1348-0421.2003.tb03403.x

Tang X, Dai J, Xie J, Zhu Y, Zhu M, Wang Z et al (2015) Enhanced antifungal activity by Ab-modified amphotericin B-loaded nanoparticles using a pH-responsive block copolymer. Nanoscale Res Lett 10(1):256. https://doi.org/10.1186/s11671-015-0969-1

Tonglairoum P, Ngawhirunpat T, Rojanarata T, Kaomongkolgit R, Opanasopit P (2015) Fabrication of a novel scaffold of clotrimazole-microemulsion-containing nanofibers using an electrospinning process for oral candidiasis applications. Colloids Surf

B: Biointerfaces 126:18–25. https://doi.org/10.1016/j.colsurfb.2014.12.009

Tonglairoum P, Woraphatphadung T, Ngawhirunpat T, Rojanarata T, Akkaramongkolporn P, Sajomsang W, Opanasopit P (2017) Development and evaluation of N-naphthyl-N, O-succinyl chitosan micelles containing clotrimazole for oral candidiasis treatment. Pharm Dev Technol 22(2):184–190. https://doi.org/10.3109/10837450.2016.1163391

Tripathi N, Watt K, Benjamin DK Jr (2012) Treatment and prophylaxis of invasive candidiasis. Semin Perinatol 36(6):416–423. https://doi.org/10.1053/j.semperi.2012.06.003

Verma P, Pathak K (2012) Nanosized ethanolic vesicles loaded with econazole nitrate for the treatment of deep fungal infections through topical gel formulation. Nanomedicine 8(4):489–496. https://doi.org/10.1016/j.nano.2011.07.004

Vyas SP, Gupta S (2006) Optimizing efficacy of amphotericin B through nanomodification. Int J Nanomedicine 1(4):417

Vallabhaneni S, Mody RK, Walker T, Chiller T (2016) The Global Burden of Fungal Diseases. Infect Dis Clin North Am 30(1):1–11. https://doi.org/10.1016/j.idc.2015.10.004

Walsh TJ, Kasai M, Francesconi A, Landsman D, Chanock SJ (1997) New evidence that Candida albicans possesses additional ATP-binding cassette MDR-like genes: implications for antifungal azole resistance. J Med Vet Mycol 35(2):133–137. https://doi.org/10.1080/02681219780001021

White TC, Marr KA, Bowden RA (1998) Clinical, cellular, and molecular factors that contribute to antifungal drug resistance. Clin Microbiol Rev 11(2):382–402. https://doi.org/10.1128/CMR.11.2.382

Willems L, Van der Geest R, De Beule K (2001) Itraconazole oral solution and intravenous formulations: a review of pharmacokinetics and pharmacodynamics. J Clin Pharm Ther 26(3):159–169. https://doi.org/10.1046/j.1365-2710.2001.00338.x

Williams DW, Kuriyama T, Silva S, Malic S, Lewis MA (2011) Candida biofilms and oral candidosis: treatment and prevention. Periodontol 55(1):250–265. https://doi.org/10.1111/j.1600-0757.2009.00338.x

Wisplinghoff H, Bischoff T, Tallent SM, Seifert H, Wenzel RP, Edmond MB (2004) Nosocomial bloodstream infections in US hospitals: analysis of 24,179 cases from a prospective nationwide surveillance study. Clin Infect Dis 39(3):309–317. https://doi.org/10.1086/421946

Yu B, Okano T, Kataoka K, Kwon G (1998) Polymeric micelles for drug delivery: solubilization and haemolytic activity of amphotericin B. J Control Release 53(1–3):131–136. https://doi.org/10.1016/S0168-3659(97)00245-9

Zazo H, Colino CI, Lanao JM (2016) Current applications of nanoparticles in infectious diseases. J Control Release 224:86–102. https://doi.org/10.1016/j.jconrel.2016.01.008

Zhang L, Pornpattananangkul D, Hu C-M, Huang C-M (2010) Development of nanoparticles for antimicrobial drug delivery. Curr Med Chem 17(6):585–594. https://doi.org/10.2174/092986710790416290

Part V

Nanoformulations for Phytopharmaceuticals

Nano-carriers for Natural Therapeutics in Management of Neuropathic Pain

16

Kuldeep Nigam, Purnam Hoshe Ruba, Pallavee Kapoor, Reema Gabrani, and Shweta Dang

Abstract

The International Association for the Study of Pain (IASP) defines neuropathic pain as "pain caused by a lesion or disease of the somatosensory nervous system, which causes unpleasant and abnormal sensation (dysaesthesia), an increased response to painful stimuli (hyperalgesia) and pain in response to a stimulus that does not normally provoke pain (allodynia)." This definition of neuropathic pain distinguishes it from other types of pain, including musculoskeletal pain, by restricting its extent to the somatosensory nervous system. In a large number of reported neurodegenerative pain cases, it has been observed that the pain would be severe and debilitating. The aim of this chapter is to bring a number of different plant therapeutics having analgesic properties in light. Plant compounds such as capsaicin, triptolide, curcumin and salicin have been widely known to protect against neuropathic pain. These compounds are most commonly found and are reported to have a variety of pharmacological effects such as an effective role in pain control. Nowadays other plant compounds such as bromelain from pineapple and ECGC from green tea, which already have multiple clinical indications, are being studied for its role in treating neuropathic pain.

Keywords

Capsaicin · Curcumin · Epigallocatechin-3-Gallate (EGCG) · Neuropathic Pain · Salicin · Triptolide

16.1 Introduction

Any lesions or damage in somatosensory system is defined as neuropathic pain (Jensen et al. 2011). Multiple conditions lead to neuropathic pain such as spinal cord injury, any sort of brain injury or multiple disease-associated pain such as diabetes, AIDS, multiple sclerosis and cancer (Fig. 16.1) (Treede et al. 2008). In a study, the estimated reports show that 6.9–10.0% of the general population suffer from neuropathic pain,which is predicted to increase in the future due to various factors (VanHecke et al. 2014) such as increasing obesity rates, growing geriatric population and improved survival rate of cancer patients being treated with advanced medical procedures (Moulin et al. 2014). Neuropathic pain could be termed as a chronic condition,

K. Nigam · P. H. Ruba · P. Kapoor · R. Gabrani · S. Dang (✉)
Department of Biotechnology, Jaypee Institute of Information Technology, Noida, India
e-mail: reema.gabrani@jiit.ac.in; shweta.dang@jiit.ac.in

S. Talegaonkar, M. Rai (eds.), *Nanoformulations in Human Health*,
https://doi.org/10.1007/978-3-030-41858-8_16

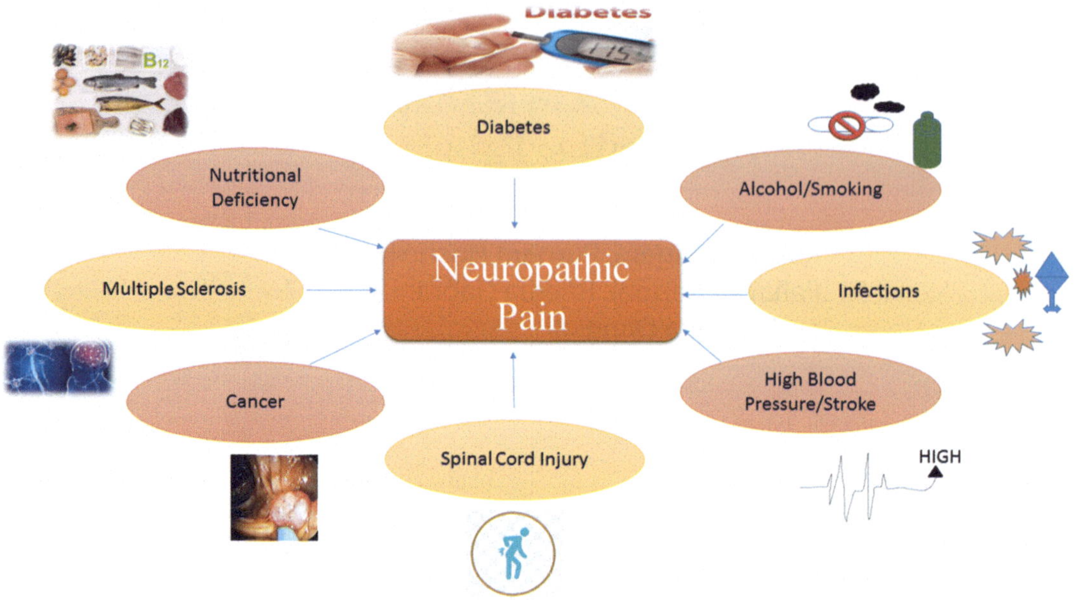

Fig. 16.1 Few listed conditions leading to neuropathic pain conditions

which embodies a significant encumbrance for patients, society and healthcare systems (Smith and Torrance 2012). The management of neuropathic pain is complex and continues to be a challenge as it is different from nociceptive pain and requires a different therapeutic approach (Finnerup et al. 2015). Various global organizations such as International Association for the Study of Pain (IASP), European Federation of Neurological Societies (EFNS), National Institute for Health and Care Excellence (NICE) and Canadian Pain Society (CPS) have published clinical practice guidelines to facilitate the assessment and treatment of neuropathic pain (Cruccu et al. 2007; Cruccu et al. 2010; Attal et al. 2010; Haanpää et al. 2011; Mailis and Taenzer 2012; Dworkin et al. 2013; Moulin et al. 2014).

The OPD treatment options are divided into three phases depending upon the complexity of the pain. The first-line treatment medications include various drug categories such as tricyclic antidepressants (e.g., amitriptyline), drug ligands for calcium channel alpha-2-delta (e.g., pregabalin and gabapentin) and serotonin–norepinephrine reuptake inhibitors commonly known as SNRIs (e.g., duloxetine). Tramadol, which belongs to opioids and SNRI class, is recommended majorly as second-line therapy for neuropathic pain treatment (Chris et al. 2017). The NICE guidelines recommend the use of tramadol specifically in rescue therapy as higher rates of withdrawal of tramadol have been observed due to adverse events compared with other treatments (NICE guidelines). Strong opioids, anti-epileptic drugs (other than gabapentinoids) and cannabinoids are commonly recommended for third-line and fourth-line treatment of neuropathic pain. Pregabalin and carbamazepine are one of the most recognized and effective medications available for trigeminal neuralgia (Cruccu and Truini 2017; Colloca et al. 2017).

However, due to the complex pathophysiology of neuropathic pain, these drugs are not completely effective in attenuating neuropathic pain and have multiple reported side effects, viz. sedation, dizziness, oedema and ataxia. This is one of the most important reasons to preferring the use of herbal medicines owing to less complication and fewer side effects than synthetic drugs (Boyd et al. 2017). Owing to the increase in the demand for medicinal plants and related compounds, the phytopharmaceutical studies and the utilization of these remedies for the treatment of neuropathic

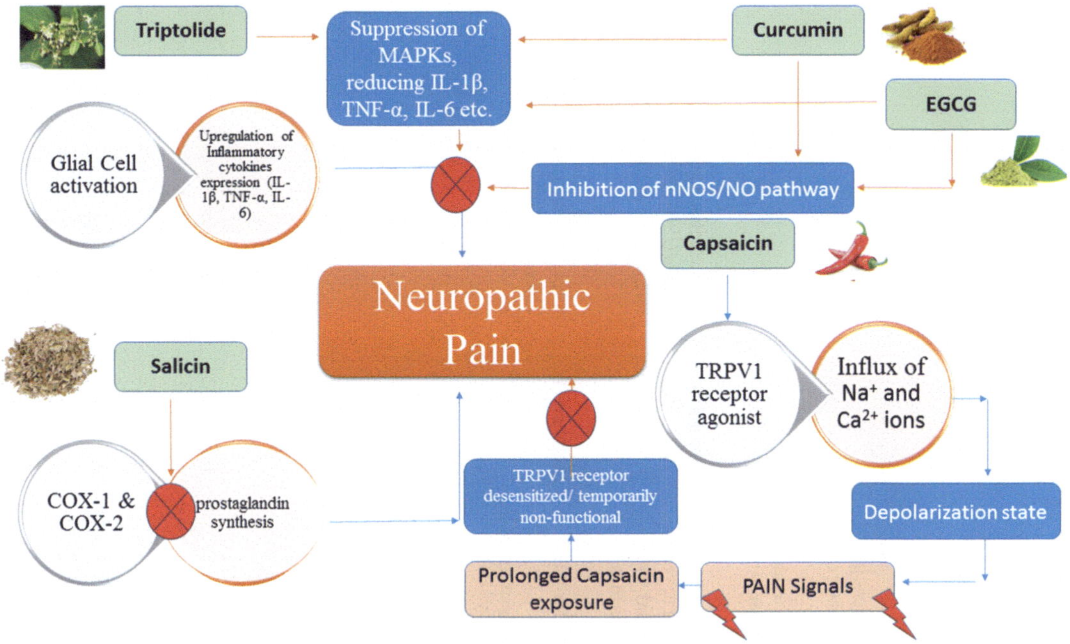

Fig. 16.2 Flowchart explaining the role of multiple phytotherapeutics in pain management

pain have been growing throughout the world (Garg and Adams 2012; Forouzanfar and Hosseinzadeh 2018).

Various plant-derived compounds are being studied for the treatment of neuropathic pain such as capsaicin that showed positive results in neuropathic pain conditions (Derry and Moore 2012). Other common plants, which are used to treat neuropathic pain, are *Acorus calamus* (sweet flag or calamus), *Artemisia dracunculus* (tarragon or estragon), *Butea monosperma* (flame of the forest), *Citrullus colocynthis* (colocynth or bitter apple), *Curcuma longa* (turmeric), *Crocus sativus* (saffron crocus or autumn crocus), *Elaeagnus angustifolia* (Russian olive), *Ginkgo biloba* (maidenhair tree), *Mitragyna speciose* (Kratom), *Momordica charantia* (bitter melon), *Nigella sativa* (black caraway, black cumin or kalonji), *Ocimum sanctum* (basil or tulasi) and *Phyllanthus amarus* (gale of the wind, stonebreaker or seed-under-leaf). Anti-oxidant activity, anti-inflammatory, antiapoptotic, neuroprotective and calcium inhibitory actions are some of the pathways that are known to be involved in pain relief through herbal medications (Fig. 16.2) (Dworkin et al. 2007; Derry and Moore 2012; Garg and Adams 2012; Daniela 2015; Diego 2017; Forouzanfar and Hosseinzadeh 2018). This chapter focuses on natural products and their nano-formulations being used in neuropathic pain. Table 16.1 lists a few important patents granted for these phytocompounds, and Table 16.2 lists some commercially available marketed products.

16.2 Capsaicin

16.2.1 Overview

Capsaicin, the active compound found commonly in genus *Capsicum* or chilli peppers, is reported to have analgesic properties. Chilli peppers are widely consumed worldwide, and the capsaicin content ranges from 0.1% to 1% from green to red varieties of peppers. The compound is reported to have high pharmacotherapeutic importance proving beneficial in multiple pain-associated conditions such as rheumatoid arthritis, post-herpetic neuralgia, post-mastectomy

Table 16.1 List of few important patents

Patent ID	Compound	Owner	Claims	Date of expiration	Reference
US6239180B1	Capsaicin (under the trade name Qutenza)	University of California	The patent is for topical patch of capsaicin (8% strength). It claims for a device for the treatment of neuropathic pain in a human patient. The device comprises a skin-adherent patch, which includes a reservoir comprising a therapeutic formulation. The formulation is continuously provided to the surface of the skin for a predetermined period of time	April, 2021	https://patents.google.com/patent/US6239180B1/en
US 6312736 B1	White willow bark extract (salicin), kava kava root extract, feverfew extract, ginger root extract, Guarana extract, and Vitamin B6	Biotech Corp	The patent claims for the herbal composition of the mentioned compounds used to relieve pain and other symptoms associated with migraines and other types of headaches.	December, 2019	https://patents.google.com/patent/US6312736B1/en?oq=US+6312736+B1
US 8765194B2	Salicin	Michelle Mills, Michael Hutsell (Inventor)	It claims a cosmetic composition for the management of pain comprising: *Salix alba* (white willow) bark extract, in an amount by weight of about 1–3% *Helichrysum gymnocephalum* flower essential oil in an amount by weight of about 0.03–1% Effective amounts of *Mentha avrensis* (menthol), camphor, *Eucalyptus* globules, *Lavandula angustifolia* (lavender) oil, *Pelargonium graveoleus* (geranium) oil, and *Mentha viridis* (spearmint) oil; and a cosmetic cream substrate.	September, 2032	https://patents.google.com/patent/US8765194B2/en?oq=US+8765194B2
US8193249B2	Triptolide	Emory University	It provides synthetic methods and compositions for the treatment of autoimmune and anti-inflammatory disorders comprising administering an effective amount of a derivative of triptolide alone or in combination or alternation with other anti-autoimmune or anti-inflammatory compounds.	June, 2022	https://patents.google.com/patent/US8193249B2/en?oq=US8193249B2

Patent ID	Compound	Owner	Claims	Date of expiration	Reference
US9623035B2	Triptolide	University of Minnesota	It claims a method for inhibiting cancer cell growth in HSP70-expressing cancer in a mammal comprising administering to the mammal a compound of formula I	May, 2030	https://patents.google.com/patent/US9623035B2/en?oq=US9623035B2
EP1330459 B1	Triptolide	Venkatesan, Snyder, Liotta, Wang (Inventor)	Triptolide analogs for the treatment of autoimmune and inflammatory disorders	October 2021	https://patents.google.com/patent/EP1330459B1/en?oq=EP1330459+B1
US9150600B2	Triptolide	University of Minnesota	It claims a method for treating cancer in a mammal, comprising administering to the mammal a compound of formula I	May, 2030	https://patents.google.com/patent/US9150600B2/en?oq=US9150600B2
US8507552B2	Triptolide	University of Minnesota	It claims a compound of formula I	May, 2030	https://patents.google.com/patent/US8507552B2/en?oq=US8507552B2
US20120309821A1	Epigallocatechin-3-gallate	National Defence Medical Centre	It claims a method for regulating immune and preventing or treating lupus erythematosus comprising administering a subject in need thereof a therapeutically effective amount of EGCG or a pharmaceutically acceptable salt or a physiologically functional derivative, together with one or more pharmaceutically acceptable carriers, diluents or excipients.	Application status is Abandoned (May 2019)	https://patents.google.com/patent/US20120309821A1/en?oq=US20120309821A1

Table 16.2 Commercially available products

S. no.	Compound name	Brand name	Product type	Manufacturer	Location	References
1	Capsaicin	Zostrix®	Ointment	Link Medical Products Pty Ltd	Warriewood, Australia	http://zostrix.com/
2	Capsaicin	Cayenne®	Capsules	Nature's Way	Wisconsin, USA	https://www.naturesway.com/Product-Catalog/Cayenne-Pepper-180-Caps
3	Capsaicin	Qutenza®	Transdermal patch	Averitas Pharma	New Jersey, USA	https://www.averitaspharma.com//
4	Capsaicin	Salonpas®	Gel based transdermal patch	Hisamitsu Pharmaceutical	Tokyo, Japan	https://us.hisamitsu/
5	Salicin	Willow Bark Extract 400 mg Capsules	Capsules	Now Foods	USA	https://www.nowfoods.com/supplements/willow-bark-extract-400-mg-capsules
6	Salicin	Willow capsules (15% salicin)	Capsules	Nature's way	Wisconsin, USA	https://www.naturesway.com/Product-Catalog/White-Willow-Bark-60-Caps
7	Salicin	White Willow Bark Extract	Capsules	*Swanson Superior Herbs*	*Fargo, North Dakota.*	https://www.swansonvitamins.com/swanson-superior-herbs-white-willow-bark-extract-500-mg-120-caps
8	Salicin	White willow bark	Capsules	Piping rock	New York, United States	https://in.pipingrock.com/white-willow-bark
9	Triptolide	Thunder god root	Capsules	Flawless herbs	USA	http://www.flawlessherbs.com/
10	Triptolide	Thunder god extract	Powder	RD health ingredients	China	http://www.health-ingredients.com/api-pharmaceuticals/thunder-god-vine-extract.html
11	EGCG	EGCG	Capsules	Now Foods	USA	https://www.nowfoods.com/supplements/egcg-green-tea-extract-400-mg-veg-capsules
12	EGCG	ECGC Green Tea	Capsule	Bluebonnet nutrition	Sugar Land, TX	https://bluebonnetnutrition.com/product/bluebonnet-nutrition-standardized-egcg-green-tea-leaf-extract-60-count/
13	EGCG	Green Tea Extract 50% EGCG Capsules	Capsules	Bulk Supplements	Henderson, USA	https://www.bulksupplements.com/green-tea-pure-extract-50-egcg-3610.html
14	EGCG	Green tea powder	Powder	Bulk Supplements	Henderson, USA	https://www.bulksupplements.com/green-tea-extract-50-egcg.html
15	Curcumin	Turmeric Curcumin	Capsules	Vimerson Health	USA	https://vimerson.com/products/turmeric-curcumin
16	Curcumin	Turmeric Force™	Capsules	New Chapter	Vermont, USA	https://www.newchapter.com/contact/
17	Curcumin	Turmeric Curcumin	Capsules	Herbal Hearts	USA	http://www.myherbalhearts.com/turmeric-200-vegetarian-capsules.html
18	Curcumin	Prosper Advanced Turmeric Curcumin	Capsules	Prosper pure life	USA	https://www.prosperpurelife.com/products/turmeric-curcumin

pain syndrome and diabetic neuropathy (Sawynok 2005; Tesfaye 2009; Backonja et al. 2010; Derry et al. 2017). The reported pathways suggest its pivotal role in effecting the primary afferent neurons, which are the peripheral part of the sensory nervous system. The versatility of capsaicin comes from its role in exhausting the substance P, the neurotransmitter for painful impulses from sensory nerve terminals, making it an important experimental tool for pain-associated studies. Multiple topical formulations are commercially available for the treatment of different neuropathic pain conditions such as post-herpetic neuralgia, musculoskeletal pain, diabetic neuropathy, osteoarthritis and rheumatoid arthritis (Watanabe et al. 1987; Sawynok 2005; Mathhews et al. 2009; Tesfaye 2009; Backonja et al. 2010).

16.2.2 Mechanism of Action

Capsaicin acts as an agonist to pain receptors transient receptor potential cation channel subfamily V member 1 (TRPV1), which is transmembrane, receptor-ion channel complex. Capsaicin acts as a ligand molecule and binds to TRPV1 receptor, resulting in the opening of the channel with a rapid influx of Na^+ and Ca^{2+} ions, which in turn leads to depolarization state. The common expression of TRPV1 is generally in A-delta and C nerve fibres, where depolarization leads to action potential sending impulses to brain and spinal cord where they are interpreted as pain signals. The immediate response is various inflammatory signals such as warming, tingling, itching, stinging, or burning sensations. Capsaicin dosing results in the induction of an initial pain sensation followed by analgesia. Prolonged high and/or repeated capsaicin exposure makes TRPV1 receptors in refractory state or desensitized state, making the receptors non-functional temporarily. This inhibition in the functionality of the receptor could be in response to thermal, mechanical, or chemical noxious stimuli. The reported evidence suggests that the process occurs when an exhaustion of neuropeptides occurs (Substance P), specifically in nerve fibres expressing TRPV1 receptors, and an increased level of Ca^{2+} ions intracellularly due to inhibition of high-voltage-activated (HVA) and low-voltage-activated (T-type) calcium channels. The delayed effect because of rapid Ca^{2+} influx in turn leads to further activation of certain calcium-dependent proteins which in turn leads to desensitization of TRPV1 (Fattori et al. 2016).

16.2.3 Pharmacokinetics of Capsaicin

Various reports assessing the pharmacokinetic profile of capsaicin suggest absorption of capsaicin majorly in stomach and entire intestinal area, ranging from 50% to 90%, with the C_{max} or mean plasma concentration reaching within one hour of oral administration. Following the absorption, the main site for the metabolism of capsaicin is liver where it produces three major metabolites such as 16-hydroxycapsaicin, 17-hydroxycapsaicinand16,17-hydroxycapsaicin and vanillin as minor metabolite. Reports suggest that cytochrome P450 (P450) enzymes are also involved in hepatic metabolism of capsaicin. Capsaicin is eliminated mainly via renal route while small amount is excreted in faeces in both unchanged and glucuronide form (O'Neill et al. 2012). The intravenous or subcutaneous administration of capsaicin shows fivefold higher levels of capsaicin in brain regions as compared to blood, whereas liver concentrations were threefold higher as compared to blood. Upon topical application, capsaicin is reported to absorb rapidly through skin. A clinical study suggested that upon topical patch treatment of capsaicin, the mean peak plasma concentration was found to be only 1.86 ng/ml, while the maximum plasma concentration reached to 17.8 ng/ml, suggesting that it is unlikely to get absorbed directly to blood upon topical administration (Sayanlar et al. 2012).

16.2.4 Nano-formulations of Capsaicin

Nagoth et al. (2015) synthesized capsaicin-capped silver nanoparticles which were 20–30 nm in size and were highly compatible with ABO blood groups in haemagglutination test, suggesting high biocompatibility and their potential role as therapeutic agent. In another study, Kaiser et al. (2015) synthesized capsaicin-loaded chitosan nanocapsule to enhance the para-cellular transport, which was earlier having low permeability, across an epithelial cell monolayer via a reversible opening of cellular tight junctions. The comparative study was performed and various physiochemical properties were assessed, comparing capsaicin-loaded chitosan nanocapsules with its free capsaicin counterpart, such as cytotoxicity towards epithelial MDCK-C7 cells, evaluating the effect on the integrity of tight junctions, membrane permeability and cellular uptake. The results exhibited that the nanocapsules modulated the interaction between capsaicin and tight junctions and were internalized by MDCK-C7 cells. Another similar study by Mrudhula et.al (2017) prepared PLGA-coated capsaicin magnetic nanoparticles (PCMN) using solvent-evaporation/co-precipitation technique and evaluated various characteristics in vitro. It was observed that the size of the nanoparticles was in the range of 10–20 nm and showed approximately 9.29% drug loading and 89.15% encapsulation efficiencies (EE %). In addition, increased solubility of capsaicin (20 ± 3% for pure capsaicin, whereas for PLGA-coated capsaicin magnetic nanoparticles, 83 ± 4.1% release after 50 h) was observed in the in vitro dissolution studies due to the nanosize of PLGA-coated capsaicin magnetic nanoparticles. Mei et al. (2015) prepared capsaicin-loaded nanoparticle gel using hot-solvent high-pressure homogenization technique and employed Box-Behnken Design during the optimization process to evaluate its properties in vitro and in vivo. The capsaicin permeability enhanced in nanoparticle-based gel was a 2.80-fold higher flux value compared to the conventional form after 24 hours. Choi et al. (2013) formulated capsaicin-loaded nanoemulsions fabricated with alginate and chitosan to examine the pharmacokinetic properties of the formulated capsaicin-loaded nanoemulsions in comparison with capsaicin control in a rat. The formulated nanoemulsions could significantly enhance the bioavailability of capsaicin (131.7 times increased bioavailability with extended half-life). Peng et al. (2015) prepared capsaicin-loaded methoxy poly (ethylene glycol)-poly(ε-caprolactone) nanoparticles using a modified emulsification solvent diffusion technique. The prepared nanoparticles had an average diameter of 82.54 ± 0.51 nm, high drug-loading capacity of 14.0% ± 0.13% and high stability than the conventional form. Xia et al. (2017) synthesized capsaicin-loaded nano-lipoidal carriers (NLCs) using modified hot melt homogenization technique to enhance permeation and attain the analgesic and anti-inflammatory effect with lower skin irritation. The capsaicin-loaded nano-lipoidal carriers and capsaicin-loaded nano-lipoidal carrier gel improved the pain onset in a dose-dependent manner and inhibited inflammation compared with capsaicin cream and capsaicin solution.

16.3 Salicin

16.3.1 Overview

Salicin belongs to the class of glycoside and acts as a precursor molecule for the synthesis of acetylsalicylic acid. Salicin is very commonly found in willow (*Salix*) barks and has reported anti-inflammatory properties in the human body. Also, Salicin is found in the bark of *Populus* spp., and the leaves of willows and other poplars. It is also used as an analgesic, antipyretic, disinfectant and antiseptic. Its action is very similar to that of aspirin. Willow bark is used as an alternative to aspirin to treat chronic headaches or back pain (Art 2009; Singh 2003).

16.3.2 Mechanism of Action

The mechanism of action of salicylic acid is identical to that of aspirin molecule. The compound inhibits cyclooxygenase enzymes (COX-1 and COX-2), which are involved in prostaglandin synthesis (Rao and Knaus 2008; Raju et al. 2015). The analgesic effect is produced via peripheral and direct CNS effects. On peripheral level, salicin is reported to act by hindering the synthesis and release of prostaglandins while centrally, it acts on hypothalamus, producing analgesia. The advantage of natural salicin over aspirin is that white willow does not interfere with coagulation, which is the major drawback of using aspirin (Vane and Botting 2003; Dissanayake et al. 2017).

16.3.3 Pharmacokinetics of Salicin

The absorption of salicin on oral administration is high and rapid. The initial metabolism of salicin to saligenin is done by intestinal flora, which is rapidly absorbed into bloodstream and transported to liver where it is initially hydrolysed into salicylic acid, and further to salicyluric acid (upon conjugation with glycine moiety) and finally to glucuronic acid. The major excretion is via renal route in the form of salicylic acid or glucuronic acid in the urine kidney (Maclagan 1879; Schmid et al. 2001; Wagner and Heide 2003). Its pharmacokinetic parameters are dependent and may vary according to specific dosage form, salicylate used, and other factors such as dissolution rate of tablet and intraluminal or gastric pH. Plasma protein binding of salicin is as high as 99.5% (with albumin) with $T_{1/2}$ or plasma half-life of around 15 minutes which is increased on increasing the doses (300–650 mg have $T_{1/2}$ of around 3.1 hours, while 1–2 g of daily doses have $T_{1/2}$ of around 5–9 hours, respectively, in the form of salicylate). Willow has a slower onset of action and an extended duration of action, where dosing is usually 60–120 mg (total salicin) daily (Lewis and Johnson 2006).

16.3.4 Nano- formulations of Salicin

Nanoparticulate delivery systems have the potential to enhance drug stability and expand the period of the therapeutic effect. Shang et al. (2018) prepared chitosan (CS)-acetylsalicylic acid (ASA) nanoparticles using interpolymer complexation method. It was observed that the developed nanoparticles exhibited a sustained and pH-dependent drug release. In addition, the preliminary pharmacokinetic studies suggested prolonged circulation of the prepared nanoparticles with higher bioavailability as compared to the crude acetylsalicylic acid. Woo et al. (2014) synthesized salicylic acid-loaded stearic acid-oleic acid nanoparticles (SONs) in cream-based formulation for topical delivery using melt emulsification method combined with ultrasonication technique. It was observed in in vitro release studies that SONs incorporated in cream showed a steady release for 24 hours, designating the integration of salicylic acid in solid matrix of SON and elongating the in vitro release. Taghizadeh and Javan (2010) prepared chitosan nanoparticles containing salicylic acid (SA) using the emulsion method. The nanoparticles were spherical with an average size of 300 nm, and the drug content ranged between 20% and 35%.

16.4 Triptolide

16.4.1 Overview

Triptolide (TP) is the therapeutically active component in *Tripterygium wilfordii* plant. Triptolide has a small molecular size of 360.406 g/mol. It also displays lipophilic properties, which makes it suitable for penetrating the blood–brain barrier. This characteristic property hence makes it a significant drug candidate against inflammatory response in the CNS. Studies have shown that repeated systemic administration of triptolide has successfully prevented and reversed neuropathic pain (Zhu et al. 2010; Wang et al. 2012; Tang et al. 2012).

16.4.2 Mechanism of Action

Triptolide shows its therapeutic potential in averting and diminishing neuropathic pain, by inhibiting immune response in the spinal dorsal horn. The activation of glial cells leads to the immune responses majorly by expressing various inflammatory cytokines from spinal dorsal horn, leading to the induction of neuropathic pain. Thus, an effective strategy to treat neuropathic pain is to target central immune activation. The triptolide extract is known to have potent anti-inflammatory and immunosuppressive effects and has been used successfully in the treatment of various inflammatory diseases. It also suppresses mitogen-activated protein kinases (MAPKs) phosphorylation that is essential for the induction and maintenance of neuropathic pain. The activation of MAPKs initiates signalling cascades and increases the synthesis of pro-inflammatory mediators. Triptolide results in the inhibition of inflammatory mediators including cytokine (interleukin-1β, tumour necrosis factor-α and interleukin-6) and chemokines. Since the exact mechanism of action of plant therapeutic is still unclear, mitogen-activated protein kinase activation and the following expression of inflammatory cytokines can be the potential targeting sites of triptolide. Triptolide-mediated decrease in the expression of the inflammatory cytokines could prevent the excitatory synaptic transmission during pain signal transduction and thus produce anti-nociception effects resulting in lowering the levels of pain (Wang et al. 2012; Jian et al. 2017).

16.4.3 Pharmacokinetics of Triptolide

A study performed on male Sprague-Dawley rats to investigate absorption, distribution, metabolism and excretion of triptolide after oral intravenous administration of single doses. It was observed that upon administration of triptolide on various doses (0.6, 1.2 and 2.4 mg/kg), the C_{max} or the maximum plasma concentration was achieved within min with the $T_{1/2}$ or elimination half-life around 16.8 to 21.7 mins. The intravenous administration of triptolide showed one-compartment model kinetics. Oral absolute bioavailability was observed to be 72.08% at the dose of 0.6 mg/kg. Triptolide was also found to be distributed rapidly, extensively metabolized in liver and eliminated via urinary and faecal routes. Within 48 hours, < 1% triptolide of the dose was obtained from the bile, urine or faeces as parent drug molecule. The metabolism of triptolide occurs in liver majorly by CYP450 (CYP3A) enzymes into 3 or 4 mono-hydroxylated metabolites (M2, M3, M4 in human live microsomes) which is then excreted out in urine, faeces and bile (Shao et al. 2007; Xu et al. 2017).

16.4.4 Nano-formulations of Triptolide

Gu et al. (2018) prepared lipid nanoparticles of triptolide for transdermal delivery to evaluate the interactions between skin and nanoparticles. Triptolide-nanostructured lipid carriers and triptolide-solid lipid nanoparticles could easily penetrate the skin by changing their structure, thermodynamic properties and components of the stratum corneum. The histopathological studies of stratum corneum suggested the possible interactions between the surfactants present in triptolide-nanostructured lipid carriers and skin where the spacing increased upon the lipid exchange between the stratum corneum and lecithin, helping in the permeation of the prepared nano-formulation.

Wang et al. (2015) prepared triptolide-polymeric micelles using methoxy poly(ethylene glycol)–block–poly(ε-caprolactone). The in vitro release profiles showed that the triptolide-polymeric micelles exhibited sustained-release action in comparison with free triptolide solution. Xiong et al. (2005) synthesized triptolide-loaded solid lipid nanoparticles, microemulsions and polymeric nanoparticles. Triptolide-loaded solid lipid nanoparticles upon transdermal delivery showed its presence 2.4 times higher as compared to triptolide solution after 12 hours of application. Similarly, triptolide-loaded polymeric nanoparticles upon oral administration showed significantly lower toxicity profiles in liver and kidney. These novel nanodrug delivery systems (NDDS) presented more powerful activity and a lower toxicity in comparison with common drug carrier forms.

16.5 Epigallocatechin-3-Gallate (EGCG)

16.5.1 Overview

The most widely consumed worldwide beverage after water is tea. Green tea is botanically called *Camellia sinensis*. It contains leaf polyphenols that contribute to the health-promoting effects. The polyphenols (known as catechins) account for 30–42% of the dry weight of the solids in brewed *Camellia sinensis*. Tea comprises of four major catechins such as epigallocatechin-3-gallate (EGCG), epigallocatechin (EGC), epicatechin-3-gallate (ECG), and epicatechin (EC). EGCG is present accounting 50–80% of the total catechines making it the main and the most abundant catechin which is known to have multiple therapeutic potentials even in the nervous system. Various in vitro investigations have suggested the involvement of EGCG in upregulating various signalling pathways, by inhibiting the inflammation and regulating oxidative stress (Tian et al. 2013). Studies showed its potential role as a neuroprotective agent to relieve the pain. Multiple experimental works have proven the protective effects of EGCG against various conditions such as spinal cord injury and control of inflammation in neurodegenerative diseases (Kuang et al. 2012; Renno et al. 2013; Raposo et al. 2015).

16.5.2 Mechanism of Action of EGCG

Anti-inflammatory and anti-oxidant properties of EGCG produce anti-nociceptive effects (Khalatbary and Ahmadvand 2011; Kuang et al. 2012). In addition, it has been observed that various EGCG derivatives can modulate neuropathic pain by reducing the NF-κB and the production of pro-inflammatory cytokines such as tumour necrosis factor-alpha (TNF-α) and interleukin-1 beta (IL-1β). EGCG has been found to suppress neuropathic pain by regulating the expression levels of particular proteins comprised in specific molecular pathways: (1) nNOS/NO (neuronal nitric oxide synthase/nitric oxide); (2) CX3CL1 (chemokine fractalkine ligand), JNK (c-Jun N-terminal kinases) and NF-κB (nuclear factor kappa-light-chain-enhancer of activated B-cells); and (3) TNF-α (tumour necrosis factor-α). Allodynia is downregulated by EGCG, which interferes with NO by inhibiting the nNOS/NO pathway (Choi et al. 2012). Chronic thermal hyperalgesia is reduced by EGCG through the regulation of the expression determinants of CX3CL1, which displayed a significant role in mediating the activity among microglia and neurons (Bosch-Mola et al. 2017). EGCG is reported to reduce pain perception by modulating c-Jun N-terminal kinases and NF-κB activities (Xavier et al. 2015; Bimonte et al. 2017).

16.5.3 Pharmacokinetics of EGCG

A study was conducted on Beagle dogs to determine the pharmacokinetics of EGCG. EGCG was administered intravenously at a dose of 25 mg/kg body weight to Beagle dogs, [3H]-EGCG was eliminated from the plasma with a half-life of nearly 6 hours. The rate of clearance was low (1.19 ml/min-kg) and was consistent with relatively slow metabolism and a mean residence time of 8.30 hours. The volume of distribution (0.59 L/kg) showed that the radioactivity was distributed to total body water. The blood/plasma ratios of the radioactivity over 24 hours were 0.61–0.77, and this tells about preferential distribution to plasma water. However, after a single oral administration of EGCG to Beagle dogs, the absorption was observed to be rapid with a maximal plasma concentration at approximately 1 hour. The elimination half-life (6.8 hours) was found to be similar to that seen after i.v. administration. The apparent bioavailability, that is, the ratio of the i.v. to the oral route of administration, was calculated to be 20% (James et al. 2001).

16.5.4 Nano-formulations of EGCG

Ramkumar et al. (2015) prepared ECGC-loaded chitosan nanoparticles using ionic-gelation method. The prepared nanoparticles were of nanometric range with high stability. While studying the release profiles, it was observed that the release was sustained following diffusion and swelling mechanisms. Amanda et al. (2019) prepared EGCG-loaded PEGylated PLGA nanoparticles using double emulsion method. In vitro and ex vivo experiments suggested EGCG nanoparticles induced disruption of tight junctions, opening blood–brain barrier (BBB). Further, the stabilization of EGCG in nanoparticles complexes and a destabilized BBB resulted in the higher therapeutic EGCG concentrations in the brain. Jia et al. (2011) prepared EGCG-loaded chitosan nanoparticles using ionic polymeric method, and particles were around 141 nm range. EGCG-loaded chitosan nanoparticles showed initial burst release following a pattern of controlled release up to a 40-h period. Jin et al. (2016) synthesized EGCG-loaded chitosan/β-lactoglobulin nanoparticles. The size of the resulting nanoparticles was observed to be between 100 and 500 nm. It was observed that the EGCG was incorporated with carboxymethyl chitosan and chitosan hydrochloride matrix and was diffused out slowly once the β-lactoglobulin layer was degraded. The sustained release pattern observed for chitosan/β-lactoglobulin nanoparticles makes it an attractive candidate for the effective delivery of EGCG. Jia et al. (2013) synthesized EGCG-loaded nanoparticles to improve EGCG stability and cellular content. The size of the nanoparticles was about 45–55 nm in diameter and it significantly increased the EGCG stability and cellular EGCG content.

16.6 Curcumin

16.6.1 Overview

Curcumin (diferuloylmethane) belongs to polyphenol class found in abundance in the rhizome region of *Curcuma longa.* It shows several different properties such as anti-oxidant, anti-inflammatory, anti-mutagenic, anti-microbial and anti-cancer properties. Several reports have suggested that the methoxy groups present on phenyl rings in curcumin structure areresponsible for having health effects. In traditional Indian and Chinese cultures, curcumin has been extensively used for combatting various pain conditions (Goel et al. 2008; Tianyu et al. 2018).

16.6.2 Mechanism of Action of Curcumin

Studies have suggested curcumin as a treatment option for diabetic neuropathy and associated pain. Various mediators such as TNF-α, superoxides and nitric oxides combining to form peroxynitrite (arising from glucose-induced oxidative injury in diabetes) results in hindering various body's molecular signalling pathways by protein nitration, DNA damage and cell death arising toxic effects on nerve cells. Often the cellular toxicity is because of high level of these nitrates in brain regions. Treatment using curcumin suggested its dual nature: nitric oxide (NO) scavenger and lowering the TNF-α levels and acting as an inhibitor for inducible nitric oxide synthases (iNOS) expression by lipopolysaccharide in the mammary glands, thus playing a pivotal role in lowering inflammation (Sharma et al. 2006).

16.6.3 Pharmacokinetics of Curcumin

The reported oral bioavailability of curcumin is very limited (around 1%) which is because of its quick metabolism in human body. In a study conducted on rats, it was observed that around 75% of curcumin and/or its metabolites were found in faeces, whereas urine had a negligible amount. In another study, oral absorption was found to be around 60% and major amount was excreted in faeces while one-third amount of curcumin was recovered unchanged. Further intravenous and intraperitoneal delivery of curcumin in rats have shown large amounts of various curcumin metabolites such as glucuronides of tetrahydrocurcumin and hexahydrocurcumin in bile (Sharma et al. 2007; Ricky et al. 2007).

16.6.4 Nano-formulations of Curcumin

Jia et al. (2018) synthesized curcumin-loaded poly-PEGMA-DMAEMA-MAO nanoparticles to investigate its effect on diabetic neuropathic pain mediated by the P2Y12 receptor on satellite glial cells in the rat dorsal root ganglia. The prepared nanoparticle-encapsulated curcumin decreased upregulated P2Y12 receptor and the expression of interleukin-1β (IL-1β) and connexin43 (Cx43) and reduced levels of phosphorylated-Akt (p-Akt) in the dorsal root ganglia of rats with diabetes mellitus. Athira and Jyothi (2014) prepared curcumin-loaded starch nanoparticles to improve cellular absorption. Curcumin-incorporated starch nanoparticles were non-toxic to normal cells, and the cellular absorption of curcumin with starch nanoparticles was significantly higher by L929 fibroblasts cells as compared to that of pure curcumin. This incorporation of curcumin in starch nanoparticles showed increasing bioavailability of curcumin in vitro. Joshi et al. (2013) developed self-nano-emulsifying drug delivery system (SNEDDS) for curcumin (which has very poor aqueous solubility). This system enhanced the bioavailability of curcumin, and the maximum plasma concentration was increased from 32.29 ng/ml (aq. curcumin suspension) to 527.01 ng/ml (curcumin-SNEDDS) in the pharmacokinetics studies on rats. Zhang et al. (2016) developed curcumin encapsulated nanoparticles for osteoarthritis-associated pain treatment. Upon oral and topical administration of curcumin nanoparticles on mice experimental models, it was observed that the developed nanoparticles were able to significantly reduce tactile hypersensitivity in response to external mechanical stimulus (von Frey tests) and other neuro-behavioural tests suggest the retention in the chondroprotective nature of curcumin perhaps due to its increased bioavailability onsite.

16.7 Conclusion

This chapter explains some phytocompounds exhibiting medicinal properties, which have been reported for the management of neuropathic pain. The pain that arises after any sort of nerve injury termed as neuropathic pain is a major chronic condition that is still problematic to treat. The conventional analgesics that are being used are non-steroidal anti-inflammatory drugs and opioids that are ineffective clinically in attenuating neuropathic pain. Opioids have many disadvantages such as it is addictive, causes seizures and respiratory depression. Tricyclic anti-depressants and anticonvulsants have also been observed to produce anti-allodynic effects in neuropathic pain. However, these drugs are reported to exhibit a wide range of adverse side effects, which limit their use for the treatment of neuropathic pain. Hence, there is a crucial need to explore for alternative medicine, which can attenuate neuropathic pain effectively with fewer or no side effects. This made the researchers to find a drug from natural sources. Plants such as *Curcuma longa, Camellia sinensis, Tripterygium wilfordii, Capsicum* species and their discussed active compounds might be useful in treating neuropathic pain. However, still more research has to be carried out to discover a potent neuropathic pain reliever of natural origin.

References

Amanda C, Miren E, Jui-Hsien C, Emma B, Marta E, Britta AK, Marta B, Carmen A, Jaume F, Eliana BS, Antoni C, Patric T, Maria LG (2019) Dual-drug loaded nanoparticles of Epigallocatechin-3-gallate (EGCG)/ ascorbic acid enhance therapeutic efficacy of EGCG in a APPswe/PS1dE9 Alzheimer's disease mice model. J Control Release 301:62–75

Art P (2009) Aspirin alternatives salicin containing herbs. Huntington Coll Health Sci 2009:1–2

Athira GK, Jyothi AN (2014) Preparation and characterization of curcumin loaded cassava starch nanoparticles with improved cellular absorption. Int J Pharm Pharm Sci 6:171–176

Attal N, Cruccu G, Baron R, Haanpää M, Hansson P, Jensen TS, Nurmikko T (2010) EFNS guidelines on the pharmacological treatment of neuropathic pain: 2010 revision. Eur J Neurol 17:1113–1e88

Backonja MM, Malan TP, Vanhove GF, Tobias JK (2010) NGX-4010, a high-concentration capsaicin patch, for the treatment of postherpetic neuralgia: a randomized, double-blind, controlled study with an open-label extension. Pain Med 11:600–608

Bimonte S, Cascella M, Schiavone V, Mehrabi-Kermani F, Cuomo A (2017) The roles of epigallocatechin-3-gallate in the treatment of neuropathic pain: an update on preclinical in vivo studies and future perspectives. Drug Des Devel Ther 11:2737–2742

Bosch-Mola M, Homs J, Álvarez-Pérez B, Puig T, Reina F, Verdú E, Boadas-Vaello P (2017) (-)-epigallocatechin-3-gallate antihyperalgesic effect associates with reduced CX3CL1 chemokine expression in spinal cord. Phytother Res 31:340–344

Boyd A, Bleakley C, Hurley DA, Gill C, Hannon-Fletcher M, Bell P, McDonough S (2017) Herbal medicinal products or preparations for neuropathic pain. Cochrane Database Syst Rev 2017(1):CD010528. https://doi.org/10.1002/14651858.CD010528.pub3. PMCID:PMC6464896

Choi JI, Kim WM, Lee HG, Kim YO, Yoon MH (2012) Role of neuronal nitric oxide synthase in the antiallodynic effects of intrathecal EGCG in a neuropathic pain rat model. Neurosci Lett 510:53–57

Choi AY, Kim CT, Park HY, Kim HO, Lee NR, Lee KE, Gwak HS (2013) Pharmacokinetic characteristics of capsaicin-loaded nanoemulsions fabricated with alginate and chitosan. J Agric Food Chem 61:2096–2102

Chris B, Deirdre AH, Chris G, Mary HF, Pamela B, Suzanne M, Adele (2017) Herbal medicinal products or preparations for neuropathic pain. Cochrane Database Syst Rev 2017:1–12

Colloca L, Ludman T, Bouhassira D, Baron R, Dickenson AH, Yarnitsky D, Freeman R, Truini A, Attal N, Finnerup NB, Eccleston C, Kalso E, Bennett DL, Dworkin RH, Raja SN (2017) Neuropathic pain. Nat Rev Dis Primers 3:1–45

Cruccu G, Truini A (2017) A review of neuropathic pain: from guidelines to clinical practice. Pain Ther 6:35–42

Cruccu G, Aziz TZ, Garcia-Larrea L, Hansson P, Jensen TS, Lefaucheur JP, Simpson BA, Taylor RS (2007) EFNS guidelines on neurostimulation therapy for neuropathic pain. Eur J Neurol 14:952–970

Cruccu G, Sommer C, Anand P, Attal N, Baron R, Garcia-Larrea L, Haanpaa M, Jensen TS, Serra J, Treede RD (2010) EFNS guidelines on neuropathic pain assessment: revised 2009. Eur J Neurol 17:1010–1018

Daniela A (2015) Pharmacological treatment of neuropathic pain: review of oral and topical therapy recommendations. Int J Clin Neurosci Mental Health 2:1–8

Derry S, Moore RA (2012) Topical capsaicin (low concentration) for chronic neuropathic pain in adults. Cochrane Database Syst 2012:1–33

Derry S, Rice AS, Cole P, Tan T, Moore RA (2017) Topical capsaicin (high concentration) for chronic neuropathic pain in adults. Cochrane Database Syst Rev 2017(1), Art. No.: CD007393. https://doi.org/10.1002/14651858.CD007393.pub4

Diego F (2017) Pharmacotherapy for neuropathic pain: a review. Pain Ther 6:25–33

Dissanayake AA, Zhang CR, Gaber MK, Nair MG (2017) Salicylic glycosides in salix mucronata with antioxidant and antiinflammatory activities. Nat Prod Commun 12:1934578X1701201126

Dworkin RH, O'Connor AB, Backonja M, Farrar JT, Finnerup NB, Jensen TS, Kalso EA, Loeser JD, Miaskowski C, Nurmikko TJ, Portenoy RK, Rice AS, Stacey BR, Treede RD, Turk DC, Wallace MS (2007) Pharmacologic management of neuropathic pain: evidence-based recommendations. Int Assoc Study Pain 132:237–251

Dworkin RH, O'Connor AB, Kent J, Mackey SC, Raja SN, Stacey BR, Levy RM, Backonja M, Baron R, Harke H, Loeser JD, Treede RD, Turk DC, Wells CD (2013) Interventional management of neuropathic pain: NeuPSIG recommendations. Pain 154:2249–2261

Fattori V, Hohmann MS, Rossaneis AC, Pinho-Ribeiro FA, Verri WA (2016) Capsaicin: current understanding of its mechanisms and therapy of pain and other preclinical and clinical uses. Molecules 21:1–33

Finnerup NB, Attal N, Haroutounian S, McNicol E, Baron R, Dworkin RH, Gilron I, Haanpää M, Hansson P, Jensen TS, Kamerman PR, Lund K, Moore A, Raja SN, Rice AS, Rowbotham M, Sena E, Siddall P, Smith BH, Wallace M (2015) Pharmacotherapy for neuropathic pain in adults: a systematic review and meta-analysis. Lancet Neurol 14:162–173

Forouzanfar F, Hosseinzadeh H (2018) Medicinal herbs in the treatment of neuropathic pain: a review. Iran J Basic Med Sci 21:347–358

Garg G, Adams JD (2012) Treatment of neuropathic pain with plant medicines. Chin J Integr Med 18:565–570

Goel A, Kunnumakkara AB, Aggarwal BB (2008) Curcumin as "Curecumin": from kitchen to clinic. Biochem Pharmacol 75:787–809

Gu Y, Yang M, Tang X, Wang T, Yang D, Zhai G, Liu J (2018) Lipid nanoparticles loading triptolide for transdermal delivery: mechanisms of penetration enhancement and transport properties. J Nanobiotechnol 16:1–14

Haanpää M, Attal N, Backonja M, Baron R, Bennett M, Bouhassira D, Cruccu G, Hansson P, Haythornthwaite JA, Iannetti GD, Jensen TS, Kauppila T, Nurmikko TJ, Rice AS, Rowbotham M, Serra J, Sommer C, Smith BH, Treede RD (2011) NeuPSIG guidelines on neuropathic pain assessment. Pain 152:14–27

James AC, Robert RS, H.-H., Sherry C, Yukihiko H (2001) The pharmacokinetics of EGCG: preclinical and clinical studies. Proc ICOS-2001 2001:103–105

Jensen TS, Ralf B, Maija H, Eija K, John DL, Andrew SCR, Rolf-Detlef T (2011) A new definition of neuropathic pain. Pain 152:2204–2205

Jia LL, Yuan GZ, Xiu HZ, Zhi GA, Xiao YS, Kun LW, Xiao LS (2011) Preparation, characterization, and *In*

Vitro evaluation of EGCG-loaded chitosan nanoparticles. Adv Mater Res 282-283:539–544

Jia Z, Shufang N, Shu W (2013) Epigallocatechin gallate (EGCG) – loaded nanoparticles decrease cholesterol content in THP-1 derived macrophages. FASEB J 2013:224–225

Jia T, Rao J, Zou L, Zhao S, Yi Z, Wu B, Gao Y (2018) Nanoparticle-encapsulated curcumin inhibits diabetic neuropathic pain involving the P2Y12 receptor in the dorsal root ganglia. Front Neurosci 11:755

Jian W, Yu Q, Ri-Sheng Y, Chun-Kui Z, Huang-Hui W, Jia-Ji L, Ting Z, Tao C, Yun-Qing L, Yu-Lin D, Jin-Lian L (2017) The synergistic effect of treatment with triptolide and MK-801 in the rat neuropathic pain model. Mol Pain 13:1–14

Jin L, Hua Y, Han-Joo Y, Hye WK, Xiaochun W, Jinhee L, Sanghoon K (2016) Synthesis and controlled-release properties of chitosan/β-Lactoglobulin nanoparticles as carriers for oral administration of epigallocatechin gallate. Food Sci Biotechnol 25:1583–1590

Joshi RP, Negi G, Kumar A, Pawar YB, Munjal B, Bansal AK, Sharma SS (2013) SNEDDS curcumin formulation leads to enhanced protection from pain and functional deficits associated with diabetic neuropathy: an insight into its mechanism for neuroprotection. Nanomedicine 9:776–785

Kaiser M, Pereira S, Pohl L, Ketelhut S, Kemper B, Gorzelanny C, Galla HJ, Moerschbacher BM, Goycoolea FM (2015) Chitosan encapsulation modulates the effect of capsaicin on the tight junctions of MDCK cells. Nature 5:1–14

Khalatbary AR, Ahmadvand H (2011) Anti-inflammatory effect of the epigallocatechin gallate following spinal cord trauma in rat. Iran Biomed J 15:31

Kuang X, Huang Y, Gu HF, Zu XY, Zou WY, Song ZB, Guo QL (2012) Effects of intrathecal epigallocatechin gallate, an inhibitor of toll-like receptor 4, on chronic neuropathic pain in rats. Eur J Pharmacol 676:51–56

Lewis M, Johnson M (2006) The clinical effectiveness of therapeutic massage for musculoskeletal pain: a systematic review. Physiotherapy 92:146–158

Maclagan T (1879) Salicin and salicylic acid. Lancet 114:179–180

Mailis A, Taenzer P (2012) Evidence-based guideline for neuropathic pain interventional treatments: spinal cord stimulation, intravenous infusions, epidural injections and nerve blocks. Pain Res Manag 17:150–158

Mei LT, Li HC, Dong SZ, Wei FZ, Yong MG, Jun SL (2015) Optimized preparation of capsaicin-loaded nanoparticles gel by Box-Behnken design. Adv Mater Res 1061-1062:359–368

Moulin D, Boulanger A, Clark AJ, Clarke H, Dao T, Finley GA, Furlan A, Gilron I, Gordon A, Morley-Forster PK, Sessle BJ, Squire P, Stinson J, Taenzer P, Velly A, Ware MA, Weinberg EL, Williamson OD (2014) Pharmacological management of chronic neuropathic pain: revised consensus statement from the Canadian Pain Society. Pain Res Manag 19:328–335

Mrudhula B, Padmamalini B, Navamoney A, Baskaran T (2017) Preparation and evaluation of PLGA-coated capsaicin magnetic nanoparticles. Pharm Res 34:1255–1263

Mathhews P, Derry S, Moore A and McQuay H (2009) Topical rubefacients for acute and chronic pain in adults. Cochrane Database Syst Rev 3: https://doi.org/10.1002/14651858.CD007403.pub2

Nagoth JA, John PPR, Antoine L (2015) Capsaicin-capped silver nanoparticles: its kinetics, characterization and biocompatibility assay. Appl Nanosci 5:403–409

O'Neill J, Brock C, Olesen AE, Andresen T, Nilsson M, Dickenson AH (2012) Unravelling the mystery of capsaicin: a tool to understand and treat pain. Pharmacol Rev 64:939–971

Peng W, Jiang XY, Zhu Y, Omari-Siaw E, Deng WW, Yu JN, Zhang WM (2015) Oral delivery of capsaicin using MPEG-PCL nanoparticles. Acta Pharmacol Sin 36:139

Raju DM, Ahsan T, Hosen SZ, Rahman MG, Emran TB, Muhammad M, Uddin N (2015) Evolution of selective COX-2 inhibitor from Alangium salviifolium: an in silico approach. J Appl Pharm Sci 5:089–093

Ramkumar P, Janakiraman K, Sivaraman G, Senthilnathan K, Meganathan V, Saravanan P (2015) Formulation and characterization of epigallocatechin gallate nanoparticles. Indo Am J Pharm Res 5:2231–6876

Rao P, Knaus EE (2008) Evolution of nonsteroidal anti-inflammatory drugs (NSAIDs): cyclooxygenase (COX) inhibition and beyond. J Pharm Pharm Sci 11:81–110

Raposo D, Morgado C, Pereira-Terra P, Tavares I (2015) Nociceptive spinal cord neurons of laminae I–III exhibit oxidative stress damage during diabetic neuropathy which is prevented by early antioxidant treatment with epigallocatechin-gallate (EGCG). Brain Res Bull 110:68–75

Renno WM, Al-Maghrebi M, AlShammari A, George P (2013) (−)-Epigallocatechin-3-gallate (EGCG) attenuates peripheral nerve degeneration in rat sciatic nerve crush injury. Neurochem Int 62:221–231

Ricky AS, William PS, Andreas JG (2007) Pharmacokinetics and pharmacodynamics of curcumin. Mol Targets Therap Uses Curcumin Health Dis 595:453–470

Sawynok J (2005) Topical analgesics in neuropathic pain. Curr Pharm Des 11:2995–3004

Sayanlar J, Guleyupoglu N, Portenoy R, Ashina S (2012) Trigeminal postherpetic neuralgia responsive to treatment with capsaicin 8% topical patch: a case report. J Headache Pain 13:587

Schmid B, Kötter I, Heide L (2001) Pharmacokinetics of salicin after oral administration of a standardised willow bark extract. Eur J Clin Pharmacol 57:387–391

Shang L, Hua M, Xile J, Yuanyuan L, Aihong P, Xuecheng Z, Yimin S (2018) Preparation and characterization of acetylsalicylic acid/chitosan nanoparticles and its antithrombotic effects. Des Monomers Polym 21:172–181

Shao F, Wang G, Xie H, Zhu X, Sun J, A J (2007) Pharmacokinetic study of triptolide, a constituent of immunosuppressive chinese herb medicine, in rats. Biol Pharm Bull 30:702–707

Sharma S, Kulkarni SK, Chopra K (2006) Curcumin, the active principle of turmeric (Curcuma longa), ameliorates diabetic nephropathy in rats. Clin Exp Pharmacol Physiol 33:940–945

Sharma RA, Steward WP, Gescher AJ (2007) Pharmacokinetics and pharmacodynamics of curcumin. In: The molecular targets and therapeutic uses of curcumin in health and disease. Springer, Boston, pp 453–470

Singh AP (2003) Salicin-A natural analgesic. Ethnobotanical Leaflets 2003:8

Smith BH, Torrance N (2012) Epidemiology of neuropathic pain and its impact on quality of life. Curr Pain Headache Rep 16:191–198

Taghizadeh SM, Javan RS (2010) Preparation and investigation of chitosan nanoparticles including salicylic acid as a model for an oral drug delivery system. e-Polymers 36:1618–7229

Tang J, Li ZH, Ge SN, Wang W, Mei XP, Wang W, Li JL (2012) The inhibition of spinal astrocytic JAK2-STAT3 pathway activation correlates with the analgesic effects of triptolide in the rat neuropathic pain model. Evid Based Complement Altern Med 2012: 1–13. https://doi.org/10.1155/2012/185167

Tesfaye S (2009) Advances in the management of diabetic peripheral neuropathy. Curr Opin Support Palliat Care 3:136–143

Tian W, Han XG, Liu YJ, Tang GQ, Liu B, Wang YQ, Xiao B, Xu YF (2013) Intrathecal epigallocatechin gallate treatment improves functional recovery after spinal cord injury by upregulating the expression of BDNF and GDNF. Neurochem Res 38:772–779

Tianyu J, Jingan R, Lifang Z, Shanhong Z, Zhihua Y, Bing W, Lin L, Huilong Y, Liran S, Chunping Z, Yun G, Shuangmei L, Hong X, Hui L, Shangdong L, and Guilin L (2018) Nanoparticle-encapsulated curcumin inhibits diabetic neuropathic pain involving the P2Y12 receptor in the dorsal root ganglia. Front Neurosci 11: 1–1

Treede RD, Troels Jensen S, Campbell JN, Cruccu G, Dostrovsky JO, Griffin JW, Hansson P, Hughes R, Nurmikko T, Jordi S (2008) Neuropathic pain: redefinition and a grading system for clinical and research purposes. Neurology 70:1630–1635

Vane JR, Botting RM (2003) The mechanism of action of aspirin. Thromb Res 110:255–258

VanHecke O, Austin SK, Khan RA, Smith BH, Torrance N (2014) Neuropathic pain in the general population: a systematic review of epidemiological studies. Pain 155:654–662

Wagner I, Heide L (2003) Salicin and treatment of rheumatic diseases. J Rheumatol 30:1125–1125

Wang W, Mei XP, Chen L, Tang J, Li JL, Wu SX, Xu LX, Li YQ (2012) Triptolide prevents and attenuates neuropathic pain via inhibiting central immune response. Pain Physician 15:995–1006

Wang C, Shan Y, Yang J, Xu X, Zhuang B, Fan Y, Xu W (2015) Inhibition of cancer using triptolide nanoparticles. J Biomed Nanotechnol 11:805–815

Woo JO, Misran M, Lee PF, Tan LP (2014) LP development of a controlled release of salicylic acid loaded stearic acid-oleic acid nanoparticles in cream for topical delivery. Sci World J 2014:1–7

Watanabe T, Kawada T, Yamamoto M, Iwai K (1987) Capsaicin, a pungent principle of hot red pepper, evokes catecholamine secretion from the adrenal medulla of anesthetized rats. Biochemical and Biochem Biophys Res Commun 142(1):259–264

Xavier X, Laura VS, Pere BV, Carlos T, Jordi A, Teresa P, Enrique V (2015) Novel epigallocatechin-3-gallate (EGCG) derivative as a new therapeutic strategy for reducing neuropathic pain after chronic constriction nerve injury in mice. PLoS One 10:1–15

Xia RW, Si QG, Xiao QN, Long JL, Xiao YY, Zhong JH, Jian QG (2017) Capsaicin-loaded nanolipoidal carriers for topical application: design, characterization, and in vitro/in vivo evaluation. Int J Nanomedicine 12:3881–3898

Xiong FL, Chen HB, Chang XL, Yang YJ, Xu HB, Yang XL (2005) Research progress of triptolide-loaded nanoparticles delivery systems. Eng Med Biol 5:4966–4969

Xu Y, Zhang YF, Chen XY, Zhong DF (2017) CYP3A4 inducer and inhibitor strongly affect the pharmacokinetics of triptolide and its derivative in rats. Acta Pharmacologica Sinic 39:1386–1392

Zhang Z, Daniel JL, Lin X, Zhiyong H, Angela W, Mahantesh N, Sun JK (2016) Curcumin slows osteoarthritis progression and relieves osteoarthritis-associated pain symptoms in a post-traumatic osteoarthritis mouse model. Arthritis Res Ther 18:128

Zhu B, Wang YJ, Zhu CF, Lin Y, Zhu XL, Wei S, Cheng XX (2010) Triptolide inhibits extracellular matrix protein synthesis by suppressing the Smad2 but not the MAPK pathway in TGF-β1-stimulated NRK-49F cells. Nephrol Dial Transplant 25:3180–3191

Comparison of Therapeutic Efficacy of Nanoformulations of Curcumin *vs* Tetrahydrocurcumin in Various Disorders

17

Vandita Kakkar, Komal Saini, Megha Saini, Manoj Kumar, Priyanka Narula, and Ishaan Duggal

Abstract

The purpose of this chapter is to consolidate the existing data on nanoformulation(s) of two folklore molecules, curcumin and tetrahydrocurcumin (THC). Latter curcuminoids have been explored extensively for their bioactive properties, including anti-inflammatory efficacy to antimicrobial, antioxidant, and chemopreventive effects. In this chapter, an attempt is made to discuss the current state of knowledge regarding the usefulness of nano-based drug delivery of curcumin and THC for various ailments. The mechanisms illustrating their in vitro and in vivo bioavailability in addition to the present clinical status of these molecules will also be considered. Different pharmaceutical nanodosage forms, viz. nanocolloidal dispersions, SMEDDS, SNEDDS, microemulsions, and nanoemulsions, will be compared, as well as the market potential of these formulations along with their predicted shelf life, efficacy, and side effects will also be covered in detail. The objective is to compare the effects of curcumin with those of THC or vice versa depending on the purpose for which it is being administered. Towards the end of the chapter, the regulatory perspective, the scope and futuristic success with these nanoformulations is discussed.

Keywords

Curcumin · Tetrahydrocurcumin · Nanodelivery systems · Bioavailability · Comparative analysis

17.1 Introduction

Curcumin and tetrahydrocurcumin (THC) have been selected as molecules of choice because of their multitargeting and pleiotropic features. The usefulness of these molecules has been proven in several disorders ranging from normal inflammation to cancer, inflammation, microbial diseases, oxidation, and others diseases (Lavor et al. 2018). These phytochemicals are evidenced to be stable, cost effective and exhibit minimal side effects, thus making them suitable candidates to be developed as therapeutics.

Turmeric is a natural plant that is well known for its medicinal properties since Vedic times in India. It has long been used as an edible spice and also is important in religious contexts. The chemical constituent of turmeric, curcumin, is a naturally occurring phytochemical with potential anti-

V. Kakkar (✉) · K. Saini · M. Saini · P. Narula · I. Duggal
Department of Pharmaceutics, University Institute of Pharmaceutical Sciences, Panjab University, Chandigarh, India

M. Kumar
HealthKart, Gurugram, India

S. Talegaonkar, M. Rai (eds.), *Nanoformulations in Human Health*,
https://doi.org/10.1007/978-3-030-41858-8_17

inflammatory effects (Hassan et al. 2019). It is a pleiotropic molecule used as an herbal medicine for the treatment of rheumatoid arthritis, chronic anterior uveitis, conjunctivitis, skin cancer, small pox, chicken pox, wound healing, urinary tract infections, liver disease, dissipating worms, regulating menstruation, dissolving gall stones, cleaning wounds, and various digestive disorders and even bacterial infections (Lal et al. 1999; Liu et al. 2017; Aggarwal et al. 2012). Turmeric contains curcuminoid in the range of 2–9%. Commercial turmeric extracts hold approximately 70–75% curcumin, with about 20% demethoxycurcumin and 5% bisdemethoxycurcumin as structural curcumin analogs (Cavaleri 2018). After per os (p.o.) dosing, curcumin undergoes metabolic O-conjugation to curcumin glucuronide and curcumin sulfate and bioreduction to THC, hexahydrocurcumin, octahydrocurcumin, and hexahydrocurcuminol (Jäger et al. 2014). Over the past three decades, in extensive preclinical studies, curcumin's therapeutic potential has been observed in numerous human disorders (Vollono et al. 2019). Additionally, curcumin has been shown to directly interact with several signaling molecules (Aggarwal et al. 2013), and positive results from preclinical studies form the basis of its evaluation in clinical trials. While the application of curcumin is hindered by its low stability and poor systemic bioavailability, it has been suggested that the biological activities of curcumin are closely related to its metabolites (Aggarwal et al. 2013).

The development of nanocarriers to solubilize or encapsulate curcumin has shown tremendous growth in the last decade. Nanocarriers provide improved solubility, stability, and selective delivery of curcumin to the target site and, hence, an improved pharmacokinetic profile. Systems developed in an attempt to resolve the compromised bioavailability of these phytochemicals (Din et al. 2017), include formulation of micro/nanoparticles (NPs) or capsules, micro/nanoemulsions, nanovesicles, lyotropic liquid vesicles, and foams. Developing these sytems help to improve the stability of these molecule against light degradation, help improve their aqueous solubility, and their permeation. In addition, they are biodegradable and biocompatibile and can encapsulate drugs with high efficiency and provide abundant surface area. Other drug delivery systems that have been reported include lyotropic liquid crystal systems, foams, micelles, hydrogels, and nanofibers (NFs). Lyotropic liquid crystal systems can be lamellar, cubic, or hexagonal mesophases and can be administered via mucosal or topical delivery (Bruschi and Ferreira 2019).

Tetrahydrocurcumin (THC) is a colorless hydrogenated metabolite of curcumin possessing physiological and pharmacological properties analogous to those of innate curcuminoids. THC exhibits excellent antioxidant activity amongst all curcuminoids (Aggarwal et al. 2014). The free radical scavenging ability of THC was significantly greater in series compared to curcumin followed by bisdemethoxycurcumin (Jäger et al. 2014). Despite the distinctive biological activities of these curcuminoids, the major limitation on their broad range of clinical applications lies in their poor bioavailability in systemic circulation in humans, which limits their therapeutic action (Aggarwal et al. 2013).

In this chapter, general comparison is made on the physicochemical profile of curcumin and THC highlighting their structural activity and challenges with respect to oral bioavailability. Further, nanotailoring approaches for both molecules and their potential to treat several ailments are also compared. The chapter ends with a brief discussion on the market potential of these molecules as nutraceuticals owing to the over sightedness of regulators.

17.2 Chemical Structure Characteristics

Curcumin, a bis-α,β-unsaturated β-diketone polyphenol obtained from the rhizome (turmeric) of the herb *Curcuma longa* is widely used as a yellow coloring agent and spice in foods. Curcumin is also known as diferuloyl methane and is a symmetric molecule. The IUPAC name of curcumin is (1E,6E)-1,7-bis(4-hydroxy-3-methoxyphenyl)-1,6-heptadiene-3,5-dione, with chemical formula $C_{21}H_{20}O_6$ and a molecular weight of 368.38. It has three chemical entities in its structure: two aromatic ring systems containing o-methoxy phenolic groups, linked by a seven-carbon linker consisting of an α,β-unsaturated β-diketone moiety (Priyadarsini 2014). The chemical structure of curcumin is given in Fig. 17.1. The diketo group exhibits keto-enol tautomerism, which can be present in different types of conformers based upon the environment. The crystal state exhibits a cis-enol configuration and is stabilized by resonance-assisted hydrogen bonding. The structure is composed of three substituted planar groups linked by two double bonds. The stability of the enol form is greater than that of the keto form by 5–8 kcals mol^{-1} in the case of nonpolar and moderately polar solvents since it is largely dependent on the polarity of the solvent. It shows extended conjugation, with a π electron cloud distributed all over the molecule. The solution phase of curcumin exhibits cis-trans isomerism, where the trans form is marginally more stable than the cis form. Since it is a hydrophobic molecule with a log *P* value of ~3.0, the calculated dipole moment (DP) of curcumin in the ground state is 10.77 D. Due to its hydrophobicity, it is almost insoluble in water and readily soluble in polar solvents like DMSO, methanol, ethanol, acetonitrile, chloroform, ethyl acetate, and others. but sparingly soluble in hydrocarbon solvents like cyclohexane and hexane. Two absorption bands are observed in the absorption spectra in the visible and UV region at 410–430 nm and 265 nm, respectively. The molar extinction coefficient value of curcumin in methanol is 55,000 $dm^3\ mol^{-1}\ cm^{-1}$ at 425 nm. It is a weak Brönsted acid with three pKa values owing to the presence of three labile protons. These pKa values were determined using both the NMR and absorption spectrometry (Priyadarsini 2014). The first pKa changes curcumin from yellow to red within a pH range of 7.5–8.5. Within this range of pH, curcumin shows increased chemical reactivity and solubility and is generally more soluble in water than the neutral form. The fully deprotonated (red) form of curcumin in alkaline pH (pH > 10) shows absorption maxima at 467 nm and a molar extinction coefficient value of 53,000 $dm^3\ mol^{-1}\ cm^{-1}$. However, the spectral changes arising due to a change in pH are difficult to differentiate between the acidic nature of the enolic OH or the phenolic OH groups, even though calculations specify that the enolic OH is the most acidic group. From 1 H-NMR studies, the pKa value for the deprotonation of the enolic proton was suggested to be

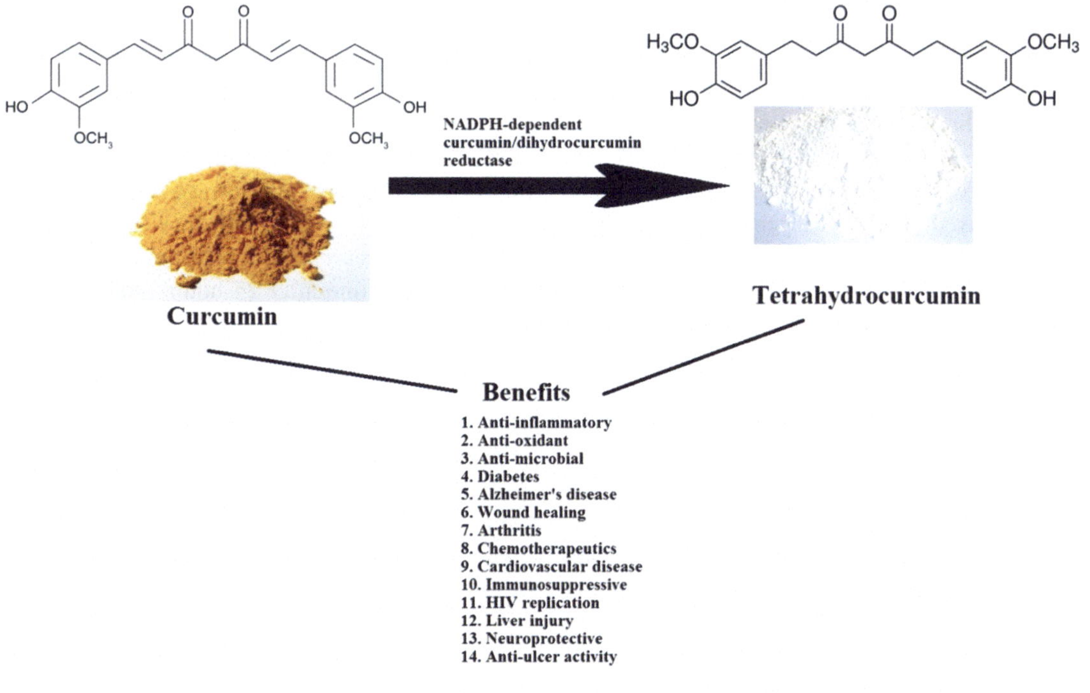

Fig. 17.1 Chemical structural comparison of curcumin and tetrahydrocurcumin (THC)

12.5 and the pKa for the phenolic protons was suggested to be 13.6 (Borsari et al. 2002). These pKa values of enolic protons still show variations compared to values calculated by other additional methods. However, in the near future it will be feasible to resolve variations in these values thanks to the accessibility of other spectroscopic methods.

THC is a metabolite of curcumin that is produced by the selective reduction of alpha-olefinic bonds to the carbonyl group in the diferuloyl backbone. THC is a colorless molecule that is attributed to the disturbance of the chromophore, α, β-unsaturated carbonyl group due to the reduction of the (=) bonds in curcumin. Several methods have been reported for the reduction of α, β-unsaturated carbonyl compounds. Catalytic reduction of curcumin is carried out by palladium (Luiza et al. 1994), hydrosilane mediated by copper (I) salt (Mori et al. 1999), and oxygen-activated palladium catalyst (Alper and Sommovigo 1992) or by raney nickel in the presence of hydrogen in organic solvents. Platinum catalysts, like PtO2, which are costly and have been utilized in curcuminoid reduction (Uehara et al. 1987), so product yields are generally moderate. On the other hand, a low yield of only 14% is obtained by hydrogenation, which is also not region-specific. In addition, this process involves the difficulty of reaction scale-up. Reduction of α, β-unsaturated ketones by hydrogenation with palladium catalysts on charcoal and barium sulfate produces 2-benzyl-1-indanones at pressures up to 5 atm show low reaction selectivity. Alternatively, THC can be derived by the hydrogenation of curcumin in a mixture of acetone and water (95:5) under pressure using a palladium on carbon catalyst. Conversion of curcumin into THC has also been reported using Marchantia polymorpha cells with a yield of 90% in 1 day (Shimoda et al. 2012).

The off-white colored THC obtained has a melting point of 96 °C. The molecular formula and molecular mass of THC are $C_{21}H_{24}O_6$ and 372.4 g/mol, respectively. The pKa value of THC is 2.98, and the molecule is nonplanar with orthogonally placed benzene rings at the ends of a heptane chain with a dihedral angle of 84.09°. The molecular geometry and H-atom locations reveal the existence of a "heptane-3,5-dione" moiety in the keto-enol form. The positioning of the molecules in the lattice is directed by O-H and O intermolecular hydrogen bonds to create two-dimensional sheets (Girija et al. 2004).

THC is more soluble and stable than curcumin at a physiological pH, as well as at basic pH, and in plasma. There is no evidence of decomposition within 2 hours, demonstrating higher stability in aqueous solutions under air (Sato et al. 2008).

17.3 Bioavailability Concerns of Curcumin and THC

One of the major problems with curcumin is its low bioavailability because it is not readily solubilized, is poorly absorbed in the gut, is quickly metabolized, and is excreted from the body. A substance is considered to have poor bioavailability if it has low intrinsic activity in the body. For example, it may show little absorption, be metabolized quickly, have inactive metabolites, or be eliminated quickly from the body (Anand et al. 2007). Undetectable or low levels of curcumin in human blood serum were found when 2 g curcumin was administered to healthy volunteers (Shoba et al. 1998). A study showed that 3.6 g curcumin administered orally gave rise to a 0.0111 μM concentration of curcumin in human plasma after 1 hour. In conjunction with the low bioavailability of curcumin in blood plasma, curcumin is not well distributed in tissue. Anand et al. (2007) reported that after oral administration of 400 mg curcumin to rats, trace levels of curcumin were found in the kidney and liver and only 1% of the curcumin was left in the stomach and small intestine after 24 hours (Anand et al. 2007).

Furthermore, a study conducted on humans with colorectal cancer that had metastasized to the liver showed no curcumin in the liver after oral administration of 450–3600 mg curcumin each day for a week (Anand et al. 2007). Curcumin's poor bioavailability has forced investigators to look for similar anticancer drugs with higher bioavailability. The poor oral absorption of curcumin in both humans and animals has increased the numerous concerns that may limit its clinical impact (Kelloff et al. 1996).

Curcumin is a biphenolic compound having hydroxyl groups at the ortho-position on the two aromatic rings that are connected by a β-diketone bridge, containing two double bonds (dienone), which can undergo Michael addition, critical for some of the effects of curcumin, but contributing to chemical instability in aqueous solution. Pharmacokinetic characterization of curcumin illustrates extensive intestinal sulfation and glucuronidation. Most clinical trials have shown negligible unconjugated curcumin plasma levels post oral dosing, suggesting that its in vivo efficacy is derived from a more bioavailable or effective metabolite (Kelloff et al. 1996). The physicochemical parameters of curcumin and THC are compared in Table 17.1.

THC, an active metabolite of curcumin, is produced by the reduction of dienone double bonds predominantly in the intestinal cells. It is resistant to hydrolysis (Pan et al. 1999), is a potent antioxidant, and possesses anti-inflammatory properties in vitro and in vivo (kidney). Due to these properties and its assumed increased bioavailability, THC has been shown to considerably increase mean and maximum life spans when constantly fed to aging mice (Pan et al. 1999). The functional significance of the dienone bridge of curcumin has also been evaluated by experiments comparing THC and curcumin. To determine the in vivo antioxidant, anti-inflammatory, and antiamyloid activity and the importance of the dienone bridge, effective blood and tissue THC and curcumin levels were studied in an acute inflammatory model and a chronic atopic dermatitis (AD) model. In the acute paradigm models, curcumin and THC were administered through different routes and the researchers examined the distinctive effects of curcumin versus THC on the drug levels in plasma and brain achieved, and effects on the neuroinflammatory responses were also observed. Curcumin metabolism and the effect of chronic dietary administration of curcumin or THC was studied in an aging APPsw transgenic mouse model of AD, and the results showed modified Aβ and inflammatory parameters (Begum et al. 2008). Few studies have been reported on THC that show it to be a better anti-oxidant, anti-inflammatory molecule and better at scavenging free-radicals compared to curcumin (Hassainasab et al. 2011). A 2-week study showed that when both THC and curcumin were incubated in human plasma, THC

Table 17.1 Physicochemical parameters of curcumin and tetrahydrocurcumin (THC)

Properties	Curcumin (Aggarwal et al. 2014)	Tetrahydrocurcumin (Aggarwal et al. 2014; Kakkar et al. 2018a, b)
IUPAC name	(1E,6E)-1,7-bis(4-hydroxy-3-methoxyphenyl)-1,6-heptadiene-3,5-dione	*1,7-bis(4-hydroxy-3-methoxyphenyl)-3,5-heptanedione*
Common name	Curcumin	Tetrahydrocurcumin/white curcumin
Empirical formula	$C_{21}H_{20}O_6$	$C_{21}H_{24}O_6$
Molecular structure	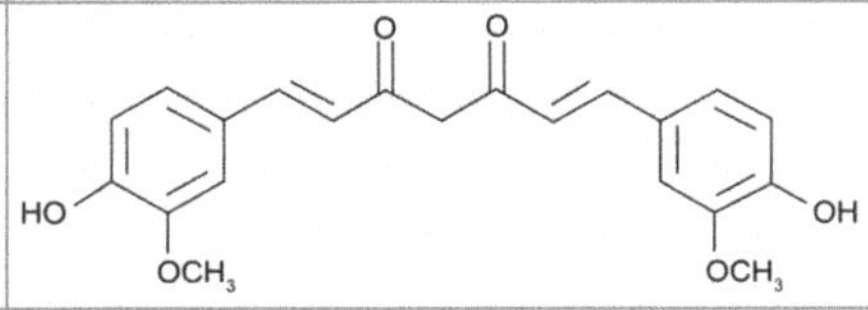	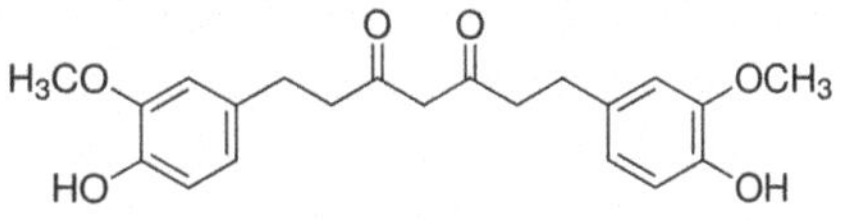
Molecular weight	368.38 g/mol	372.41 g/mol
Appearance	Yellow	Off-white powder
Melting point	183 °C	95–97 °C
Packaging storage	Preserve in tightly closed container	Preserve in tightly closed container
Solubility	Soluble in ethanol, DMSO, methanol, acetic acid	Freely soluble in methanol Soluble in acetone, glacial acetic acid
Water solubility	0.1 mg/mL	0.0056 mg/mL
Log *P*	3.29	2.98
Pka	9.06	9.31
Half-life	7 h	813 min

was reported to be more stable than curcumin with respective recovery rates of 67–77% and 35–45%. The latter is attributed to higher saturation, making it more water soluble, compared to curcumin (Hassainasab et al. 2011). Curcumin is found to be less stable in culture medium than THC by in vitro studies with half-lives of 186 and 813 minutes, respectively (Saradhi et al. 2010). It has been reported that THC is also more readily absorbed in the gastrointestinal tract. Hence, it has been proposed that THC is responsible for curcumin's pharmacological affects in vivo (Kang et al. 2014). Several molecular targets of THC have been identified, including targets that make it effective against cancers. THC activates the antioxidant enzymes NADPH:quinone reductase, glutathione peroxidase, and glutathione S-transferase. Kang et al. (2014) showed that MCF-7 breast cancer cells exhibited mitochondrial apoptosis and G2/M phase arrest in vitro when treated in a dose-dependent manner with 15–112.5 μM THC. The effect is due to increased protein expression of Bax and caspases-3 and -9 due to THC (Kang et al. 2014). Furthermore, THC shows chemopreventive abilities by retarding the development of aberrant crypt foci in the colon (Kim et al. 1998). THC also inhibits colon carcinogenesis by decreasing cancer cell proliferation and inhibiting phosphorylation of ERK1/2 (Lai et al. 2011), making it a better alternative to curcumin. THC was also found to be a stronger anti-angiogenic agent, whereas curcumin was found to have stronger antiproliferation properties when HepG2 cells were treated with both of them (Yoysungmoen et al. 2008). THC effectively increases leukemic cell death through autophagy. In a study by Wu et al. (2014), it was demonstrated that THC inhibits the metastasis of fibrosarcoma by lowering levels of *Matrix metallopeptidases* MMP-2 and MMP-9 in HT1080 cells (Wu et al. 2014).

Phytochemicals derived from natural plants exhibit chemical diversity, with flexible chemical and biological properties exhibiting macromolecular specificity and less toxicity. These make them favorable leads in the discovery of novel drugs. Despite their several advantages, pharmaceutical companies are hesitant to invest more in natural product-based drug discovery and drug delivery systems and are more inclined to instead explore the available chemical compound libraries to discover novel drugs (Pan et al. 2013).

17.4 Nanotailoring Approaches of Curcumin and THC

On the basis of almost decade-long experience with nanobased delivery systems for curcumin and THC, it was evident that these phytochemicals hold an excellent level of therapeutic potential for neurodegenerative diseases, cancer, inflammation not relating to the skin but in general, and several other ailments (Kakkar et al. 2011, 2012, 2013, 2018b; Kakkar and Kaur 2011). Nanotechnology is indeed being used to discover innovative ways to develop these molecules as therapeutic agents, owing to its ability to reduce the therapeutically effective dose and improve its solubility and permeation, thereby enhancing the overall bioavailability of the molecules.

NPs have the ability to increase the bioavailability and solubility of lipophilic compounds such as curcumin/THC in drug delivery systems. Nanobased systems can lead to improved therapeutic effects by encapsulating drugs and protecting them from enzymatic degradation, result in a controlled release and an extended blood circulation time. They can modify the pharmacokinetic profile of drugs, decrease their toxicity, and limit their nonspecific uptake (Patra et al. 2018). Therefore, over the last two decades, there have been tremendous advancements in their involvement as nanocarriers.

Nanotechnology when applied to the field of medicine is referred to as nanomedicine. Nanomedicine involves the use of nanomaterials for the diagnosis, monitoring, control, prevention, and treatment of diseases (Tinkle et al. 2014). Nanomaterials have unique physicochemical properties due to their small size. These properties make them highly useful in drug development, but some concerns pertaining to their safety have been reported. Nanoformulations possess a different pattern of pharmacokinetics, such as absorption, distribution, elimination, and metabolism of the encapsulated drugs, can easily cross the biological barriers, and reduce the amount of doseto be administered, thus reducing the chancing of side effects (Tinkle et al. 2014; Bleeker et al. 2013).

The term nanoparticle is an umbrella word that comprises several delivery systems, i.e., liposomes, polymeric NPs, micelles, nanogels, niosomes, cyclodextrins, dendrimers, silvers, and solid lipids, as useful alternatives for delivering therapeutically effective concentrations of poorly water soluble molecules, i.e., curcumin (Zhao et al. 2016). These systems thus improve their solubility, stability, bioavailability, and metabolism to result in therapeutically effective concentrations for the treatment of cancers, wound healing, Alzheimer's disease, status epilepticus, ischemia, inflammatory diseases, and many more (Negar et al. 2014).

The field of delivery systems has undergone rapid growth in recent years in terms of the targeted delivery of therapeutics or phytochemicals in the treatment of various ailments (Obeid et al. 2017). Minimal toxicity and side effects, reasonable economies, and good therapeutic potential are the reasons for exploring these phytochemicals for their therapeutic use. Curcumin and THC in their natural forms suffer from issues such as low bioavailability and low solubility, leading to poor absorption in the body. In addition, there are issues pertaining to target-specific delivery, tonic effectiveness, and probable adverse effects of drugs in addition to the poor physiological stability of curcumin. Hence, taking into account these issues, new drug delivery systems for targeting drugs to specific body parts might resolve these critical issues. Thus the role of nanotechnology in advanced medicine/drug formulations, targeted delivery, and controlled drug release can be significantly enhanced.

A number of different types of drug delivery systems have been successfully used in recent years; however, owing to certain challenges, the development of an innovative technology needs to be achieved for successful and targeted drug delivery (Martinho et al. 2011). Figure 17.2 illustrates various molecular targets by which cur-

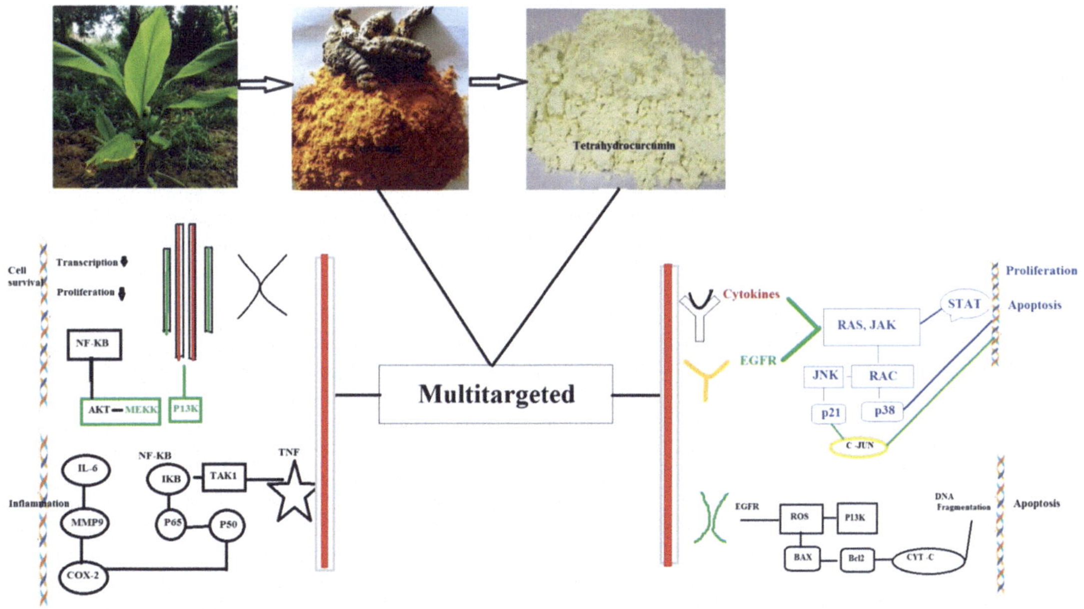

Fig. 17.2 Potential targets of curcumin and tetrahydrocurcumin. Cytokines (IL-1,2,5,6,12,16,17), ROS reactive oxygen species, HO-1 heme oxygenase 1, JNK c-Jun N-terminal kinases, COX-2 cyclooxygenase-2, TNF tumor necrosis factor, NF-Kβ nuclear factor-kappaβ, EGFR epidermal growth factor receptor, STAT signal transducers and activators of transcription, BAX bcl-2-like protein 4

cumin and THC exhibit their therapeutic activities.

The role of these nanobased drug delivery systems in several disorders is summarized in Table 17.2.

17.4.1 Ulcers

Mouth ulcers are painful round or oval sores that occur on mucous membranes of the oral cavity. The general causes of mouth ulcers include nutritional deficiencies like iron, vitamins, especially $B_{12}$and C, poor oral hygiene, infections, stress, indigestion, mechanical injury, food allergies, hormonal imbalance, and skin disease, for example. Mouth ulcers (also referred as aphthous ulcers) can be painful when eating, drinking, or brushing teeth (Daddy et al. 2013; Shashy and Ridley 2000).

THC has been shown to be beneficial in the treatment of disorders like mouth ulcers. Rramaswamy et al. (2018b) prepared PVP-THC composite NF using an electrospinning method, and these NFs have been found to be a potential buccal drug delivery system with higher drug entrapment efficiency. The prepared NF mat showed a drug release of around 91% of the loaded THC within the first 5 minutes of dissolution evaluation, which might be suitable for a buccal delivery system with a higher dissolution rate (Rramaswamy et al. 2018a, b, c).

Curcumin, which shows excellent wound-healing, anticarcinogenic, and antibacterial activities, has also shown effects in mouth ulcers. Thorat et al. (2015) formulated a thermoreversible mucoadhesive gel (TMG) containing curcumin for curing mouth ulcers. With an increase in the concentration of mucoadhesive agent, mucoadhesive force significantly increased. In vitro release showed that formulations delivered the drug for about 4 hours. This showed that the residence time and contact area of curcumin at ulcers could be enhanced along with a sustained release. The authors concluded that a TMG of curcumin can

Table 17.2 Nano-mediated carriers for curcumin and THC for various disorders

Sr. No.	Disease	Drug	Formulation	Route of administration	Reference
1	Mouth ulcers	Curcumin	Thermoreversible mucoadhesive gel	Buccal route	Thorat et al. (2015)
		Tetrahydrocurcumin	Nanofibers	Buccal drug delivery system	Rramaswamy et al. (2018b)
2	HIV	Curcumin	Nanoparticles	Oral	Sankar et al. (2013)
			Silver nanoparticles	Oral	Sharma et al. (2017)
			Nanoparticles	Oral	Gandapu et al. (2011)
		Tetrahydrocurcumin	Vaginal nanomicrobicide	Vaginal	Mirani et al. (2019)
3	Diabetic	Curcumin	SNEDDS	Oral	Joshi et al. (2013)
			Liposomes	Intraperitoneal	Yekollu et al. (2011)
4	Alzheimer's disease	Curcumin	Solid lipid nanoparticles	Oral	Kakkar and Kaur (2011)
			Solid lipid nanoparticles	Oral	Kakkar et al. (2013)
			Nanoparticles	Oral	Ramassamy et al. (2012)
			Nanoparticles	Oral	Cheng et al. (2015)
			Nanoparticles	Oral	Ray et al. (2011)
			Magnetic nanoparticles	Intraperitoneal	Jaruszewski et al. (2014)
			Nanoparticles	Oral	Doggui et al. (2013)
			Nanoparticles	i.v.	Sandhir et al. (2014)
5	Cardiovascular diseases	Curcumin	Nanoparticles	Oral	Wang et al. (2012)
			Nanoparticles	Oral	Carlson et al. (2014)
			Nanoparticles	Oral	Pramanik et al. (2012)
			Nanoparticles	Oral	Deveza et al. (2012)

(continued)

Table 17.2 (continued)

Sr. No.	Disease	Drug	Formulation	Route of administration	Reference
6	Inflammatory diseases	Curcumin	Nanoparticles	Intervention	Singh et al. (2013)
			Nanoparticles	Topical	Beloqui et al. (2014)
			Nano-exosomes	Topical	Shukla et al. (2014)
			Nanoparticles	Topical	Sun et al. (2010)
			Nanoparticulate hydrogel	Topical	Chaudhary et al. (2014)
			Nanoparticles	Oral	Gugulothu et al. (2014)
			Nanoparticles	Oral	Singh et al. (2014)
			Nanoparticles	Topical	Arora et al. (2015)
			Nanoparticles	Topical	Rachmawati et al. (2013)
			Nanoparticles	Topical	Janesirisakule et al. (2013)
			Nanoparticles	Topical	Suwannateep et al. (2013)
			Liposomes	Topical	Castangia et al. (2014)
			Nanoparticles	Topical	Suwannateep et al. (2012)
		Tetrahydrocurcumin	Nanoparticles	Topical	Kakkar et al. (2018a, b)
			Nanofibers	Topical	Rramaswamy et al. (2018c)
7	Antimicrobial activity and wound healing	Curcumin	Nanovesicles	Topical	Dogra et al. (2015)
			Hydrogel	Topical	Gong et al. (2013)
			Nanoparticles	Topical	Krausz et al. (2015)
			Nanoparticles	Topical	Krausz et al. (2015)
			Nanoparticles	Topical	Chereddy et al. (2013)
			Nanofilm	Topical	Li et al. (2012)
			Nanoparticles	Topical	Dai et al. (2017)
		Tetrahydrocurcumin	Nanofibers	Topical	Rramaswamy et al. (2018a)
			Nanofibers	Topical	Goto et al. (2019)
8	Gastrointestinal tract	Curcumin	Solid lipid nanoparticles	Oral	Ji et al. (2016)
		Tetrahydrocurcumin	Liquid THC-SMEDDS	Oral	Sermkaew et al. (2013)
			THC-SEFDDS	Oral	Setthacheewakul et al. (2011)
9	Hepatotoxicity	Curcumin	Nanoparticles	Oral	Marslin et al. (2018)
10	Colorectal cancer	Curcumin	Micelles	i.v.	Gou et al. (2011)
			Nanoparticles	Oral	Udompornmongkol and Chiang (2015)
			Nanoparticles	Oral	Lotfi-Attari et al. (2017)
			Nanoparticles	Oral	Prajakta et al. (2009)
11	Breast cancer	Curcumin	Nanoparticles	Oral	Yallapu et al. (2010)
			Nanoparticles	Oral	Mirakabad et al. (2016)
			Nanoparticles	Oral	Farajzadeh et al. (2018)
			Nanoparticles	Oral	Shutava et al. (2009)
12	Lung cancer	Curcumin	Liposomes	Oral	Ibrahim et al. (2018)
			Nanoparticles	Oral	Lee et al. (2014)
			Nanoparticles	Oral	Yin et al. (2013)
			Nanoparticles	Oral	Khan et al. (2018)
			Nanoparticles	Oral	Kakkar et al. (2012)
13	Malaria	Curcumin	Liposomes	Oral	Coma-cros et al. (2018)
			Nanoparticles	Oral	Nayak et al. (2010), Isacchi et al. (2012), Alam et al. (2016), Akhtar et al. (2012)
14	Osteoporosis	Curcumin	Gold nanoparticles	Oral	Heo et al. (2014)
15	Cystic fibrosis	Curcumin	Nanoparticles	Oral	Cartiera et al. (2010)

be a principal candidate for mouth ulcer treatment (Thorat et al. 2015).

17.4.2 Human Immunodeficiency Virus (HIV)

Acquired immunodeficiency syndrome (AIDS) is a communicable disease caused by infection by the human immunodeficiency virus (HIV). According to recent reports of the Joint United Nations Programme on HIV/AIDS (UNAIDS) in 2015, 34 million people currently live with HIV around the world (UN Joint Programme 2016). Etiologically, sexual transmission is the principal form of HIV spread and is confirmed to be the chief cause in 80% of the total reported cases. This type of transmission of HIV is frequent in females (52% of total infected) due to the absence of women-dependent prophylactic approaches (Ariën et al. 2011).

Currently available treatment is a regimen known as highly active antiretroviral therapy (HAART) (Neves et al. 2010). There are five major types of antiretroviral drugs presently approved for the treatment of AIDS. These are reverse transcriptase inhibitors that contain nucleoside reverse transcriptase inhibitors (NRTIs), nucleotide reverse transcriptase inhibitors (NtRTIs) and nonnucleotide reverse transcriptase inhibitors (NNRTIs), protease inhibitors (PIs), fusion inhibitors, and integrase inhibitors (Wong et al. 2010). The latter act in different phases of the viral life cycle (Gupta and Jain 2010).

Curcumin formulations have shown to be advantageous in treating HIV infection. Formulations releasing curcumin after softening the polymer implants have dual functions of causing minimal implant neuroinflammation and utilizing a novel localized curcumin delivery model (Potter et al. 2014). Sankar et al. (2013) showed that curcumin nanoformulations caused a reduction in arsenic-induced oxidative damage to the brain with significant enhancement in enzymatic and nonenzymatic anti-oxidants (glutathione content (GSH), superoxide dismutase (SOD), catalase, glutathione (GSH) peroxidase, and glutathione (GSH) reductase) and resulted in a decrease in lipid peroxidation (LPO) (Sankar et al. 2013). They reported a simple and direct poly(*N*-isopropyl acrylamide)–based nose-to-brain delivery of curcumin nanoformulation.

Sharma et al. (2017) fabricated curcumin-stabilized silver nanoparticles (Cur-AgNPs) that caused a reduction in the extent of replication of HIV by inhibiting NF-κB nuclear translocation and the expression of proinflammatory cytokines (Sharma et al. 2017).

Gandapu et al. (2011) revealed superior anti-HIV activity of nanocurcumin (IC(50) < 1.75 μM) compared to sol–curcumin (IC(50) = 5.1 μM) by preparing apotransferrin (Apo Tf)–tagged curcumin NPs to improve uptake in T cells through sol–oil chemistry via transferrin-mediated endocytosis. This was attributed to the inhibition of HIV-1-induced expression of Topo II α, IL-1β, COX-2, and others and blockage in the gag region for the synthesis of viral cDNA (Gandapu et al. 2011).

Mirani et al. (2019) designed a THC-based vaginal microbicide as a potential substitute for condoms for unprotected sexual intercourse–associated HIV prevention. It was observed to be stable with a coitus-independent release rate and displayed rapid time-independent intracellular uptake. The results indicate that THC could be an excellent prophylactic agent for HIV/AIDS (Mirani et al. 2019).

17.4.3 Diabetes

Diabetes mellitus is a condition that exhibits high blood glucose levels. It is one of the most prevalent metabolic and chronic disease affecting more than 415 million adults in the world. Over time, ineffective or absent insulin in a person may cause damage to tissues, leading to the development of disabling complications such as renal failure, cardiovascular disease, ketoacidosis, stroke, nerve damage, lower limb amputation, and retinopathy (Wonga et al. 2017). Improved therapeutic outcomes have been reported through NPs and lipid/liposome-based delivery of curcumin for diabetes-related ailments as well as heart, kidney, and liver disease (Maradana et al. 2013).

Self-nanoemulsifying drug delivery systems containing curcumin for diabetic neuropathy were developed and evaluated by Joshi et al. (2013) in male Sprague–Dawley rats (Joshi et al. 2013). Their study showed a greater neuroprotective function as confirmed by a change in the expressions of the evaluated parameters (NF-κB, COX-2, IKK-β, iNOS, IL-6, and TNF-α). Reductions in C-reactive protein levels, IL-6, and tumor necrosis factor (TNF) were observed in streptozotocin-induced diabetic rats using a PLGA-curcumin nanoformulation. Considerable lessening of plasma triglycerides and total cholesterol in addition to high-density lipoprotein (HDL) cholesterol enhancement were also observed (Devadasu et al. 2011).

Yekollu et al. (2011) reported a targeted inflammatory approach for type 2 diabetes by preparing curcumin-loaded liposomes for improved insulin resistance in a leptin-deficient (ob/ob) mouse model. Proinflammatory pathways were inhibited in hepatic TNF, inducible nitric oxide (NO) synthase-producing dendritic cells, as well as adipose tissue macrophages (ATMs) (Yekollu et al. 2011). There were no direct study reports on the effects of THC on alleviating diabetes.

17.4.4 Neurodegenerative Disorders

Several strategic approaches to bypassing the blood-brain barrier (BBB) have been explored and reported by researchers across the globe. In one study, the authors functionalized NPs using apolipoprotein E (ApoE)-originated peptides (141–150 residues) to reach targeting (Re et al. 2011).

One neurodegenerative disease is Alzheimer's disease, which involves progressive neurodegeneration and is characterized by the presence of amyloid-β (Aβ) accumulation and intraneuronal neurofibrillary tangles (Apetz et al. 2014; Tsai et al. 2014). Curcumin can be used as a targeting moiety for amyloid pathology, so delivering its bioavailable form has received considerable attention. Further, being fluorescent in nature, it can be used for both therapeutic and diagnostic purposes (Lee et al. 2013).

The effect of curcumin-loaded solid lipid nanoparticles (SLNs) in an $AlCl_3$ mouse model of Alzheimer's disease was demonstrated by the authors (Kakkar and Kaur 2011). The SLNs revealed a 97% and 73% rate of recovery in lipid peroxidation (LPO) and acetylcholinesterase (AchE) with a dose of 50 mg/kg, respectively. Morris water maze (MWM) experiment observations showed much better upgrading using SLNs administered orally (50 mg/kg and 1 mg/kg, respectively) (Kakkar and Kaur 2011). We further confirmed, via confocal microscopy, the presence of fluorescent NPs in the plasma and brain representing the efficient penetration of oral SLNs across the gut wall and BBB. The AUC for SLNs was 8.1 times higher compared to the AUC of free curcumin. Also, a 30-fold increase in curcumin accumulation in the brain was assigned to curcumin loaded SLNs in comparison to free curcumin (Kakkar et al. 2013).

Ramassamy et al. (2012) reported the neuronal uptake and neuroprorective effects of developed biodegradable PLGA–curcumin nanoformulations. They reported the prevention of induction of the redox-sensitive transcription factor Nrf2 in the presence of H_2O_2, to offer protection to neurons against damage caused by the use of free radical generation in Alzheimer's disease (Ramassamy et al. 2012). In another study, a NanoCurc™ formulation showed a lowering of H_2O_2 levels, an increase in GSH levels, and reduced levels of caspase 3 and caspase 7 activity in athymic mouse brain, suggesting a potential redox intracellular environment and proposing it as a potential product for Alzheimer's disease treatment (Ray et al. 2011).

Similarly, another study reported the reversal of neurotoxicity induced by acrolein using PLGA-based curcumin nanoformulations. This reversal was attributed to the restoration of γ-glutamylcysteine synthetase (GCH) expression, ROS, and reactive nitrogen species levels but had no effect on the decrease of glutathione (GSH) and on the elevation of protein carbonyls (Doggui et al. 2013).

A research study reporting on the usefulness of superparamagnetic iron oxide conjugated with curcumin demonstrated its ability to be detected in the amyloid plaques in Tg2576 mouse brains using ex vivo magnetic resonance imaging (MRI) (Cheng et al. 2015). The researchers observed the accumulation and colocalization of NPs in mouse brain in the presence of amyloid plaques in immunohistochemical examination. In essence, their formulation could be used effectively for the noninvasive diagnosis of Alzheimer's disease via MRI over positron emission tomography (PET) scan imaging. Some researchers have used anti-amyloid antibody-conjugated, and curcumin/dexamethasone-loaded gadolinium/magnetic NPs for early analysis, efficient targeting, and as therapeutic agents of cerebrovascular amyloid (Jaruszewski et al. 2014).

Attenuation of 3-nitropropionic-acid (NPA)-induced Huntington's disease (HD) in rats was illustrated by another curcumin SLN formulation due to increased complex II activity, which restored the GSH and SOD. Involvement of ameliorated mitochondrial dysfunctions in HD was attributed to the lowering of mitochondrial swelling, LPO, protein carbonyls, and ROS (Sandhir et al. 2014). To the best of our knowledge there are no reports on the usefulness of THC in AD.

17.4.5 Cardiovascular Diseases

Cardiovascular disease generally refers to conditions that involve narrowed or blocked blood vessels that can lead to a heart attack, chest pain (angina), or stroke. The current nanobased research explores new technologies and treatment strategies curbing the limitations of conventional therapies for consolidating future pharmacological, clinical, and therapeutic prospects in this area (Khodabandehloo et al. 2016; Kumari et al. 2016; Kaushik et al. 2014; Ali et al. 2011). Curcumin's role in the prevention and cure of cardiovascular illness has been reported; however, no such reports for THC exist to date.

A self-assembled curcumin loaded in amphiphilic carbomethyl-hexanol chitosan nanomatrix was reported by Wang et al. (2012). They demostrated an.efficient therapeutic approach to inhibit the migration and growth of vascular smooth muscle cells (VSMCs) via a low-dose sustained elution of demethoxycurcumin (DMC), through a self-assembled amphiphilic carbomethyl-hexanol chitosan (CHC) nanomatrix. Further they reported the cellular internalization and controlled cytotoxic effect of DMC-CHC nanoparticles over the VSMCs. Pluronic loaded nanocurcumin formulation diminished the severe cardiotoxicity caused by doxorubicin hydrochloride (DOX) by reducing apoptosis and ROS levels (Carlson et al. 2014). Pramanik et al. (2012) further illustrated that the nanocurcumin formulation could overcome multidrug resistance (MDR) in cancer cells and ameliorate doxorubicin-associated cardiomyopathy due to a decline in DOX-induced intracellular oxidative stress (an indicator of total GSH levels and GSH peroxidase activity) in cardiac tissue. Angiogenesis plays a fundamental role in atherosclerosis and other cardiovascular diseases worldwide (Deveza et al. 2012). Curcumin in poly(ester amine) NPs revealed novel anti-angiogenesis therapy by inhibiting angiogenesis in a transgenic zebra fish model (Ding et al. 2014).

17.4.6 Inflammatory Diseases

Inflammation is one of the body's defensive biological reactions to several harmful infections and is elucidated in most of the disorders. Curcumin and its nanoformulations have shown to have several intrinsic properties like anti-inflammatory, anti-oxidative, and neuro-protective properties (Aggarwal et al. 2014).

Curcumin nanoformulations revealed subdued lipopolysaccharide (LPS)-induced inflammation in rat model (Singh et al. 2013) independently of the administered concentration. No adverse effects were observed as measured by blood as well as brain lactic acid concentrations, kidney function, or neuronal apoptosis. In another study, the author showed the ability of a PLGA-Eudragit®S100-based nanoformulation of curcumin to decrease the secretion of TNF-α by

LPS-activated macrophages (J774 cells) (Beloqui et al. 2014). The results of in vivo studies showed a drop in neutrophil infiltration and TNF-α discharge in a murine dextran sulfate sodium–induced colitis model representing an appropriate treatment mode for inflammatory bowel disease (IBD) (Beloqui et al. 2014).

In another study by Shukla et al. (2014), LPS-induced lung- and liver-associated injury in rats was inhibited by the nanoemulsion of curcumin due to its ability to minimize the migration of neutrophils, a reduction in levels of TNF-α, and finally oxidative stress. Curcumin delivery mediated by exosomes was also found to be competent in myeloid cells activation in septic shock mouse model induced by LPS (Sun et al. 2010).

Chaudhary et al. (2014) prepared a nanocarrier transdermal gel of curcumin for localized inflammation, and it was found to be a nonirritant (skin irritation scored 0.49) and safe for human use (Chaudhary et al. 2014). Reduction in IL-1β expression and serum proinflammatory cytokines (IL-6, TNF-α, and IL-1β), inflammation (cytokine IL-10), and suppressed NF-κB activation and IκBα degradation levels was established by curcumin-loaded SLNs signifying sepsis treatment (Wang et al. 2015). In another study therapeutic efficacy was achieved using a combination of celecoxib and curcumin in nano form in rats in an ulcerative colitis model (Gugulothu et al. 2014). Curcumin SLNs have also been tested for hepatoprotection (Singh et al. 2014). This was confirmed by examining (i) the extent of liver damage and repair, (ii) concentrations of alanine aminotransferase (ALT) and aspartate aminotransferase (AST), (iii) OS markers (malondialdehyde, SOD, and reduced GSH), and (iv) TNF-α, in a carbon tetrachloride-induced hepatic injury rat model.

Curcumin SLNs also hold potential for the treatment of rheumatoid arthritis that is a chronic inflammatory disease occurring in joints and cartilages. A study by Arora et al. (2015) confirmed the utility of curcumin SLNs in complete Freund's adjuvant-induced arthritis rat model (Arora et al. 2015). The results in arthritic rat model showed a significant boost in (i) white blood cell count, (ii) oxidative-nitrosative stress, (iii) TNF-α and C-reactive protein, (iv) cyclic citrullinated peptide antibody levels, and (v) radiological alterations, hence showing protective effects.

Rachmawati et al. (2013) prepared a NP complex of β-cyclodextrin–curcumin for improving permeability across skin model tissue by 1.8 times in gel form compared to free CUR gel (Rachmawati et al. 2013). No improved penetration across pig skin dermis via hair follicles was observed in a study by Janesirisakule et al. (2013), who prepared a curcumin PVA nanoformulation (Janesirisakule et al. 2013). Ethyl cellulose and methylcellulose blended curcumin NPs have been utilized for the efficient transportation of curcumin into porcine ear skin (Suwannateep et al. 2013). Castangia et al. (2014) formulated biocompatible curcumin-loaded phospholipid vesicles that showed their efficacy in phorbol ester 12-O-tetradecanoylphorbol-13-acetate (TPA)-induced lesions as well as inflammation (Castangia et al. 2014). This finding was subsequently further verified by a wide spectrum of re-epithelialization in TPA-damaged skin. Another study showed that encapsulated curcumin NPs enter into the skin and later slow down the UVB-irradiation-induced radical formation more than curcumin that is present in free form (Suwannateep et al. 2012).

AD or eczema is a chronic inflammatory itchy disease that starts early in life. Kakkar et al. (2018a, b) prepared THC-loaded lipidic NPs using a microemulsification technique. It was found that THC-SLNs gel showed significantly better ($p \leq 0.001$) activity than free THC in gel. Because inflammation is innate to all skin disorders, the developed product opens up new therapeutic avenues for several skin diseases (Kakkar et al. 2018a, b).

Rramaswamy et al. (2018a, b, c) developed a simple composite electrospun NF made of cellulose acetate phthalate (CAP)-polyethylene glycol (PEG) loaded with THC. It was found that the formulated THC-loaded CAP + PEG NF showed an anomalous mechanism, demonstrating both diffusion and swelling controlled modes. The drug release extended up to 12 hours with a final cumulative release of 94.24% (Rramaswamy et al. 2018c).

17.4.7 Antimicrobial Activity and Wound Healing

Wound healing represents a dynamic set of coordinated physiological processes observed in response to tissue injury. Several natural products are known to accelerate the process of wound healing (Bhaskar Rao et al. 2015). Curcumin has been well known for centuries as a home therapy that has antimicrobial properties (Moghadamtousi et al. 2014). Additionally, the wound healing activity of curcumin aids in increased granulation tissue formation, collagen deposition, tissue remodeling, and wound contraction (Akbik et al. 2014). Nanoformulations of THC and curcumin have shown equivalent therapeutic efficacy in wound healing animal models in our lab. We can thus forsee these molecules to reach the market once the clinical studies have been performed (Kakkar et al. 2018a, b).

Dogra et al. (2015) prepared curcumin nanovesicles for binding efficacy to the surface of bacteria and showed a decline from 5 log CFU mL^{-1} to an untraceable level, suggesting a new process for controlling microbial growth, cross contamination, and biofilm formation (Dogra et al. 2015).

Gong et al. (2013) prepared a curcumin-loaded biodegradable in situ gel that supported tissue adhesiveness to release curcumin in a sustained mode for wound healing treatment (Gong et al. 2013). In vivo wound healing activity was studied in the epidermis, and an increase in collagen content, granulation, wound maturity, and catalase content was established by this gel formulation, and a decrease in SOD was observed.

Krausz et al. (2015) reported the dose-dependent inhibition of methicillin-resistant *S. aureus* (MRSA) and *P. aeruginosa* by curcumin-encapsulated NPs (Krausz et al. 2015). A murine wound model showed MRSA growth inhibition and enhancement of wound healing activity. One combination of curcumin NPs with a silver and chitosan formulation was efficient in eliminating parasites from stool and intestine in *Giardia lamblia* cyst rat model (Said et al. 2012). The treatment produced no signs of undesired toxicity.

Chereddy et al. (2013) prepared PLGA NPs encapsulating curcumin that could potentially greatly accelerate wound healing. PLGA–curcumin NPs showed twofold higher wound healing activity in a mouse model in comparison with PLGA or curcumin. Histology and reverse transcription polymerase chain reaction (RT-PCR) studies confirmed that PLGA–curcumin NPs exhibited higher re-epithelialization, granulation tissue formation, and anti-inflammatory potential. PLGA NPs offered various benefits for the encapsulated curcumin, such as protection from light degradation and enhanced water solubility, and showed a sustained release of curcumin over a period of 8 days. As a result, the study demonstrated the additive effect of lactic acid from PLGA and encapsulated curcumin for the active healing of wounds (Chereddy et al. 2013).

Li et al. (2012) studied the curcumin nanoformulation-loaded methoxy poly(ethylene glycol)-graft-chitosan film (curcumin-MPEG-chitosan film) and its applicability that showed the effectiveness of curcumin-MPEG chitosan film in wound healing (Li et al. 2012). In another study, Dai et al. (2017) presented a simple methodology to engineer a smart integrated system that could act as a mechanically competent carrier to topically deliver bioactive curcumin to wounds to improve healing (Dai et al. 2017).

In the case of THC, Rramaswamy et al. (2018a, b, c) developed THC-loaded polycaprolactone (PCL)- PEG composite electrospun NF and hybridized as a transdermal patch for wound healing. As a result, a transdermal NF patch showed that the formulated NF mats with the specific polymeric and drug ratios could be used to hybridize the prepared NFs as transdermal patches (Rramaswamy et al. 2018a).

Goto et al. (2019) prepared freeze-dried Sac/SDACNF (1:1) pellets containing a THC/HP-β-CD complex for increasing the antioxidant activity of the drug by increasing its solubility. In particular, freeze-dried Sac/SDACNF (1:1) pellets can be used as an effectual wound dressing biomaterial to deliver THC that is complexed with HP- β-CD. It has been suggested that freeze-dried Sac/SDACNF (1:1) pellets containing the THC/HP-β-CD complex has the potential for use as a new transdermal therapeutic system, from the perspective of wound healing activity with a slow release of the THC and the usability of pellets (Goto et al. 2019).

17.4.8 Gastrointestinal Tract

When coming in contact with our gastrointestinal tract, NPs can cause drastic changes to our cells, tissues, and organs because they are prone to be "influenced" by these nanomaterials in largely undiscovered ways (Karavolos and Holban 2016). Owing to the low aqueous solubility of lipophilic drugs, oral delivery of such compounds is a challenging task. In such cases, the oral absorption of lipophilic drugs can be improved by using a self-emulsifying drug delivery system (SEDDS) to design formulations. Sermkaew et al. (2013) prepared self-microemulsifying floating tablets of THC. The optimized formulation showed good floating behavior along with more controlled drug release in comparison to other formulations. The authors illustrated the potential use of a new solid self-microemulsifying system for oral delivery of THC (Sermkaew et al. 2013). Similarly, Setthacheewakul et al. (2011) prepared floating pellets of THC with 70% mixtures of two surfactants, Cremophor EL and Labrasol (1:1), and 30% mixtures of oil/ Labrafac PG and Capryol 90 (1:1) with silicon dioxide, Compritol®ATO888, pregelatinized starch, sodium starch glycolate, and microcrystalline cellulose, for example. These floating pellets may give a useful solid lipid-based dosage form of THC and other hydrophobic compounds for oral delivery (Setthacheewakul et al. 2011).

Ji et al. (2016) formulated the SLNs of curcumin with Brij 78 and TPGS to inhibit a P-glycoprotein efflux pump. Their i n vivo pharmacokinetic study revealed AUC0→t for Cur-SLNs to be 12.27-folds greater than curcumin suspension and the relative bioavailability of Cur-SLNs was 942.53%. They showed Tmax and t1/2 of curcumin for Cur-SLNs were delayed compared to the suspensions ($p < 0.01$). Further, in situ intestinal absorption study revealed that the effective permeability (Peff) value of curcumin for SLNs was significantly improved ($p < 0.01$) compared to curcumin solution. It was concluded that the Cur-SLNs with TPGS and Brij78 could improve the oral bioavailability and intestinal absorption of curcumin effectively (Ji et al. 2016).

17.4.9 Hepatotoxicity

The liver is the second major organ that infiltrates and biotransforms all received chemicals and fluids. Liver diseases are generally caused by toxic chemicals, excessive intake of alcohol, infections, and autoimmune disorders. Hepatotoxicity due to drug intake appears to be a common contributing factor. Phytochemicals have shown significant hepatoprotective effects and are generally preferred over allopathic medications owing to their economics, better cultural acceptability, improved compatibility with the human body, and minimal side effects (Kumar and Mohan 2015).

Marslin et al. (2018) reported the usefulness of PLGA- and PLA-encapsulated curcumin NPs in protecting Wistar rats against carbon tetrachloride (CCl_4)-induced subacute hepatotoxicity. Nanoformulations were found to be very effective in terms of the behavioral, biochemical, and histochemical examination of liver (Marslin et al. 2018).

In another study, Pari and Amali (2005) studied the effects of THC and curcumin against chloroquine (CQ)-induced toxicity. They reported that THC, being a metabolic product of curcumin, has greater effects in terms of attenuation of CQ-induced lipid peroxidation than curcumin (Pari and Amali 2005).

17.4.10 Various Cancers

17.4.10.1 Colorectal Cancer

With more than 1.8 million new cases and resulting in almost 861,000 deaths in 2018, colorectal cancer is among the most common cancer affecting humans (WHO 2018). While treatment approaches like surgery, chemotherapy, radiotherapy, immunotherapy, and photothermic therapy have resulted in lower mortality rates following cancer, but chemotherapy-associated side effects occur generally due to their harmful effects on healthy tissue cells. Moreover, it has also been observed that cancer cells have the ability to develop resistance to chemotherapy and radiotherapy over time (Yallapu et al. 2015). Thus, herbal drugs like curcumin and their nanoformulations have now emerged as a plausible option with added advantages of fewer or less severe side effects. Gou et al. (2011) incorporated curcumin into biodegradable monomethoxy poly(ethylene glycol) poly(lactide) copolymer (MPEG-PLA) micelles, and this resulted in improvements in the pharmacokinetic parameters and efficient inhibition of tumor cell-induced angiogenesis compared to that of free curcumin (Gou et al. 2011). In a different study, curcumin encapsulated in chitosan and gum arabic NPs using an emulsification solvent diffusion method imparted potent anticolorectal cancer activities against HCT116 and HT29 cell lines (Udompornmongkol and Chiang 2015).

Additionally, in another study, curcumin and chrysin were co-encapsulated in PEGylated PLGA NPs and their synergistic inhibitory effects against Caco-2 cancer cells were investigated. It was revealed by Rt-PCR that curcumin, chrysin, and their combinations could inhibit human telomerase reverse transcriptase (hTERT) gene expression (Lotfi-Attari et al. 2017). Prajakta et al. (2009) designed pH-sensitive polymeric NPs of curcumin using Eudragit® S100 for the treatment of colon cancer. It was determined that the IC50, i.e. the concentration of the drug moiety per formulation required to kill 50% of the cells in a given period, was 5 M for polymeric NPs compared to 50 M for free curcumin, thereby indicating the better cytotoxic action of polymeric NPs in comparison to plain curcumin (Prajakta et al. 2009). While a lot of work has already been done on curcumin in colorectal cancer, THC remains unexplored, and little data are available on its nanoformulations in cancer treatment.

17.4.10.2 Breast Cancer

With one in eight women in the United States (USA) predicted to develop breast cancer, this cancer is a concern to the vast majority of the female population. Breast cancer is the second largest cause of cancer-related deaths in women (Liu and Chen 2013). Though drugs including doxorubicin, etoposide, and paclitaxel are commercially available, their use is associated with high recurrence rate, low survival rates, and a significant decrease in quality of life after treatment. As a result, complementary and alternative medicines have been explored that could produce positive results without the associated side effects. Curcumin offers a good option for treating the cancer owing to its low nonspecific danger to normal cells. Curcumin affects different biochemical pathways responsible for the proliferation and survival of malignant cells by acting on different molecular targets. It is involved in blocking NF-κB activation, which is associated with the proliferation, invasion, and potentiation of apoptosis (Reuter et al. 2011). Yallapu et al. (2010) prepared poly(lactic-*co*-glycolide)-loaded curcumin NPs that showed a substantial increase in cellular uptake performed in cisplatin-resistant A2780CP ovarian and metastatic MDA-MB-231 breast cancer cells compared to plain curcumin (Yallapu et al. 2010). Mirakabad et al. (2016) compared the cytotoxic effects of curcumin with PLGA-PEG-encapsulated curcumin NPs and observed their greater cytotoxicity against MCF-7 breast cancer lines compared to curcumin perse (Mirakabad et al. 2016).

Furthermore, Farajzadeh et al. (2018) prepared curcumin- and metformin-encapsulated PLGA/PEG NPs using the double emulsion method and the combination was found to exhibit superior anticancer properties in comparison to individual drugs. A synergistic action between the two drugs was recorded as the combination exhibited hTERT to a greater degree than either free drug (Farajzadeh et al. 2018). Zeighamian et al. (2016) fabricated curcumin-encapsulated poly(N-isopropylacrylamideco-methacrylic acid) (PNIPAAm–MAA) NPs using a free radical mechanism and showed an increased cytotoxic effect on the MCF-7 cell line, which powerfully inhibited the growth of the breast cancer cell population, in comparison with the curcumin in free form (Zeighamian et al. 2016). Newer approaches, including the layer-by-layer deposition of polyelectrolytes (polystyrene sulfonate/polyallylamine hydrochloride, polyglutamic acid/

poly-l-lysine, dextran sulfate/protamine sulfate, and carboxymethyl cellulose/gelatin loaded with curcumin), can establish to be advantageous in the treatment of breast cancer and in the blockage of hepatocyte growth factor-induced signaling in the breast cancer cell line, MDA-MB-231 (Shutava et al. 2009). Though there are few reports on the anticancer effects of THC, efficacy of nanoformulations of THC are not available.

17.4.10.3 Lung Cancer

Lung cancer is the most common cancer in men and is among the four main cancers in women. It is an aggressive and progressively deadly disease with few treatment options and poor overall survival rates. While systemic chemotherapy does show some promise, it is associated with unavoidable toxicity without satisfactory treatment effects. Therefore, it is important to identify potential drugs and explore more efficient therapeutic strategies for the treatment of lung cancer.

Ibrahim et al. (2018) prepared lipid-based curcumin-loaded liposomes (marinosomes) utilizing a modified thin drug-lipid film hydration method supplemented by extrusion or sonication. These marinosomes exhibit high physicochemical and oxidative stability and showed effective anticancer effects on A549 and HUVEC cells (Ibrahim et al. 2018). In another study, Lee et al. (2014) synthesized curcumin micellar nanoparticles (Cur-NPs) using a homogenization method and subsequently evaluated their cytotoxic effects against non-small-cell lung cancer, human lung carcinoma (A549), and human lung adenocarcinoma (Calu-3). They reported that Cur-NPs were superior to raw curcumin in killing lung cancer cells (Lee et al. 2014). Yin et al. (2013) fabricated curcumin-loaded NPs using amphilic methoxy poly(ethylene glycol)–polycarbonate block copolymers using in vitro studies to show that the NPs had significant effects on A549 cells compared to plain drug (Yin et al. 2013). In a study report on biodegradable curcumin-loaded poly(lactic-co-glycolic acid) PLGA NPs fabricated using a solvent evaporation technique a significant lowering of increased levels of hypoxia-inducible factor (HIF)-1α and nuclear p65 proved their efficacy (Khan et al. 2018). Kakkar et al. (2012) synthesized curcumin-loaded NPs and found them to have potent action in the A549 cancer cell line because there was a several-fold reduction in IC50 values (Kakkar et al. 2012). While it is believed that THC shows anticancer actions similar to curcumin, not much work has been reported or published in this area.

17.4.11 Malaria

The World Health Organization (WHO) estimates that around 219 million people have been infected with malaria and about a half million deaths happen because of it in 2017 (Potter et al. 2014). Malaria is a parasitic infection caused by different species of *Plasmodium* and transmitted via the bites of infected mosquitoes. Coma-cros et al. (2018) fabricated curcumin-loaded Eudragit nutriosomes, and these nutrisomes enhanced the survival of all *Plasmodium yoelii* in comparison to free drug (Coma-cros et al. 2018). Nayak et al. (2010) prepared a parenteral formulation incorporating curcumin-based SLNs, which caused a twofold increase in antimalarial activity over free curcumin (Nayak et al. 2010). Several other formulations, like curcumin-encapsulated PEGylated liposomes, curcumin-based phenylalanine–α,β-dehydrophenylalanine nanotubes, and chitosan-bound curcumin nanoformulations, have also shown promise as antimalarial agents (Isacchi et al. 2012; Alam et al. 2016; Akhtar et al. 2012).

17.4.12 Osteoporosis

Osteoporosis is a condition associated with a weakening of bones where the bones become fragile and likely to break. Curcumin and its nanoformulations have shown promise as anti-osteoporotic agents. Heo et al. (2014) synthesized cyclodextrin-conjugated gold NPs self-assembled with curcumin to slow down the osteoclast formation of bone marrow-derived macrophages by suppressing the receptor activator of NF-κB ligand-induced signaling pathways

(Heo et al. 2014). It was determined that this formulation improved bone density and could be a promising anti-osteoporotic agent. THC has been relatively unexplored and little work has been done to evaluate its anti-osteoporotic activity.

17.4.13 Cystic Fibrosis

Cystic fibrosis is associated with retention of ΔF508-CFTR in the endoplasmic reticulum and absence of CFTR Cl(−) channels due to mutations in the gene encoding the cystic fibrosis transmembrane conductance regulator (CFTR). Curcumin has shown potential in treating this life-threatening disease (Egan et al. 2004; Lipecka et al. 2006). Cartiera et al. (2010) designed a PLGA-based curcumin nanoparticle formulation that was found to be effective against symptoms of cystic fibrosis in two different mouse strains (Cartiera et al. 2010). Additionally, it was established that a formulation with a merging of PLGA-*b*-PEG-triphenylphosphonium could target mitochondria and be used in mitochondrial-associated diseases (Sharma et al. 2012).

17.5 Clinical Status of Curcumin and THC

Extensive research data accumulated over the past half-century indicate that curcumin, a component of the golden spice turmeric, can modify multiple cell signaling pathways. The nutraceutical has been found to have pharmacokinetic action, be safe, and be effective against numerous diseases in humans.

Human clinical trials show safety, tolerability, and nontoxicity of curcumin at high doses (Vogel and Pelletier 1815). It was found that the administration of curcumin at a dose as high as 8 g/day in combination with gemcitabine was safe and well tolerated in patients with pancreatic cancer (Kanai et al. 2011). Curcumin has been reported to hold therapeutic promise against a wide range of human diseases as per the clinical trial reports conducted so far and to be effective against hepatic conditions, chronic arsenic exposure, and alcohol intoxication. In these clinical trials, curcumin was used either alone or in combination with other agents such as quercetin, gemcitabine, piperine, docetaxel, soy isoflavones, bioperine, sulfasalazine, mesalamine, prednisone, lactoferrin, N-acetylcysteine, and pantoprazole. The multitargeting potential of curcumin has been a mystery for scientists. However, abundant lines of evidence have indicated curcumin's ability in human subjects to modulate multiple cell signaling molecules such as proinflammatory cytokines (TNF-α, IL-1β, IL-6), apoptotic proteins, NF-κB, cyclooxygenase (COX)-2, STAT3, IKKβ, endothelin-1, malondialdehyde (MDA), C-reactive protein (CRP), prostaglandin E2, GST, PSA, VCAM1, GSH, pepsinogen, phosphorylase kinase (PhK), transferrin receptor, total cholesterol, transforming growth factor (TGF)-β, triglyceride, creatinine, HO1, antioxidants, AST, and ALT.

Although curcumin has shown efficacy against numerous human ailments, its poor bioavailability due to poor absorption, rapid metabolism, and rapid systemic elimination often limits its therapeutic efficacy (Anand et al. 2007). Thus, abundant efforts have been made to improve curcumin's bioavailability by altering these features. The most common approach to increasing the bioavailability of curcumin is by the use of adjuvants that can block the metabolic pathway of curcumin. Piperine, a known inhibitor of hepatic and intestinal glucuronidation, when combined with curcumin enhanced the bioavailability of curcumin in healthy human subjects (Shoba et al. 1998). The serum levels of curcumin in humans were either undetectable or very low upon administration of a dose of 2 g curcumin alone. Piperine is known to increase the curcumin bioavailability by 2000% via simultaneous administration of 20 mg piperine with curcumin. It produced much higher concentrations within 30 minutes to 1 hour after drug treatment. Several methods have been employed to increase curcumin bioavailability in humans such as the use of NPs (Sasaki et al. 2011), liposomes (Gota et al. 2010), phospholipid complexes (Cuomo et al. 2011), and structural analogs (Anand et al. 2007). Meriva, a patented phytosome complex of curcumin with soy phosphatidylcholine, has better bioavailability compared to curcumin. A study on the absorption capacity of a curcuminoid mixture and Meriva was examined in a randomized, double-blind, crossover human study (Cuomo et al. 2011). It was observed that the total curcuminoid absorption was about 29 times higher for the Meriva mixture in comparison with a corresponding curcuminoid mixture alone. The phospholipid formulation has been reported to increase the absorption of demethoxylated curcuminoids much more compared to the curcumin (Cuomo et al. 2011). Altering curcumin with the noncurcuminoid components of turmeric has also been shown to greatly improve curcumin bioavailability (Antony et al. 2008), as observed in clinical studies on people with health problems.

The health-promoting efficacy of lipidated curcumin was evaluated in healthy middle-aged applicants (40–60 years old). The study comprised participants who were given either lipidated curcumin (80 mg/day) or placebo for 4 weeks. It was observed that curcumin, but not placebo, produced a reduction in salivary amylase and in the plasma levels of triglycerides, beta amyloid, ALT, and soluble intercellular adhesion molecule1 (sICAM-1). In addition, increased salivary radical scavenging capacities, activities in plasma catalase, myeloperoxidase, and nitric oxide production were also reported in these participants. These studies predicted the health-promoting effects of lipidated curcumin in healthy middle-aged people (Disilvestro et al. 2012). Recent reports revealed the inhibitory action of Theracurmin, a highly absorptive curcumin, against alcohol intoxication in humans when dispersed with colloidal NPs (Sasaki et al. 2011).

17.6 Regulatory Aspects of Nanobased Products

Though nanotechnology-based formulations are being marketed under the banner of nutraceuticals, there is still a long way to go to develop them as drugs with known therapeutic efficacy. Based on the existing database on curcumin and THC, it is clear that, although curcumin has shown its efficacy against all the investigated disorders, THC still needs to be explored in chronic conditions. It is a more stable molecule than curcumin and is expected to demonstrate a superior in vitro–in vivo correlation once all study protocols are suitably tested.

Regulatory agencies are required to take tangible measures to set up a standardized international board to promote recent guidelines, developing new procedures, improving the regulation of safety-assessment procedures governing the approval of nanobased phytoproducts, and regulating new products entering the market. Nevertheless, for successful commercialization, consumers must also be educated about the advantages versus risks of these nanoceuticals. In vitro and in vivo animal studies have shown an increase in the bioavailability and therapeutic potential of nanoceuticals (Kakkar et al. 2018a, b).

However, it is important to execute additional in vivo efficacy studies in order to assess the toxicity and safety aspects of these nano-encapsulated nutraceuticals in the human body and in the environment. A reform once drafted by the FDA may pave a clear path for marketing safe nanoceuticals to reach consumers for subsequent use.

17.7 Conclusion and Remarks on Future Directions

Undoubtedly, the nanoformulations of curcumin and THC are better candidates with greater therapeutic effects and represent candidates for development as drugs. It seems that only multidisciplinary efforts can raise the status of these promising traditional molecules to that of therapeutics from one of being just prophylactic agents against different diseases. Therefore, the promise of nanotechnology-based medicine may become a reality if sufficient effort is devoted it by researchers. Considering the high cost and long period of new drug development, as well as the high drug attrition rate, an urgent task of pharmaceutical companies is to investigate new directions of drug research and development. Consequently, additional attention in the field of drug discovery has been paid to nutraceuticals, which as a source of new compounds for drugs will emerge as a worldwide trend in the pharmaceutical industry. Human trials need to be conducted to establish the effectiveness of curcumin and THC in clinical applications as an improved therapeutic modality for the treatment of different diseases.

References

Aggarwal BB, Gupta SC, Patchva S, Koh W (2012) Discovery of curcumin, a component of golden spice, and its miraculous biological activities. Clin Exp Pharmacol Physiol 39(3):283–299

Aggarwal BB, Gupta SC, Patchva S (2013) Therapeutic roles of curcumin: lessons learned from clinical trials. AAPS J 15(1):195–218

Aggarwal BB, Deb L, Prasad S (2014) Curcumin differs from tetrahydrocurcumin for molecular targets, signaling pathways and cellular responses. Molecules 20(1):185–205

Akbik D, Ghadiri M, Chrzanowski W, Rohanizadeh R (2014) Curcumin as a wound healing agent. Life Sci 116(1):1–7

Akhtar F, Rizvi MM, Kar SK (2012) Oral delivery of curcumin bound to chitosan nanoparticles cured Plasmodium yoelii infected mice. Biotechnol Adv 30(1):310–320

Alam S, Panda JJ, Mukherjee TK, Chauhan VS (2016) Short peptide based nanotubes capable of effective curcumin delivery for treating drug resistant malaria. J Nanobiotechnol 14:26

Ali I, Rahis-Uddin Salim K, Rather MA, Wani WA, Haque A (2011) Advances in nano drugs for cancer chemotherapy. Curr Cancer Drug Targets 11(2):135–146

Alper H, Sommovigo M (1992) Mild reduction of a, β -unsaturated ketones and aldehydes with an oxygen-activated palladium catalyst. Tetrahedron 34:59–62

Anand P, Kunnumakkara AB, Newman RA, Aggarwal BB (2007) Bioavailability of curcumin: problems and promises. Mol Pharm 4(6):807–818

Antony B, Merina B, Iyer VS, Judy N, Lennertz K, Joyal S (2008) A pilot cross-over study to evaluate human oral bioavailability of BCM-95CG (Biocurcumax), a novel bioenhanced preparation of curcumin. Indian J Pharm Sci 70(4):445–449

Apetz N, Munch G, Govindaraghavan S, Gyengesi E (2014) Natural compounds and plant extracts as therapeutics against chronic inflammation in Alzheimer's diseased translational perspective. CNS Neurol Disord Drug Targets 13(7):1175–1191

Ariën K, Jespers V, Vanham G (2011) HIV sexual transmission and microbicides. Rev Med Virol 21:110–133

Arora R, Kuhad A, Kaur IP, Chopra K (2015) Curcumin loaded solid lipid nanoparticles ameliorate adjuvant-induced arthritis in rats. Eur J Pain 19(7):940–952

Begum AN, Jones MR, Lim GP, Morihara T, Kim P, Heath DD, Rock CL, Pruitt MA, Yang F, Hudspeth B, Hu S, Faull KF, Teter B, Cole GM, Frautschy SA (2008) Curcumin structure-function, bioavailability, and efficacy in models of neuroinflammation and Alzheimer's disease. J Pharmacol Exp Ther 326(1):196–208

Beloqui A, Coco R, Memvanga PB, Ucakar B, des Rieux A, Preat V (2014) pH-sensitive nanoparticles for colonic delivery of curcumin in inflammatory bowel disease. Int J Pharm 473(1–2):203–212

Bhaskar Rao A, Prasad E, Deepthi SS, Haritha V, Ramakrishna S, Madhusudan K, Surekha MV, Venkata Rao YS (2015) Wound healing: a new perspective on glucosylated tetrahydrocurcumin. Drug Des Dev Ther 13(9):3579–3588

Bleeker EA, de Jong WH, Geertsma RE, Groenewold M, Heugens EH, Koers-Jacquemijns M (2013) Considerations on the EU definition of a nanomaterial: science to support policy making. Regul Toxicol Pharmacol 65:119–125

Borsari M, Ferrari E, Grandi R, Saladini M (2002) Curucminoids as potential new iron-chelating agents: spectroscopic, polarographic and potentiometric study on their Fe(III) complexing ability. Inorg Chim Acta 328:61–68

Bruschi ML, Ferreira SBS (2019) Improving the bioavailability of curcumin: is micro/nanoencapsulation the key? Ther Deliv 10(2):83–86

Carlson LJ, Cote B, Alani AW, Rao DA (2014) Polymeric micellar co-delivery of resveratrol and curcumin to mitigate *in vitro* doxorubicin-induced cardiotoxicity. J Pharm Sci 103(8):2315–2322

Cartiera MS, Ferreira EC, Caputo C, Egan ME, Caplan MJ, Saltzman WM (2010) Partial correction of cystic fibrosis defects with PLGA nanoparticles encapsulating curcumin. Mol Pharm 7(1):86–93

Castangia I, Nácher A, Caddeo C, Valenti D, Fadda AM, Díez-Sales O, Ruiz-Saurí A, Manconi M (2014) Fabrication of quercetin and curcumin bionanovesicles for the prevention and rapid regeneration of full-thickness skin defects on mice. Acta Biomater 10(3):1292–1300

Cavaleri F (2018) Presenting a new standard drug model for turmeric and its prized extract, curcumin. Int J Inflamm 2018:5023429

Chaudhary H, Kohli K, Kumar V (2014) A novel nano-carrier transdermal gel against inflammation. Int J Pharm 465(1–2):175–816

Cheng KK, Chan PS, Fan S, Kwan SM, Yeung KL, Wang YX, Chow AHL, Wu EX, Baum L et al (2015) Curcumin-conjugated magnetic nanoparticles for detecting amyloid plaques in Alzheimer's disease mice using magnetic resonance imaging (MRI). Biomaterials 44:155–172

Chereddy KK, Coco R, Memvanga PB, Ucakar B, des Rieux A, Vandermeulen G (2013) Combined effect of PLGA and curcumin on wound healing activity. J Control Release 171(2):208–215

Coma-Cros EM, Biosca A, Lantero E, Manca ML, Caddeo C, Gutiérrez L, Ramírez M, Borgheti-Cardoso LN, Manconi M, Fernàndez-Busquets X (2018) Antimalarial activity of orally administered curcumin incorporated in Eudragit®-containing liposomes. Int J Mol Sci 19(5):1361

Cuomo J, Appendino G, Dern AS, Schneider E, McKinnon TP, Brown MJ (2011) Comparative absorption of a standardized curcuminoid mixture and its lecithin formulation. J Nat Prod 74(4) :664–669

Daddy H, Khalik NIBA, Taib H, Pohchi A, Hassan A, Alam MK (2013) Novel material in the treatment of minor oral recurrent aphthous stomatitis. Int Med J 20:392–394

Dai X, Liu J, Zheng H, Wichmann J, Hopfner U, Sudhop S, Prein C, Shen Y, Machens HG, Schillin AF (2017) Nano-formulated curcumin accelerates acute wound healing through Dkk-1-mediated fibroblast mobilization and MCP-1-mediated anti-inflammation. NPG Asia Mater 9:e368

Devadasu VR, Wadsworth RM, Kumar MN (2011) Protective effects of nanoparticulate coenzyme Q10 and curcumin on inflammatory markers and lipid metabolism in streptozotocin-induced diabetic rats: a possible remedy to diabetic complications. Drug Deliv Transl Res 1(6):448–455

Deveza L, Choi J, Yang F (2012) Therapeutic angiogenesis for treating cardiovascular diseases. Theranostics 2(8):801–814

Din FU, Aman W, Ullah I, Qureshi OS, Mustapha O, Shafique S, Zeb A (2017) Effective use of nanocarriers as drug delivery systems for the treatment of selected tumors. Int J Nanomedicine 12:7291–7309

Ding Q, Niu T, Yang Y, Guo Q, Luo F, Qian Z (2014) Preparation of curcumin-loaded poly(ester amine) nanoparticles for the treatment of anti-angiogenesis. J Biomed Nanotechnol 10(4):632–641

Disilvestro RA, Joseph E, Zhao S, Joshua B (2012) Diverse effects of a low dose supplement of lipidated curcumin in healthy middle aged people. Nutr J 11(1):79

Doggui S, Belkacemi A, Paka GD, Perrotte M, Pi R, Ramassamy C (2013) Curcumin protects neuronal-like cells against acrolein by restoring Akt and redox signaling pathways. Mol Nutr Food Res 57(9):1660–1670

Dogra N, Choudhary R, Kohli P, Haddock JD, Makwana S, Horev B, Vinokur Y, Droby S, Rodov V (2015) Polydiacetylene nanovesicles as carriers of natural phenylpropanoids for creating antimicrobial foodcontact surfaces. J Agric Food Chem 63(9):2557–2565

Egan ME, Pearson M, Weiner SA, Rajendran V, Rubin D, Glockner-Pagel J (2004) Curcumin, a major constituent of turmeric, corrects cystic fibrosis defects. Science 304(5670):600–602

Farajzadeh R, Pilehvar-Soltanahmadi Y, Dadashpour M, Javidfar S, Lotfi-Attari J, Sadeghzadeh H, Shafiei-Irannejad V, Zarghami N (2018) Nano-encapsulated metformin-curcumin in PLGA/PEG inhibits synergistically growth and hTERT gene expression in human breast cancer cells. Artif Cells Nanomed Biotechnol 46(5):917–925

Gandapu U, Chaitanya RK, Kishore G, Reddy RC, Kondapi AK (2011) Curcumin-loaded apotransferrin nanoparticles provide efficient cellular uptake and effectively inhibit HIV-1 replication *in vitro*. PLoS One 6(8):e23388

Girija CR, Begum NS, Syed AA, Thiruvenkatam V (2004) Hydrogenbonding and C-H-π interactions in 1,7-bis(4-hydroxy-3- methoxyphenyl)heptane-3,5-dione(tetrahydrocurcumin). Acta Crystallogr C 60(8):0611–0613

Gong C, Wu Q, Wang Y, Zhang D, Luo F, Zhao X, Wei Y, Qian Z (2013) A biodegradable hydrogel system containing curcumin encapsulated in micelles for cutaneous wound healing. Biomaterials 34(27):6377–6387

Gota VS, Maru GB, Soni TG, Gandhi TR, Kochar N, Agarwal MG (2010) Safety and pharmacokinetics of a solid lipid curcumin particle formulation in osteosarcoma patients and healthy volunteers. J Agric Food Chem 58(4):2095–2099

Goto M, Ifuku S, Azuma K, Arima H, Kaneko S, Iohara D, Hirayama F, Anraku M (2019) Preparation and evaluation of freeze dried surface-deacetylated chitin nanofiber/sacran pellets for use as an extended-release excipient. Int J Biol Macromol 124:888–894

Gou M, Men K, Shi H, Xiang M, Zhang J, Song J, Long J, Wan Y, Luo F, Zhao X, Qian Z (2011) Curcumin-loaded biodegradable polymeric micelles for colon cancer therapy *in vitro* and *in vivo*. Nanoscale 3(4):1558–1567

Gugulothu D, Kulkarni A, Patravale V, Dandekar P (2014) pHsensitive nanoparticles of curcumin-celecoxib combination: evaluating drug synergy in ulcerative colitis model. J Pharm Sci 103(2):687–696

Gupta U, Jain NK (2010) Non-polymeric nano-carriers in HIV/AIDS drug delivering and targeting. Adv Drug Deliv Rev 62:478–490

Hassainasab A, Hashimoto Y, Tomita-Yokotani K, Kobayashi M (2011) Discovery of the curcumin metabolic pathway involving a unique enzyme in an intestinal microorganism. Proc Natl Acad Sci U S A 108(16):6615–6620

Hassan F, Rehman MS, Khan MS, Ali MA, Javed A, Nawaz A, Yang C (2019) Curcumin as an alternative epigenetic modulator: mechanism of action and potential effects. Front Genet 10(514):1–16

Heo DN, Ko WK, Moon HJ, Kim HJ, Lee SJ, Lee JB (2014) Inhibition of osteoclast differentiation by gold nanoparticles functionalized with cyclodextrin curcumin complexes. ACS Nano 8(12):12049–12062

Ibrahim S, Tagami T, Kishi T, Ozeki T (2018) Curcumin marinosomes as promising nano-drug delivery system for lung cancer. Int J Pharm 540(1–2):40–49

Isacchi B, Bergonzi MC, Grazioso M, Righeschi C, Pietretti A, Severini C (2012) Artemisinin and artemisinin plus curcumin liposomal formulations: enhanced antimalarial efficacy against Plasmodium berghei-infected mice. Eur J Pharm Biopharm 80(3):528–534

Jäger R, Lowery RP, Calvanese AV, Joy JM, Purpura M, Wilson JM (2014) Comparative absorption of curcumin formulations. Nutr J 13:11

Janesirisakule S, Sinthusake T, Wanichwecharungruang S (2013) Nanocarrier with self-antioxidative property for stabilizing and delivering ascorbyl palmitate into skin. J Pharm Sci 102(8):2770–2779

Jaruszewski KM, Curran GL, Swaminathan SK, Rosenberg JT, Grant SC, Ramakrishnan S, Lowe VJ, Poduslo JF, Kandimalla KK (2014) Multimodal nanoprobes to target cerebrovascular amyloid in Alzheimer's disease brain. Biomaterials 35(6):1967–1976

Ji H, Tang J, Li M, Ren J, Zheng N, Wu L (2016) Curcumin-loaded solid lipid nanoparticles with Brij78 and TPGS improved in vivo oral bioavailability and in situ intestinal absorption of curcumin. Drug Deliv 23:459–470

Joshi RP, Negi G, Kumar A, Pawar YB, Munjal B, Bansal AK, Sharma SS et al (2013) SNEDDS curcumin formulation leads to enhanced protection from pain and functional deficits associated with diabetic neuropathy: an insight into its mechanism for neuroprotection. Nanomedicine 9(6):776–785

Kakkar V, Kaur IP (2011) Evaluating potential of curcumin loaded solid lipid nanoparticles in aluminium induced behavioural, biochemical and histopathological alterations in mice brain. Food Chem Toxicol 49:2906–2913

Kakkar V, Singh S, Singla D, Kaur IP (2011) Exploring solid lipid nanoparticles to enhance the oral bioavailability of curcumin. Mol Nutr Food Res 55(3): 495–503

Kakkar V, Bhushan S, Kumar GS, Kaur IP (2012) Enhanced apoptotic effect of curcumin loaded solid lipid nanoparticles. Mol Pharm 9(12):3411–3421

Kakkar V, Mishra AK, Chuttani K, Kaur IP (2013) Proof of concept studies to confirm the delivery of curcumin loaded solid lipid nanoparticles (C-SLNs) to brain. Int J Pharm 448:354–359

Kakkar V, Kumar M, Saini K (2018a) Nanoceuticals governance and market review. Environ Chem Lett 16(4):1293–1300

Kakkar V, Kaur IP, Kaur AP, Saini K, Singh KK (2018b) Topical delivery of tetrahydrocurcumin lipid nanoparticles effectively inhibits skin inflammation: in vitro in vivo study. Drug Dev Ind Pharm 44(10):1701–1712

Kanai M, Yoshimura K, Asada M, Imaizumi A, Suzuki C, Matsumoto S (2011) A phase I/II study of gemcitabine-based chemotherapy plus curcumin for patients with gemcitabine resistant pancreatic cancer. Cancer Chemother Pharmacol 68(1):157–164

Kang N, Wang MM, Wang YH, Zhang ZN, Cao HR, Lv YH, Yang Y, Fan PH, Qiu F, Gao XM (2014) Tetrahydrocurcumin induces G2/M cell cycle arrest and apoptosis involving p38 MAPK activation in human breast cancer cells. Food Chem Toxicol 67:193–200

Karavolos M, Holban A (2016) Nanosized drug delivery systems in gastrointestinal targeting: interactions with microbiota. Pharmaceuticals 9(4):62

Kaushik A, Jayant RD, Sagar V, Nair M (2014) The potential of magneto-electric nanocarriers for drug delivery. Expert Opin Drug Deliv 11(10):1635–1646

Kelloff GJ, Crowell JA, Hawk ET, Steele VE, Lubet RA, Boone CW, Covey JM, Doody LA, Omenn GS, Greenwald P, Hong WK, Parkinson DR, Bagheri D, Baxter GT, Blunden M, Doeltz MK, Eisenhauer KM, Johnson K, Knapp GG, Longfellow DG, Malone WF, Nayfield SG, Seifried HE, Swall LM, Sigman CC (1996) Strategy and planning for chemopreventive drug development: clinical development plan: II. J Cell Biochem Suppl 26:54–71

Khan MN, Haggag YA, Lane ME, McCarron PA, Tambuwala MM (2018) Polymeric nano-encapsulation of curcumin enhances its anti-cancer activity in breast (MDA-MB231) and lung (A549) cancer cells through reduction in expression of HIF-1α; and nuclear p65 (Rel A). Curr Drug Deliv 15:286

Khodabandehloo H, Zahednasab H, Hafez AA (2016) Nanocarriers usage for drug delivery in cancer therapy. Iran J Cancer Prev 9(2):e3966

Kim JM, Araki S, Kim DJ, Park CB, Takasuka N, Baba-Toriyama H, Ota T, Nir Z, Khachik F, Shimidzu N, Tanaka Y, Osawa T, Uraji T, Murakoshi M, Nishino H, Tsuda H (1998) Chemopreventative effects of carotenoids and curcumins on mouse colon carcinogenesis after 1,2-dimethylhydrazine initiation. Carcinogenesis 19(1):81–85

Krausz AE, Adler BL, Cabral V, Navati M, Doerner J, Charafeddine RA, Chandra D, Liang H, Gunther L, Clendaniel A, Harper S, Friedman JM, Nosanchuk JD, Friedman AJ (2015) Curcumin-encapsulated nanoparticles as innovative antimicrobial and wound healing agent. Nanomedicine 11(1):195–206

Kumar SC, Mohan S (2015) Fabrication, characterization and evaluation of hepatoprotective activity drug loaded flavono nanoparticle delivery system. J Phytopharmacol 4(2):90–96

Kumari P, Ghosh B, Biswas S (2016) Nanocarriers for cancer-targeted drug delivery. J Drug Target 24(3):179–191

Lai CS, Wu JC, Yu SF, Badmaev V, Nagabhushanam K, Ho CT, Pan MH (2011) Tetrahydrocurcumin is more effective than curcumin in preventing azoxymethane-induced colon carcinogenesis. Mol Food Nutr Res 55(12):1819–1828

Lal B, Kapoor AK, Asthana OP, Agrawal PK, Prasad R, Kumar P, Srimal RC (1999) Efficacy of curcumin in the management of chronic anterior uveitis. Phytother Res 13(4):318–322

Lavor EM, Fernandes AWC, Teles RBA (2018) Essential oils and their major compounds in the treatment of chronic inflammation: a review of antioxidant potential in preclinical studies and molecular mechanisms. Oxidative Med Cell Longev 2018:1–23

Lee WH, Loo CY, Bebawy M, Luk F, Mason RS, Rohanizadeh R (2013) Curcumin and its derivatives: their application in neuropharmacology and neuroscience in the 21st century. Curr Neuropharmacol 11:338–378

Lee WH, Ong HX, Loo CY, Traini D, Young P, Luk F, Mary B, Rohanizadeh R (2014) Synthesis of curcumin nanoparticles for lung cancer therapy. J Aerosol Med Pulm Drug Deliv 27:A1–A27

Li X, Nan K, Li L, Zhang Z, Chen H (2012) In vivo evaluation of curcumin nanoformulation loaded methoxy poly(ethylene glycol)-graft-chitosan composite film for wound healing application. Carbohydr Polym 88:84–90

Lipecka J, Norez C, Bensalem N, Baudouin-Legros M, Planelles G, Becq F (2006) Rescue of DeltaF508-CFTR (cystic fibrosis transmembrane conductance regulator) by curcumin: involvement of the keratin 18 network. J Pharmacol Exp Ther 317(2):500–505

Liu D, Chen Z (2013) The effect of curcumin on breast cancer cells. J Breast Cancer 16(2):133–137

Liu XF, Hao JL, Xie T, Mukhtar NJ, Zhang W, Malik TH, Lu CW, Zhou DD (2017) Curcumin, A potential therapeutic candidate for anterior segment eye diseases: a review. Front Pharmacol 14(8):66

Lotfi-Attari J, Pilehvar-Soltanahmadi Y, Dadashpour M, Alipour S, Farajzadeh R, Javidfar S, Zarghami N (2017) Co-delivery of curcumin and chrysin by polymeric nanoparticles inhibit synergistically growth and hTERT gene expression in human colorectal cancer cells. Nutr Cancer 69(8):1290–1299

Luiza A, Holleben V, Zucolotto M, Zini CA, Oliveira ER (1994) Selective reduction of a, ß- unsaturated ketones. Tetrahedron 50:973–978

Maradana MR, Thomas R, O'Sullivan BJ (2013) Targeted delivery of curcumin for treating type 2 diabetes. Mol Nutr Food Res 57(9):1550–1556

Marslin G, Prakash J, Qi S, Franklin G (2018) Oral delivery of curcumin polymeric nanoparticles ameliorates CCl4-induced subacute hepatotoxicity in Wistar rats. Polymers 10(5):541

Martinho N, Damgé C, Reis CP (2011) Recent advances in drug delivery systems. J Biomater Nanobiotechnol 2:510

Mirakabad FS, Akbarzadeh A, Milani M, Zarghami N, Taheri-Anganeh M, Zeighamian V, Badrzadeh F, Rahmati-Yamchi M (2016) A comparison between the cytotoxic effects of pure curcumin and curcumin-loaded PLGA-PEG nanoparticles on the MCF-7 human breast cancer cell line. Artif Cells Nanomed Biotechnol 44(1):423–430

Mirani A, Kundaikar H, Velhal S, Patel V, Bandivdekar A, Degani M, Patravale V (2019) Tetrahydrocurcumin-loaded vaginal nanomicrobicide for prophylaxis of HIV/AIDS: in silico study, formulation development, and in vitro evaluation. Drug Deliv Transl Res 9(4):828–847

Moghadamtousi SZ, Kadir HA, Hassandarvish P, Tajik H, Abubakar S, Zandi K (2014) A review on antibacterial, antiviral, and antifungal activity of curcumin. BioMed Res Int 2014:186864

Mori A, Fujita A, Kajiro H, Nishihara Y, Hiyama T (1999) Conjugate reduction of α, β-unsaturated ketones with hydrosilane mediated by copper (I) salt. Tetrahedron 55(15):4573–4582

Nayak AP, Tiyaboonchai W, Patankar S, Madhusudhan B, Souto EB (2010) Curcuminoids-loaded lipid nanoparticles: novel approach towards malaria treatment. Colloids Surf B Biointerfaces 81(1):263–273

Negar G, Alizadeh AM, Ashkani-Esfahani S (2014) Nanotechnology-applied curcumin for different diseases therapy. Biomed Res Int 394264:1–23

Neves JD, Amiji MM, Bahia MF, Sarmento B (2010) Nanotechnology-based system for the treatment and prevention of HIV/AIDS. Adv Drug Deliv Rev 62:458–447

Obeid MA, Al Qaraghuli MM, Alsaadi M, Alzahrani AR, Niwasabutra K, Ferro VA (2017) Delivering natural products and biotherapeutics to improve drug efficacy. Ther Deliv 8(11):947–956

Pan MH, Huang TM, Lin JK (1999) Biotransformation of curcumin through reduction and glucuronidation in mice. Drug Metab Dispos 27(4):486–494

Pan SY, Zhou SF, Gao SH, Yu ZL, Zhang SF, Tang MK, Sun JN, Ma DL, Han YF, Fong WF, Ko KM (2013) New perspectives on how to discover drugs from herbal medicines: CAM's outstanding contribution to modern therapeutics. Evid Based Complement Alternat Med 627375:25

Pari L, Amali DR (2005) Protective role of tetrahydrocurcumin (THC) an active principle of turmeric on chloroquine induced hepatotoxicity in rats. J Pharm Pharm Sci 8(1):115–123

Patra JK, Das G, Fraceto LF, Campos E, Rodriguez-Torres M, Acosta-Torres LS, Shin HS, Diaz-Torres LA, Grillo R, Swamy MK, Sharma Sand Habtemariam S (2018) Nano based drug delivery systems: recent developments and future prospects. J Nanobiotechnol 16(1):71

Potter KA, Jorfi M, Householder KT, Foster EJ, Weder C, Capadona JR (2014) Curcumin-releasing mechanically adaptive intracortical implants improve the proximal neuronal density and blood–brain barrier stability. Acta Biomater 10(5):2209–2222

Prajakta D, Ratnesh J, Chandan K, Suresh S, Grace S, Meera V, Vandana P (2009) Curcumin loaded pH-sensitive nanoparticles for the treatment of colon cancer. J Biomed Nanotechnol 5:445–455

Pramanik D, Campbell NR, Das S, Gupta S, Chenna V, Bisht S, Sysa-Shah P, Bedja D, Karikari C, Steenbergen C, Gabrielson KL, Maitra A, Maitra A (2012) A composite polymer nanoparticle overcomes multidrug resistance and ameliorates doxorubicin-associated cardiomyopathy. Oncotarget 3(6): 640–650

Priyadarsini K (2014) The chemistry of curcumin: from extraction to therapeutic agent. Molecules 19(12):20091–20112

Rachmawati H, Edityaningrum CA, Mauludin R (2013) Molecular inclusion complex of curcumin-beta-cyclodextrin nanoparticle to enhance curcumin skin permeability from hydrophilic matrix gel. AAPS PharmSciTech 14(4):1303–1312

Ramassamy C, Doggui S, Sahni JK, Arseneault M, Dao L (2012) Neuronal uptake and neuroprotective effect of curcumin-loaded PLGA nanoparticles on the human SK-N-SH cell line. J Alzheimers Dis 30(2):377–392

Ray B, Bisht S, Maitra A, Maitra A, Lahiri DK (2011) Neuroprotective and neurorescue effects of a novel polymeric nanoparticle formulation of curcumin (NanoCurc) in the neuronal cell culture and animal model: implications for Alzheimer's disease. J Alzheimers Dis 23(1):61–77

Re F, Cambianica I, Zona C, Sesana S, Gregori M, Rigolio R, La Ferla B, Nicotra F, Forloni G, Cagnotto A, Salmona M, Masserini M, Sancini G (2011) Functionalization of liposomes with ApoE-derived peptides at different density affects cellular uptake and drug transport across a blood–brain barrier model. Nanomedicine 7(5):551–559

Reuter S, Gupta SC, Park B, Goel A, Aggarwal BB (2011) Epigenetic changes induced by curcumin and other natural compounds. Genes Nutr 6(2):93–108

Rramaswamy R, Mani G, Venkatachalam S, Venkata RY, Lavanya JS, Choi EY (2018a) Tetrahydro curcumin loaded PCL-PEG electrospun transdermal nanofiber patch: preparation, characterization, and in vitro diffusion evaluations. J Drug Deliv Sci Technol 44:342–348

Rramaswamy R, Mani G, Jang HT (2018b) Fabrication of buccal dissolving tetrahydro curcumin loaded polyvidone fiber mat: synthesis, characterization, and in vitro evaluations. J Appl Pharm Sci 8(08):026–031

Rramaswamy R, Mani G, Venkatachalam S, Venkata Yasam R, Rajendran JCB, Hyun Tae J (2018c) Preparation and characterization of tetrahydrocurcumin-loaded cellulose acetate phthalate/polyethylene glycol electrospun nanofibers. AAPS PharmSciTech 19(7):3000–3008

Said DE, Elsamad LM, Gohar YM (2012) Validity of silver, chitosan, and curcumin nanoparticles as anti-Giardia agents. Parasitol Res 111(2):545–554

Sandhir R, Yadav A, Mehrotra A, Sunkaria A, Singh A, Sharma S (2014) Curcumin nanoparticles attenuate neurochemical and neurobehavioral deficits in experimental model of Huntington's disease. NeuroMolecular Med 16(1):106–118

Sankar P, Telang AG, Kalaivanan R, Karunakaran V, Suresh S, Kesavan M (2013) Oral nanoparticulate curcumin combating arsenic-induced oxidative damage in kidney and brain of rats. Toxicol Ind Health 32(3):410–421

Saradhi UVRV, Ling Y, Wang J, Chiu M, Schwartz EB, Fuchs JR, Chan KK, Liu Z (2010) A liquid chromatography-tandem mass spectrometric method for quantification of curcuminoids in cell medium and mouse plasma. J Chromatogr B 878:3045–3051

Sasaki H, Sunagawa Y, Takahashi K, Imaizumi A, Fukuda H, Hashimoto T (2011) Innovative preparation of curcumin for improved oral bioavailability. Biol Pharm Bull 34(5):660–665

Sato K, Iki N, Takahashi T, Hoshino H (2008) Evaluation of stability against oxidation and acid dissociation properties for tetrahydrocurcumin in aqueous solution. Bunseki Kagaku 57(4):257–263

Sermkaew N, Wiwattanawongsa K, Ketjinda W, Wiwattanapatapee R (2013) Development, characterization and permeability assessment based on Caco-2 monolayers of self-microemulsifying floating tablets of tetrahydrocurcumin. AAPS PharmSciTech 14(1):321–331

Setthacheewakul S, Kedjinda W, Maneenuan D, Wiwattanapatapee R (2011) Controlled release of oral tetrahydrocurcumin from a novel self-emulsifying floating drug delivery system (SEFD). AAPS PharmSciTech 12(1):152–164

Sharma RK, Cwiklinski K, Aalinkeel R, Reynolds J (2017) Immunomodulatory activities of curcumin-stabilized silver nanoparticles: efficacy as an antiretroviral therapeutic. Immunol Investig 46(8):833–846

Sharma A, Soliman GM, Al-Hajaj N, Sharma R, Maysinger D, Kakkar A (2012) Design and Evaluation of Multifunctional Nanocarriers for Selective Delivery of Coenzyme Q10 to Mitochondria. Biomacromolecules 13(1):239–252

Shashy R, Ridley M (2000) Aphthous ulcers: a difficult clinical entity. Am J Otolaryngol 21(6):389–393

Shimoda K, Kubota N, Hirano H, Matsumoto M, Hamada H, Hamada H (2012) Formation of tetrahydrocurcumin by reduction of curcumin with cultured plant cells of Marchantia polymorpha. Nat Prod Commun 7(4):529–530

Shoba G, Joy D, Joseph T, Majeed M, Rajendran R, Srinivas PS (1998) Influence of piperine on the pharmacokinetics of curcumin in animals and human volunteers. Planta Med 64(4):353–356

Shukla P, Dwivedi P, Gupta PK, Mishra PR (2014) Optimization of novel tocopheryl acetate nanoemulsions for parenteral delivery of curcumin for therapeutic intervention of sepsis. Expert Opin Drug Deliv 11(11):1697–1712

Shutava TG, Balkundi SS, Vangala P, Steffan JJ, Bigelow RL, Cardelli JA, O'Neal DP, Lvov YM (2009) Layer-by-layer-coated gelatin nanoparticles as a vehicle for delivery of natural polyphenols. ACS Nano 3(7):1877–1885

Singh AK, Jiang Y, Gupta S, Younus M, Ramzan M (2013) Antiinflammatory potency of nano-formulated puerarin and curcumin in rats subjected to the lipopolysaccharide-induced inflammation. J Med Food 16(10):899–911

Singh N, Khullar N, Kakkar V, Kaur IP (2014) Attenuation of carbon tetrachloride-induced hepatic injury with curcumin-loaded solid lipid nanoparticles. BioDrugs 28(3):297–312

Sun D, Zhuang X, Xiang X, Liu Y, Zhang S, Liu C, Barnes S, Grizzle W, Miller D, Zhang HG (2010) A novel nanoparticle drug delivery system: the anti-inflammatory activity of curcumin is enhanced when encapsulated in exosomes. Mol Ther 18(9):1606–1614

Suwannateep N, Wanichwecharungruang S, Haag SF, Devahastin S, Groth N, Fluhr JW, Lademann J, Meinke MC (2012) Encapsulated curcumin results in prolonged curcumin activity in vitro and radical scavenging activity ex vivo on skin after UVB-irradiation. Eur J Pharm Biopharm 82(3):485–490

Suwannateep N, Wanichwecharungruang S, Fluhr J, Patzelt A, Lademann J, Meinke MC (2013) Comparison of two encapsulated curcumin particular systems contained in different formulations with regard to in vitro skin penetration. Skin Res Technol 19(1):1–9

Thorat YS, Sarvagod AM, Kulkarni SV, Hosmani AH (2015) Treatment of mouth ulcer by curcumin loaded thermoreversible mucoadhesive gel: a technical note. Int J Pharm Pharm Sci 7(10):399–402

Tinkle S, McNeil SE, Stefan Mühlebach S, Bawa R, Borchard G, Barenholz Y, Tamarkin L, Desai N (2014) Nanomedicines: addressing the scientific and regulatory gap. Ann N Y Acad Sci 1313(1):35–56

Tsai CH, Yen YH, Yang JPW (2014) Finding of polysaccharideepeptide complexes in cordyceps militaris and evaluation of its acetylcholinesterase inhibition activity. J Food Drug Anal 23:63–70

Udompornmongkol P, Chiang BH (2015) Curcumin-loaded polymeric nanoparticles for enhanced anti-colorectal cancer applications. J Biomater Appl 30(5):537–546

Uehara SI, Yasuda I, Akiyama K, Morita H, Takeya K, Itokawa H (1987) Diarylheptanoids from the rhizomes of Curcuma xanthorrhiza and Alpinia fficinarum (pharmacognosy, chemical). Chem Pharm Bull 35(8):3298–3304

UN Joint Programme on HIV/AIDS (UNAIDS) (2016) Global report: UNAIDS report on the global AIDS epidemic

Vogel A, Pelletier J (1815) Examen chimique de la racine de Curcuma. J Pharm 1:289–300

Vollono L, Falconi M, Gaziano R, Iacovelli F, Dika E, Terracciano C, Bianchi L, Campione E (2019) Potential of curcumin in skin disorders. Nutrients 11(9):2169

Wang YJ, Lin HY, Wu CH, Liu DM (2012) Forming of demethoxycurcumin nanocrystallite-chitosan nanocarrier for controlled low dose cellular release for inhibition of the migration of vascular smooth muscle cells. Mol Pharm 9(8):2268–2279

Wang J, Wang H, Zhu R, Liu Q, Fei J, Wang S (2015) Anti-inflammatory activity of curcumin-loaded solid lipid nanoparticles in IL-1beta transgenic mice subjected to the lipopolysaccharide-induced sepsis. Biomaterials 53:475–483

WHO (2018) Cancer fact sheet. WHO Media Centre. IARC, France

Wong HL, Chattopadhyay N, Wu XY, Bendayan R (2010) Nanotechnology application for improved delivery of antiretroviral drugs to the brain. Adv Drug Deliv Rev 62:503–517

Wonga CY, Al-Salami H, Dassa CR (2017) Potential of insulin nanoparticle formulations for oral delivery and diabetes treatment. J Control Release 264: 247–275

Wu JC, Tsai ML, Lai CS, Wang YJ, Ho CT, Pan MH (2014) Chemopreventative effects of tetrahydrocurcumin on human diseases. Food Funct 5(1): 12–17

Yallapu MM, Gupta BK, Jaggi M, Chauhan SC (2010) Fabrication of curcumin encapsulated PLGA nanoparticles for improved therapeutic effects in metastatic cancer cells. J Colloid Interface Sci 351:19–29

Yallapu MM, Nagesh PK, Jaggi M, Chauhan SC (2015) Therapeutic applications of curcumin nanoformulations. AAPS J 17:1341–1356

Yekollu SK, Thomas R, O'Sullivan B (2011) 60Targeting curcusomes to inflammatory dendritic cells inhibits NF-kappaB and improves insulin resistance in obese mice. Diabetes 11:2928–2938

Yin H, Zhang H, Liu B (2013) Superior anticancer efficacy of curcumin-loaded nanoparticles against lung cancer. Acta Biochim Biophys Sin 45(8):634–640

Yoysungmoen P, Wirachwong P, Changtam C, Suksamrarn A, Patumraj S (2008) Anticancer and anti-angiogenic effects of curcumin and tetrahydrocurcumin on implanted hepatocellular carcinoma in nude mice. World J Gastroenterol 14(13):2003–2009

Zeighamian V, Darabi M, Akbarzadeh A, Rahmati-Yamchi M, Zarghami N, Badrzadeh F, Salehi R, Mirakabad FS, Taheri-Anganeh M (2016) PNIPAAm-MAA nanoparticles as delivery vehicles for curcumin against MCF-7 breast cancer cells. Artif Cells Nanomed Biotechnol 44(2):735–742

Zhao K, Li D, Shi C, Ma X, Rong G, Kang H, Wang X, Sun B (2016) Biodegradable polymeric nanoparticles as the delivery carrier for drug. Curr Drug Deliv 13(4):494–499

Phytonanomedicines as Topical Alternatives for the Treatment of Skin Cancer

18

Pooja Dalal, Varsha Kadian, and Rekha Rao

Abstract

The global incidence of skin cancer has increased dramatically in recent years. It is viewed as the most widespread form of malignant disease in the world, particularly in the United States. Surgery or radiotherapy has taken the first place among the treatment modalities for skin tumors. However, to improve patient compliance and to lessen undesirable scars and surgical expenses, especially where malignant growth has spread over maximum body parts, the topical route for anticancer moieties has been investigated by researchers. Further, this mode of delivery of anticancer moieties is an appealing approach for circumventing side effects and for improving therapeutic benefits and drug targeting. In the last few years, efforts of the scientific community have been toward the discovery of effective and new chemopreventive agents from natural origin. Literature reports show that a multitude of phytoconstituents have been investigated (in vitro and in vivo) for their potential to prevent carcinogenesis via diverse cellular as well as molecular approaches. One of the most active research domains relates to nanomedicine, which applies nanotechnology to highly precise medical interventions, including cancer. Nanomedicine possesses a broad potential to enhance the selective targeting of neoplastic cells by preferential delivery of agents to tumors, owing to the improved permeability and drug retention. Nanocarriers can also ameliorate the solubility of poorly soluble drugs, enhance the bioavailability, increase drug half-life by controlling immunogenicity, and enhance pharmacokinetics and reduce drug metabolism. They can also allow an adjustable release of therapeutic agents and the simultaneous administration of two or more drugs. By administering the drug doses, it is also possible to reduce related side effects and improve the patients' compliance. The present chapter will briefly discuss conventional modalities for the treatment of skin cancer. The aim of this chapter is to furnish a comprehensive account of the nanomedicine-based approaches that can be applied to vanquish the skin barrier. Nanocarrier-based delivery systems have been reviewed in the context of their utility for the topical delivery of anticancer drugs. An account of phytoagents for the treatment and prevention of skin cancers has also been provided.

P. Dalal · V. Kadian · R. Rao (✉)
Department of Pharmaceutical Sciences, Guru Jambheshwar University of Science & Technology, Hisar, Haryana, India

S. Talegaonkar, M. Rai (eds.), *Nanoformulations in Human Health*,
https://doi.org/10.1007/978-3-030-41858-8_18

Keywords

Nanomedicines · Natural agents · Cytotoxicity · Bioactives · Dermal application · Apoptosis · Keratinocytes

18.1 Introduction

Skin cancer represents the most challenging public health issue worldwide that has led to the greatest economic loss to humans (Torre et al. 2018). It is chiefly categorized into non-melanoma (NM) and melanoma (MM) (Katalinic et al. 2003). Among these, MM is the harshest form of cancer developed from melanocytes, located at the bottom epidermis. This layer protects the skin from environmental factors. Although less commonly found, among the various skin cancers, it has a larger mortality rate (Strickland et al. 2015; Penta et al. 2018). As per current reports, every year approximately 48,000 deaths occur worldwide due to melanoma. The mortality associated with it is 90%, with a survival rate of fewer than 10 years (Garbe et al. 2010; Eggermont et al. 2014). Another type of skin cancer, NM, is further categorized into BCC (basal cell carcinoma) and SCC (squamous cell carcinoma), both originating from the epidermis. In the Caucasians, the incidences of NM are found greater (by as much as 18–20 times) in comparison to MM (Leiter et al. 2014; Apalla et al. 2017). The risks associated with BCC include age, genetic disorder, and gender [Gorlin-Goltz syndrome, Fitzpatrick skin types I and II] (Didona et al. 2018). Howbeit, UV rays act as the key factor in triggering BCC pathology. Basal cell carcinoma usually develops on sun-exposed skin areas (Apalla et al. 2017). On the other hand, squamous cell carcinoma is known by the multiplication of squamous cells possessing metastasizing property. Squamous cell carcinoma is also known to have a notable feature of relapse, which depends on tumor lesion depth, size, perineural invasion, the immune capacity of the patient, and its anatomical position. Risk factors include Fitzpatrick skin (types I and II), human papillomavirus (types 16, 18, and 31), and genetic disorders, viz., albinism and xeroderma pigmentosum (Steward and Brown 2013). However, the most important risk factors are sunlight and UV radiations (Hennings et al. 1993; Calzavara-Pinton et al. 2015). Commonly, SCC flourishes on specific regions of the skin having direct exposure to sunlight (Leiter et al. 2014; Apalla et al. 2017).

Skin cancer is a multistage disorder comprising initiation, promotion stage, and progression (Fig. 18.1) (Hennings et al. 1993; Cadet et al. 2005). The initiation of this disease is stimulated after exposure to a carcinogen, like UV rays, resulting in damage either by photons, via DNA alteration, proteins, or membranes through reactive oxidative stress (Kvam and Tyrrell 1997). In case DNA damage is not repaired, the cell encounters permanent genetic modifications and develops the tendency for autonomous growth (Brash et al. 1991). Next comes the promotion stage in which initiated cells are continually exposed to compounds that provoke selective proliferation of clonal cells in a benign tumor with time. Regenerative proliferation, UV radiation, oxidative stress, and chronic inflammation promote skin tumor (Rundhaug and Fischer 2010). Eventually, during the progression stage, the benign tumor engages in more genetic mutations and becomes progressively invasive, leading to a malignant tumor with a capacity to metastasize (Hennings et al. 1993). The exponential growth of tumor during this stage depends on the intake of nutrition and oxygen supply via angiogenesis (a process in which new blood vessels originate from existing vascular bodies) (Naumov et al. 2006). Epidemiological reports throughout the world have also advocated that UV exposure of skin is the major environmental carcinogen, responsible for the development of both MM and NM. Exposure of the skin to both ultraviolet A (320–400 nm) and B (280–320 nm) radiation has been reported to cause immunosuppression and DNA damage. In comparison to UVA, UVB has been found to be more lethal, which acts as a complete carcinogen (Miller and Weinstock 1994). An in-depth understanding of the etiological parameters is crucial for prevent-

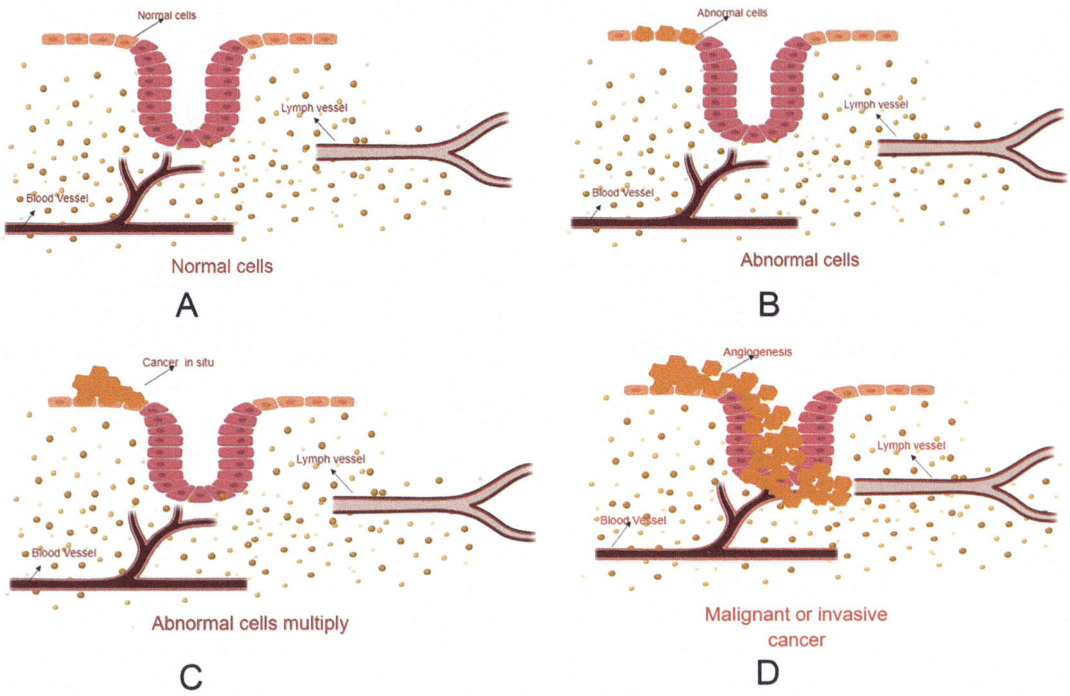

Fig. 18.1 Skin cancer proliferation

ing skin cancer (Fabbrocini et al. 2010). Individuals with a family history of genetic syndromes are vulnerable to specific types of skin cancers. Around 10% of patients having melanoma possess a positive family history (Azoury and Lange 2014). Ionizing radiation, chemical carcinogens, environmental pollutants, and work-associated exposures have been associated with skin cancer (Table 18.1) (Saladi and Persaud 2005). The increase in incidence and poorer progress of melanoma with higher age may be partially due to the accumulation of cellular damage with time and reduced immune surveillance and host defense (Azoury and Lange 2014). Inorganic arsenic exposure via drinking water is a major concern, particularly because it is a strong multi-site carcinogen for humans. The combination of arsenic and UVB treatments results in proapoptotic and anti-proliferative effects by stimulating both caspase pathways in skin cells (Fabbrocini et al. 2010). Several RNA and DNA viruses are also carcinogenic. HPV (human papillomavirus), hepatitis viruses B and C, EBV (Epstein-Barr virus), and KSHV

Table 18.1 Most common causes reported for skin cancer

UV radiation	Chemicals	Viruses
ROS (generate reactive oxygen species) Oxidative DNA damage Activate oncogenes and tumor suppressor genes Cell growth-regulating signaling moieties' alteration Modify the antiapoptotic proteins, cell cycle regulatory proteins, proapoptotic proteins, transcription factors, various protein kinases, inflammatory enzymes, and growth factor signaling pathways	PAH (polycyclic aromatic hydrocarbons) Arsenic	HPV (human papilloma virus) Kaposi's sarcoma-associated herpes virus HTLV-1 (human T-cell leukemia virus type 1)

Abbreviations: *DNA* deoxyribonucleic acid; *HPV* human papilloma virus; *HTLV*-1 human T-cell leukemia virus type 1; *PAH* polycyclic aromatic hydrocarbons; *ROS* reactive oxygen species; *UV* ultraviolet

(Kaposi's sarcoma herpes virus) are the best examples of oncogenic viruses (Swamy et al. 2019). In spite of preventive measurements taken, informative campaigns for prior detection of melanoma, and newer targeted therapies, its incidence still follows an ascending curve worldwide (Coricovac et al. 2018).

18.2 Conventional Treatment Modalities Available for Skin Cancer

Early recognition of skin cancer may help in its effective treatment. Although there are various treatment modalities used conventionally for the management of skin cancer, there is no standard treatment available for skin tumors. The choice of treatment approach should include functional results, low cost, and good efficacy of treatment. In view of this, the biomedical community has been widely using multiple treatment modalities such as conventional treatment like surgery, chemotherapy, and radiation therapy, immunotherapy, photodynamic therapy, chemical peel, targeted therapy. However, due to patient morbidity post treatment, variation in cure rates and use of cosmetics, outcomes vary widely to the abovementioned treatment options. Standard treatment modalities have also been reported here.

Surgery is the primary mode of treatment reported for most skin cancers (Potenza et al. 2018). Small skin tumors can be excised surgically. For this, the tumor can be removed with a curette (an instrument having a sharp and ring-shaped tip) and cauterized, frozen (using liquid nitrogen), or killed (using low-dose radiation) (Lipke 2006). Rarely, when basal cell/squamous cell carcinoma has invaded beyond the skin, tumors are surgically removed. The patients are further treated with radiation and chemotherapy. Similarly, melanoma tumors have to be removed surgically, before they proliferate into other regions (Joyce 2017). Selection of surgical procedure depends on the size and location of the lesion. Surgical procedures are used to cure basal cell or squamous cell carcinoma and actinic keratosis including curettage and electrodessication, Mohs surgery, reconstructive surgery, and cryosurgery. During simple excision, the tumor and some of the surrounding normal tissues are cut and removed from the skin (Potenza et al. 2018). In case of a large tumor, an incision is made, and the skin from other body parts is used to close the wound. This is known as skin grafting. This also helps in healing as well as reducing scars (Shimizu and Kishi 2012). To numb the affected area, the patients are given local anesthesia. For shave excision, tumor growth is peeled off from the skin surface using a tool like a sharp razor (Lipke 2006). The advantages of standard surgical excision include a low risk of infection and less hematoma formation. Unlike other destructive or topical treatments modalities, histologic investigation of the excised tumor specimen can be performed. Standard surgical excision is a faster operation than Mohs surgery. Mohs surgery is preferred in particular conditions where skin grafting or tissue rearrangement is required for the closure of excision. Lack of absolute surgical margin assessment accounts for the greater relapse noticed with SSE in comparison to Mohs surgery.

Another technique, curettage and electrodesiccation, is usually approved for small squamous cell carcinomas. The surgeon scrapes off, either a part or full lesion after local anesthesia with a curette, and burns the tumor, employing an electrocautery needle to stop bleeding and kill any remains of cancer cells. The surgeon repeats this procedure a few times, to ensure that no tumor remains. This technique is appropriate, predominantly, for superficial invasive SCC. Yet, it is not recommended for aggressive squamous cell carcinoma, present in high-risk sites, such as the genitalia, eyelids, ears, and lips around the face since this procedure leaves a hypopigmented scar (Goldman 2002).

Frederic Mohs (1930) designed Mohs surgery to remove skin tumors while preserving completely healthy tissues. In this technique, tumors are removed from the skin, layer by layer. This surgery is often used on visible sites, like the neck and head or hands. It is also helpful in recurrent skin cancers. This procedure requires local anesthesia and leaves a scar. Mohs surgery possesses the highest treatment rate. It is especially employed for squamous cell cancers (bigger than 2 cm, around 4/5 inch) with imperfectly defined edges, for cancers that have recurred after other treatments, for cancers that are growing along the nerves under the skin, and for cancers on the genital area or face. This treatment approach is time-consuming and more complex than other surgeries. Although expensive, Mohs surgery is reported as a safe technique (Kauvar et al. 2015).

As reported earlier, skin cancer surgery results in disfigurement or scarring, especially in wide excisions or when the surgery is carried out on the head, face, hands, or neck. Hence, a reconstructive facial or surgeon specialist may form part of the physician's team as treatment might affect a patient's quality of life (Potenza et al. 2018).

Cryosurgery is a technique that employs an instrument and liquid nitrogen to freeze as well as destroy the abnormal cells in situ. This technique may be repeated again and again as per need. The treated area may swell, blister, and scar. This is usually used for precancerous lesions or small skin cancers. Laser surgery uses a laser beam to produce bloodless cuts in skin tissue or to remove tumor. Easy and inexpensive to administer, cryosurgery may be a suitable alternative for patients having an intolerance or bleeding disorders to anesthesia. Nevertheless, it possesses a lower success rate in comparison to the surgical options (Yiu et al. 2007). A low-cost treatment option, cryosurgery is rarely used for small, well-defined low-risk BCCs, when surgery and radiation have to be avoided. The successful outcome of the technique depends on the operator, and the recurrence frequency is high for BCC. Cryosurgery takes longer healing times as compared to sutured wounds; besides severe scarring, there is no histologic evidence of complete tumor removal (Kauvar et al. 2015).

Photodynamic therapy (PDT) comprises the application of a photosensitizing agent combined with irradiation on the skin. In this technique, a light-sensitive drug is applied directly over the skin tumor. After 78 hours, the treated skin is exposed to blue light, which activates the medication, resulting in targeting of cancer cells. This treatment option is often chosen for actinic keratosis. Further, patients remain photosensitive for 24–48 hours after treatment with PDT. Tumor clearance rates are lower than those with other treatment options. No histologic validation of complete tumor removal is seen. Patients feel burning and pain during photodynamic therapy. In addition, edema and erythema develop immediately and last for 1 week. Other side effects associated with this technique are blistering, crusting, bleeding, and weeping. The treatment rates for photodynamic therapy are comparatively lower than surgery. Over surgery, it shows better cosmesis. This technique is comparatively safer for healthy skin tissues (Kauvar et al. 2015). Radiation therapy is a commonly used cancer treatment modality that uses high-energy X-rays to destroy cancer cells or stop their growth. A radiation treatment regimen usually consists of a fixed number of treatments required over a fixed time interval. Several treatments may be required for the complete elimination of cancer. There are two modes of radiation therapy: internal and external. Internal radiation sends radiation via a machine outside the body, as a source of radiation. However, external radiation therapy utilizes a radioactive substance as a source of radiation to destroy cancer cells. The mode of radiation therapy chosen depends on the type of skin cancer; external radiation therapy is employed to treat BCC and SCC of the skin. A radiation oncologist specializes in giving radiation therapy to manage cancer. Radiation therapy may be preferred to surgery for skin cancers that are located in the eyelid, the ear, or the tip of the nose. This therapy avoids scarring as well as reoccurrence of cancer after surgery. Radiation therapy is often given as adjuvant therapy for Merkel cell cancer (stage I and II disease). Radiation therapy is not allowed for people having nevoid basal cell carcinoma. Other side effects from radiation include skin infections, rashes, itchy skin, redness, or change in the skin color. These side effects may be prevented by topically applying an antibiotic or corticosteroid. Radiation therapy is not the first treatment choice in young patients because of the associated risk of long-term complications (Strojan 2010).

Radiation treatment modality is applied as the primary or adjuvant mode of therapy for nonmelanoma squamous carcinoma (Kauvar et al. 2015).

Chemotherapy is another widely used cancer treatment option that utilizes drug moieties to stop the growth of cancerous cells, either by stopping their division or by killing them. During chemotherapy via oral/parenteral route, the drugs enter the systemic circulation and can reach cancer cells throughout the body. In regional chemotherapy, the drug is kept directly in the target organ which predominantly affects cancer cells (like CSF (cerebrospinal fluid), abdomen). Chemotherapy for BCC, SCC, and actinic keratosis is usually given via topical route. This further depends upon cancerous condition being treated, for example, topical fluorouracil (5-FU) is given to treat BCC. Topical drugs are generally applied every day for several weeks. These may result in irritation, inflammation, stinging, burning, and redness during treatment. However, topical therapy rules out the probability of scar formation. Sometimes, chemotherapy is combined with radiation therapy and surgery (Wilson and Schuchter 2016).

In immunotherapy treatment, the patient's immune system is used to fight against cancer. This is also known as biologic therapy or biotherapy. Substances produced by the body or immunotherapy drugs such as imiquimod and interferons are used to restore the natural defense mechanism of the skin against cancer. Interferon may be given by means of injection to cure squamous cell carcinoma (SCC) of the skin. Topical imiquimod cream has been reported to treat some BCC of the skin (Lugowska et al. 2018).

Chemabrasion is a chemical peel procedure adopted to improve outer skin conditions. In this procedure, a chemical solution is applied on the skin, and as a result, top layers of the cell get dissolved. This technique may be used for the treatment of actinic keratosis (PDQ Adult Treatment Editorial Board 2002).

In laser treatment, a narrow light beam (high intensity) is employed to kill precancer cells located in the outer region of the skin (Zipser et al. 2010).

18.3 Nanomedicine as Alternative for Topical Management of Skin Cancer

Some prominent anticancer phytoagents have been discussed in this chapter. Examples include apigenin, α-santalol, β-carotene, curcumin, caffeic acid, daidzein, eugenol, emodin, ferulic acid, epigallocatechin-3-gallate, genistein, resveratrol, silymarin, vitamin C, kaempferol, and quercetin. These bioactives have been considered potentially effective to improve cancer treatment or chemoprevention through multiple mechanisms. Development of an appropriate delivery system is an important aspect for anticancer natural moieties, owing to their poor solubility, bioavailability, and stability (Abirami et al. 2014). Besides these, sustained delivery, reduced side effects, proper distribution, and safeguard from metabolic degradation are other advantages provided by these delivery systems. Their multifunctionality and targeting ability can further resolve other challenges associated with cancer therapy. The most widely explored phytochemical agents include alkaloids and a variety of polyphenols, for improvement in their efficacy. A variety of novel formulations have been explored for the development of an optimized delivery system for skin cancer. The application of nanotechnology for the development of novel delivery system includes carriers such as nanosponges, polymeric nanoparticles, solid lipid nanoparticles (SLNs), nanolipid carriers, dendrimers, magnetic nanoparticles, polymer micelles, carbon nanotubes, liposomes, and phytosomes (Fig. 18.2). These nanocarriers aid in augmenting the therapeutic utility of herbal moieties by addressing the abovementioned challenges. Various nanoformulations comprising herbal bioactives have been tabulated below (Table 18.2).

In topical delivery, drug penetration via the stratum corneum (SC) is of paramount importance to assess the therapeutic action of the drug moiety. Furthermore, drug transport to the epidermis is crucial for agents possessing poor efficacy. Here, transport features of the drug moiety via the skin are considered critical. These features are governed by the drug's physicochemical

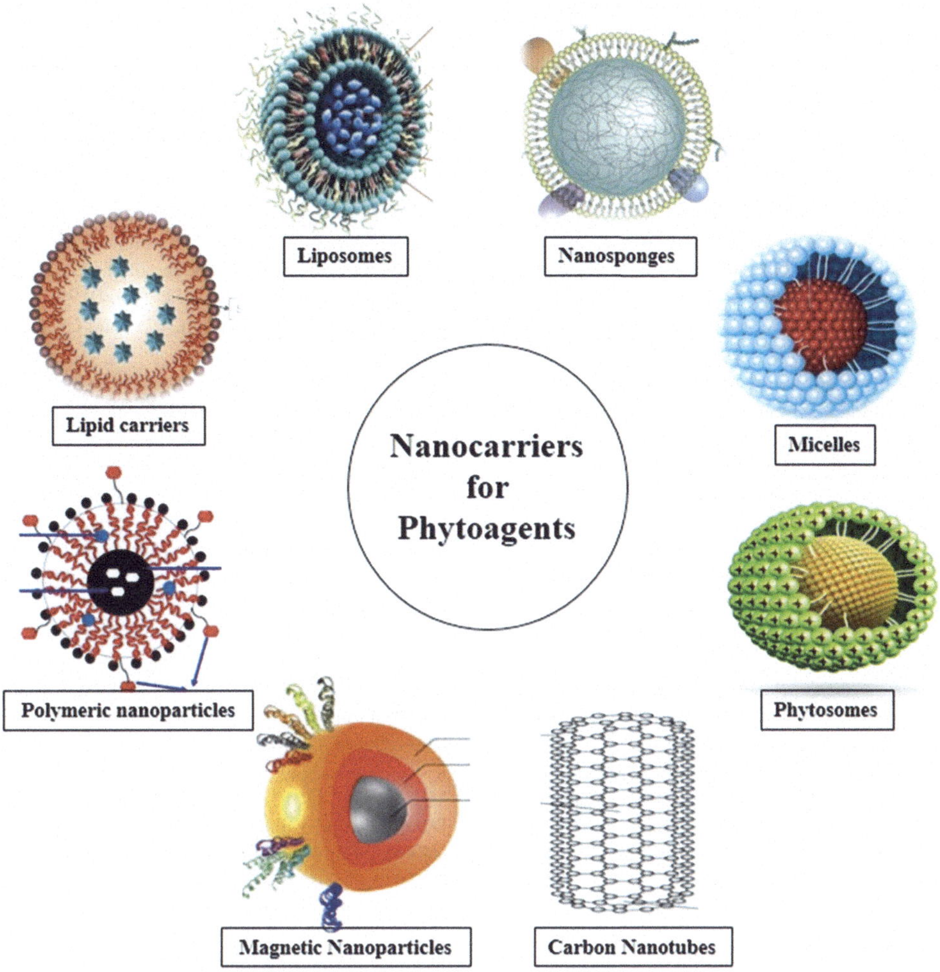

Fig. 18.2 Nanomedicines as novel delivery system

properties (lipophilicity and molecular weight) and can be tailored to achieve local effect. Hence, appropriate crafting of the formulation is vital for topical delivery of drug molecules (Conte et al. 2014).

18.3.1 Nanosponges

Cyclodextrin (CD)-based nanosponges (NS) are innovative nanocarriers obtained via cross-linking of cyclodextrin in three-dimensional architectures. CD-NS are highly porous nanostructures either amorphous or crystalline fabricated with different cross-linkers. A variety of cross-linkers, which are commonly employed for crafting nanosponges, include an active carbonyl compound, like diphenyl carbonate, triphosgene, carbonyldiimidazole, or organic dianhydrides (Chilajwar et al. 2014). The dimension of the polymer mesh, polarity, and release of entrapped moiety can be easily tailored by modifying the type of cross-linker and degree of cross-linking (Sherje et al. 2017). Nanosponges can be loaded with a wide variety of drugs (hydrophilic and hydrophobic). These tiny spongy structures circulate throughout the body to reach the target site, subsequently stick on its surface, and finally release the drug contents in a predictable fashion (Bolmal et al. 2013). The prolonged-release property of these carriers offers retention of topical actives on the skin, resulting in their better

Table 18.2 Nanofomulations comprising phytochemical actives for skin cancer

Sr. no.	Nanosystems	Phytochemical actives	References
1	Liposomes	5-Aminolevulinic acid, ursolic acid, paclitaxel, quercetin, curcumin, vincristine, berberine	Pierre et al. (2001), Harmand et al. (2003), Zhigaltsev et al. (2005), Yuan et al. (2006), Chen et al. (2012a), Flaten et al. (2013) and Ma et al. (2013)
2	Solid lipid nanoparticles	Camptothecin, quercetin, retinoic acid, naringenin, methotrexate, curcumin, resveratrol, paclitaxel, indirubin	Yang and Zhu (2002), Dhawan et al. (2011), Akanda et al. (2015), Ji et al. (2016), Battaglia et al. (2017), Rompicharla et al. (2017), Wang et al. (2017), Xu et al. (2018) and Rahiminejad et al. (2019)
3	Nanostructured lipid carriers	Docetaxel, lutein, coenzyme Q10	Liu et al. (2011), Mitri et al. (2011) and Chen et al. (2013)
4	Polymeric nanoparticles	Curcumin, paclitaxel, berberine, vincristine, ferulic acid, apigenin, resveratrol, luteolin, EGCG, piperine	Bisht et al. (2007), Wang et al. (2010), Chang et al. (2011), Chen et al. (2012b), Merlin et al. (2012), Das et al. (2013a), Sanna et al. (2013), Majumdar et al. (2014), Siddiqui et al. (2014) and Pentak (2016)
5	Magnetic nanoparticles	Camptothecin, quercetin	Castillo et al. (2014) and Kumar et al. (2014)
6	Phytosomes	Naringenin, silibinin, curcumin, sinigrin, quercetin, luteolin, mitomycin	Maiti et al. (2006), Flaig et al. (2007), Kidd (2009), Hou et al. (2012), Rasaie et al. (2014), Sabzichi et al. (2014) and Mazumder et al. (2016)
7	Carbon nanotubes	Paclitaxel, doxorubicin	Sobhani et al. (2011) and Verma et al. (2013)
8	Micelles	Paclitaxel, honokiol, β-lapachone, luteolin, doxorubicin, curcumin	Singla et al. (2002), Wei et al. (2009), Blanco et al. (2010), Dong et al. (2010), Qiu et al. (2013) and Kumari et al. (2016)
9	Nanosponges	Camptothecin, resveratrol, paclitaxel, curcumin, imiquimod	Swaminathan et al. (2010), Ansari et al. (2011), Minelli et al. (2012), Mognetti et al. (2012), Darandale and Vavia (2013), Bastiancich et al. (2014), Gigliotti et al. (2016), Gholibegloo et al. (2019) and Pushpalatha et al. (2019)

therapeutic performance. Nanosponges can also be incorporated into a variety of topical formulations such as cream, lotion, ointment, gel, and emulgel. Another important feature of these nanocarriers is their tendency to enhance aqueous solubility for poorly soluble drugs (Thakre et al. 2016).

Nanosponges can also be used to deliver anticancer agents for the treatment of tumors. It was claimed that these nanocarriers are three to five times more efficacious at retarding tumor growth in comparison to direct injection of the drug substances. These tiny nanostructures are filled with an anticancer compound and exposed to a targeting peptide that binds to surface receptors on tumor cells. When nanosponges encounter tumors, they stick to their surface and release their cargo. Hence, such targeted delivery results in more effective treatment with the same dose of the drug and lesser side effects (Singh et al. 2016). Camptothecin, a potent antitumor plant alkaloid, possesses a limited therapeutic efficacy owing to its lactone ring instability, poor aqueous solubility, and serious side effects. As reported earlier, CD-NS have been employed earlier to protect the labile groups, to enhance the solubility of poorly soluble moieties, and to control the drug release. Therefore, Swaminathan and his coworkers encapsulated camptothecin in cyclodextrin nanosponges to address challenges associated with it (Swaminathan et al. 2010; Singh et al. 2016).

18.3.2 Polymeric Nanoparticles

Over the past decade, polymeric nanoparticles (PN) have been proposed widely for topical drug delivery, where these nanoformulations have proved their worth. The advantages of these nanocarriers include reduction in adverse side effects associated with drug's systemic toxicity and enhanced retention of the drug in the skin (Stevanovic and Uskokovic 2009; Zhao et al. 2009, 2010; Kolenyak dos Santos et al. 2013). PN can also be referred to as nanospheres or nanocapsules, depending upon their composition. The features defining the nature of PN are governed by the type of polymer, surface charge, and size. A variety of biodegradable and synthetic polymers can be chosen for crafting PN, e.g., natural polymers, such as chitosan, and synthetic polymers, like polyglycolides (PGA), polylactides (PLA), poly(lactide-co-glycolides) (PLGA), and polyanhydrides. Research scientists have explored a combination of polymer technology and nanotechnology for skin cancer management.

In nanocapsules, the oil promotes formation of a vesicular structure, resulting in the reservoir-based delivery system, while absence of oil in nanospheres articulates matrix-organized polymeric chains (Magenheim and Benita 1991; Soppimath et al. 2001). Drugs are entrapped via mixing in the polymer solution (Hu and Zhang 2012) or dispersing them or chemically adsorbing them in the polymer matrix (Guterres et al. 2007). Polymeric nanoparticles have accomplished a significant place in the treatment of chronic hyperproliferative diseases, providing scientists with promising tools to overcome major current issues associated with contemporary topical chemotherapy (Kolenyak dos Santos et al. 2013).

Ourique and his research team (2011) investigated the fabrication and characterization of hydrogels comprising tretinoin lipid-core polymeric nanocapsules for topical application. Tretinoin is reported for the topical treatment of skin cancer. Although effective topically, tretinoin in dermatological products is associated with skin irritation. It is also unstable in the presence of air, heat, and light. Hence, the entrapment of tretinoin in nanoparticles resulted in its photostability, and prolonged its residence time in the skin, by retarding its permeation to the systemic circulation. As a result, side effects associated with this moiety were also reduced. The skin permeation studies demonstrated that drug-encapsulated lipid-core polymeric nanocapsules facilitated controlled permeation into the skin. Therefore, this prepared tretinoin system was reported worth for topical delivery for the treatment of skin diseases (Ourique et al. 2011).

18.3.3 Solid Lipid Nanoparticles and Nanolipid Carriers

At the beginning of 1990s, SLNs (solid lipid nanoparticles) were introduced as an alternative mode of delivery system to liposomes, polymeric NP, and emulsions. No toxic organic solvents are required for the fabrication of SLNs. SLNs present good physical stability to labile drugs by protecting them against degradation and allowing easy control over their release. Further, this system is biocompatible and biodegradable with low toxicity. Additionally, the production as well as sterilization of SLNs on a large scale is relatively easy (Mehnert and Mäder 2012; Cappellano et al. 2019). Due to the lipophilic nature of the skin, SLN favors skin permeation and penetration. Furthermore, SLN also possesses a targeting feature, which results in their high skin accumulation (Maia et al. 2000; Souto et al. 2004). Recent fabrication techniques have been proposed to encapsulate drug moieties within this lipophilic cargo for augmented topical application. Visualization of their distribution via confocal microscopy illustrated deep penetration up to 60 mm with the help of tape-stripping (for removal of SC) (Lee et al. 2011), penetration of larger nanoparticles up to >200 nm, while normal SC can only allow the penetration of nanoparticles up to 600 Daltons. The enhancement in the penetration advocated improved drug retention in the skin (Naik et al. 2004).

A variety of SLN-based delivery systems have been reported for cytotoxic agents such as idarubicin, doxorubicin, camptothecin, PTX, 7-ethyl-10hydroxy-20(S)-CPT, retinoic acid, cholesterylbutyrate, flurodooxyuridine (FudR), and ETP (Wei et al. 2015). Xu et al. crafted SLNs of silibinin comprising phosphatidylcholine and TPGS (tocopheryl polyethylene glycol succinate) by employing the thin-film hydration technique and evaluated these on MDA-MB-231 breast cancer cells. Here, the results exhibited higher cellular uptake of SLNs (twice higher than that of free silibinin). These were supported by similar observations in cell viability, migration, and invasion assays. An interesting result by this group was the suppression of the migratory and invasive potential of MDA-MB-231 cells at 20 mg/mL concentration of SLNPs. This might have occurred via downregulation of the MMP-9 and Snail pathways (Xu et al. 2013; Khan and Gurav 2018).

The solid lipid matrix in SLNs may lead to some problems, since this system is prone to crystallization, resulting in low encapsulation and expulsion of a drug during storage. To address these limitations, the second generation of nanoparticles termed "nanostructured lipid carriers" (NLCs) was developed (Luiza Ribeiro de Souza et al. 2012). These nanosystems are engineered by the intercalation of liquid and solid lipid phases, subsequently resulting in the formation of disorganized matrix and encapsulation of the active moieties (Muller et al. 2004; Pardeike et al. 2009). Similar to the SLNs, NLCs can also be administered by pulmonary, intravenous, and oral routes. Besides these, these nanolipidic systems have also been found appropriate for dermal delivery, since their application on the skin surface resulted in occlusive film formation, controlled release profile, low toxicity, and biodegradability. Moreover, owing to their small size, SLNs and NLCs ensure contact with the SC, enabling enhanced drug penetration into the skin (Agrawal et al. 2010; Obeidat et al. 2010; Luiza Ribeiro de Souza et al. 2012).

Palombo and coworkers (2007) observed that topical application of lutein improved its concentration in the skin layers, and lowered its peroxidation, with enhanced hydration, elasticity, and skin protection (Fang et al. 2008). Mitri et al. (2011) demonstrated that this moiety is effective in skin cancer, owing to its role in the prevention of inflammation and erythema (by UV rays). This group prepared two different NLCs, the first comprising glyceryl tripalmitate and capric/caprylic triglyceride as solid and liquid lipids, respectively, and the second composed of carnauba wax and capric/caprylic triglyceride. The prepared NLCs were named as NLC1 and NLC2, respectively. From release evaluation, this group noted the release of 12.12% (NLC1) and 7.38% (NLC2), after 24 hours. This research team also assessed the percent penetration of lutein into the pig's ear dermis, recording penetration of 19% (NLC1) and 11% (NLC2), after 24 hours (Mitri et al. 2011; Kolenyak dos Santos et al. 2013).

18.3.4 Dendrimers

Dendrimers are nanostructures comprising multiple channels (having functionalizable terminal groups) branching out from the central cavity. These novel nanosystems can accumulate multiple therapeutic agents, either via conjugation to functional end groups (Svenson 2009) or entrapment inside the central core or multiple units between dendrimers' architecture. Controlled depolymerization of these structures results in highly tunable drug release profiles. Dendrimers comprising polyamidoamine can be modulated to enhance biocompatibility and improve tumor targeting (Berciano-Guerrero et al. 2014). Owing to their unique physical characteristics like monodispersity, water encapsulation ability, and solubility, these macromolecular structures are highly helpful in the engineering of topical delivery vehicles for a variety of drugs. The prominent features of dendrimers are mainly dominated by the functional groups present on their molecular surface; howbeit, there are some examples of dendrimers possessing internal functionality. A well-defined nanoarchitecture with large internal volume is present in dendrimer (Abdel-Rahman and Al-Abd 2013). Malar and his coworkers crafted dendrosomal capsaicin (CAP) nanoformulations by esterification technique and evaluated these for in vitro anticancer potential on HEp2, VERO, and MCF-7 cell lines. The results exhibited that the prepared dendrimers possessed remarkable cytotoxicity on VERO cells (IC50 of 1.25 μg/mL) and MCF7 and HEp2 cells (IC50 of

0.62 μg/mL) (Malar and Bavanilathamuthiah 2015).

18.3.5 Magnetic Nanoparticles

Magnetic nanoparticles (MNPs), particularly iron oxide (also called magnetite) NPs and their multi-functionalized counterparts, are a vital class of nanocarriers that have fascinated the scientific community for their potential utilities in drug delivery. Recent advancements in fabrication and surface modification techniques for these nanoparticles may revolutionize present clinical therapeutic technologies and diagnostics. The well-known surface chemistry of magnetite MNPs allows entrapping of a wide variety of functional moieties, for imaging and targeting ligands. It is also possible to finely tune the physical features of MNPs, such as shape, size, magnetism, and crystallinity (Khan and Gurav 2018).

The basic criterion behind the fabrication of magnetic nanoparticles is the fact that the drug moiety is either entrapped into magnetic nanospheres or conjugated on their surface or implanted in the form of magnetically active disk. The drug release can be controlled utilizing a powerful magnetic field in the target (tumor area). Magnetic materials receive their magnetic response to a magnetic field from materials such as magnetite, nickel, iron, samarium-cobalt, and cobalt and neodymium-iron-boron. Potential treatment of cancer involves attachment of MNPs to the tumor cells, enabling them to be captured and taken out of the body. This treatment has been evaluated in the laboratory, taking mice as an animal model (Scarberry et al. 2008; Huang and Hainfeld 2013). Magnetic nanoparticles can also be used for cancer detection. For this, a microfluidic chip having magnetic nanoparticles can be inserted in blood. These MNPs are generally entrapped inside owing to an externally applied magnetic field, as the blood is free to flow through. The MNPs are coated with antibodies for targeting proteins or cancer cells. For melanoma, several studies have been performed and reported using this carrier (Ito et al. 2003; Balivada et al. 2010).

Verma and his collaborators prepared MNPs of quercetin (QUR) via nebulization and assessed their cytotoxicity potential in lung cancer cell line (A549). This group coated the surface of MNPs with PLGA to augment the drug dispersion in an aqueous medium, enhance its stability (against oxidation), and ensure biocompatibility. The biocompatibility of QUR MNPs was checked by carrying in vitro and in vivo evaluation studies. The results showed remarkable retardation in the number of viable A549 cells for quercetin-loaded MNPs. The results of this research advocated QUR-loaded MNPs promising in lung cancer (Verma et al. 2013).

18.3.6 Polymer Micelles

The promising potential of the polymeric micelles as prospective drug delivery carriers in anticancer therapy has been an interesting topic of discussion among research scientists for decades. Polymer micelles are spherical nanoconstructs (from 10 to 100 nm), prepared from self-assembly of amphiphilic-surfactant molecules in an aqueous environment. A polymeric micelle essentially composed of an inner hydrophobic core thus encapsulates a hydrophobic drug, while the corona is comprised of the hydrophilic portion of the block copolymer. Some inherent features of polymeric micelles, which make them an attractive choice as a carrier for anticancer drugs, include (1) nano-size range, (2) stable in plasma, (3) in vivo longevity, and (4) augmented permeability. The pathological characteristics of the tumor cells allowed their passive targeting to tumor cells (Kedar et al. 2010). The corona serves the dual role of stabilization of the polymeric micelles against recognition by RES (reticuloendothelial system) and drug targeting by attaching specific ligands (recognizing the tumor sites). Drug release can be tailored by appropriate application of heat or ultrasound or other external stimuli. Hence, polymeric micelles possess promising active as well as passive targeting potential to the tumor tissues (Rapoport 2007).

The activation of the polymer micelles in the tumor tissue prevents the drug release in the blood during circulation, hence retarding the drug toxicity to normal cells (Lu et al. 2013). The major breakthrough was noted in the early 1990s by Kataoka and his research team, who fabricated doxorubicin-conjugated block copolymer micelles (Kwon et al. 1997; Kataoka et al. 2000).

18.3.7 Carbon Nanotubes

Carbon nanotubes (CNTs) were firstly discovered by Iijima in 1991 (Iijima 1991; Sinha and Yeow 2005). Carbon nanotubes can be grouped as SWNT (single-walled), which essentially composed of a layer of cylinder graphene, or MWNT (multi-walled) comprising several concentric graphene sheets (Sinha and Yeow 2005). Over the last decade, carbon nanotubes have been extensively investigated in almost every cancer treatment, including lymphatic-targeted chemotherapy, drug delivery, photodynamic therapy, thermal therapy, and gene therapy. Carbon nanotubes as drug delivery vehicles have demonstrated promising potential in targeting specific cancer cells with a lower dosage than conventional drugs (Srinivasan 2008). Moreover, this modality do not harm healthy cells and have shown reduced side effects.These nanoparticles have been reported to enhance the efficacy of chemotherapy in melanoma cells as well (Chaudhuri et al. 2009; Bei et al. 2010). Chaudhuri and his coworkers showed that an SWNT loaded with doxorubicin triggered melanoma cell death in a dose-dependent manner (in vitro) and abolished tumor growth studied in a xenograft melanoma model.

A variety of approaches have been employed to entrap drug moieties to the sidewalls of functionalized CNTs by noncovalent or covalent attachment (Wu et al. 2005; Zhang et al. 2010; Kakran and Li 2012). Liu and his collaborators utilized PEGylated NGO (nanoscale graphene oxide) as a nanocarrier to entrap anticancer agents via noncovalent interactions and assessed its cellular uptake (Liu et al. 2008). Ali-Boucetta and his research group investigated the noncovalent interaction of doxorubicin (an anticancer drug) with CNTs and evaluated its cytotoxic potential (Ali-Boucetta et al. 2008). These research works illustrated that GO derivatives and CNTs can be employed as efficient nanovehicles for delivering water-insoluble aromatic molecules. Howbeit, the cytotoxicity and cellular uptake of camptothecin, on entrapment in GO and CNTs have not been checked in this investigation. Sahoo and his coworkers used the PVA-functionalized MWCNTs and GO to administer camptothecin, while such similar works have not been reported in the literature. This group investigated the cytotoxic potential and the drug loading of camptothecin-loaded CNT- and GO-based nanosystems and compared their efficacy (Sahoo et al. 2011).

18.3.8 Liposomes

Liposomes are nanolipid cargos formed by self-assembly of phospholipids in an aqueous environment. They resemble biological membranes in their structure. These are engineered using phospholipids, possessing a hydrophilic head and hydrophobic tail (Xi and Guo 2007). Water-soluble moieties can be encapsulated in the aqueous core, whereas the hydrophobic drugs can be retained in their lipid bilayers (Cappellano et al. 2019). Owing to their lipidic structure, they are easily absorbed by the liver and taken up by macrophages, resulting in a decrease in their efficiency. This can be escaped by coating liposomal lipid surface with appropriate ligands like monosialoganglioside or by incorporating polyvinylpyrrolidone polyacrylamide lipids, cholesterol, phospholipid distearoylphosphatidylcholine, or glucuronic acid lipids into liposomes. The polar end has phosphoric atom attached to a hydrophilic molecule. Liposome augments the biodistribution, bioavailability, solubility, and in vivo and in vitro stability of entrapped moieties and altered pharmacokinetics. In the similar way, liposome-based delivery systems can enhance the therapeutic utility of herbal moieties (Saraf 2010).

Liposomes have been explored extensively for the temporal and spatial delivery of anticancer agents. The first FDA-approved liposomal product is liposomal doxorubicin (Doxil®) for Kaposi's sarcoma, ovarian cancer, and refractory breast cancer. Liposomes have been employed to entrap chemotherapeutic agents, siRNA, and immunocytokines to enhance treatment potential for melanoma (Bei et al. 2010).

Wang et al. fabricated folic acid-conjugated PEGylated liposomes of vincristine (FA-PEG-LS/VCR), specifically for multidrug-resistant cancer. Thin-flim extrusion and hydration techniques were employed for fabrication and their cytotoxicity was investigated on KBv200 cells (multidrug-resistant variants), a human epidermoid nasopharyngeal carcinoma cell lines. In vivo antitumor activities were accessed and evaluated by tumor growth inhibition (apoptosis assessment studies and tumor growth inhibition by TUNEL). The obtained results demonstrated that the IC50 value of the PEGylated folic acid-conjugated VCR liposomes was found to be 23.99 nM and 363.08 nM for PEG-LS/VCR and 1.10 μM for free VCR. The in vivo studies suggested that the folic acid conjugation remarkably strengthened the antitumor potential of the PEGylated liposomes of VCR and also depicted a higher apoptosis index in the TUNEL analysis (Terminal deoxynucleotidyl transferase-mediated dUTP nick-end labeling). Vincristine liposomes have also been commercialized as Marqibo (trade name of the drug) (Wang et al. 2013).

18.3.9 Phytosomes

Phytosomes are phospholipid-derived delivery systems, explored for delivery of herbal drug. Mixing the phytoactive constituents at appropriate molar ratios with phosphatidylcholine (natural phospholipid) results in the synthesis of phytosomes. The phospholipid-substrate interaction can be due to the formation of hydrogen bonds between the polar functional groups and polar head of phospholipids on the substrate. This phytolipid-based delivery system bridges the novel and conventional delivery systems. These are herbal formulations with better absorption properties. This novel delivery system also exhibits better pharmacokinetic therapeutic profiles in comparison to conventional extracts from medicinal plants. In aqueous environments, phytosomes attain micellar liposomal-like architecture. In phytosomes, the bioactive molecule is attached to the polar head portion of phospholipids, hence becoming an integral structure of the membrane (Kumar et al. 2017).

Ochi et al. entrapped two plant-derived anticancer compounds, silibinin and glycyrrhizic acid, in nanophytosomes to enhance their poor bioavailability and examined their effects on (hepatocellular carcinoma) HCC cell lines (HepG2) (Ochi et al. 2016). Silibinin is a natural bioactive extracted from silymarin and has been known to possess anticancer potential (Ramakrishna et al. 2011). Another bioactive glycyrrhizic acid extracted from *Glycyrrhiza glabra* (*L.*) possesses anticancer activity (Verschoyle et al. 2008). In vitro release investigation depicted a sustained-release behavior with 88% (w/w) of glycyrrhizic acid and 14% (w/w) of silibinin over 48 hours. Cell viability analysis using HepG2 cell lines exhibited that co-encapsulated nanophytosomes of glycyrrhizic acid and silibinin were three times more potent than individual glycyrrhizic acid (75% w/v) and silibinin (25% w/v). Hence, phytosomes enhanced the bioavailability of silibinin, and this phytosome technology is capable of providing co-encapsulated systems, which resulted in the enhancement of therapeutic effects of silibinin by synergistic action with glycyrrhizic acid (Ochi et al. 2016). Recent studies have shown that the capability of silibinin against prostate cancer was found augmented on its combination with other potential anticancer agents like mitoxantrone (Flaig et al. 2007), doxorubicin (Tyagi et al. 2002) carboplatin and cisplatin (Dhanalakshmi et al., 2003).

18.4 Natural Agents for Prevention and Treatment of Skin Cancer

A summary of various herbal bioactives along with their sources and anticancer activities have been illustrated in Table 18.3. Some important bioactives have been discussed in detail below.

Table 18.3 Phytochemical actives reported for skin cancer

Sr. no.	Natural agents	Category	Common sources	Reported activities	References
1	Apigenin	Flavonoids	Parsley, celery, celeriac, and chamomile	Apoptosis, anti-proliferative	Srivastava and Gupta (2007)
2	Allyl sulfides	Sulfides	Garlic	Anti-proliferative	Srinivasan et al. (2007) and Srivastava and Gupta (2007)
3	α-Santalol	Sesquiterpenes	Sandalwood oil	Apoptosis	Arasada et al. (2008)
4	β-Carotene	Carotenoids	Carrots, spinach, kale, pepper, pumpkin, sweet potatoes, and cantaloupe	Apoptosis, anti-metastatic	Palozza et al. (2003)
5	Berberine	Alkaloids	Goldenseal, *Coptis* or goldenthread, Oregon grape, barberry, and tree turmeric	Apoptosis, anti-proliferative, anti-metastatic	Shen et al. (2016)
6	Curcumin	Phenols	Turmeric	Apoptosis, anti-proliferative	Li et al. (2016)
7	Capsaicin	Phenols	Red chili peppers and jalapenos	Apoptosis	Oyagbemi et al. (2010)
8	Caffeic acid	Phenolic acids	Coffee	Apoptosis, cell cycle arrest	Kang et al. (2008)
9	Daidzein	Isoflavonoids	Soybeans	Anti-metastatic	Lee et al. (2011)
10	Eugenol	Phenols	Cloves, nutmeg, cinnamon, bay leaves, and basil	Apoptosis, anti-proliferative	Jaganathan and Supriyanto (2012)
11	Emodin	Hydroxyanthraquinones	Aloe vera	Anti-proliferative	Muto et al. (2007), Subramaniam et al. (2013) and Yaoxian et al. (2013)
12	Ferulic acid	Phenols	Rice and maize Bran	Apoptosis, anti-proliferative	Srinivasan et al. (2007)
13	Epigallocatechin-3-gallate	Flavonoids	Green tea	Apoptosis, anti-proliferative, cell cycle arrest	Nihal et al. (2010)
14	Fucoxanthin	Xanthophylls	Brown seaweeds and diatoms	Apoptosis, anti-proliferative, anti-metastatic	Kumar et al. (2014)
15	Genistein	Flavonoids	Soybean	Apoptosis, anti-proliferative, anti-metastatic	Wei et al. (1998), Sarkar and Li (2002) and Rusin et al. (2010)
16	Honokiol	Neolignan biphenols	Magnolia plant	Apoptosis, cell cycle arrest	Hahm and Singh (2007)
17	Indole-3-carbinol	Organosulfurs	Cabbage	Apoptosis, cell cycle arrest	Kim et al. (2006, 2011)

(continued)

Table 18.3 (continued)

Sr. no.	Natural agents	Category	Common sources	Reported activities	References
18	Kaempferol	Flavonoids	Grapes, tomatoes, broccoli, tea, and ginkgo biloba	Apoptosis, anti-proliferative	Calderon-Montano et al. (2011) and Chen and Chen (2013)
19	Luteolin	Flavonoids	Carrots, peppers, celery, oliver	Apoptosis	Iwashita et al. (2000) and Nakashima et al. (2010)
20	Lycopene	Acyclic carotenoids	Watermelon, papaya, tomato, guava, grapefruit, apricot, and peaches	Apoptosis, cell cycle arrest	Chiang et al. (2007) and Wu and Kubota (2008)
21	Myricetin	Flavonoids	Walnuts	Apoptosis	Jung et al. (2008) and Kim et al. (2010)
22	Norathyriol	Xanthones	Mango	Apoptosis, cell cycle arrest	Li et al. (2012)
23	Piperine	Alkaloids	Black pepper and long pepper	Anti-proliferative, cell cycle arrest	Rather and Bhagat (2018)
24	Quercetin	Flavonols	Apple, tomatoes, tea, grapes, ginkgo, and St John's wort	Apoptosis	Lin et al. (2011)
25	Resveratrol	Polyphenol stilbenes	Grapes, peanuts, mulberries, and red wine	Apoptosis, anti-metastatic	Ndiaye et al. (2011)
26	Silymarin and silibinin	Polyphenol flavonoids	Milk thistle	Apoptosis, cell cycle arrest	Dhanalakshmi et al. (2004a, b)
27	Ursolic acid	Terpenoids	Basil	Anti-proliferative, anti-metastatic, cell cycle arrest	Es-Saady et al. (1996) and Harmand et al. (2003)
28	Vitamin A	Vitamins	Carrot, eggs, milk, and cheese	Anti-proliferative, anti-metastatic	Fan et al. (2010) and Bettoli et al. (2013)
29	Vitamin C	Vitamins	Citrus fruits, broccoli, green pepper, tomatoes, strawberries, and melons	Apoptosis, anti-proliferative, anti-metastatic	Chambial et al. (2013)
30	Vitamin D	Vitamins	Salmon, mackerel, bluefish, cod liver oil, mushrooms, egg yolks, and yeasts	Anti-proliferative	Tang et al. (2012)

18.4.1 Apigenin

Apigenin
is a natural product belonging to flavone class, which is frequently found in celery, tea, oranges, parsley, onions, and thyme (Shukla and Gupta 2010). It serves multiple physiological roles, for instance, strong antioxidant, anti-inflammatory, antiviral, and antibacterial activities and reduction in blood pressure (Ali et al. 2017). The anticancer action of apigenin has been examined in vitro in different cell lines, viz., neck and head squamous cell carcinoma cells, liver cells, and melanoma cells. It has been known to display UVB radiation protective action on human keratinocytes (evaluated in vitro) and on mice skin (evaluated in vivo). The mechanism involved is hindering cell survival as well as proliferation via the nuclear factor kappa-light-chain-enhancer (NF-κB) of activated β cells and mitogen-activated protein kinase (MAPK) routes (Das et al. 2013b).

18.4.2 α-Santalol

Alpha-santalol is a natural sesquiterpene, derived from the oil of sandalwood. Accumulated evidences advocate that this agent extracted from natural sources shows various medicinal activities, like antibacterial, anti-inflammatory, antidiabetic, and anticancer. Cancer and antitumor preventive properties of this herbal moiety have been involved in cell death induction via cell cycle arrest and apoptosis in different cancer models. Further, a significant reduction in inflammatory markers has been reported with α-santalol application in skin tissue models (Bommareddy et al. 2019).

18.4.3 β-Carotene

The most commonly studied carotenoid among the abundantly available carotenoids in human food is β-carotene. Some of its dietary sources include carrots, spinach, kale, pepper, pumpkin, sweet potatoes, and cantaloupe. It is capable of inducing apoptosis in melanoma cells (in vitro) by stimulating caspase-3, caspase-8, and caspase-9, through a caspase cascade (Palozza et al. 2003). As per studies of Guruvayoorappan and Kuttan, the antineoplastic mechanism of β-carotene in melanoma (murine) may include the regulation of p53, Bcl-2, and caspase-3, which subsequently triggers apoptosis. In another investigation by this research group (Guruvayoorappan and Kuttan 2007), the effect of β-carotene on tumor-expressed specific angiogenesis (influencing tumor growth) was also explored.

18.4.4 Curcumin

Curcumin, a vital component of turmeric, is obtained from a powdered rhizome of *Curcuma longa* abundantly used in Unani, Ayurveda, and Siddha medicines. Long back, it was reported to possess anti-inflammatory, anticarcinogenic, antioxidant, anticoagulant, antimutagenic, and antiinfective properties (Li et al. 2016). Recently, it was demonstrated that the anti-melanoma potential of curcumin was found dependent on the opening of mPTP (mitochondrial permeability transition pore), as displayed by curcumin in melanoma (in vitro) (Qiu et al. 2014). Curcumin has the capacity to trigger apoptosis, which is independent of p53 activity in melanoma cells (in a dose- and time-dependent fashion). Melanoma cells when treated with curcumin led to inhibition of the NF-κB pro-survival pathway and activation of the death receptor Fas-associated protein. The tolerability and safety of curcumin make it a promising candidate for the prevention of skin cancer (Bush et al. 2001).

18.4.5 Caffeic Acid

Caffeic acid (CA) is a potential polyphenolic moiety, widely present in fruits, coffee, and vegetables. This bioactive possesses potential anti-inflammatory, antioxidant, and anticancer potential (Fernandez et al. 1998; Moon et al. 2009). Yang and his research team reported that

CA remarkably inhibited the formation of a colony, and EGF triggered a neoplastic transformation of human keratinocyte cells (malignant) (Yang et al. 2013). The topical application of CA on the dorsal portion of UV-induced skin cancer in mice model stopped the cancer incidence (Esmaeili et al. 2016). The MAPK signaling pathway includes several other pathways, among which Ras-Raf-MEK-extracellular signal-regulated kinase (ERK) 1/2 cascade is the most abundant in human cancers. This molecular mechanism regulates many other vital functions of cell-like growth and proliferation (McCubrey et al. 2007). It also suppresses ERK1/2 functions (in vitro) and results in chemotherapeutic actions against UV-induced skin cancer (Esmaeili et al. 2016). In addition to MAPK, it was also found to enhance the expression of COX-2 and Fyn kinase in UV-triggered skin cancer (Kang et al. 2008).

18.4.6 Daidzein

Daidzein is a naturally dried isoflavonic phytoestrogen (Cassidy 2003). It is predominantly obtained from the leguminous plants such as mung bean and soybean. It is the major bioactive component used in traditional Chinese medicine Gegen, which is commonly applied for the treatment of acute dysentery, fever, diabetes, diarrhea, liver injury, cardiac dysfunctions, etc. (Wong et al. 2011). It also possesses several other biological properties independent of the ER such as anticancer, anti-inflammation, protection of the skin, and inhibition of oxidative damage of nerves. The beneficial properties are majorly due to immune response regulation (Wei et al. 2012), inhibition of proliferation, and scavenging of oxygen, free radicals, and so on. Some derivatives of daidzein include 7, 3′, 4′-THIF, which also show anticancer potential and efficacy in non-melanoma skin cancer (UVB induced) both in vitro and in vivo. The metabolite binds to MKK4 and cots directly to stop their activity, which further notably subdues the expression of UVB-induced COX-2 (cyclooxygenase 2) and, finally, curbing the number, elongation, and volume of tumors (Lee et al. 2011).

18.4.7 Eugenol

Eugenol is a volatile phenolic component of clove essential oil derived from *Eugenia caryophyllata* leaves and buds, found in India, Madagascar, and Indonesia. It (phenylpropanoid) is a pale yellow oil, with a molecular weight 164.2 g/mol and a spicy aroma. This bioactive is a weak acid and is easily soluble in organic solvents. It is commonly extracted from nutmeg, clove oil, basil, and bay and cinnamon leaf. It is known to possess several pharmacological properties, like antioxidant, anesthetic, antihelmintic, antimicrobial, anticarcinogenic, anti-inflammatory, antifumigant, and insect-repellent properties. Eugenol and its derivatives exhibited its activity against skin tumors, melanoma, gastric cancer, prostate cancer, and leukemia through oncogene regulation and caspase-dependent pathway, which is reviewed extensively by Jaganathan and Supriyanto (2012).

18.4.8 Emodin

Emodin belongs to a member of natural bioactives known as anthraquinones. Emodin is identified in 17 plant families worldwide but primarily found in three plant families Fabaceae, Polygonaceae, and Rhamnaceae (Harborne et al. 1989). Chemically 1,3,8-trihydroxy-6-methylanthraquinone, emodin is present in the root, bark, vegetative (stem, foliage), and reproductive organs (fruit, flower, pods, seeds) and is also produced by lichens. It has antibacterial, vasorelaxant, antitumor, and diuretic effects (Koyama et al. 1988; Zhou and Chen 1988; Huang et al. 1992). It triggers growth inhibition in cancerous cells but not affecting normal cells (Muto et al. 2007; Subramaniam et al. 2013; Yaoxian et al. 2013) and modified cellular redox status in time- and dose-dependent fashion (Yen et al. 2000; Srinivasan 2008; Kuo et al. 2009). The photo-protective action of emodin against the UV region of the solar radiation (290–400 nm) has also been demonstrated (Chang et al. 1999). Emodin is highly efficacious in pancreatitis, myocarditis, asthma, atherosclerosis, arthritis, glomerulonephritis, chronic obstructive lung disease, hepatitis, and Alzheimer's disease (Shrimali et al. 2013; Xue et al. 2010). Several studies reported that emodin-induced apoptosis was shown by (ROS) reactive oxygen species generated from semiquinone (Jing et al. 2002; Su et al. 2005); howbeit, there was also a report that emodin-induced apoptosis was ROS-independent (Chen et al. 2002).

18.4.9 Ferulic Acid

Ferulic acid has gained much importance in the Chinese medicine, as it is among one of the effective components in Chinese herbs like *Angelica sinensis*, *Cimicifuga heracleifolia*, and *Lignsticum chuangxiong* (Sakai et al. 1999). It exhibits a wide range of pharmacological activities including antiallergic, antioxidant, anticarcinogenic, hepatoprotective, antiviral, anti-inflammatory, antithrombotic, and vasodilatory. It also helps to increase the viability of sperms (Graf 1992; Ou and Kwok 2004). As free radicals play a vital role in cancer, the anticancer properties of some antioxidants are attributed to their capacity in free radical scavenging. Kaul and Khanduja (1998) demonstrated that topical application of polyphenols (tannic acid, ellagic acid, ferulic acid, and caffeic acid) simultaneously with mezerein or phorbol-12-myristate-13-acetate resulted in remarkable protection for 7,12-dimethylbenz[a]anthracene-triggered skin Ty6 tumors in mice (Rundlöf et al. 2000). Most of its therapeutic potential is ascribed to its anti-inflammatory and antioxidant activity (Srinivasan et al. 2007).

18.4.10 Epigallocatechin -3-allate

Epigallocatechin-3-gallate (EGCG) is another plant-derived stable and water-soluble member of flavonoid family, known as flavan-3-ols. These are widely available in tea, red wine, strawberry, and cocoa, with green tea reported as the major source (Corcoran et al. 2012). EGCG induces apoptosis and causes cell cycle arrest in melanoma (Hs-294T and A374), alone and in combination with vorinostat (in vitro) (Nihal et al. 2010; Zhang et al. 2000). Treatment with interferon and EGCG combination has also displayed synergistic anti-proliferative behavior in vitro against human melanoma cells and in vivo in a mice melanoma model (Nihal et al. 2009). The mechanisms with which EGCG exerts these actions include decrease in apoptosis-inhibiting proteins, or cell survival-promoting proteins (D1, Bcl-2, and cdk2 (cyclin-dependent kinase 2) the upregulation of Bax (Bcl-2-associated X protein) and pro-apoptosis protein. The triggering of caspase-3, caspase-7, and caspase-9; and the triggering of tumor suppressor proteins (p21WAF1/CIP1, p16INK4a, and p2KP1) by EGCG are also responsible for therapeutic outcomes (Nihal et al. 2005).

18.4.11 Genistein

Genistein is a soybean-derived bioactive, which has long been used as a dietary supplement for cardiovascular disorders, osteoporosis, and cancers (Wei et al. 2002, 2003; Singh et al. 2014). It is an abundantly available phytoestrogen moiety in soybeans and known to possess potent anti-inflammatory, antioxidant, and anti-proliferative effects (Wei et al. 1998; Sarkar and Li 2002; Sarkar et al. 2009; Rusin et al. 2010). Cancer chemopreventive actions of genistein have been exhibited in various malignancies, including neuroblastoma and breast cancer, as well as both non-melanoma and melanoma cancers (Afaq and Katiyar 2011; Ji et al. 2012). It has been shown to retard tumor proliferation, exert anti-angiogenesis effect and reduce metastasis, induce cell cycle arrest (Rusin et al. 2010), and improve cell apoptosis. The delivery of genistein retarded UV-induced sunburns in humans, protecting them from photoaging as well as UV-induced skin cancer (Wei et al. 2003). Moreover, genistein also possesses beneficial effects against melanoma cells. It interferes with cell cycles, inhibits tumor growth, and shows metastasis in a xenograft model (Ji et al. 2012). Inhibition of melanoma cell cycle by genistein was ascribed by targeting p21, p53, and Chk2 (checkpoint kinase) (Rauth et al. 1997; Casagrande and Darbon 2000; Darbon et al. 2000).

18.4.12 Kaempferol

Kaempferol (flavonoid) is abundantly found in a wide variety of dietary components like strawberries, tea, carrot, green chili, brinjal, pumpkin, propolis, broccoli, apples, grapefruit, onions, and beans (Corcoran et al. 2012; Albishi et al. 2013). Epidemiological reports have evidenced a positive relationship between consumption of high kaempferol in food and retardation in the incidence of various cancers (ovarian, lung, pancreatic, and gastric) and cardiovascular disorders. Kaempferol adopts several possible mechanisms for inhibiting cell proliferation and promoting apoptosis (Chen and Chen 2013). It has also been found to block the progression of choroidal melanoma cell cycle in the G2/M phase (Casagrande and Darbon 2001). Chao et al. had crafted submicron emulsion systems for the transdermal administration of kaempferol and observed that the use of a suitable carrier could remarkably influence the flux obtained, amount of drug deposition in the skin, and lag time (Chao et al. 2012).

18.4.13 Quercetin

Quercetin is identified by the presence of OH groups on positions 3, 5, 7, 3′, and 4′ of its flavonol skeleton. It is found insoluble in cold water, slightly soluble in hot water, and soluble in alcohol (Kelly 2011). It is commonly present in the human diet and is available in plants in glycosidic forms, like rhamnosides, galactosides, glucosides, or arabinosides (Hollman et al. 1997; Erlund 2004). The major sources of quercetin include tomatoes, grapes, apples, tea, and ginkgo (Kelly 2011). Onions are also known to contain good amounts of quercetin (Erlund 2004; Kelly 2011). Other sources are dark chocolate, cloves, capers, oregano, and black elderberries (Asensi et al. 2011). It seems to be one of the promising therapeutic flavonoids in terms of its biological potential (Lin et al. 2011). The anticancer potential of quercetin is mainly attributed to its anti-inflammatory and antioxidant activity. Quercetin acts via above-cited mechanisms. It reduces the viability and improves the apoptosis of UVB-irradiated B16F10 melanoma cells by various mechanisms: it enhances the levels of ROS, triggers the imbalance of calcium homeostasis, depolarizes mitochondrial membrane potential, attenuates MEK-ERK signaling, and modulates the ratio of Bax, Bcl-2, and Bim expression favoring of cell death elicitation (Rafiq et al. 2015). It also offers photoprotection against melanogenesis via a regulatory action on the Nrf2-ARE pathway (Chaiprasongsuk et al. 2016). Further, quercetin inhibits migration of melanoma cells in an experimentally activated set-up receptor tyrosine kinase c-Met, known to participate in the procurement of metastatic phenotypes (Cao et al. 2015).

18.4.14 Resveratrol

Resveratrol (trans-3, 5, 4′-trihydroxystilbene) is found in berries, grapes, red wine, peanuts, and various other plants. The major source of resveratrol is grapevine skin, where it protects the plant from bacterial infections (Delmas et al. 2006). It has shown to possess strong anticancer property via anti-inflammatory, anti-proliferative, and antioxidant potential (Ndiaye et al. 2011) and is a strong scavenger for ROS (Kowalczyk et al. 2009). It also arrests melanoma proliferation (in vitro), inhibiting cell divisions at the G1/S transition, and triggers apoptosis targeting Bcl-2-associated X protein, B-cell lymphoma 2, and caspase-9 and caspase-3 (Wu et al. 2015). Via suppression of STAT3 and β-catenin-pathway, resveratrol retarded the levels of a protein survivin, which is an essential requirement for the survival of melanoma cells. Additionally, this compound has anti-migratory effects mediated by the deactivation of the proto-oncogenic Akt (Bhattacharya et al. 2011).

18.4.15 Silymarin

Silymarin is a flavonolignan obtained from seeds (and also from fruits) of *Silybum marianum* (milk thistle or bank thistle), belonging to the Compositae family (Pandey 1990). This compound used so far particularly as hepatoprotectant was shown to have other interesting pharmacological activities, e.g., cancer-protective and anticancer and hypocholesterolemic activity (Gazak et al. 2007). These activities have been due to the antioxidant potential of silymarin, like chain-breaking antioxidant, scavenger of reactive oxygen species, and scavenger of phenylglyoxylic ketyl radicals. Reports of several clinical investigations evidenced the chemotherapeutic potential of silymarin on a variety of tumors including skin cancer (Luper 1998; Deep and Agarwal 2010). Further, Katiyar et al. demonstrated that this bioactive assures UV rays triggered skin cancer in a photocarcinogenesis mouse model (Katiyar et al. 1997; Vaid and Katiyar 2010; Afaq and Katiyar 2011). Additionally, silymarin arrests UVB-induced skin edema and sunburn, reduces catalase activity, instigates apoptotic cell formation, and triggers COX and ornithine decarboxylase articulation. The similar defensive effects were also demonstrated by silymarin on UVB-affected skin. Multiplying cell nuclear antigen, apoptotic sunburn cells and thymidine dimer-positive cells were found reduced using silymarin (Dhanalakshmi et al. 2004a, b).

18.4.16 Vitamin C

The major sources of vitamin C include citrus fruits, broccoli, green pepper, tomatoes, strawberries, and melons. Vitamin C has been most commonly used in the prevention and treatment of a large number of diseases such as atherosclerosis, diabetes, cataracts, common cold, macular degeneration, glaucoma, stroke, cancer, heart diseases, and so on. It probably acts by induction of apoptosis and via inhibition of cell growth and proliferation in cancer (Chambial et al. 2013). Apoptosis induction by this vitamin occurs by pro-oxidant activities, which can be blocked by a potent antioxidant N-acetyl-L-cysteine. It is known to possess antioxidant property, but its anticancer potential in melanoma cells has been related to oxidative stress, instead of the caspase-8 pathway (Kang et al. 2003). According to Neena et al., a low amount of ascorbate led to melanoma cell death, which was concentration-dependent. Another study suggested mechanism for the anticancer property of this vitamin encompasses angiogenesis. Vitamin C stifles the expression of VEGF (vascular endothelial growth factor) in melanoma cells, hence allowing it to extinguish angiogenic activities and bringing about tumor relapse (Kim et al. 2011).

18.5 Conclusion

Skin cancer is a frightening disorder, and its prevalence has been growing over the last three decades and is one of the largest health care issues for humans worldwide. The development of resistance with radiotherapy and chemotherapy is commonly observed in skin cancer. Hence, the development of the most effective novel eco-friendly, safe, and efficient treatment modality is the need of the hour. Plants being a reservoir of numerous chemical entities provide a suitable line for cancer research. In this scenario, phytochemicals may serve as a promising alternative against skin cancer. They are known to be reliable, easily available, cheap, and globally acceptable options as the natural bioactive-based anticancer therapies. Over the last 25 years, approximately 65% of anticancer moieties introduced have been obtained from natural sources, mainly plants. A variety of plant constituents from vegetables and fruits such as flavonoids, tannins, and terpenoids have displayed promising anticancer potential. Epidemiological evidence has reported an inverse relationship between skin cancer and dietary phytochemicals. These natural agents enhance the expression of cyclines, antioxidant enzymes, Bax proteins, p53, p21, and CDKs. They also scavenge ROS and modify different signaling routes like Notech-1, NF-κB,

EGFR, STAT, ERK/MAPK, P13K/AKt/mTOR, and β-catenin. Additionally, they prevent the articulation of oncogenes like Fos genes, c-Myc, and H-ras and downregulate Bcl-xl and Bcl-2. Further, anti-metastasis, antioxidation, anti-angiogenesis, anti-inflammation, and modification of cancer stem cells are the versatile protective phenomena involved in anticarcinogenic effects of most of the phytochemicals. These phytochemicals can be expected to prove a revolutionary in the prevention and treatment of skin cancer in the future. The skin serves as the prime barrier toward environmental hazards and hence needs to differentiate and proliferate endlessly at a high rate. The anti-proliferative action of phytoconstituents needs to specially target proliferative tumor cells to reduce adverse consequences to the skin. Thus, the topical route may serve as a perfect model of delivery for phytoagents. However, the research community has been facing newer challenges in skin delivery, and therefore, extensive studies are being undertaken to fabricate nanomedicine-based delivery systems. In addition, most of the phytoactive compounds suffer from limitations such as poor solubility and low bioavailability. In this regard, nanodelivery-based platforms surmount the abovementioned challenges. Further, these systems offer advantages such as lower toxicity, good biocompatibility, prolongation of drug circulation time, scope of surface modification, and multiple drug loading, all making major contribution to their enhanced utility. The challenges associated with the development of nano-drug delivery formulations include the scale-up possibilities and the feasibility of attaining these systems to achieve numerous therapeutic and biological applications.

To date, in vitro and epidemiologic evidence support the chemoprotective action of phytoagents in skin cancer. However, evaluations are required to further evaluate their bioavailability and pharmacokinetics clinically. For topical delivery, issues regarding augmented skin penetration, drug retention, stability of the final product, and treatment time need to be investigated to translate the research to fruitful commercial products. A gap exists and research activities to develop tumor-targeted nanodelivery system of phytotherapeutic agents may prove efficacious in the management of skin cancer. A synergistic combination of herbal agents with synthetic drugs could increase drug circulation times, yielding better efficacy, reducing toxicity, and providing coordinated drug release, leading to clinical trials and finally reaching the bedside. Novel formulations targeting strategies and their evaluation, matching international standards, will pave the way for functionalizing phytochemical agents for skin cancer.

References

Abdel-Rahman MA, Al-Abd AM (2013) Thermoresponsive dendrimers based on oligoethylene glycols: design, synthesis and cytotoxic activity against MCF-7 breast cancer cells. Eur J Med Chem 69:848–854

Abirami A, Halith SM, Pillai KK, Anbalagan C (2014) Herbal nanoparticle for anticancer potential-a review. World J Pharm Pharm Sci 3(8):2123–2132

Afaq F, Katiyar SK (2011) Polyphenols: skin photoprotection and inhibition of photocarcinogenesis. Mini Rev Med Chem 11(14):1200–1215

Agrawal Y, Petkar KC, Sawant KK (2010) Development, evaluation and clinical studies of Acitretin loaded nanostructured lipid carriers for topical treatment of psoriasis. Int J Pharm 401(1–2):93–102

Akanda MH, Rai R, Slipper IJ, Chowdhry BZ, Lamprou D, Getti G, Douroumis D (2015) Delivery of retinoic acid to LNCap human prostate cancer cells using solid lipid nanoparticles. Int J Pharm 493(1–2):161–171

Albishi T, John JA, Al-Khalifa AS, Shahidi F (2013) Antioxidative phenolic constituents of skins of onion varieties and their activities. J Funct Foods 5(3):1191–1203

Ali F, Rahul, Naz F, Jyoti S, Siddique YH (2017) Health functionality of apigenin: a review. Int J Food Prop 20(6):1197–1238

Ali-Boucetta H, Al-Jamal KT, McCarthy D, Prato M, Bianco A, Kostarelos K (2008) Multiwalled carbon nanotube–doxorubicin supramolecular complexes for cancer therapeutics. Chem Commun 4:459–461

Ansari KA, Vavia PR, Trotta F, Cavalli R (2011) Cyclodextrin-based nanosponges for delivery of resveratrol: in vitro characterisation, stability, cytotoxicity and permeation study. AAPS PharmSciTech 12(1):279–286

Apalla Z, Nashan D, Weller RB, Castellsague X (2017) Skin cancer: epidemiology, disease burden, pathophysiology, diagnosis, and therapeutic approaches. Dermatol Ther 7(1):5–19

Arasada BL, Bommareddy A, Zhang X, Bremmon K, Dwivedi C (2008) Effects of α-santalol on proapoptotic caspases and p53 expression in UVB irradiated mouse skin. Anticancer Res 28(1A):129–132

Asensi M, Ortega A, Mena S, Feddi F, Estrela JM (2011) Natural polyphenols in cancer therapy. Crit Rev Clin Lab Sci 48(5–6):197–216

Azoury SC, Lange JR (2014) Epidemiology, risk factors, prevention, and early detection of melanoma. Surg Clin North Am 94(5):945–962

Balivada S, Rachakatla RS, Wang H, Samarakoon TN, Dani RK, Pyle M et al (2010) A/C magnetic hyperthermia of melanoma mediated by iron (0)/iron oxide core/shell magnetic nanoparticles: a mouse study. BMC Cancer 10(1):119

Bastiancich C, Scutera S, Alotto D, Cambieri I, Fumagalli M, Casarin S et al (2014) Cyclodextrin-based nanosponges as a nanotechnology strategy for imiquimod delivery in pathological scarring prevention and treatment. J Nanopharm Drug Deliv 2(4):311–324

Battaglia L, Muntoni E, Chirio D, Peira E, Annovazzi L, Schiffer D et al (2017) Solid lipid nanoparticles by coacervation loaded with a methotrexate prodrug: preliminary study for glioma treatment. Nanomedicine 12(6):639–656

Bei D, Meng J, Youan B-BC (2010) Engineering nanomedicines for improved melanoma therapy: progress and promises. Nanomedicine 5(9):1385–1399

Berciano-Guerrero MA, Montesa-Pino A, Castaneda-Penalvo G, Munoz-Fernandez L, Rodriguez-Flores J (2014) Nanoparticles in melanoma. Curr Med Chem 21(32):3701–3716

Bettoli V, Zauli S, Virgili A (2013) Retinoids in the chemoprevention of non-melanoma skin cancers: why, when and how. J Dermatol Treat 24(3):235–237

Bhattacharya S, Darjatmoko SR, Polans AS (2011) Resveratrol modulates the malignant properties of cutaneous melanoma via changes in the activation and attenuation of the anti-apoptotic proto-oncogenic protein Akt/PKB. Melanoma Res 21(3):180

Bisht S, Feldmann G, Soni S, Ravi R, Karikar C, Maitra A, Maitra A (2007) Polymeric nanoparticle-encapsulated curcumin ("nanocurcumin"): a novel strategy for human cancer therapy. J Nanobiotechnol 5(1):3

Blanco E, Bey EA, Khemtong C, Yang S-G, Setti-Guthi J, Chen H et al (2010) β-Lapachone micellar nanotherapeutics for non–small cell lung cancer therapy. Cancer Res 70(10):3896–3904

Bolmal UB, Manvi FV, Rajkumar K, Palla SS, Paladugu A, Reddy KR (2013) Recent advances in nanosponges as drug delivery system. Int J Pharm Sci Nanotechnol 6:1934–1944

Bommareddy A, Brozena S, Steigerwalt J, Landis T, Hughes S, Mabry E et al (2019) Medicinal properties of alpha-santalol, a naturally occurring constituent of sandalwood oil. Nat Prod Res 33(4):527–543

Brash DE, Rudolph JA, Simon JA, Lin A, McKenna GJ, Baden HP et al (1991) A role for sunlight in skin cancer: UV-induced p53 mutations in squamous cell carcinoma. Proc Natl Acad Sci 88(22):10124–10128

Bush JA, Cheung K-JJ Jr, Li G (2001) Curcumin induces apoptosis in human melanoma cells through a Fas receptor/caspase-8 pathway independent of p53. Exp Cell Res 271(2):305–314

Cadet J, Sage E, Douki T (2005) Ultraviolet radiation-mediated damage to cellular DNA. Mutat Res 571(1–2):3–17

Calderon-Montano JM, Burgos-Morón E, Pérez-Guerrero C, López-Lázaro M (2011) A review on the dietary flavonoid kaempferol. Mini Rev Med Chem 11(4):298–344

Calzavara-Pinton P, Ortel B, Venturini M (2015) Non-melanoma skin cancer, sun exposure and sun protection. Giornale Italiano Di Dermatologia e Venereologia: Organo Ufficiale, Societa Italiana Di Dermatologia e Sifilografia 150(4):369–378

Cao H-H, Cheng C-Y, Su T, Fu X-Q, Guo H, Li T et al (2015) Quercetin inhibits HGF/c-Met signaling and HGF-stimulated melanoma cell migration and invasion. Mol Cancer 14(1):103

Cappellano G, Comi C, Chiocchetti A, Dianzani U (2019) Exploiting PLGA-based biocompatible nanoparticles for next-generation tolerogenic vaccines against auto immune disease. Int J Mol Sci 20(1):204

Casagrande F, Darbon J-M (2000) P21CIP1 is dispensable for the G2 arrest caused by genistein in human melanoma cells. Exp Cell Res 258(1):101–108

Casagrande F, Darbon J-M (2001) Effects of structurally related flavonoids on cell cycle progression of human melanoma cells: regulation of cyclin-dependent kinases CDK2 and CDK1. Biochem Pharmacol 61(10):1205–1215

Cassidy (2003) Potential risks and benefits of phytoestrogen-rich diets. Int J Vitam Nutr Res 73(2):120–126

Castillo PM, de la Mata M, Casula MF, Sánchez-Alcázar JA, Zaderenko AP (2014) PEGylated versus non-PEGylated magnetic nanoparticles as camptothecin delivery system. Beilstein J Nanotechnol 5(1):1312–1319

Chaiprasongsuk A, Onkoksoong T, Pluemsamran T, Limsaengurai S, Panich U (2016) Photoprotection by dietary phenolics against melanogenesis induced by UVA through Nrf2-dependent antioxidant responses. Redox Biol 8:79–90

Chambial S, Dwivedi S, Shukla KK, John PJ, Sharma P (2013) Vitamin C in disease prevention and cure: an overview. Indian J Clin Biochem 28(4):314–328

Chang L-C, Sheu H-M, Huang Y-S, Tsai T-R, Kuo K-W (1999) A novel function of emodin: enhancement of the nucleotide excision repair of UV-and cisplatin-induced DNA damage in human cells. Biochem Pharmacol 58(1):49–57

Chang C-H, Huang W-Y, Lai C-H, Hsu Y-M, Yao Y-H, Chen T-Y et al (2011) Development of novel nanoparticles shelled with heparin for berberine delivery to treat Helicobacter pylori. Acta Biomater 7(2):593–603

Chao Y, Huang C-T, Fu L-T, Huang Y-B, Tsai Y-H, Wu P-C (2012) The effect of submicron emulsion systems on transdermal delivery of kaempferol. Chem Pharm Bull 60(9):1171–1175

Chaudhuri P, Soni S, Sengupta S (2009) Single-walled carbon nanotube-conjugated chemotherapy exhibits increased therapeutic index in melanoma. Nanotechnology 21(2):025102

Chen AY, Chen YC (2013) A review of the dietary flavonoid, kaempferol on human health and cancer chemoprevention. Food Chem 138(4):2099–2107

Chen Y-C, Shen S-C, Lee W-R, Hsu F-L, Lin H-Y, Ko C-H, Tseng S-W (2002) Emodin induces apoptosis in human promyeloleukemic HL-60 cells accompanied by activation of caspase 3 cascade but independent of reactive oxygen species production. Biochem Pharmacol 64(12):1713–1724

Chen H, Wu J, Sun M, Guo C, Yu A, Cao F et al (2012a) N-trimethyl chitosan chloride-coated liposomes for the oral delivery of curcumin. J Liposome Res 22(2):100–109

Chen J, Li S, Shen Q (2012b) Folic acid and cell-penetrating peptide conjugated PLGA–PEG bifunctional nanoparticles for vincristine sulfate delivery. Eur J Pharm Sci 47(2):430–443

Chen S, Liu W, Wan J, Cheng X, Gu C, Zhou H et al (2013) Preparation of Coenzyme Q10 nanostructured lipid carriers for epidermal targeting with high-pressure microfluidics technique. Drug Dev Ind Pharm 39(1):20–28

Chiang H-S, Wu W-B, Fang J-Y, Chen D-F, Chen B-H, Huang C-C et al (2007) Lycopene inhibits PDGF-BB-induced signaling and migration in human dermal fibroblasts through interaction with PDGF-BB. Life Sci 81(21–22):1509–1517

Chilajwar SV, Pednekar PP, Jadhav KR, Gupta GJ, Kadam VJ (2014) Cyclodextrin-based nanosponges: a propitious platform for enhancing drug delivery. Expert Opin Drug Deliv 11(1):111–120

Conte C, Caldera F, Catanzano O, D'Angelo I, Ungaro F, Miro A et al (2014) β-cyclodextrin nanosponges as multifunctional ingredient in water-containing semisolid formulations for skin delivery. J Pharm Sci 103(12):3941–3949

Corcoran MP, McKay DL, Blumberg JB (2012) Flavonoid basics: chemistry, sources, mechanisms of action, and safety. J Nutr Gerontol Geriatr 31(3):176–189

Coricovac D, Dehelean C, Moaca E-A, Pinzaru I, Bratu T, Navolan D, Boruga O (2018) Cutaneous melanoma—a long road from experimental models to clinical outcome: a review. Int J Mol Sci 19(6):1566

Darandale SS, Vavia PR (2013) Cyclodextrin-based nanosponges of curcumin: formulation and physicochemical characterization. J Incl Phenom Macrocycl Chem 75(3–4):315–322

Darbon J-M, Penary M, Escalas N, Casagrande F, Goubin-Gramatica F, Baudouin C, Ducommun B (2000) Distinct Chk2 activation pathways are triggered by genistein and DNA-damaging agents in human melanoma cells. J Biol Chem 275(20):15363–15369

Das S, Das J, Paul A, Samadder A, Khuda-Bukhsh AR (2013a) Apigenin, a bioactive flavonoid from Lycopodium clavatum, stimulates nucleotide excision repair genes to protect skin keratinocytes from ultraviolet B-induced reactive oxygen species and DNA damage. J Acupunct Meridian Stud 6(5):252–262

Das S, Das J, Samadder A, Paul A, Khuda-Bukhsh AR (2013b) Efficacy of PLGA-loaded apigenin nanoparticles in Benzo [a] pyrene and ultraviolet-B induced skin cancer of mice: mitochondria mediated apoptotic signalling cascades. Food Chem Toxicol 62:670–680

Deep G, Agarwal R (2010) Antimetastatic efficacy of silibinin: molecular mechanisms and therapeutic potential against cancer. Cancer Metastasis Rev 29(3):447–463

Delmas D, Lançon A, Colin D, Jannin B, Latruffe N (2006) Resveratrol as a chemopreventive agent: a promising molecule for fighting cancer. Curr Drug Targets 7(4):423–442

Dhanalakshmi S, Agarwal P, Glode,LM, Agarwal R (2003) Silibinin sensitizes human prostate carcinoma DU145 cells to cisplatin-and carboplatin-induced growth inhibition and apoptotic death. International Journal of Cancer, 106(5):699–705

Dhanalakshmi S, Mallikarjuna GU, Singh RP, Agarwal R (2004a) Dual efficacy of silibinin in protecting or enhancing ultraviolet B radiation-caused apoptosis in HaCaT human immortalized keratinocytes. Carcinogenesis 25(1):99–106

Dhanalakshmi S, Mallikarjuna GU, Singh RP, Agarwal R (2004b) Silibinin prevents ultraviolet radiation-caused skin damages in SKH-1 hairless mice via a decrease in thymine dimer positive cells and an up-regulation of p53-p21/Cip1 in epidermis. Carcinogenesis 25(8):1459–1465

Dhawan S, Kapil R, Singh B (2011) Formulation development and systematic optimization of solid lipid nanoparticles of quercetin for improved brain delivery. J Pharm Pharmacol 63(3):342–351

Didona D, Paolino G, Bottoni U, Cantisani C (2018) Non melanoma skin cancer pathogenesis overview. Biomedicine 6(1):6

Dong P, Wang X, Gu Y, Wang Y, Wang Y, Gong C et al (2010) Self-assembled biodegradable micelles based on star-shaped PCL-b-PEG copolymers for chemotherapeutic drug delivery. Colloids Surf A Physicochem Eng Asp 358(1–3):128–134

Eggermont AM, Spatz A, Robert C (2014) Cutaneous melanoma. Lancet 383(9919):816–827

Erlund I (2004) Review of the flavonoids quercetin, hesperetin, and naringenin. Dietary sources, bioactivities, bioavailability, and epidemiology. Nutr Res 24(10):851–874

Esmaeili F, Rajabnejhad S, Partoazar AR, Mehr SE, Faridi-Majidi R, Sahebgharani M et al (2016) Anti-inflammatory effects of eugenol nanoemulsion as a topical delivery system. Pharm Dev Technol 21(7):887–893

Es-Saady D, Simon A, Ollier M, Maurizis JC, Chulia AJ, Delage C (1996) Inhibitory effect of ursolic acid on B16 proliferation through cell cycle arrest. Cancer Lett 106(2):193–197

Fabbrocini G, Triassi M, Mauriello MC, Torre G, Annunziata MC, De Vita V et al (2010) Epidemiology of skin cancer: role of some environmental factors. Cancers 2(4):1980–1989

Fan J, Eastham L, Varney ME, Hall A, Adkins NL, Sollars VE et al (2010) Silencing and re-expression of retinoic acid receptor beta2 in human melanoma. Pigment Cell Melanoma Res 23(3):419–429

Fang J-Y, Fang C-L, Liu C-H, Su Y-H (2008) Lipid nanoparticles as vehicles for topical psoralen delivery: solid lipid nanoparticles (SLN) versus nanostructured lipid carriers (NLC). Eur J Pharm Biopharm 70(2):633–640

Fernandez MA, Saenz MT, Garcia MD (1998) Natural products: anti-inflammatory activity in rats and mice of phenolic acids isolated from Scrophularia frutescens. J Pharm Pharmacol 50(10):1183–1186

Flaig TW, Gustafson DL, Su L-J, Zirrolli JA, Crighton F, Harrison GS et al (2007) A phase I and pharmacokinetic study of silybin-phytosome in prostate cancer patients. Investig New Drugs 25(2):139–146

Flaten GE, Chang TT, Phillips WT, Brandl M, Bao A, Goins B (2013) Liposomal formulations of poorly soluble camptothecin: drug retention and biodistribution. J Liposome Res 23(1):70–81

Garbe C, Peris K, Hauschild A, Saiag P, Middleton M, Spatz A et al (2010) Diagnosis and treatment of melanoma: European consensus-based interdisciplinary guideline. Eur J Cancer 46(2):270–283

Gazak R, Walterova D, Kren V (2007) Silybin and silymarin-new and emerging applications in medicine. Curr Med Chem 14(3):315–338

Gholibegloo E, Mortezazadeh T, Salehian F, Ramazani A, Amanlou M, Khoobi M (2019) Improved curcumin loading, release, solubility and toxicity by tuning the molar ratio of cross-linker to β-cyclodextrin. Carbohydr Polym 213:70–78

Gigliotti CL, Minelli R, Cavalli R, Occhipinti S, Barrera G, Pizzimenti S et al (2016) In vitro and in vivo therapeutic evaluation of camptothecin-encapsulated β-cyclodextrin nanosponges in prostate cancer. J Biomed Nanotechnol 12(1):114–127

Goldman G (2002) The current status of curettage and electrodesiccation. Dermatol Clin 20(3):569–578. https://doi.org/10.1016/S0733-8635(02)00022-0

Graf E (1992) Antioxidant potential of ferulic acid. Free Radic Biol Med 13(4):435–448

Guruvayoorappan C, Kuttan G (2007) β-Carotene down-regulates inducible nitric oxide synthase gene expression and induces apoptosis by suppressing bcl-2 expression and activating caspase-3 and p53 genes in B16F-10 melanoma cells. Nutr Res 27(6):336–342

Guterres SS, Alves MP, Pohlmann AR (2007) Polymeric nanoparticles, nanospheres and nanocapsules, for cutaneous applications. Drug Target Insights 2:147–157, 117739280700200000

Hahm E-R, Singh SV (2007) Honokiol causes G0-G1 phase cell cycle arrest in human prostate cancer cells in association with suppression of retinoblastoma protein level/phosphorylation and inhibition of E2F1 transcriptional activity. Mol Cancer Ther 6(10):2686–2695

Harborne JB, Dey PM, Lea PJ (1989) Methods in plant biochemistry. Academic Press, London

Harmand P-O, Duval R, Liagre B, Jayat-Vignoles C, Beneytout J-L, Delage C, Simon A (2003) Ursolic acid induces apoptosis through caspase-3 activation and cell cycle arrest in HaCat cells. Int J Oncol 23(1):105–112

Hennings H, Glick AB, Greenhalgh DA, Morgan DL, Strickland JE, Tennenbaum T, Yuspa SH (1993) Critical aspects of initiation, promotion, and progression in multistage epidermal carcinogenesis. Proc Soc Exp Biol Med 202(1):1–8

Hollman PC, Van Trijp JM, Mengelers MJ, De Vries JH, Katan MB (1997) Bioavailability of the dietary antioxidant flavonol quercetin in man. Cancer Lett 114(1–2):139–140

Hou Z, Li Y, Huang Y, Zhou C, Lin J, Wang Y et al (2012) Phytosomes loaded with mitomycin C–soybean phosphatidylcholine complex developed for drug delivery. Mol Pharm 10(1):90–101

Hu C-MJ, Zhang L (2012) Nanoparticle-based combination therapy toward overcoming drug resistance in cancer. Biochem Pharmacol 83(8):1104–1111

Huang HS, Hainfeld JF (2013) Intravenous magnetic nanoparticle cancer hyperthermia. Int J Nanomedicine 8:2521

Huang H-C, Chang J-H, Tung S-F, Wu R-T, Foegh ML, Chu S-H (1992) Immunosuppressive effect of emodin, a free radical generator. Eur J Pharmacol 211(3):359–364

Iijima S (1991) Helical microtubules of graphitic carbon. Nature 354(6348):56

Ito A, Tanaka K, Kondo K, Shinkai M, Honda H, Matsumoto K et al (2003) Tumor regression by combined immunotherapy and hyperthermia using magnetic nanoparticles in an experimental subcutaneous murine melanoma. Cancer Sci 94(3):308–313

Iwashita K, Kobori M, Yamaki K, Tsushida T (2000) Flavonoids inhibit cell growth and induce apoptosis in B16 melanoma 4A5 cells. Biosci Biotechnol Biochem 64(9):1813–1820

Jaganathan SK, Supriyanto E (2012) Antiproliferative and molecular mechanism of eugenol-induced apoptosis in cancer cells. Molecules 17(6):6290–6304

Ji J-L, Huang X-F, Zhu H-L (2012) Curcumin and its formulations: potential anti-cancer agents. Anticancer Agents Med Chem 12(3):210–218

Ji P, Yu T, Liu Y, Jiang J, Xu J, Zhao Y et al (2016) Naringenin-loaded solid lipid nanoparticles: preparation, controlled delivery, cellular uptake, and pulmonary pharmacokinetics. Drug Des Devel Ther 10:911

Jing X, Ueki N, Cheng J, Imanishi H, Hada T (2002) Induction of apoptosis in hepatocellular carcinoma cell lines by emodin. Jpn J Cancer Res 93(8):874–882

Joyce KM (2017) Surgical management of melanoma. In: Ward WH, Farma JM (eds) Cutaneous melanoma: etiology and therapy. Retrieved from http://www.ncbi.nlm.nih.gov/books/NBK481850/

Jung SK, Lee KW, Byun S, Kang NJ, Lim SH, Heo Y-S et al (2008) Myricetin suppresses UVB-induced skin cancer by targeting Fyn. Cancer Res 68(14):6021–6029

Kakran M, Li L (2012) Carbon nanomaterials for drug delivery. In: Key engineering materials, vol 508. Trans Tech Publications, Switzerland. pp 76–80

Kang JS, Cho D, Kim Y-I, Hahm E, Yang Y, Kim D et al (2003) L-Ascorbic acid (vitamin C) induces the apoptosis of B16 murine melanoma cells via a caspase-8–independent pathway. Cancer Immunol Immunother 52(11):693–698

Kang NJ, Lee KW, Shin BJ, Jung SK, Hwang MK, Bode AM et al (2008) Caffeic acid, a phenolic phytochemical in coffee, directly inhibits Fyn kinase activity and UVB-induced COX-2 expression. Carcinogenesis 30(2):321–330

Katalinic A, Kunze U, Schäfer T (2003) Epidemiology of cutaneous melanoma and non-melanoma skin cancer in Schleswig-Holstein, Germany: incidence, clinical subtypes, tumour stages and localization (epidemiology of skin cancer). Br J Dermatol 149(6):1200–1206

Kataoka K, Matsumoto T, Yokoyama M, Okano T, Sakurai Y, Fukushima S et al (2000) Doxorubicin-loaded poly (ethylene glycol)–poly (β-benzyl-l-aspartate) copolymer micelles: their pharmaceutical characteristics and biological significance. J Control Release 64(1–3):143–153

Katiyar SK, Korman NJ, Mukhtar H, Agarwal R (1997) Protective effects of silymarin against photocarcinogenesis in a mouse skin model. J Natl Cancer Inst 89(8):556–565

Kaul A, Khanduja L (1998) Polyphenols inhibit promotional phase of tumorigenesis: relevance of superoxide radicals. Nutr Cancer 32(2):81–85

Kauvar ANB, Cronin T, Roenigk R, Hruza G, Bennett R (2015) Consensus for nonmelanoma skin cancer treatment: basal cell carcinoma, including a cost analysis of treatment methods. Dermatol Surg 41(5):550–571. https://doi.org/10.1097/DSS.0000000000000296

Kedar U, Phutane P, Shidhaye S, Kadam V (2010) Advances in polymeric micelles for drug delivery and tumor targeting. Nanomedicine 6(6):714–729

Kelly GS (2011) Quercetin. Altern Med Rev 16(2):172–195

Khan T, Gurav P (2018) PhytoNanotechnology: enhancing delivery of plant based anti-cancer drugs. Front Pharmacol 8:1002

Kidd PM (2009) Bioavailability and activity of phytosome complexes from botanical polyphenols: the silymarin, curcumin, green tea, and grape seed extracts. Altern Med Rev 14(3):226–246

Kim D-S, Jeong Y-M, Moon S-I, Kim S-Y, Kwon S-B, Park E-S et al (2006) Indole-3-carbinol enhances ultraviolet B-induced apoptosis by sensitizing human melanoma cells. Cell Mol Life Sci 63(22):2661–2668

Kim W, Yang HJ, Youn H, Yun YJ, Seong KM, Youn B (2010) Myricetin inhibits Akt survival signaling and induces Bad-mediated apoptosis in a low dose ultraviolet (UV)-B-irradiated HaCaT human immortalized keratinocytes. J Radiat Res 51(3):285–296

Kim HN, Kim H, Kong JM, Bae S, Kim YS, Lee N et al (2011) Vitamin C down-regulates VEGF production in B16F10 murine melanoma cells via the suppression of p42/44 MAPK activation. J Cell Biochem 112(3):894–901. https://doi.org/10.1002/jcb.22997

Kolenyak dos Santos F, Helena Oyafuso M, Priscila Kiill C, Palmira Daflon-Gremiao M, Chorilli M (2013) Nanotechnology-based drug delivery systems for treatment of hyperproliferative skin diseases-a review. Curr Nanosci 9(1):159–167

Kowalczyk MC, Walaszek Z, Kowalczyk P, Kinjo T, Hanausek M, Slaga TJ (2009) Differential effects of several phytochemicals and their derivatives on murine keratinocytes in vitro and in vivo: implications for skin cancer prevention. Carcinogenesis 30(6):1008–1015

Koyama M, Kelly TR, Watanabe KA (1988) Novel type of potential anticancer agents derived from chrysophanol and emodin. Some structure-activity relationship studies. J Med Chem 31(2):283–284

Kumar SR, Priyatharshni S, Babu VN, Mangalaraj D, Viswanathan C, Kannan S, Ponpandian N (2014) Quercetin conjugated superparamagnetic magnetite nanoparticles for in-vitro analysis of breast cancer cell lines for chemotherapy applications. J Colloid Interface Sci 436:234–242

Kumar AB, Habbu P, Hullatti P, Kumar RS (2017) Phytosomes as novel drug delivery system for herbal medicine-A review. Sys Rev Pharm 8(1):5

Kumari P, Swami MO, Nadipalli SK, Myneni S, Ghosh B, Biswas S (2016) Curcumin delivery by poly (Lactide)-based co-polymeric micelles: an in vitro anticancer study. Pharm Res 33(4):826–841

Kuo T-C, Yang J-S, Lin M-W, Hsu S-C, Lin J-J, Lin H-J et al (2009) Emodin has cytotoxic and protective effects in rat C6 glioma cells: roles of Mdr1a and nuclear factor κB in cell survival. J Pharmacol Exp Ther 330(3):736–744

Kvam E, Tyrrell RM (1997) Induction of oxidative DNA base damage in human skin cells by UV and near visible radiation. Carcinogenesis 18(12):2379–2384

Kwon G, Naito M, Yokoyama M, Okano T, Sakurai Y, Kataoka K (1997) Block copolymer micelles for drug delivery: loading and release of doxorubicin. J Control Release 48(2–3):195–201

Lee DE, Lee KW, Byun S, Jung SK, Song N, Lim SH et al (2011) 7, 3′, 4′-Trihydroxyisoflavone, a metabolite of the soy isoflavone daidzein, suppresses ultraviolet B-induced skin cancer by targeting Cot and MKK4. J Biol Chem 286(16):14246–14256

Leiter U, Eigentler T, Garbe C (2014) Epidemiology of skin cancer. In: Sunlight, vitamin D and skin cancer. Springer, New York, NY. pp 120–140

Li J, Malakhova M, Mottamal M, Reddy K, Kurinov I, Carper A et al (2012) Norathyriol suppresses skin cancers induced by solar ultraviolet radiation by targeting ERK kinases. Cancer Res 72(1):260–270

Li H, Gao A, Jiang N, Liu Q, Liang B, Li R et al (2016) Protective effect of curcumin against acute ultraviolet B irradiation-induced photo-damage. Photochem Photobiol 92(6):808–815

Lin Y-S, Tsai P-H, Kandaswami CC, Cheng C-H, Ke F-C, Lee P-P et al (2011) Effects of dietary flavonoids, luteolin, and quercetin on the reversal of epithelial–mesenchymal transition in A431 epidermal cancer cells. Cancer Sci 102(10):1829–1839

Lipke MM (2006) An armamentarium of wart treatments. Clin Med Res 4(4):273–293. Retrieved from https://www.ncbi.nlm.nih.gov/pmc/articles/PMC1764803/

Liu Z, Robinson JT, Sun X, Dai H (2008) PEGylated nanographene oxide for delivery of water-insoluble cancer drugs. J Am Chem Soc 130(33):10876–10877

Liu D, Liu Z, Wang L, Zhang C, Zhang N (2011) Nanostructured lipid carriers as novel carrier for parenteral delivery of docetaxel. Colloids Surf B: Biointerfaces 85(2):262–269

Lu LY, Ou N, Lu Q-B (2013) Antioxidant induces DNA damage, cell death and mutagenicity in human lung and skin normal cells. Sci Rep 3:3169

Lugowska I, Teterycz P, Rutkowski P (2018) Immunotherapy of melanoma. Contemp Oncol 22(1A):61–67. https://doi.org/10.5114/wo.2018.73889

Luiza Ribeiro de Souza A, Priscila Kiill C, Kolenyak dos Santos F, Marielli da Luz G, Rocha e Silva H, Chorilli M, Palmira Daflon Gremiao M (2012) Nanotechnology-based drug delivery systems for dermatomycosis treatment. Curr Nanosci 8(4):512–519

Luper S (1998) A review of plants used in the treatment of liver disease: part 1. Altern Med Rev 3(6):410–421

Ma X, Zhou J, Zhang C-X, Li X-Y, Li N, Ju R-J et al (2013) Modulation of drug-resistant membrane and apoptosis proteins of breast cancer stem cells by targeting berberine liposomes. Biomaterials 34(18):4452–4465

Magenheim B, Benita S (1991) Nanoparticle characterization: a comprehensive physicochemical approach. STP Pharma Sci 1(4):221–241

Maia CS, Mehnert W, Schäfer-Korting M (2000) Solid lipid nanoparticles as drug carriers for topical glucocorticoids. Int J Pharm 196(2):165–167

Maiti K, Mukherjee K, Gantait A, Saha BP, Mukherjee PK (2006) Enhanced therapeutic potential of naringenin-phospholipid complex in rats. J Pharm Pharmacol 58(9):1227–1233

Majumdar D, Jung K-H, Zhang H, Nannapaneni S, Wang X, Amin AR et al (2014) Luteolin nanoparticle in chemoprevention: in vitro and in vivo anticancer activity. Cancer Prev Res 7(1):65–73

Malar C, Bavanilathamuthiah (2015) Dendrosomal capsaicin nanoformulation for the in vitro anti-cancer effect on HEp 2 and MCF - 7 cell lines. Int J Appl Bioeng 9:30–35. https://doi.org/10.18000/ijabeg.10133

Mazumder A, Dwivedi A, Du Preez JL, Du Plessis J (2016) In vitro wound healing and cytotoxic effects of sinigrin–phytosome complex. Int J Pharm 498(1–2):283–293

McCubrey JA, Steelman LS, Chappell WH, Abrams SL, Wong EW, Chang F et al (2007) Roles of the Raf/MEK/ERK pathway in cell growth, malignant transformation and drug resistance. Biochim Biophys Acta (BBA)-Mol Cell Res 1773(8):1263–1284

Mehnert W, Mäder K (2012) Solid lipid nanoparticles: production, characterization and applications. Adv Drug Deliv Rev 64:83–101

Merlin JJ, Prasad NR, Shibli SMA (2012) Ferulic acid loaded poly-d, l-lactide-co-glycolide nanoparticles: systematic study of particle size, drug encapsulation efficiency and anticancer effect in non-small cell lung carcinoma cell line in vitro. Biomed Prev Nutr 2(1):69–76

Miller DL, Weinstock MA (1994) Nonmelanoma skin cancer in the United States: incidence. J Am Acad Dermatol 30(5):774–778

Minelli R, Cavalli R, Ellis L, Pettazzoni P, Trotta F, Ciamporcero E et al (2012) Nanosponge-encapsulated camptothecin exerts anti-tumor activity in human prostate cancer cells. Eur J Pharm Sci 47(4):686–694

Mitri K, Shegokar R, Gohla S, Anselmi C, Müller RH (2011) Lipid nanocarriers for dermal delivery of lutein: preparation, characterization, stability and performance. Int J Pharm 414(1–2):267–275

Mognetti B, Barberis A, Marino S, Berta G, De Francia S, Trotta F, Cavalli R (2012) In vitro enhancement of anticancer activity of paclitaxel by a Cremophor free cyclodextrin-based nanosponge formulation. J Incl Phenom Macrocycl Chem 74(1–4):201–210

Moon MK, Lee YJ, Kim JS, Kang DG, Lee HS (2009) Effect of caffeic acid on tumor necrosis factor-alpha-induced vascular inflammation in human umbilical vein endothelial cells. Biol Pharm Bull 32(8):1371–1377

Muller RH, Radtke M, Wissing SA (2004) Solid lipid NPs and nanostructured lipid carriers. In: Encyclopedia of nanoscience and nanotechnology. American Scientific Publishers, Stevenson Ranch

Muto A, Hori M, Sasaki Y, Saitoh A, Yasuda I, Maekawa T et al (2007) Emodin has a cytotoxic activity against human multiple myeloma as a Janus-activated kinase 2 inhibitor. Mol Cancer Ther 6(3):987–994

Naik A, Kalia YN, Guy RH, Fessi H (2004) Enhancement of topical delivery from biodegradable nanoparticles. Pharm Res 21(10):1818–1825

Nakashima S, Matsuda H, Oda Y, Nakamura S, Xu F, Yoshikawa M (2010) Melanogenesis inhibitors from the desert plant Anastatica hierochuntica in B16 melanoma cells. Bioorg Med Chem 18(6):2337–2345

Naumov GN, Akslen LA, Folkman J (2006) Role of angiogenesis in human tumor dormancy: animal models of the angiogenic switch. Cell Cycle 5(16):1779–1787

Ndiaye M, Philippe C, Mukhtar H, Ahmad N (2011) The grape antioxidant resveratrol for skin disorders: promise, prospects, and challenges. Arch Biochem Biophys 508(2):164–170

Nihal M, Ahmad N, Mukhtar H, Wood GS (2005) Anti-proliferative and proapoptotic effects of (−)-epigallocatechin-3-gallate on human melanoma: possible implications for the chemoprevention of melanoma. Int J Cancer 114(4):513–521

Nihal M, Ahsan H, Siddiqui IA, Mukhtar H, Ahmad N, Wood GS (2009) (−)-Epigallocatechin-3-gallate (EGCG) sensitizes melanoma cells to interferon induced growth inhibition in a mouse model of human melanoma. Cell Cycle 8(13):2057–2063

Nihal M, Roelke CT, Wood GS (2010) Anti-melanoma effects of vorinostat in combination with polyphenolic antioxidant (−)-epigallocatechin-3-gallate (EGCG). Pharm Res 27(6):1103–1114

Obeidat WM, Schwabe K, Müller RH, Keck CM (2010) Preservation of nanostructured lipid carriers (NLC). Eur J Pharm Biopharm 76(1):56–67

Ochi MM, Amoabediny G, Rezayat SM, Akbarzadeh A, Ebrahimi B (2016) In vitro co-delivery evaluation of novel pegylated nano-liposomal herbal drugs of silibinin and glycyrrhizic acid (nano-phytosome) to hepatocellular carcinoma cells. Cell J (Yakhteh) 18(2):135

Ou S, Kwok K-C (2004) Ferulic acid: pharmaceutical functions, preparation and applications in foods. J Sci Food Agric 84(11):1261–1269

Ourique AF, Melero A, da Silva C d B, Schaefer UF, Pohlmann AR, Guterres SS et al (2011) Improved photostability and reduced skin permeation of tretinoin: development of a semisolid nanomedicine. Eur J Pharm Biopharm 79(1):95–101

Oyagbemi AA, Saba AB, Azeez OI (2010) Capsaicin: a novel chemopreventive molecule and its underlying molecular mechanisms of action. Indian J Cancer 47(1):53

Palombo P, Fabrizi G, Ruocco V, Ruocco E, Fluhr J, Roberts R, Morganti P (2007) Beneficial long-term effects of combined oral/topical antioxidant treatment with the carotenoids lutein and zeaxanthin on human skin: A double-blind, placebo-controlled study. Skin Pharmacology and Physiology, 20(4):199–210

Palozza P, Serini S, Torsello A, Di Nicuolo F, Maggiano N, Ranelletti FO et al (2003) Mechanism of activation of caspase cascade during β-carotene-induced apoptosis in human tumor cells. Nutr Cancer 47(1):76–87

Pandey GP (1990) Hepatogenic effect of some indigenous drugs on experimental liver damage. PhD thesis, College of Veterinary Science & Animal Husbandry

Pardeike J, Hommoss A, Müller RH (2009) Lipid nanoparticles (SLN, NLC) in cosmetic and pharmaceutical dermal products. Int J Pharm 366(1–2):170–184

PDQ Adult Treatment Editorial Board (2002) Skin Cancer Treatment (PDQ®): Patient Version. In: PDQ Cancer Information Summaries. Retrieved from http://www.ncbi.nlm.nih.gov/books/NBK65824/

Penta D, Somashekar BS, Meeran SM (2018) Epigenetics of skin cancer: interventions by selected bioactive phytochemicals. Photodermatol Photoimmunol Photomed 34(1):42–49

Pentak D (2016) In vitro spectroscopic study of piperine-encapsulated nanosize liposomes. Eur Biophys J 45(2):175–186

Pierre MBR, Tedesco AC, Marchetti JM, Bentley MVL (2001) Stratum corneum lipids liposomes for the topical delivery of 5-aminolevulinic acid in photodynamic therapy of skin cancer: preparation and in vitro permeation study. BMC Dermatol 1(1):5

Potenza C, Bernardini N, Balduzzi V, Losco L, Mambrin A, Marchesiello A et al (2018) A review of the literature of surgical and nonsurgical treatments of invasive squamous cells carcinoma. Biomed Res Int 2018:1–9. https://doi.org/10.1155/2018/9489163

Pushpalatha R, Selvamuthukumar S, Kilimozhi D (2019) Cyclodextrin nanosponge based hydrogel for the transdermal co-delivery of curcumin and resveratrol: development, optimization, in vitro and ex vivo evaluation. J Drug Delivery Sci Technol 52:55–64

Qiu L-Y, Yan L, Zhang L, Jin Y-M, Zhao Q-H (2013) Folate-modified poly (2-ethyl-2-oxazoline) as hydrophilic corona in polymeric micelles for enhanced intracellular doxorubicin delivery. Int J Pharm 456(2):315–324

Qiu Y, Yu T, Wang W, Pan K, Shi D, Sun H (2014) Curcumin-induced melanoma cell death is associated with mitochondrial permeability transition pore (mPTP) opening. Biochem Biophys Res Commun 448(1):15–21

Rafiq RA, Quadri A, Nazir LA, Peerzada K, Ganai BA, Tasduq SA (2015) A potent inhibitor of phosphoinositide 3-kinase (PI3K) and mitogen activated protein (MAP) kinase signalling, quercetin (3, 3′, 4′, 5, 7-pentahydroxyflavone) promotes cell death in ultraviolet (UV)-B-irradiated B16F10 melanoma cells. PLoS One 10(7):e0131253

Rahiminejad A, Dinarvand R, Johari B, Nodooshan SJ, Rashti A, Rismani E et al (2019) Preparation and investigation of indirubin-loaded SLN nanoparticles and their anti-cancer effects on human glioblastoma U87MG cells. Cell Biol Int 43(1):2–11

Ramakrishna Y, Goda H, Baliga MS, Munshi AK (2011) Decreasing cariogenic bacteria with a natural, alternative prevention therapy utilizing phytochemistry (plant extracts). J Clin Pediatr Dent 36(1):55–64

Rapoport N (2007) Physical stimuli-responsive polymeric micelles for anti-cancer drug delivery. Prog Polym Sci 32(8–9):962–990

Rasaie S, Ghanbarzadeh S, Mohammadi M, Hamishehkar H (2014) Nano phytosomes of quercetin: a promising formulation for fortification of food products with antioxidants. Pharma Sci 20(3):96

Rather RA, Bhagat M (2018) Cancer chemoprevention and piperine: molecular mechanisms and therapeutic opportunities. Front Cell Dev Biol 6:10

Rauth S, Kichina J, Green A (1997) Inhibition of growth and induction of differentiation of metastatic melanoma cells in vitro by genistein: chemosensitivity is regulated by cellular p53. Br J Cancer 75(11):1559

Rompicharla SVK, Bhatt H, Shah A, Komanduri N, Vijayasarathy D, Ghosh B, Biswas S (2017) Formulation optimization, characterization, and evaluation of in vitro cytotoxic potential of curcumin loaded solid lipid nanoparticles for improved anticancer activity. Chem Phys Lipids 208:10–18

Rundhaug JE, Fischer SM (2010) Molecular mechanisms of mouse skin tumor promotion. Cancers 2(2):436–482

Rundlöf T, Olsson E, Wiernik A, Back S, Aune M, Johansson L, Wahlberg I (2000) Potential nitrite scavengers as inhibitors of the formation of N-nitrosamines in solution and tobacco matrix systems. J Agric Food Chem 48(9):4381–4388

Rusin A, Krawczyk Z, Grynkiewicz G, Gogler A, Zawisza-Puchałka J, Szeja W (2010) Synthetic derivatives of genistein, their properties and possible applications. Acta Biochim Pol 57(1):23–34

Sabzichi M, Hamishehkar H, Ramezani F, Sharifi S, Tabasinezhad M, Pirouzpanah M et al (2014) Luteolin-loaded phytosomes sensitize human breast carcinoma MDA-MB 231 cells to doxorubicin by suppressing Nrf2 mediated signalling. Asian Pac J Cancer Prev 15(13):5311–5316

Sahoo NG, Bao H, Pan Y, Pal M, Kakran M, Cheng HKF et al (2011) Functionalized carbon nanomaterials as nanocarriers for loading and delivery of a poorly water-soluble anticancer drug: a comparative study. Chem Commun 47(18):5235–5237

Sakai S, Kawamata H, Kogure T, Mantani N, Terasawa K, Umatake M, Ochiai H (1999) Inhibitory effect of ferulic acid and isoferulic acid on the production of macrophage inflammatory protein-2 in response to respiratory syncytial virus infection in RAW264. 7 cells. Mediat Inflamm 8(3):173–175

Saladi RN, Persaud AN (2005) The causes of skin cancer: a comprehensive review. Drugs Today 41(1):37–54

Sanna V, Siddiqui IA, Sechi M, Mukhtar H (2013) Resveratrol-loaded nanoparticles based on poly (epsilon-caprolactone) and poly (d, l-lactic-co-glycolic acid)–poly (ethylene glycol) blend for prostate cancer treatment. Mol Pharm 10(10):3871–3881

Saraf S (2010) Applications of novel drug delivery system for herbal formulations. Fitoterapia 81(7):680–689

Sarkar FH, Li Y (2002) Mechanisms of cancer chemoprevention by soy isoflavone genistein. Cancer Metastasis Rev 21(3–4):265–280

Sarkar FH, Li Y, Wang Z, Kong D (2009) Cellular signaling perturbation by natural products. Cell Signal 21(11):1541–1547

Scarberry KE, Dickerson EB, McDonald JF, Zhang ZJ (2008) Magnetic nanoparticle- peptide conjugates for in vitro and in vivo targeting and extraction of cancer cells. J Am Chem Soc 130(31):10258–10262

Shen R, Kim JJ, Yao M, Elbayoumi TA (2016) Development and evaluation of vitamin E D-α-tocopheryl polyethylene glycol 1000 succinate-mixed polymeric phospholipid micelles of berberine as an anticancer nanopharmaceutical. Int J Nanomedicine 11:1687

Sherje AP, Dravyakar BR, Kadam D, Jadhav M (2017) Cyclodextrin-based nanosponges: a critical review. Carbohydr Polym 173:37–49

Shimizu R, Kishi K (2012) Skin graft. Plast Surg Int 2012. https://doi.org/10.1155/2012/563493

Shrimali D, Shanmugam MK, Kumar AP, Zhang J, Tan BK, Ahn KS, Sethi G (2013) Targeted abrogation of diverse signal transduction cascades by emodin for the treatment of inflammatory disorders and cancer. Cancer Lett 341(2):139–149

Shukla S, Gupta S (2010) Apigenin and cancer chemoprevention. In: Bioactive foods in promoting health. Elsevier, Cleveland, Ohio, USA. pp 663–689

Siddiqui IA, Bharali DJ, Nihal M, Adhami VM, Khan N, Chamcheu JC et al (2014) Excellent anti-proliferative and pro-apoptotic effects of (−)-epigallocatechin-3-gallate encapsulated in chitosan nanoparticles on human melanoma cell growth both in vitro and in vivo. Nanomedicine 10(8):1619–1626

Singh M, Suman S, Shukla Y (2014) New enlightenment of skin cancer chemoprevention through phytochemicals: in vitro and in vivo studies and the underlying mechanisms. BioMed Res Int 2014. pp 1–18

Singh D, Soni GC, Prajapati SK (2016) Recent advances in nanosponges as drug delivery system: a review. Eur J Pharm Med Res 3:364–371

Singla AK, Garg A, Aggarwal D (2002) Paclitaxel and its formulations. Int J Pharm 235(1–2):179–192

Sinha N, Yeow J-W (2005) Carbon nanotubes for biomedical applications. IEEE Trans Nanobioscience 4(2):180–195

Sobhani Z, Dinarvand R, Atyabi F, Ghahremani M, Adeli M (2011) Increased paclitaxel cytotoxicity against cancer cell lines using a novel functionalized carbon nanotube. Int J Nanomedicine 6:705

Soppimath KS, Aminabhavi TM, Kulkarni AR, Rudzinski WE (2001) Biodegradable polymeric nanoparticles as drug delivery devices. J Control Release 70(1–2):1–20

Souto EB, Wissing SA, Barbosa CM, Müller RH (2004) Development of a controlled release formulation based on SLN and NLC for topical clotrimazole delivery. Int J Pharm 278(1):71–77

Srinivasan C (2008) Carbon nanotubes in cancer therapy. Curr Sci 94(3):300

Srinivasan M, Sudheer AR, Menon VP (2007) Ferulic acid: therapeutic potential through its antioxidant property. J Clin Biochem Nutr 40(2):92–100

Srivastava JK, Gupta S (2007) Antiproliferative and apoptotic effects of chamomile extract in various human cancer cells. J Agric Food Chem 55(23):9470–9478

Stevanovic M, Uskokovic D (2009) Poly (lactide-co-glycolide)-based micro and nanoparticles for the controlled drug delivery of vitamins. Curr Nanosci 5(1):1–14

Steward WP, Brown K (2013) Cancer chemoprevention: a rapidly evolving field. Br J Cancer 109(1):1

Strickland LR, Pal HC, Elmets CA, Afaq F (2015) Targeting drivers of melanoma with synthetic small molecules and phytochemicals. Cancer Lett 359(1):20–35

Strojan P (2010) Role of radiotherapy in melanoma management. Radiol Oncol 44(1):1–12. https://doi.org/10.2478/v10019-010-0008-x

Su Y-T, Chang H-L, Shyue S-K, Hsu S-L (2005) Emodin induces apoptosis in human lung adenocarcinoma cells through a reactive oxygen species-dependent mitochondrial signaling pathway. Biochem Pharmacol 70(2):229–241

Subramaniam A, Shanmugam MK, Ong TH, Li F, Perumal E, Chen L et al (2013) Emodin inhibits growth and induces apoptosis in an orthotopic hepatocellular carcinoma model by blocking activation of STAT3. Br J Pharmacol 170(4):807–821

Svenson S (2009) Dendrimers as versatile platform in drug delivery applications. Eur J Pharm Biopharm 71(3):445–462

Swaminathan S, Pastero L, Serpe L, Trotta F, Vavia P, Aquilano D et al (2010) Cyclodextrin-based nanosponges encapsulating camptothecin: physicochemical characterization, stability and cytotoxicity. Eur J Pharm Biopharm 74(2):193–201

Swamy MK, Patra JK, Rudramurthy GR (2019) Medicinal plants: chemistry, pharmacology, and therapeutic applications. CRC Press. Boco Raton.

Tang JY, Fu T, Lau C, Oh DH, Bikle DD, Asgari MM (2012) Vitamin D in cutaneous carcinogenesis: part I. J Am Acad Dermatol 67(5):803–8e1

Thakre AR, Gholse YN, Kasliwal RH (2016) Nanosponges: a novel approach of drug delivery system. J Med Pharm Allied Sci 78(92):78

Torre LA, Trabert B, DeSantis CE, Miller KD, Samimi G, Runowicz CD et al (2018) Ovarian cancer statistics, 2018. CA Cancer J Clin 68(4):284–296

Tyagi AK, Singh RP, Agarwal C, Chan DC, Agarwal R (2002) Silibinin strongly synergizes human prostate carcinoma DU145 cells to doxorubicin-induced growth inhibition, G2-M arrest, and apoptosis. Clin Cancer Res 8(11):3512–3519

Vaid M, Katiyar SK (2010) Molecular mechanisms of inhibition of photocarcinogenesis by silymarin, a phytochemical from milk thistle (Silybum marianum L. Gaertn.). Int J Oncol 36(5):1053–1060

Verma NK, Crosbie-Staunton K, Satti A, Gallagher S, Ryan KB, Doody T et al (2013) Magnetic core-shell nanoparticles for drug delivery by nebulization. J Nanobiotechnol 11(1):1

Verschoyle RD, Greaves P, Patel K, Marsden DA, Brown K, Steward WP, Gescher AJ (2008) Evaluation of the cancer chemopreventive efficacy of silibinin in genetic mouse models of prostate and intestinal carcinogenesis: relationship with silibinin levels. Eur J Cancer 44(6):898–906

Wang J, Liu W, Tu Q, Wang J, Song N, Zhang Y et al (2010) Folate-decorated hybrid polymeric nanoparticles for chemically and physically combined paclitaxel loading and targeted delivery. Biomacromolecules 12(1):228–234

Wang C, Feng L, Yang X, Wang F, Lu W (2013) Folic acid-conjugated liposomal vincristine for multidrug resistant cancer therapy. Asian J Pharm Sci 8(2):118–127

Wang W, Zhang L, Chen T, Guo W, Bao X, Wang D et al (2017) Anticancer effects of resveratrol-loaded solid lipid nanoparticles on human breast cancer cells. Molecules 22(11):1814

Wei H, Bowen R, Zhang X, Lebwohl M (1998) Isoflavone genistein inhibits the initiation and promotion of two-stage skin carcinogenesis in mice. Carcinogenesis 19(8):1509–1514

Wei H, Zhang X, Wang Y, Lebwohl M (2002) Inhibition of ultraviolet light-induced oxidative events in the skin and internal organs of hairless mice by isoflavone genistein. Cancer Lett 185(1):21–29

Wei H, Saladi R, Lu Y, Wang Y, Palep SR, Moore J et al (2003) Isoflavone genistein: photoprotection and clinical implications in dermatology. J Nutr 133(11):3811S–3819S

Wei Z, Hao J, Yuan S, Li Y, Juan W, Sha X, Fang X (2009) Paclitaxel-loaded Pluronic P123/F127 mixed polymeric micelles: formulation, optimization and in vitro characterization. Int J Pharm 376(1–2):176–185

Wei J, Bhatt S, Chang LM, Sampson HA, Masilamani M (2012) Isoflavones, genistein and daidzein, regulate mucosal immune response by suppressing dendritic cell function. PLoS One 7(10):e47979

Wei T, Chen C, Liu J, Liu C, Posocco P, Liu X et al (2015) Anticancer drug nanomicelles formed by self-assembling amphiphilic dendrimer to combat cancer drug resistance. Proc Natl Acad Sci 112(10):2978–2983

Wilson MA, Schuchter LM (2016) Chemotherapy for melanoma. Cancer Treat Res 167:209–229. https://doi.org/10.1007/978-3-319-22539-5_8

Wong KH, Li GQ, Li KM, Razmovski-Naumovski V, Chan K (2011) Kudzu root: traditional uses and potential medicinal benefits in diabetes and cardiovascular diseases. J Ethnopharmacol 134(3):584–607

Wu M, Kubota C (2008) Effects of high electrical conductivity of nutrient solution and its application timing on lycopene, chlorophyll and sugar concentrations of hydroponic tomatoes during ripening. Sci Hortic 116(2):122–129

Wu W, Wieckowski S, Pastorin G, Benincasa M, Klumpp C, Briand J-P et al (2005) Targeted delivery of amphotericin B to cells by using functionalized carbon nanotubes. Angew Chem Int Ed 44(39):6358–6362

Wu Z, Liu B, Liu J, Zhang Q, Liu J, Chen N et al (2015) Resveratrol inhibits the proliferation of human melanoma cells by inducing G1/S cell cycle arrest and apoptosis. Mol Med Rep 11(1):400–404

Xi J, Guo R (2007) Studies on molecular interactions between puerarin and PC liposomes. Chin Sci Bull 52(19):2612–2617

Xu P, Yin Q, Shen J, Chen L, Yu H, Zhang Z, Li Y (2013) Synergistic inhibition of breast cancer metastasis by silibinin-loaded lipid nanoparticles containing TPGS. Int J Pharm 454(1):21–30

Xu W, Bae EJ, Lee M-K (2018) Enhanced anticancer activity and intracellular uptake of paclitaxel-containing solid lipid nanoparticles in multidrug-resistant breast cancer cells. Int J Nanomedicine 13:7549

Xue J, Ding W, Liu Y (2010) Anti-diabetic effects of emodin involved in the activation of PPARγ on high-fat diet-fed and low dose of streptozotocin-induced diabetic mice. Fitoterapia 81(3):173–177

Yang SC, Zhu JB (2002) Preparation and characterization of camptothecin solid lipid nanoparticles. Drug Dev Ind Pharm 28(3):265–274

Yang Y, Li Y, Wang K, Wang Y, Yin W, Li L (2013) P38/NF-κB/snail pathway is involved in caffeic acid-induced inhibition of cancer stem cells-like properties and migratory capacity in malignant human keratinocyte. PLoS One 8(3):e58915

Yaoxian W, Hui Y, Yunyan Z, Yanqin L, Xin G, Xiaoke W (2013) Emodin induces apoptosis of human cervical cancer hela cells via intrinsic mitochondrial and extrinsic death receptor pathway. Cancer Cell Int 13(1):71

Yen G-C, Duh P-D, Chuang D-Y (2000) Antioxidant activity of anthraquinones and anthrone. Food Chem 70(4):437–441

Yiu W, Basco MT, Aruny JE, Cheng SW, Sumpio BE (2007) Cryosurgery: a review. Int J Angiol 16(1):1–6. Retrieved from https://www.ncbi.nlm.nih.gov/pmc/articles/PMC2732998/

Yuan Z, Chen L, Fan L, Tang M, Yang G, Yang H et al (2006) Liposomal quercetin efficiently suppresses growth of solid tumors in murine models. Clin Cancer Res 12(10):3193–3199

Zhang G, Miura Y, Yagasaki K (2000) Induction of apoptosis and cell cycle arrest in cancer cells by in vivo metabolites of teas. Nutr Cancer 38(2):265–273

Zhang L, Xia J, Zhao Q, Liu L, Zhang Z (2010) Functional graphene oxide as a nanocarrier for controlled loading and targeted delivery of mixed anticancer drugs. Small 6(4):537–544

Zhao Y, Moddaresi M, Jones SA, Brown MB (2009) A dynamic topical hydrofluoroalkane foam to induce nanoparticle modification and drug release in situ. Eur J Pharm Biopharm 72(3):521–528

Zhao Q-H, Zhang Y, Liu Y, Wang H-L, Shen Y-Y, Yang W-J, Wen L-P (2010) Anticancer effect of realgar nanoparticles on mouse melanoma skin cancer in vivo via transdermal drug delivery. Med Oncol 27(2):203–212

Zhigaltsev IV, Maurer N, Akhong Q-F, Leone R, Leng E, Wang J et al (2005) Liposome-encapsulated vincristine, vinblastine and vinorelbine: a comparative study of drug loading and retention. J Control Release 104(1):103–111

Zhou XM, Chen QH (1988) Biochemical study of Chinese rhubarb. XXII. Inhibitory effect of anthraquinone derivatives on Na+-K+-ATPase of the rabbit renal medulla and their diuretic action. Yao Xue Xue Bao= Acta Pharmaceutica Sinica 23(1):17

Zipser MC, Mangana J, Oberholzer PA, French LE, Dummer R (2010) Melanoma after laser therapy of pigmented lesions—circumstances and outcome. Eur J Dermatol 20(3):334–338. https://doi.org/10.1684/ejd.2010.0933

Part VI

Nanoformulations: Other Applications

19 Advances in Nanocarrier-Based Delivery of Therapeutic Peptides

Srishti Mittal, Vanshika Singh, and Shweta Dang

Abstract

There have been rapid developments in the field of peptide therapeutics since the advent of insulin therapy in the 1920s. Conventionally, like other drugs, peptides/proteins were also delivered intravenously, but due to low patient compliance, other modes of delivery like oral and nasal were explored. The oral route being the most sought-after mode of drug delivery has its own set of challenges when it comes to the delivery of peptides, high proteolytic activity, and acidic pH conditions in GI tract, to name a few. Another upcoming yet challenging mode is intranasal route. The nasal route has been used for brain targeting as it circumvents the blood-brain barrier; the drug/peptide can also cross the nasal epithelium to reach systemic circulation directly. This chapter focuses on the mechanism of intranasal mode of delivery, nanocarriers used to enhance the efficacy of delivery, and the peptides that have been developed and patented.

Srishti Mittal and Vanshika Singh contributed equally with all other contributors.

S. Mittal · V. Singh · S. Dang (✉)
Department of Biotechnology, Jaypee Institute of Information Technology, Noida, India
e-mail: shweta.dang@jiit.ac.in

Keywords

Intranasal · Nanocarriers · Peptides · Therapeutics · Blood-brain barrier · Bioavailability

19.1 Introduction

Peptides, by definition, are a class of compounds which comprise two or more amino acids that are linked in such a way that the carboxyl group of one amino acid is joined to the amino group of the next amino acid by the bond -CO-NH-, known as a peptide bond. Peptides are a class of molecules that prevail in between the molecular weight range of proteins and small molecules yet have distinct biochemical structure and therapeutic applications (Lau and Dunn 2018).

Peptides have been used in various therapeutic indications since insulin therapy first arrived in the 1920s. With the advancement of technology, there have been rapid developments in the field of protein and peptide pharmacology. With the use of recombinant DNA technology, large-scale manufacture of peptides has become feasible. This has led to large-scale commercialization of peptides (Agarwal and Rupenthal 2013). Peptides being intrinsic signaling molecules for many physiological pathways can therapeutically intervene natural pathways (Lau and Dunn 2018) (Fig. 19.1).

S. Talegaonkar, M. Rai (eds.), *Nanoformulations in Human Health*,
https://doi.org/10.1007/978-3-030-41858-8_19

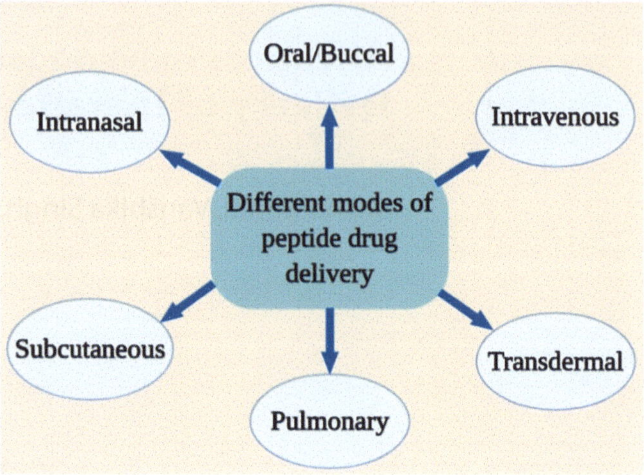

Fig. 19.1 Different modes of peptide drug delivery

The presence of protein- and peptide-degrading enzymes in the body is abundant; therefore, delivering peptide or protein-based drugs via other routes is not as efficient. A number of pathways have been adopted for the delivery of therapeutic peptides to the human body, some of them being intravenous, intrathecal, oral, transdermal (Dillon et al. 2019), and intranasal. The choice of mode of delivery of peptides is largely limited to injectable owing to low bioavailability via the oral route. Peptides are mostly delivered intravenously; however, delivery via intranasal or intrathecal routes has also been explored for some conditions like Parkinson's disease, Alzheimer's (Gaudreault and Mousseau 2019), major depressive disorder, etc. However, the action of mucociliary clearance, enzymatic degradation, and poor olfactory region deposition lowers the therapeutic efficiency of the administered drug (Shah and Shao 2017; Sonvico et al. 2018). But the drug's efficiency via intranasal route can be enhanced by using the drug in conjugation with certain carrier particles and absorption-enhancing agents (Bourganis et al. 2018) (Table 19.1).

Table 19.1 Different modes of delivery of therapeutic peptides

Peptide	Mode of delivery	References
Ocreotide	Oral	Tuvia et al. (2012)
Salmon calcitonin	Oral	Anselmo et al. (2018)
Leuprolide	Oral	Iqbal et al. (2012)
Insulin (buccal films)	Buccal (oral mucosal surface)	Anselmo et al. (2018)
Teriparatide	Transdermal	Anselmo et al. (2018)
Abaloparatide	Transdermal	Yates et al. (2014)
Insulin (dry powder inhalers)	Inhalation (pulmonary)	Anselmo et al. (2018)
Api137	Subcutaneous	Knappe et al. (2019)
Leuprolide	Intravenous	Hu et al. (2015)

In view of the various hindrances that come in the way of delivery to the brain via intranasal route, researchers tried to explore various options that would help to improve the process of drug delivery and thereby have better therapeutic efficacy (Phukan et al. 2016). To address this issue, partition-based formulations in addition to particle size are being tried in the field of pharmacy. This has led to the development of nanoparticulate drug delivery systems (Phukan et al. 2016). Particles with their size ranging from 10 to 1000 nm and having colloidal nature are termed as nanoparticles. Dissolving, attaching, or entrapping the drug in the polymer matrix is some of the ways by which these nanoparticles can be designed as efficient drug delivery systems. Different forms of nanoparticles can be designed via these methods like liposomes, dendrimers, polymeric nanoparticles, and solid-lipid nanoparticles, to name a few (Phukan et al. 2016).

Table 19.2 Commercially available peptides and the medical condition they treat

Company	Product(s)	Peptide	Medical condition
Novartis AG (Switzerland)	Neoral®/ Sandimmune®	Cyclosporine	Immunosuppression
Ferring Pharmaceuticals (Switzerland)/ Generic (e.g. Actavis Labs FL Inc., NJ, USA)	DDAVP® Tablets DDAVP® Melt Minrin®	Desmopressin acetate hydrate	Central diabetes insipidus, primary nocturnal enuresis
Mitsubishi Tanabe Pharma Corporation (Japan)	Ceredist® Ceredist OD®	Taltirelin hydrate	Spinocerebellar degeneration
Theranaturals Inc. (ID, USA)	Reduced L-Glutathione	Glutathione	AIDS-related cachexia/cystic fibrosis
Acatavis, Inc. (NJ, USA)/Ironwood Pharma, Inc. (MA, USA)	Linzess® (USA) Constella® (Europe)	Linaclotide	Irritable bowel syndrome, chronic idiopathic constipation
ANI Pharmaceuticals, Inc. (MN, USA)	Vancocin®	Vancomycin HCl	Infection
Biocon Ltd. (India)	Koolistin®	Colistin sulfate	Infection

To overcome the efficiency-limiting characteristics of the nasal cavity (e.g., poor mucosal permeability, rapid physical clearance mechanism, high enzymatic activity), various conventional and non-conventional approaches such as introducing a chemical modification to the drug molecule, auxiliary agent utilization either as co-administration agents or as formulation components, and new formulation development are used (Bourganis et al. 2018). This chapter focuses on the mechanism of the intranasal mode of delivery, nanocarriers used to enhance the efficacy of delivery, and the peptides that have been developed and patented (Table 19.2).

19.2 Intranasal Mode of Delivery

Intranasal mode of drug delivery has been practiced since ancient times. It has been prevalent in the Ayurvedic system of Indian medicine and was popularly known as "NASAYA KARMA" (Kushwaha et al. 2011). Nasal mucosa, a potent administration route, helps to achieve higher and faster levels of drug absorption. This is because of the neutral pH of the nasal mucosa and comparatively lesser enzymatic degradation in comparison to the oral mode of delivery. Oral mode of delivery is one of the most conventional drug administration methods; it has its own drawbacks like enzymatic activity, highly variable pH, hepatic first-pass effect, etc. Intranasal mode of delivery allows drugs comprising proteins and peptides that are active in low doses and show lesser bioavailability orally to achieve better administration rates.

Nasal administration of compounds has been long practiced. Psychotropic drugs and other hallucinogens were snorted by natives of South America since ages. This practice is still prevalent among abusers of heroin and cocaine (Wadell 2002). In the nasal route of administration, drugs are insufflated through the external nares.

Disorders of the central nervous system (CNS) like multiple sclerosis (Schirmer et al. 2019), Alzheimer's disease, Parkinson's disease, and epilepsy are on the rise because of the changing lifestyle and aging population. These disorders show a variety of clinical and pathological outcomes but in totality result in alteration of neural functions and gradual loss of neural tissue (Bourganis et al. 2018). The complexity of the CNS and the ostensible multifactorial pathogenic mechanism makes effective treatment of such disorders a challenge despite major advances in both the understanding of the pathogenesis of neurological disorders and drug delivery research. Presently available drugs mainly target to lessen the neurodegeneration but have failed to reverse the disease state and restore normal neural condition and function (Bourganis et al. 2018).

Acquired metabolic and congenital disorders like osteoporosis and diabetes mellitus require long-term therapy by protein- and peptide-based

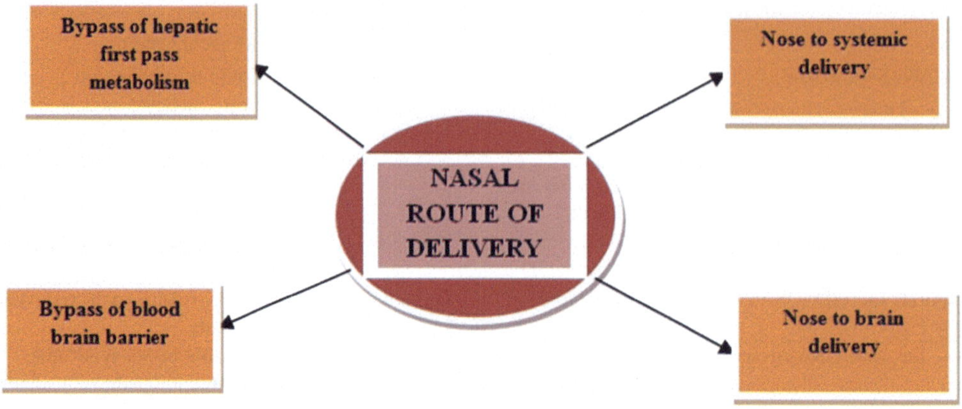

Fig. 19.2 Nasal route of delivery of peptide drugs

pharmaceuticals. But the hepatic first-pass effect (Raza et al. 2019) and degradation by proteolytic enzymes call for daily injections to maintain efficacy. For this reason, research has been directed toward finding new delivery modes, some of them being ocular, pulmonary, buccal, rectal, and nasal (Ahsan et al. 2001). Out of these, nasal route of delivery is preferred over the other routes due to the ease of administration and high patient compliance (Fig. 19.2).

19.2.1 Nose Anatomy

A nasal cavity in humans (volume: 15–20 ml) and animals has two major functions of breathing and olfaction. Apart from these, nasal cavity also performs the physiological functions of resonance of produced sounds, heating and humidification of inhaled air before it reaches the lungs, filtration of particles, immunological activities, and mucociliary clearance (Wadell 2002). The median septum divides the nose into two symmetrical halves. Each of these halves extends posteriorly to the nasopharynx and opens out exteriorly to the face through nostrils. The respiratory region, the anterior and posterior vestibules, and the olfactory regions are the three main areas of the nasal cavity (Illum 2004). The lateral wall consists of a convoluted structure which is referred to as the nasal labial folds or conchae (Bakary et al. 2019). This highly folded structure further consists of the inferior, median, and superior turbinates which vastly increases the surface area to about 150 cm^2. The respiratory region covers about 85% of this area in humans (Wadell 2002).

The nostrils are protected by the skin on the outside, while the nasal cavity anteriorly is lined by stratified squamous (Firat et al. 2018) and transitional epithelium. The epithelial tissue is highly vascularized and provides a potential channel for drug delivery. The highly vascular respiratory epithelium present in the posterior part of the nasal cavity is ciliated, columnar, and stratified. It consists of five main types of cells: ciliated columnar cells, non-ciliated columnar cells, goblet cells, basal cells, and a small number of neurosecretory cells are also present in the basement membrane. The columnar cells are covered with microvilli, which help to increase the surface area by many folds. About 20% of the total cells present in the lower concha are ciliated which helps to transport mucous toward the nasopharynx, while non-ciliated cells comprise about 60–70% of the respiratory mucosa, are high in metabolic activity, and are involved in the transport of fluids in and out of the cells. The goblet cells comprise about 10% of the mucosa in the turbinate area, contain plentiful of secretory granules filled with mucin, and produce secretion that forms the mucous layer. Being poorly differentiated, the basal cells replace other epithelial cells, acting as stem cells (Wadell 2002).

19.2.2 Pathway of Transport

It is believed that a combination of pathways involving cerebrospinal fluid, lymphatic system, gastrointestinal tract, and vascular system are responsible for the transport of molecules through the nasal cavity. An overview of the pathways involved in intranasal transport of therapeutics to the CNS is explained further. It has been well documented that systemic, olfactory, and trigeminal nerve pathways are the major routes through which nose-to-brain transport occurs. The common benefits that these pathways offer are that they avoid clearance due to enzymatic degradation mechanisms. It is the physiochemical property of the drug that dictates which pathway it would be transported by (Hanson and Frey 2008).

19.2.2.1 Systemic Pathway

This pathway is an indirect route for a nose-to-brain delivery. In this, the drug is absorbed from vascularized nasal respiratory epithelium and the lymphatic system. Systemic pathway mainly favors the transcellular delivery of lipophilic substances which have the ability to get readily absorbed in the bloodstream, thereby crossing the blood-brain barrier and entering the brain parenchyma. This pathway is the least studied, with prevalent research only in animal models such as rats, rabbits, and swine (Bourganis et al. 2018).

19.2.2.2 Olfactory Pathway

The olfactory pathway further bifurcates into neuronal and epithelial routes. Other categorizations are done on the basis of the extracellular or intracellular destiny of the delivered drug. Incorporation of the drug containing formulation into the olfactory sensory neuron is done by endocytotic or pinocytotic mechanism (Michael Danielsen and Hansen 2016) for the neuronal route. The drug is then intracellularly transported in the axon to the olfactory bulb, from where it is distributed throughout the CNS. Delivery via axonal pathway is rather time-consuming, but it also depends on factors such as the substance transported, the species, the axonal diameter, etc.

Delivery of therapeutics to the brain via the olfactory region can also take place by the olfactory epithelium. In this pathway, the drug requires only minutes upon administration to reach the olfactory bulb and other parts of the brain, which is much faster than the axonal pathway. Both intracellular and extracellular mechanisms are involved in transport across the olfactory mucosa (Bourganis et al. 2018).

19.2.2.3 Trigeminal Pathway

The trigeminal nerve route which innervates both the respiratory and olfactory mucosa serves as a channel for the delivery of drugs to the brain stem and other structures connected to it. It is a much less explored pathway, utilizing many branches of the trigeminal nerve (Okada et al. 2018) which is the largest cranial nerve. Its main function is to convey thermosensory and chemosensory information to the ocular, nasal, and oral mucosae. Transport via this pathway might occur either extracellularly or intracellularly (Bourganis et al. 2018).

19.2.2.4 Lymphatic Pathway

The lamina propria (olfactory region's submucosal area) (Ladel et al. 2018) clears the drug either by the method of absorption into olfactory blood vessels or into the olfactory lymphatic vessels, draining the substance deep into the lymph nodes present in the cervical region in the neck. Another way of transporting the drug could be through the extracellular pathway wherein the olfactory nerve passes from the lamina propria to the olfactory bulb present in the brain (Bourganis et al. 2018).

19.2.3 Advantages and Disadvantages

The intranasal route of drug delivery has emerged as a potential route for delivering drugs into systemic circulation as well as the brain. The nasal mucosa has a large absorption area (150 cm^2) which is highly vascularized and permeable to most of the therapeutics. Nasal delivery also offers additional benefits over the oral mode of delivery, some of them being rapid onset of action, high patient compliance, avoidance of gastrointestinal degradation due to acidic pH or presence of proteolytic enzymes, non-invasive administration, avoidance of hepatic first-pass effect, etc. (Shah and Shao 2017). The intranasal route can be exploited to accentuate the delivery of therapeutics to the brain as this method of delivery bypasses the blood-brain barrier.

However, this mode of drug delivery suffers from certain limitations like low permeability of the nasal mucosa to hydrophilic molecules (especially those having molecular weight over several thousand Daltons), small applicable volume per dose, the short residence time of the drug formulation due to mucociliary clearance (Whitsett 2018), enzymatic degradation, etc.

To overcome these challenges associated with the nasal route, nanoparticles are being developed which enhances the efficacy of the drug.

19.3 Nanoparticles for Intranasal Delivery

With constant advancements in technology, there have been plenty of developments in the field of drug delivery methods. As there is evident enzymatic degradation in both the oral and intranasal routes of delivery, the necessity of developing an efficient delivery system that protects the peptide drug from harsh environment and aids in heightening its absorption without altering biological activity has risen. Nanocarriers or nanoparticles, as we commonly call them, are a promising approach (Chen et al. 2016) which can be integrated with the therapeutic molecule to achieve desired results (Fig. 19.3).

In a study conducted by Shahnaz et al., thiolated chitosan nanoparticles (Rahbarian et al. 2018) were developed for the efficient delivery of leuprolide (Shahnaz et al. 2012). Leuprolide is an efficient treatment option for prostate cancer and disorders related to endocrine system malfunction such as fibroids in the uterus, central precocious puberty in minors, and endometriosis. Its synthetic variant leuprolide acetate (nanopeptide) acts as a substitute of the luteinizing hormone-releasing hormone (Nian et al. 2019). Since the treatment for these disorders requires constant drug administration via injections, it is not patient compliant. To overcome this challenge, the intranasal method of drug delivery was adopted and thiolated chitosan nanoparticles were developed. To prepare the nanoparticles, ionic interaction between thiolated (chitosan-TGA) and unmodified chitosan was allowed with sodium tripolyphosphate. The prepared nanoparticles were observed to have a mean size of 252 ± 82 nm and zeta potential equal to +10.9 ± 4 mV. The thiolated(chitosan-TGA) nanoparticles were compared to chitosan nanoparticles without any modification. It was observed that the transport

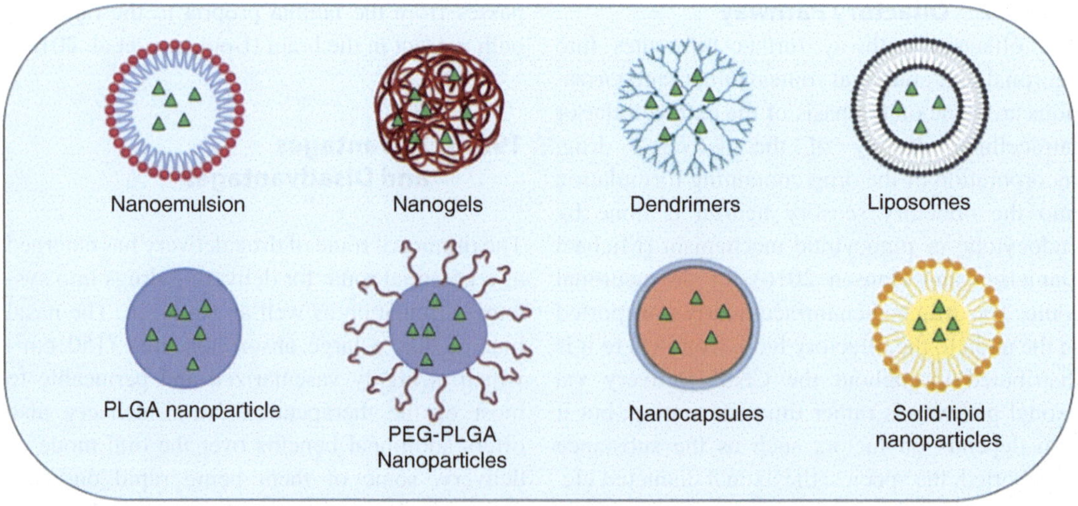

Fig. 19.3 Different types of nanoparticles used in peptide drug delivery

of unmodified nanoparticles and thiolated nanoparticles across porcine nasal mucosa was increased by 2- and 5.2-fold as compared to leuprolide solutions. Also, the nasal bioavailability of thiolated nanoparticles was about 19.6% in comparison to leuprolide solution 2.8% according to $AUC_{(0-6)}$. A fourfold increase in elimination half-life was also observed for thiolated nanoparticles as compared to leuprolide solution. Therefore, this approach sustains the drug in the body for a longer time duration and enhances its bioavailability (Shahnaz et al. 2012).

In another study conducted by Yadav et al. in Sprague-Dawley rats, the comparative biodistribution of cyclosporine A was done by intranasal administration of drug using oil in water nanoemulsion. For this purpose, flaxseed oil (omega-3 fatty acid rich) was used which is known to play a major role in the functioning of the brain. Cyclosporin A is an immunosuppressive agent and is hydrophobic in nature (Yadav et al. 2015). It has also been demonstrated to be a potential anti-inflammatory agent, and being a neuroprotective agent, it mainly targets the brain (Guada et al. 2016). The cyclosporine A nanoemulsion was prepared by using ultrasonication and was studied for encapsulation efficiency of the drug, size of the globule formed, and zeta potential. The hydrodynamic diameter of Cyclosporin A-nanoemulsion was observed to be 272 ± 12 nm having a zeta potential of 57 ± 10 mV, percentage drug encapsulation of 88 ± 13% and CsA loading concentration of 25 mg/mL. Upon administering intranasally, CsA nanoemulsion resulted in an increase in blood-to-brain concentration from 1.03 to 10 from 30 min to 240 min, while other approaches did not show efficient brain targeting with the blood-to-brain ratio reaching up to the maximum value of 0.713 at 120 min for Cyclosporin A solution when administered intranasally. The result suggests that intranasally delivered nanoemulsion has proven to provide elevated brain-to-blood drug concentration and can be adopted as a suitable delivery system (Yadav et al. 2015).

Zhao et al. developed phospholipid-based gelatin nanoparticles encapsulating basic fibroblast growth factor. In Parkinson's disease, basic fibroblast growth factor and brain-derived neurotrophic factor expression are found to be reduced in the dopaminergic neurons of substantia nigra pars compacta (Cookson 2017). It was found that in basic fibroblast growth factor null mutant mice, dopaminergic neurons die of neurotoxicity whereas neurons were preserved in basic fibroblast growth factor overexpressing mice. This indicates dopaminergic neuron protection efficiency of basic fibroblast growth factor from neurotoxicity. Water-in-water emulsion followed by freeze-drying method was used for the preparation of lipid nanocarrier molecules made up of gelatin having particle size 143 ± 1.14 nm and zeta potential equal to −38.2 ± 1.2 mV. These gelatin nanostructured lipid carriers were compared to gelatin nanoparticles on the basis of the dopaminergic neuron amount. In basic fibroblast growth factor-gelatin nanostructured lipid carrier group administered intranasally, the number of dopaminergic neurons was observed to be 3000.38 ± 331.03 ng/g tissue weight, while in the basic fibroblast growth factor-gelatin nanoparticle group administered intranasally, it was found to be 1020 ± 141.3 ng/g tissue weight. This suggests that the former were effective in enhancing the brain delivery of basic fibroblast growth factor, which is a significant neuroprotective agent via the intranasal route (Zhao et al. 2013). Another peptide drug, urocortin, was integrated with odorranalectin-conjugated poly(ethylene glycol)-poly(lactic-co-glycolic acid) nanoparticles, and studies were conducted on hemiparkinsonian rats. Urocortin being a peptide related to corticotropin-releasing factor has been shown to be efficient in providing sustained restoration of nigrostriatal function (Md et al. 2015). The nanoparticles were designed to have a diameter between 80 nm and 90 nm, and they had a zeta potential of −24.7 ± 1.5 mV. The resulting nanoparticles upon delivering intranasally to hemiparkinsonian rats have shown to accentuate the brain uptake and neuroprotective effects of urocortin (Wen et al. 2011).

In a case of developing alginate nanoparticles, Haque et al. synthesized and evaluated alginate nanoparticles carrying the antidepressant drug Venlafaxine following the intranasal delivery route. It can be used as a treatment option for patients suffering from major depressive disorder. Venlafaxine was chosen because it inhibits neuronal reuptake of central serotonin and norepinephrine increasing their level in the synaptic clefts present in the brain (Gallagher et al. 2015). The prepared Venlafaxine alginate nanoparticle had a particle size of 173.7 ± 2.5 nm and positive zeta potential of +37.4 ± 1.74 mV with a loading capacity of 26.74 ± 1.40%. Fluorescence microscopic studies were performed to determine the efficacy of nanoparticle delivery to the brain with Rodamine-123 as the marker molecule. Venlafaxine was observed to reach a brain concentration of 742.5 ± 32.50 ng/mL upon administration via alginate nanoparticles intranasally, while it was observed to be 396.97 ± 29.17 ng/mL upon intranasal administration via solution. The above-stated results indicate better drug absorption by using alginate nanoparticles (Haque et al. 2014).

Polymeric nanoparticles developed by Godfrey et al. aim to deliver leucine-enkephalin hydrochloride to the brain. The peptide delivered is used as a pain therapeutic (Boumrah et al. 2015). Nanoparticle administration of leucine-enkephalin hydrochloride exhibited an accentuated anti-nociceptive response in assays of ongoing and evoked pain in contrast to animals dosed with leucine-enkephalin hydrochloride alone. The peptide was formulated with N-palmitoyl-N-monomethyl-N,N-dimethyl-N,N,N-trimethyl-6-O-glycolchitosan into a mixture of single (30–40 nm) and aggregated (100–200 nm) nanoparticles (NMO127). No plasma exposure to the drug indicates the capability of the drug to exclusively target the brain. Animal behavioral data pointed out the potentiality of NMO127 at a dose of 7.5 mg kg^{-1} to reverse hypersensitivity in inflammation-induced hypersensitivity. It also relieved neuropathic pain in the case of nerve injuries. The peptide encapsulation in the nanoparticle has been proven to be instrumental in the distribution of peptide to the thalamus and cortex and reduction in off-target effects (Godfrey et al. 2017). Another group comprising Kumar M. et al. developed leucine-enkephalin-loaded N-trimethyl chitosan nanoparticles and evaluated for brain targeting of the peptide. Mean particle size and zeta potential were found to be 443 ± 23 nm and +15 ± 2 mV. It was observed that the permeability of the peptide released from the nanoparticle was around 35-fold higher than the leucine-enkephalin solution (Kumar et al. 2013).

In a study conducted by Mansoor et al., assessment of synthetic bovine parainfluenza virus type 3 peptide motifs and solubilized BPI3V proteins encapsulated in PLGA nanoparticles to induce humoral immune response was conducted. To overcome the deficiencies of conventional vaccines, use of adjuvants for vaccine delivery was proposed. Majority of the particles produced were spherical in shape having a size less than 330 nm with a zeta potential of −23 mV. Upon administration, it was observed that there was an increase in IgG response after immunization with BPI3V or BPI3V motifs nanoparticles compared to empty nanoparticles. The response was sustained for over 57 days of study probably due to slow release of the antigen (Mansoor et al. 2014).

Liu et al. studied PEG-PCL nanoparticles carrying lactoferrin. A natural iron-binding protein, lactoferrin, plays an essential role in Alzheimer's disease, Parkinson's disease, amyotrophic lateral sclerosis, etc. Lactoferrin's receptors have the property of overexpressing respiratory epithelial cells and neurons which was utilized to facilitate the drug delivery from nose to brain (Legrand 2016). NAP(NAPVSIPQ) which is an 8 amino acid neuropeptide currently in Phase II clinical trials was used as a model drug. The nanoparticles had an average diameter of 70–90 nm and lactoferrin conjugation efficiency of 22.6%. The biodistribution of Coumarin-6 was used as an indicator for determining the results of intranasal administration of lactoferrin-loaded nanoparticles. It was observed that there was an increase in the accumulation of fluorescence tracer embedded in lactoferrin nanoparticle in parts of the brain like cerebellum, hippocampus, olfactory bulb, and olfactory tract. The results indicated that the nanoparticles helped in higher transmucosal transport and better brain targeting efficiency (Liu et al. 2013). In an attempt to transport levodopa, a drug used in the treatment of

Parkinson's disease, Sharma et al. formulated nanoparticles made up of chitosan and loaded them with levodopa, incorporating it into a thermo reversible gel. Due to the extensive metabolism of levodopa, it exhibits low oral bioavailability so it is co-administered with carbidopa which is an amino acid decarboxylase inhibitor preventing the degradation of levodopa. Results suggested that with 90 mg of drug, the nanoparticle size was 164.5 nm and it had a zeta potential of 28.3 mV. From the experiments conducted, it was found that CNL exhibited higher drug recovery in the brain (74.7 ± 2.27%) than levodopa in saline. It can be inferred that because of the high adhesion of chitosan with mucin in the nasal mucosal tissue such results have been obtained. This clearly proves that the use of chitosan can reduce the clearance time of formulation, thereby increasing the residence time for better drug absorption (Sharma et al. 2013).

Oppong-Damoah et al. synthesized bovine serum albumin nanoparticles carrying the peptide oxytocin. Oxytocin, a nine amino acid longneuropeptide, is synthesized in the paraventricular and supraoptic nuclei of the hypothalamus. The posterior pituitary gland releases it into the blood circulation, but it also has neurotransmitter like properties and acts at an identified oxytocin receptor throughout much of the brain in mammals. Though known for being a uterine contraction-causing hormone during parturition, recent studies have shown that it also plays a role in social behavior, social recognition, altruism, and social comfort as a brain neurotransmitter. This recent finding has led to the therapeutic use of oxytocin as a potent drug for treating central nervous system disorders like fragile X-syndrome, Dravet syndrome, and altruism spectrum disorder. Nanoparticles were developed for the efficient delivery of oxytocin since it is not able to permeate the blood-brain barrier, which leads to lesser bioavailability. These nanoparticles were labeled with fluorescein isothiocyanate, and their transport across the blood-brain barrier was examined by determining the effect of the absence or presence of the cell barrier and the effect of time. It was observed that there was no significant difference in the transport of fluoresceinisothiocyanate present in the nanoparticles that targeted the brain because of the cellular barrier at any point in time. The resistance provided by the cellular barrier at the first sampling point was 107.28 ± 31.7 ohm.cm^2 (at $t = 60$ min), and it was observed to be 127.22 ± 28 ohm.cm^2 (at $t = 240$ min), at the end of the experiment. The resistance of the cellular barrier was found to be 5.03 ± 1.8 ohm.cm^2 (at $t =$ n60 min) and 10.8 ± 2 ohm.cm^2 (at $t = 240$ min), at the end of the experiment without the cellular barrier. These results indicated that the brain-targeting nanoparticles swiftly surpass the blood-brain barrier, believably via active transport across the barrier (Oppong-Damoah et al. 2019).

Vaccines based on peptides have the capability of overcoming the limitations of their classical counterparts; their use, however, is impeded due to the shortage of adjuvants and carriers fit for human use. Nevagi et al. developed a self-adjuvanting peptide-carrying system, based on the ionic interactions between a peptide antigen conjugated with artificially designed anionic alpha-poly (L-glutamic acid) and cationic trimethyl chitosan. The antigen bearing a preserved B-cell epitope which was acquired from group A streptococcus bacteria and a common T-helper epitope was coupled with alpha-poly-(L-glutamic acid), using cycloaddition. Chitosan is an environment-friendly natural polymer which is non-toxic in nature and has mucoadhesive properties. It is recognized by several receptors present in antigen-presenting cells like C type lectin receptors mannose receptors and toll-like receptor 2, and it is shown to have self-adjuvanting ability, improving the immunogenicity of the peptide-based vaccine. The chitosan nanoparticles were synthesized and checked for size, zeta potential, and morphology. The smallest size of the nanoparticles was found to be 201±8 nm with a zeta potential of +36 mV. During the study, it was shown that nanoparticles in the size range of 50–200 nm were taken up effectively by the M-cells further internalizing by receptor-mediated endocytosis in dendritic cells. Also, the positively charged nanoparticles easily gained access to the antigen-presenting cells taking into account the negatively charged membranes of these cells, which was evident from several reports. Therefore, the positive zeta potential of the nanoparticles played an important role in their uptake. Further, it was proven that these nanoparticles affected increased IgA and IgG antibody titers even at low antigen concentrations compared to earlier reports and exhibited protection against group A streptococcus infection. Thus, proving to be a highly promising strategy for the delivery of peptide antigens (Nevagi et al. 2018).

Kubek et al. developed polylactide nanoparticles having thyrotropin-releasing hormone, which were proven to hinder the kindling seizure development in terms of clonus duration, after discharge duration and behavioral stages. Thyrotropin-releasing hormone is an endogenous neuropeptide, which is acknowledged as being an anticonvulsant in animal models and numerous recalcitrant epileptic patients. However, its duration of action is circumscribed by the blood-brain barrier and quick tissue metabolism. To rectify this problem, the method of intranasal delivery of the neuropeptide in sustained-release biodegradable nanoparticles was developed. This ensured enhanced bioavailability of the neuropeptide in the CNS. Solvent evaporation method using double emulsion process was used for the preparation of Poly(L-lactic acid-D-lactic acid) nanoparticles with or without thyrotropin-releasing hormone. Transmission electron microscopy analysis revealed that an average diameter of 108 ± 12 nm was observed for the thyrotropin-releasing hormone containing nanoparticles, and it was 102 ± 12 nm for the blank nanoparticles, showing consistency in the shape and size of the nanoparticles. The availability and distribution of these nanoparticles were evaluated by staining with the lipophilic Nile red stain and then visualizing them under fluorescence microscope. It was observed that nanoparticles in the 80–100 nm size range loaded with the fluorescent dye when delivered contiguous to the olfactory neuroepithelium can be efficiently transferred from the nose to brain. These nanoparticles are internalized by the cells efficiently, cross the epithelial lining barriers, penetrate deep into the tissues, and seem to have negligible ciliotoxicity (Kubek et al. 2009).

In another study conducted by Kaur et al., thyrotropin-releasing hormone analogues were synthesized and encased in environment-friendly poly-lactide-co-glycolide nanoparticles, which were coated with the mucoadhesive polymer chitosan. Nanoparticles (unloaded) were prepared by oil-in-water emulsion-solvent evaporation method, while the drug-loaded nanoparticles were prepared by the water-in-oil-in-water double emulsion method, and these nanoparticles were conjugated with chitosan. The mean diameter of the unloaded nanoparticles was found to be 110.97 ± 9.7 nm, and for the unloaded chitosan nanoparticles, it was 163.6 ± 8.0 nm. The increase in the size of the nanoparticles can be associated with the formation of the chitosan layer over the unloaded poly-lactide-co-glycolide nanoparticles, thus demonstrating fruitful surface modification. In addition, a change in zeta potential was observed, going from less than zero to more than zero which in turn proved to be the successful adhesion of chitosan over the nanoparticles. The unloaded nanoparticles had a zeta potential of −32.22 mV while the chitosan poly-lactide-co-glycolide nanoparticles had a zeta potential of 20.29 mV. Thus, thyrotropin-releasing hormone may provide a novel therapeutic approach option that can fairly hinder or conceivably avert epileptogenesis, where more traditional therapies have not been very effective (Kaur et al. 2018).

Gao et al. evaluated vasoactive intestinal peptide which acts as a neuroprotective peptide and is incorporated into the poly (ethylene glycol)-poly (lactic acid) nanoparticles having wheat germ agglutinin modification. The vasoactive intestinal peptide is a 28 amino acid neuropeptide which is widespread in the central and peripheral nervous system. It exhibits diverse biological functions including smooth muscle relaxation, anti-inflammatory functions, regulation of cell growth, etc. It can also be used in the treatment of neurological disorders like Alzheimer's disease. In the study, nanoparticles were investigated for their potential as a promising drug delivery sys-

Table 19.3 Peptide drugs with properties of nanoparticles carrying them

Carrier type and base materials	Particle size	Surface-modifying agents or additives	Peptide drug	References
Liposomes				
Phosphatidylethanol-based lipids	50–250 nm	None	Porcine insulin	Kisel et al.
Soyalecithin/Chol	190 nm	WGA, TL, or UEA1-N-Glut-PE conjugates	Insulin	Zhang et al.
Poly(alkyl(meth)acrylates)				
P(IBC)	85 nm	Pluronic acid	Human insulin	Mesiha et al.
P(St)/hydrophilic polymer chains	400–1250 nm	None	Salmon calcitonin	Sakuma et al.
Polyesters/polyanhydrides				
DEAPA-co-PVAg-PLLA	200–500 nm	None	Recombinant human insulin	Simon et al.
PLGA	250 nm	None	TRH	Kawashima et al.
Polysaccharides				
Chitosan	269–688 nm	Tripolyphosphate	Porcine insulin	Ma et al.
Chitosan	643 nm	Sodium alginate	Ovalbumin.	Borges et al.

tem. The size of wheat germ agglutinin-modified vasoactive intestinal peptide nanoparticle was 100–120 nm and had a spherical shape. The results indicated that the peptide was efficiently entrapped (encapsulation efficiency: 70%) by poly (ethylene glycol)-poly (lactic acid) nanoparticle. Despite this, PEG-PLA nanoparticles showed low bioavailability, as a result of which wheat germ agglutinin was used as an alternative which in turn enhanced the peptide-loaded nanoparticles and nasal mucosa binding. WGA-modified nanoparticles were efficient and proved to be a potential mode of peptide delivery (Gao et al. 2007) (Table 19.3).

19.4 Conclusion

Nose-to-brain drug delivery is a very intriguing and appealing topic and holds a lot of potential for further research and development. It surmounts a lot of limitations that other modes of delivery like intravenous and oral possess. Delivery of therapeutic agents to the brain for the treatment of neurological disorders is a very challenging task due to the presence of various biochemical and dynamic barriers like the blood-brain barrier and the blood-cerebrospinal fluid barrier. The intranasal route of delivery delivers the therapeutic directly to the nasal mucosa which leads to the olfactory and trigeminal pathways of the brain. These are the most exposed areas of the central nervous system; therefore, it becomes very easy for the drug to reach the brain and show immediate response. Using nanocarriers for this purpose enhanced the drug-targeting efficiency, resulting in sustained release and better absorption. Various types of nanoparticles carrying different peptide drugs were administered intranasally, and it was observed that the nanoparticles had better uptake and absorption by the nasal mucosa and the drug showed sustained-release profile and higher bioavailability. Conjugating the nanoparticles to certain polymers like chitosan, which is mucoadhesive in nature, enhanced the residence time of the nanoparticles in the nasal cavity and lessened their mucociliary clearance. Thus, intranasal route of delivery is a very efficient method of drug delivery, especially for neurological disorders, where the drug is required to reach the brain directly. Recent advances in nanotechnology have improved the nose-to-brain delivery and can facilitate therapy for CNS disorders.

References

Agarwal P, Rupenthal IV (2013) Injectable implants for the sustained release of protein and peptide drugs. Drug Discov Today 18(7–8):337–349

Ahsan F, Arnold J, Meezan E, Pillion DJ (2001) Enhanced bioavailability of calcitonin formulated with alkylglycosides following nasal and ocular administration in rats. Pharm Res 18:1742–1746

Anselmo A, Gokarn Y, Mitragotri S (2018) Non-invasive delivery strategies for biologics. Nat Rev Drug Discov 18(1):19–40. https://doi.org/10.1038/nrd.2018.183

Bakary R, Enany E, Karkoura A, Abumandour M, Gafaar S (2019) Histological characterizations of the nasal conchae of the dog Canis Iupus. Alex J Vet Sci 60(2):42. https://doi.org/10.5455/ajvs.23184

Boumrah Y, Humbert L, Phanithavong M, Khimeche K, Dahmani A, Allorge D (2015) In vitro characterization of potential CYP- and UGT-derived metabolites of the psychoactive drug 25B-NBOMe using LC-high resolution MS. Drug Test Anal 8(2):248–256. https://doi.org/10.1002/dta.1865

Bourganis V, Kammona O, Alexopoulos A, Kiparissides C (2018) Recent advances in carrier mediated nose-to brain delivery of pharmaceutics. Eur J Pharm Biopharm (128):1–74

Chen G, Roy I, Yang C, Prasad P (2016) Nanochemistry and nanomedicine for nanoparticle-based diagnostics and therapy. Chem Rev 116(5):2826–2885. https://doi.org/10.1021/acs.chemrev.5b00148

Cookson M (2017) Parkinson's disease. In: Disease-modifying targets in neurodegenerative disorders. Elsevier, Amsterdam, pp 157–174. https://doi.org/10.1016/b978-0-12-805120-7.00007-5

Dillon C, Hughes H, O'Reilly N, Allender C, Barrow D, McLoughlin P (2019) Dissolving microneedle based transdermal delivery of therapeutic peptide analogues. Int J Pharm 565:9–19. https://doi.org/10.1016/j.ijpharm.2019.04.075

Firat A, Onerci-Celebi O, Tuncel A, Ergun M, Hayran M (2018) Microscopic study of human nasal cavity microanatomy using semi-thin resin embedding and methylene blue staining. J Histotechnol 42(1):13–18. https://doi.org/10.1080/01478885.2018.1550848

Gallagher H, Gallagher R, Butler M, Buggy D, Henman M (2015) Venlafaxine for neuropathic pain in adults. Cochrane Database Syst Rev. https://doi.org/10.1002/14651858.cd011091.pub2

Gao X, Wu B, Zhang Q, Chen J, Zhu J, Zhang W, Rong Z, Chen H, Jiang X (2007) Brain delivery of vasoactive intestinal peptide enhanced with the nanoparticles conjugated with wheat germ agglutinin following intranasal administration. J Control Release 121:156–167

Gaudreault R, Mousseau N (2019) Mitigating Alzheimer's disease with natural polyphenols: a review. Curr Alzheimer Res 16(6):529–543. https://doi.org/10.2174/1567205016666190315093520

Godfrey L, Iannitelli A, Garrett N, Moger J, Imbert I, King T, Porreca F, Soundararajan R, Lalatsa A, Schätzlein A, Uchegbu I (2017) Nanoparticulate peptide delivery exclusively to the brain produces tolerance free, analgesia. J Control Release 270:135. https://doi.org/10.1016/j.jconrel.2017.11.041

Guada M, Beloqui A, Alhouayek M, Muccioli G, Dios-Viéitez M, Préat V, Blanco-Prieto M (2016) Cyclosporine A-loaded lipid nanoparticles in inflammatory bowel disease. Int J Pharm 503(1–2):196–198. https://doi.org/10.1016/j.ijpharm.2016.03.012

Hanson L, Frey W (2008) Intranasal delivery bypasses the blood-brain barrier to target therapeutic agents to the central nervous system and treat neurodegenerative disease, BMC Neurosci, 9(3):S5. Available: https://doi.org/10.1186/1471-2202-9-s3-s5

Haque S, Md S, Sahni JK, Ali J, Baboota S (2014) Development and evaluation of brain targeted intranasal alginate nanoparticles for treatment of depression. J Psychiatr Res 48:1–12

Hu Q, van Gaal E, Brundel P, Ippel H, Hackeng T, Rijcken C et al (2015) A novel approach for the intravenous delivery of leuprolide using core-cross-linked polymeric micelles. J Control Release 205:98–108. https://doi.org/10.1016/j.jconrel.2014.12.023

Illum L (2004) Is nose-to-brain transport of drugs in man a reality? J Pharm Pharmacol 56:3–17

Iqbal J, Shahnaz G, Perera G, Hintzen F, Sarti F, Bernkop-Schnürch A (2012) Thiolated chitosan: development and in vivo evaluation of an oral delivery system for leuprolide. Eur J Pharm Biopharm 80(1):95–102. https://doi.org/10.1016/j.ejpb.2011.09.010

Kaur S, Manhas P, Swami A, Bhandari R, Sharma KK, Jain R, Kumar R, Pandey SK, Kuhad A, Sharma RK, Wangoo N (2018) Bioengineered PLGA-chitosan nanoparticles for brain targeted intranasal delivery of antiepileptic TRH analogues. Chem Eng J 346:630. https://doi.org/10.1016/j.cej.2018.03.176

Knappe D, Schmidt R, Adermann K, Hoffmann R (2019) Continuous subcutaneous delivery of proline-rich antimicrobial peptide Api137 provides superior efficacy to intravenous administration in a mouse infection model. Front Microbiol 10:2283. https://doi.org/10.3389/fmicb.2019.02283

Kubek M, Domb A, Veronesi M (2009) Attenuation of kindled seizures by intranasal delivery of neuropeptide-loaded nanoparticles. Neurotherapeutics 6(2):359–371

Kumar M, Pandey R, Patra K, Jain S, Soni M, Dangi J, Madan J (2013) Evaluation of neuropeptide loaded trimethyl chitosan nanoparticles for nose to brain delivery. Int J Biol Macromol 61:189–119

Kushwaha KS, Keshari RV, Rai AK (2011) Advances in nasal trans-mucosal drug delivery. J Appl Pharm Sci 07:21–28

Ladel S, Flamm J, Zadeh A, Filzwieser D, Walter J, Schlossbauer P et al (2018) Allogenic Fc domain-facilitated uptake of IgG in nasal lamina propria: friend or foe for intranasal CNS delivery? Pharmaceutics 10(3):107. https://doi.org/10.3390/pharmaceutics10030107

Lau JL, Dunn MK (2018) Therapeutic peptides: historical perspectives, current development trends, and future directions. Bioorg Med Chem 26:2700–2707

Legrand D (2016) Overview of lactoferrin as a natural immune modulator. J Pediatr 173:S10–S15. https://doi.org/10.1016/j.jpeds.2016.02.071

Liu Z, Jiang M, Kang T, Miao D, Gu G, Song Q, Yao L, Hu Q, Tu Y, Pang Z, Chen H, Jiang X, Gao X, Chen J (2013) Lactoferrin-modified PEG-co-PCL nanoparticles for enhanced brain delivery of NAP peptide following intranasal administration. Biomaterials 34:3870–3881

Mansoor F, Earley B, Cassidy J, Markey B, Foster C, Doherty S, Welsh M (2014) Intranasal delivery of nanoparticles encapsulating BPI3V proteins induces an early humoral immune response in mice. Res Vet Sci 96:551–557

Md S, Mustafa G, Baboota S, Ali J (2015) Nanoneurotherapeutics approach intended for direct nose to brain delivery. Drug Dev Ind Pharm 41(12):1922–1934. https://doi.org/10.3109/03639045.2015.1052081

Michael Danielsen E, Hansen G (2016) Small molecule pinocytosis and clathrin-dependent endocytosis at the intestinal brush border: two separate pathways into the enterocyte. Biochim Biophys Acta Biomembr 1858(2):233–243. https://doi.org/10.1016/j.bbamem.2015.11.022

Nevagi RJ, Khalil ZG, Hussein WM, Powell J, Batzloff MR, Capon RJ, Good MF, Skwarczynski M, Toth I, (2018) Polyglutamic acid-trimethyl chitosan-based intranasal peptide nano-vaccine induces potent immune responses against group A streptococcus. Acta Biomaterialia 80:278–287

Nian D, Shi P, Sun J, Ren L, Hao X, Han J (2019) Application of luteinizing hormone-releasing hormone–ferrosoferric oxide nanoparticles in targeted imaging of breast tumors. J Int Med Res 47(4):1749–1757. https://doi.org/10.1177/0300060519834457

Okada Y, Sumioka T, Ichikawa K, Sano H, Nambu A, Kobayashi K et al (2018) Sensory nerve supports epithelial stem cell function in healing of corneal epithelium in mice: the role of trigeminal nerve transient receptor potential vanilloid 4. Lab Invest 99(2):210–230. https://doi.org/10.1038/s41374-018-0118-4

Oppong-Damoah A, Zaman R, D'Souza M, Murnane K (2019) Nanoparticle encapsulation increases the brain penetrance and duration of action of intranasal oxytocin. Horm Behav 108:20–29

Phukan K, Nandy M, Sharma R, Sharma H (2016) Nanosized drug delivery systems for direct nose to brain targeting: a review. Recent Pat Drug Deliv Formul 10:156–164

Rahbarian M, Mortazavian E, Dorkoosh F, Rafiee Tehrani M (2018) Preparation, evaluation and optimization of nanoparticles composed of thiolated triethyl chitosan: a potential approach for buccal delivery of insulin. J Drug Delivery Sci Technol 44:254–263. https://doi.org/10.1016/j.jddst.2017.12.016

Raza A, Sime F, Cabot P, Maqbool F, Roberts J, Falconer J (2019) Solid nanoparticles for oral antimicrobial drug delivery: a review. Drug Discov Today 24(3):858–866. https://doi.org/10.1016/j.drudis.2019.01.004

Schirmer L, Velmeshev D, Holmqvist S, Kaufmann M, Werneburg S, Jung D et al (2019) Neuronal vulnerability and multilineage diversity in multiple sclerosis. Nature 573(7772):75–82. https://doi.org/10.1038/s41586-019-1404-z

Shah D, Shao J (2017) Nasal delivery of proteins and peptides. Glob J Pharm Pharm Sci 1(4). ISSN:2573–2250. https://doi.org/10.19080/GJPPS.2017.01.555569

Shahnaz G, Vetter A, Barthelmes J, Rahmat D, Laffleur F, Iqbal J, Perera G, Schlocker W, Dunnhaput S, Augustijns P, Bernkop-Schnurch A (2012) Thiolated chitosan nanoparticles for the nasal administration of leuprolide: bioavailability and pharmacokinetic characterization. Int J Pharm 428:164–170

Sharma S, Lohan S, Murthy RSR (2013) Formulation and characterization of intranasal mucoadhesive nanoparticulates and thermo-reversible gel of levodopa for brain delivery. Drug Dev Ind Pharm, Early Online: 1–10

Sonvico F, Clementino A, Buttini F, Colombo G, Pescina S, Guterres S, Pohlmann A, Nicoli S (2018) Surface-modified nanocarriers for nose-to-brain delivery: from bioadhesion to targeting. Pharmaceutics 10(1):1–34

Tuvia S, Atsmon J, Teichman SL, Katz S, Salama P, Pelled D, Landau I, Karmeli I, Bidlingmaier M, Strasburger CJ, Kleinberg DL, Melmed S, Mamluk R (2012) Oral octreotide absorption in human subjects: comparable pharmacokinetics to parenteral octreotide and effective growth hormone suppression. J Clin Endocrinol Metab 97(7):2362–2369. https://doi.org/10.1210/jc.2012-1179

Wadell C (2002) In-vitro studies on factors influencing permeability and implications on absorption. Faculty Pharm 278:55

Wen Z, Yan Z, Hu K, Pang Z, Cheng X, Guo L, Zhang Q, Jiang X, Fang L, Lai R (2011) Odorranalectin-conjugated nanoparticles: preparation, brain delivery and pharmacodynamic study on Parkinson's disease following intranasal administration. J Control Release 151:131–138

Whitsett J (2018) Airway epithelial differentiation and mucociliary clearance. Ann Am Thorac Soc 15(Supplement_3):S143–S148. https://doi.org/10.1513/annalsats.201802-128aw

Yadav S, Gattacceca F, Panicucci R, Amiji M (2015) Comparative biodistribution and pharmacokinetic analysis of cyclosporine-A in the brain upon intranasal or intravenous administration in an oil-in-water nanoemulsion formulation. Mol Pharm 12(5):1523–1533. Available: https://doi.org/10.1021/mp5008376

Yates J, Alexandersen P, Krogsaa A, Nedergaard B, Clarkin M, Hattersley G et al (2014) A transdermal patch delivering the PTHrP1-34 analog, abaloparatide (BA058), dose-dependently increases spine and hip bmd compared to placebo. Bone Abstr. https://doi.org/10.1530/boneabs.3.pp351

Zhao YZ, Li X, Lu CT, Lin MN, Chen LJ, Xiang Q, Zhang M, Jon RR, Jiang X, Shen XT, Li XK, Cai J (2013) Gelatin nanostructured lipid carriers-mediated intranasal delivery of basic fibroblast growth factor enhances recovery in hemiparkinsonian rats. Nanomedicine 10:755–764

Emerging Nanotechnology in Chronic Respiratory Diseases

20

Parijat Pandey, Meenu Mehta, Shakti Shukla, Ridhima Wadhwa, Gautam Singhvi, Dinesh Kumar Chellappan, Saurabh Satija, Gaurav Gupta, Rajendra Awasthi, Parteek Prasher, Philip M. Hansbro, Kamal Dua, and Harish Dureja

Abstract

A large population, including people of all age groups, is suffering from chronic respiratory diseases worldwide. Asthma, chronic obstructive pulmonary disease, occupational lung diseases, cystic fibrosis, etc. are the most common of these diseases and are noncurable with conventional and currently available therapies. Nanotechnology is emerging as a great therapeutic promise in different spheres including drug delivery systems and is becoming the technology of choice nowadays. The administration of drugs via inhalation helps in avoiding the first-pass metabolism by targeted delivery to the affected site. It has been observed that there is a huge diversity in nanotechnology being used in pulmonary diseases, and thus safety assessment is a challenging as well as important task. The present review focuses on some of the major emerging nanotechnologies for chronic pulmonary diseases and includes some of the latest studies in the field of nanomedicines.

Authors Parijat Pandey and Meenu Mehta Sharing First Authorship in Equal Contributuion

P. Pandey
Shri Baba Mastnath Institute of Pharmaceutical Sciences and Research, Baba Mastnath University, Rohtak, India

M. Mehta
Centenary Institute, Royal Prince Alfred Hospital, Camperdown, NSW, Australia

Discipline of Pharmacy, Graduate School of Health, University of Technology Sydney, Ultimo, NSW, Australia

S. Shukla
Priority Research Centre for Healthy Lungs, Hunter Medical Research Institute (HMRI) & School of Biomedical Sciences and Pharmacy, University of Newcastle, Callaghan, NSW, Australia

R. Wadhwa
Faculty of Life Sciences and Biotechnology, South Asian University, Akbar Bhawan, Chanakyapuri, New Delhi, India

Centenary Institute, Royal Prince Alfred Hospital, Camperdown, NSW, Australia

Discipline of Pharmacy, Graduate School of Health, University of Technology Sydney, Ultimo, NSW, Australia

G. Singhvi
Department of Pharmacy, Birla Institute of Technology and Science (BITS), Pilani, India

D. K. Chellappan
Department of Life Sciences, School of Pharmacy, International Medical University, Bukit Jalil, Kuala Lumpur, Malaysia

S. Talegaonkar, M. Rai (eds.), *Nanoformulations in Human Health*, https://doi.org/10.1007/978-3-030-41858-8_20

Keywords

Chronic respiratory disease · Asthma · Nanotechnology · Liposomes · Dendrimers

20.1 Chronic Respiratory Diseases

Chronic respiratory diseases (CRDs) affect millions of individuals globally and are considered as the most common inflammatory diseases. The World Health Organization (WHO) estimates that approximately 328 million people live with chronic obstructive pulmonary disease (COPD) and approximately three million individuals die each year due to COPD. COPD is currently the third leading cause of mortality worldwide (Cruz 2007). In addition, the WHO also estimates the prevalence of asthma globally, which stands at around 235 million. Moreover, asthma is also the most common respiratory disease in children, and around 250,000 asthmatics die due to the disease (Asher and Pearce 2014). These two most common CRDs significantly affect the quality of life of the patients, notably reductions in physical activity, difficulties in breathing, and increased mucus production and cough (Celli and Mac Nee 2004). CRDs also exert enormous economic and social burden on patients and their families, as well as the healthcare system in terms of treatment cost and hospitalizations. Moreover, the cost attributed to disability-adjusted life years and loss of productivity also runs in billions (Guarascio et al. 2013).

COPD is characterized by progressive airflow limitation with poor reversibility, which is primarily related to inflammation of the lungs in response to noxious particles and gases (TO 2018). The precise definition of COPD has been proposed by The Global Burden of Obstructive Lung Disease (GOLD) as "COPD is a common, preventable and treatable disease that is characterized by persistent respiratory symptoms and airflow limitation that is due to airway and/or alveolar abnormalities, usually caused by significant exposure to noxious particles or gases" (Gold: https://goldcoped.org/). The major symptoms associated with COPD include chronic cough, increased mucus production/secretion, and progressive dyspnea (breathlessness). COPD is often defined as a complex and heterogeneous lung condition that includes a number of pathological manifestations, mainly chronic bronchi-

S. Satija
School of Pharmaceutical Sciences, Lovely Professional University, Phagwara, Punjab, India

Discipline of Pharmacy, Graduate School of Health, University of Technology Sydney, Ultimo, NSW, Australia

G. Gupta
School of Pharmacy, Suresh Gyan Vihar University, Jaipur, India

R. Awasthi
Amity Institute of Pharmacy, Amity University, Noida, Uttar Pradesh, India

P. Prasher
Department of Chemistry, University of Petroleum and Energy Studies, Dehradun, India

P. M. Hansbro
School of Life Sciences, University of Technology Sydney, Sydney, NSW, Australia

Centenary Institute, Royal Prince Alfred Hospital, Camperdown, NSW, Australia

Priority Research Centre for Healthy Lungs, Hunter Medical Research Institute (HMRI) & School of Biomedical Sciences and Pharmacy, University of Newcastle, Callaghan, NSW, Australia

K. Dua
Centenary Institute, Royal Prince Alfred Hospital, Camperdown, NSW, Australia

Priority Research Centre for Healthy Lungs, Hunter Medical Research Institute (HMRI) & School of Biomedical Sciences and Pharmacy, University of Newcastle, Callaghan, NSW, Australia

Discipline of Pharmacy, Graduate School of Health, University of Technology Sydney, Ultimo, NSW, Australia

School of Pharmaceutical Sciences, Shoolini University, Bajhol, Sultanpur, Solan, Himachal Pradesh, India

H. Dureja (✉)
Department of Pharmaceutical Sciences, Maharshi Dayanand University, Rohtak, India

tis, and emphysema (enlarged airspaces and loss of lung elasticity). These pathological aspects vary to a greater extent between different COPD patients. Thus, the treatments need to be optimized based upon the clinical presentation of COPD patients, as well as the risk factors that are primarily implicated in the development of the disease. Cigarette smoke is the most important risk factor for COPD, which is a global trend, whereas air pollution and occupational exposure to chemical dust and fumes also contribute significantly to the development and progression of the disease in low- and middle-income countries (Barnes 2003; Kc et al. 2018). Most importantly, COPD patients often exhibit frequent episodes of increased symptoms that may require changes in medication and hospitalizations. These episodic worsening of disease is termed as acute exacerbations of COPD (AECOPD), which are the most important predictors of mortality and morbidity in COPD patients. AECOPD could be caused by bacterial or viral infections or noninfectious causes (air pollution, allergens, etc.) (Sapey and Stockley 2006).

Asthma is considered as a chronic disease that primarily affects the proximal airways. Asthma is characterized by periodic symptoms, variable airflow obstruction, and chronic inflammation of airways and lung tissues, e.g., airway smooth muscles (Bateman et al. 2008). Of particular interest is airway inflammation that results in a variety of asthma-specific pathological conditions. Also, asthma patients have been categorized into different clinical subtypes which are based up on the predominance of the type of inflammatory cells in the pulmonary samples, such as sputum and bronchial biopsies (Wenzel et al. 1999; Simpson et al. 2006). Utilizing inflammatory cells for categorizing asthmatics, the patients are classified into four inflammatory subtypes, i.e., neutrophilic, eosinophilic, mixed granulocytic, and paucigranulocytic (Simpson et al. 2006). Moreover, adaptive immune response in asthma is further categorized as type I or type II responses. Type I immune response constitutes delayed hypersensitivity and increased production of interleukin (IL)-2 and interferon (IFN)-γ. On the other hand, type II responses are mediated by B-cell leading to humoral immunity and increased production of IL-4, IL-5, IL-9, and IL-13 (Mosmann and Coffman 1989).

Current therapies focus on reducing the symptoms of these CRDs. Targeting the inflammatory and pathological mechanisms involved in asthma and COPD will potentially reduce the burden of these chronic diseases (Dua et al. 2019). However, another major challenge remains when considering the optimal delivery of therapeutic compounds in the complex structures of the lung. For example, lung defense mechanism involves resistance and removal of any inhaled foreign particle by various physicochemical mechanisms, such as mucociliary clearances (Newman 2017). In addition, the poor delivery of these therapeutic compounds is further increased by the poor adherence to medications and/or inappropriate inhaler device techniques followed by patients with CRDs (Hickey 2014). Hence, more innovative and effective routes of drug delivery are urgently required to treat these CRDs. There are several benefits of using the inhalation route of drug delivery. The major comparison of inhalation route of drug delivery with other major routes is represented in Fig. 20.1.

20.2 Pathophysiology of COPD and Asthma

The major aspect of pathophysiology of COPD includes the progressive, nonreversible airflow limitation, which is largely attributed to both small airway disease (SAD) and emphysema. Both SAD and emphysema in COPD patients may commence at different stages of the disease history, as well as may greatly vary in terms of severity and its contribution to overall airflow limitation. Recent reports also highlighted that ~50% of small airways are effectively obliterated even before any observable clinical symptoms may appear (Koo et al. 2018). This is simultaneously accompanied by more detectable symptoms of increased mucus production in the large airways, which later manifests as chronic cough. Emphysema is a condition characterized by irreversible enlargement of lung air sacs, along with

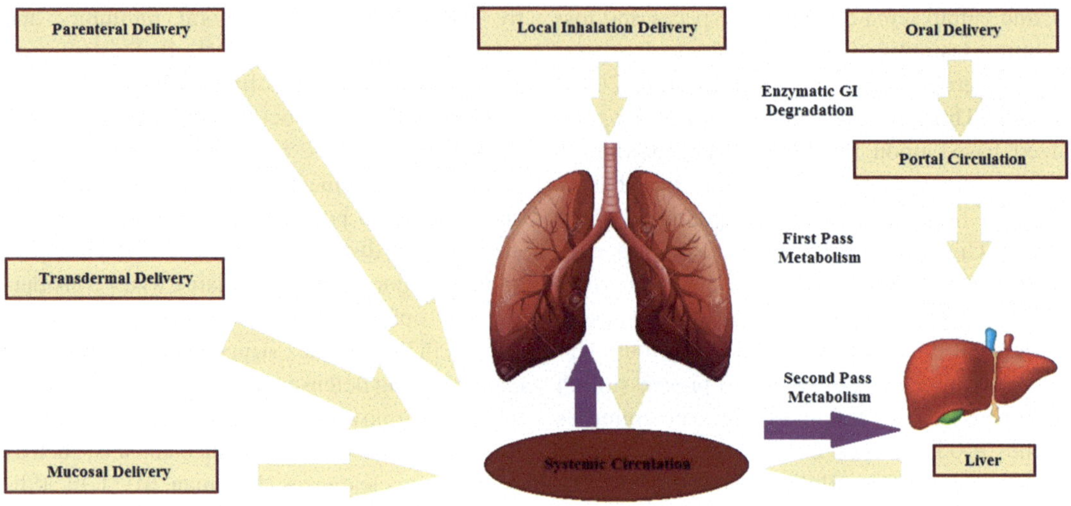

Fig. 20.1 Inhalation route of drug delivery

the destruction of alveolar sans fibrosis. Also, destruction of parenchymal tissues is also observed (Pahal and Sharma 2019). Collectively, these pathophysiological processes result in significantly decreased lung function and increased risk of frequent bacterial/viral infections, which is termed as acute exacerbations (AE) (Agustí and Celli 2017). Small airway narrowing is also attributed to an increase in lymphoid follicle formation, as well as collagen deposition around the airways.

Asthma is another important chronic inflammatory disease that is characterized by the hyperresponsiveness of the airways resulting in repeated wheezing, breathlessness, tightness of chest, and cough. Chronic inflammation is a major feature of asthma, which involves infiltration of immune cells (neutrophils, eosinophils, lymphocytes, mast cells, etc.) that then lead to hallmark structural changes in asthma including hypertrophy of the smooth muscle layer, subbasement fibrosis, destruction of elastic fiber, hyperplasia of goblet cells and glandular submucosa, edema, and desquamation of epithelium in airways (National asthma: https://www.ncbi.nlm.nih.gov/books/NBK7223/). Again, asthma is a heterogeneous disease, and the concept of personalized medicine should be the way forward for both prevention and treatment (Pavord et al. 2018).

20.3 Drug Delivery in Respiratory Diseases

In recent times, inhalation therapy has been an important route for targeting respiratory diseases via reduction in localized symptoms including airway inflammation and constriction. Several inhalation devices have been used such as nebulizers, dry powder inhalers (DPI), pressurized metered dose inhalers (pMDI), and soft mist inhalers that can lower the dose with therapeutic equivalence and reduce the systematic side effects associated with oral or intravenous delivery (Winkler et al. 2004). Drug deposition via inhalation is determined by particle size, aerosol velocity, and inspiratory flow. Drugs given via the inhalation route include corticosteroids, beta-sympathomimetics, muscarinic antagonists, and antibiotics (Dozor 2010) and are commonly prescribed in asthma and chronic obstructive pulmonary disease (COPD). Inhaled corticosteroids have an anti-inflammatory effect and are effective against asthma, but their role is conflicted in COPD. Glucocorticosteroids have been the major therapy for asthma, while PDE4 inhibitors, NFκB inhibitors, MAPK p38 inhibitors, ß2-agonists, and corticosteroids have been important therapeutics for COPD (Barnes 2011). However, they did not reduce the disease progression and inflammation which manifests the need for potential therapeutics to reduce the pathology of the disease.

Inhalation therapy is advantageous as there is increased bioavailability of the drug since lungs have restricted intracellular and extracellular drug metabolizing enzymes (Loira-Pastoriza et al. 2014). It also reduces nonreversible tissue damage caused by cytotoxicity of drugs. There is a reduction in dose, high absorption leading to rapid action (Loira-Pastoriza et al. 2014; Ruge et al. 2013).

The bio-barriers such as mucus, macrophages, and ciliated cells limit the drug localization, penetration, and absorption. For effective drug delivery to lungs, drugs should be localized to the target site, should be able to penetrate through mucus, and escape the bio-barriers (Dua et al. 2019; Hamman et al. 2005). It is an important need to identify new therapies against different respiratory diseases including COPD, asthma, lung cancer, and pulmonary infections (Hamman et al. 2005). Some of the important instances highlighting the novel drug delivery systems are as follows.

Chennakesavulu et al. worked on the delivery of liposome encapsulating budesonide and colchicine against idiopathic pulmonary fibrosis. In vivo studies on adult male Wistar rats showed reduced systemic absorption when inhalation route was used, and these liposomal dry powders were stable for 6 months (Chennakesavulu et al. 2018). Further, a successful synthesis and delivery through DPI has been reported for saturated egg phosphatidylcholine (EPC) and cholesterol liposome encapsulated with ketotifen fumarate, an antiasthmatic drug in COPD/asthma (Joshi and Misra 2001). Polymeric micelles of polyethylene glycol (PEG) and 1,2-distearoyl-sn-glycero-3-phosphoethanolamine (DSPE) encapsulating budesonide fabricated via co-precipitation method delivered to COPD rat model have been found to have better dissolution compared to budesonide. Furthermore, it has shown a decrease in inflammatory cells in bronchoalveolar lavage fluid (BALF) (Sahib et al. 2011). Researchers have assessed BSA nanoparticles encapsulated with DOX for the regeneration of the extracellular matrix (ECM) for emphysema. In vivo studies showed a significant decrease in MMPs in lungs for up to 4 weeks in rat model. Therefore, elastic tissue regeneration could be significant for the unmet need for COPD treatment (Parasaram et al. 2016).

The drawbacks associated with generating inhalable drugs, namely, formulation and deposition difficulties, can mostly be overcome by using nanoparticles. Since nearly all the drugs can be encapsulated but nanoparticles can additionally be modified on the surface to enhance bioavailability or to help penetrate the mucus layer (van Rijt et al. 2014), although, due to the relatively small size, nanoparticles can easily penetrate into the systemic circulation and sometimes open a door for adverse side effects (Kuzmov and Minko 2015).

20.4 Role of Nanoformulations in Respiratory Disease

There is a need for confined and prolonged drug release in the lungs, which is more anticipated in targeting. The lipid-based formulations in nanocarriers, solid lipid nanocarriers (SLNs) and nanostructured lipid nanocarriers, (NLCs) became an attractive strategy for delivery of poorly soluble drugs (Kuzmov and Minko 2015). The structure of some of these nanoformulations is shown in the Fig. 20.2.

SLNs are aqueous dispersions prepared using solid lipids consisting of triglycerides and phospholipids. As the composition for the preparation of SLNs includes physiologically compatible lipids, these preparations are less toxic and highly adequate for delivery of therapeutics by the respiratory route. The components used in SLN help in conserving the optimal surface tension at the alveolar surface and reduction of friction at lung tissue. Due to the low toxicity and utilization of physiologically compatible lipids, SLN-based formulations have endured as the prevailing drug delivery system (Paranjpe and Müller-Goymann 2014; Beloqui et al. 2016; Dua et al. 2019).

SLN-based formulations hold numerous benefits such as avoidance of organic solvents in the process of preparation and high drug loading,

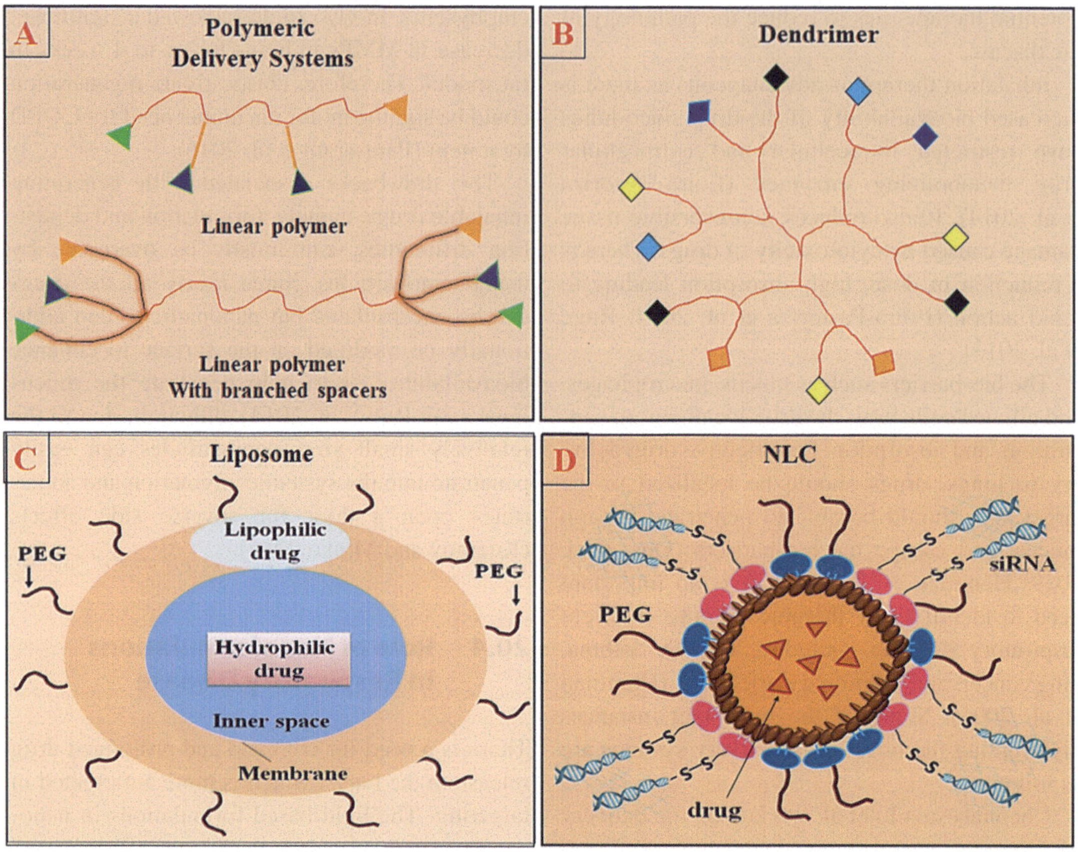

Fig. 20.2 Structure of some of the nanoformulations used in the treatment of respiratory diseases. (Adapted from Kuzmov and Minko 2015)

improve the drug stability with minimum interaction with the external environment, and provide controlled release of the drug and drug targeting. SLN-based formulations exhibit certain drawbacks such as aggregation on storage, gelation propensity, polymorphic transitions of lipids, and low amalgamation of the drug due to the formation of the perfect crystalline lattice of lipid. Some efforts were made to overcome these issues with the newer generation of lipidic nanocarriers including nanostructured lipid nanocarriers, lyotropic liquid crystalline nanoparticles, and lipidic nanospheres (Girdhar et al. 2018; Singhvi et al. 2018).

Nanostructured lipid carriers are among the second-generation lipid nanocarriers developed with a combination of liquid lipids and solid lipids. The liquid lipid is enclosed into a solid lipid matrix which prevents coalescence and strongly immobilizes the drug. In NLCs, the liquid oil is blended with solid lipid to impart the imperfections in crystal order of solids. The additional liquid lipid increases the entrapment efficiency and decreases the drug leaching on storage (Khosa et al. 2018).

SLNs and NLCs have been explored for respiratory diseases. These lipidic nanocarriers provide drug targeting and prolonged release (Dua et al. 2018). Islan et al. reported encapsulation of levofloxacin-based SLN- and NLC-based formulations for the treatment of recurrent infection caused by *Pseudomonas aeruginosa*, particularly in cystic fibrosis. SLNs were prepared using myristyl myristate (Crodamol™ MM), Pluronic F68 using ultrasonication method. Crodamol™ GTCC-LQ oil was added to 3% weight of lipid in case of NLC formulation. SLN-based formulation showed entrapment efficiency of

20.1 ± 1.4%, whereas 55.9 ± 1.6% was observed in NLC-based formulation. The report reveals controlled drug release in case of NLC-based formulation in comparison to SLN-based formulation. DNase enzyme was amalgamated into NLC-based formulation, to improve the antibiotic diffusion by decreasing the viscoelasticity of mucus which was observed in the lungs of cystic fibrosis condition. The results demonstrated that formulation showed resilient antibacterial activity against gram-negative bacteria *Pseudomonas aeruginosa* and gram-positive bacteria *Staphylococcus aureus*. In vitro antimicrobial assay of levofloxacin-loaded NLCs showed complete destruction of the biofilm of *Pseudomonas aeruginosa* which is the most pertinent pathogen in cystic fibrosis (Islan Germán et al. 2016).

Rosiere and his colleagues developed paclitaxel loaded SLNs. The SLN surface was modified when coating with a folate grafted copolymer of polyethylene glycol and chitosan (F-PEG-HTCC). The prepared formulation showed 99.0 ± 0.3% encapsulation efficiency with 4.6 ± 0.1% drug loading, and particle size was found to be 249 ± 36 nm (0.31 particle size distribution). The in vitro studies were performed in M109-HiFR cells, and results showed a decreased inhibitory concentration (60 nanomolar) with paclitaxel-loaded in F-PEG-HTCC-coated SLNs compared to free taxol (340 nanomolar). The in vivo studies revealed an increase in localization of paclitaxel in tumor tissue and minimal systemic absorption by pulmonary delivery in case of F-PEG-HTCC-coated SLNs. The F-PEG-HTCC-coated SLNs were distributed throughout the lung tumor after pulmonary delivery regardless of blood vessels. The F-PEG-HTCC-coated SLNs exhibited high antiproliferative activity compared to PEG-HTCC-coated SLNs. It was expected due to increased uptake of F-PEG-HTCC-coated SLN by multiple pathways. It is concluded from the study that the folate receptor was found to exhibit an important role in drug targeting with the antiproliferative activity (Rosière et al. 2018).

In an investigation, phosphodiesterase type 5 inhibitor, sildenafil citrate, was loaded in SLN-based formulation for the treatment of pulmonary hypertension. SLN-based formulation was developed for pulmonary delivery of sildenafil citrate to overcome high first-pass metabolism, low oral bioavailability (40%), and short half-life (3–5 hours). The developed lipid-based formulation was investigated for their potential to retain their properties after nebulization and autoclaving. The prepared formulation exhibited encapsulation efficiency in the range of 88–100% with sustained release of the payload for over 24 hours. The results showed no alteration in SLN properties after nebulization with a jet nebulizer and autoclaving for 20 minutes at 120 °C. The SLN-based dispersion was evaluated for interaction with mucin, which was determined by turbidimetrically. Results showed an increased size and zeta potential which indicated the adherence of mucin on the surface of SLNs (Makled et al. 2017).

In a study, methyl α-d-mannopyranoside surface modified SLN formulation of rifampicin showed improved targeting toward macrophages. Mannose was used for surface modification to increase internalization due to mannose receptors located on infected alveolar macrophages. Cytotoxicity and cell internalization were studied on J774 murine macrophage cell line. MTT (3-(4,5 di-methylthiazol-2-yl)-2,5-diphenyltetrazolium bromide) assay results demonstrated dose-dependent cytotoxicity, and the cell viability was reduced by <80% after 24 hours. Cell internalization study results exhibited quick uptake of mannosylated SLNs by macrophages. The cell internalization was observed under confocal microscopy with blue stained nuclei in J774 cell monolayer. The results detailed active targeting was achieved in case of SLNs coated with methyl α-d-mannopyranoside (Maretti et al. 2017).

Vieira and co-authors reported the improvement of tuberculosis management by mucoadhesive chitosan coated SLNs loaded with rifampicin. These chitosan coated SLNs were evaluated for mucoadhesive property and permeability in alveolar epithelial cells A549. Results showed significant permeation in the case of chitosan-coated SLNs compared to nonmucoadhesive SLNs (Vieira et al. 2018).

Sastre et al. developed tobramycin loaded NLCs for *Pseudomonas aeruginosa* infections associated with cystic fibrosis. Hot melt homogenization technique was utilized for the preparation of NLC. In vitro release studies showed a biphasic drug release profile characterized by an initial burst release followed by a sustained and progressive release of tobramycin. It is expected that initial high release can contribute to inhibiting the biofilm growth and later sustained release can provide prolonged lung exposures. Such a biphasic release pattern can reduce the number of dose and dosing intervals. The cell viability studies indicated that there was no decrease in viability after treatment with tobramycin NLC dispersion. There was no effect of the mucolytic agents on NLCs dispersion which was studied on an artificial mucus barrier. In vivo pulmonary administration of infrared dye-labeled lipid nanoparticles by Penn century® device showed an extensive distribution in the lungs for 48 hours (Moreno-Sastre et al. 2016).

SLN-based formulation was utilized for delivery of protein plasmid (pEGFP) and doxorubicin for lung cancer. A target-based approach was utilized for delivery of gene and drug, by modifying the surface of SLNs using transferrin ligands. The particle size of the optimized nanoformulation was 267 nm with a zeta potential of +42 mV. In vitro transfection efficiency of the developed formulation was estimated on adenocarcinoma cell line (A549 cells). Transferrin coated SLNs with doxorubicin and protein plasmid exhibited higher transfection efficiency compared to SLNs without transferrin coating and naked plasmid protein. In vivo antitumor efficiency was observed in mice bearing A549 tumor. The transferrin-coated SLNs with a combination of doxorubicin and plasmid (gene) demonstrated higher antitumor efficacy with a smaller tumor volume compared to noncoated SLNs (Han et al. 2014).

For concurrent delivery of anti-cancer drugs and siRNA specifically for lung cancer, NLC-based formulations were reported. The objective of co-delivery was to overcome multidrug resistance by siRNA and the drug was used to induce cell death. In order to resolve multidrug resistance, two siRNAs were evaluated, including siRNA targeting the responsible MRP1 mRNA drug efflux transporters and SiRNA targeting BCL2 mRNA, suppressing cellular anti-apoptotic defences. The prepared NLCs were compared with intravenous injection and inhalation. The inhalation therapy showed improved lung accumulation whereas intravenous injection led to accumulation in liver, lung, kidney, and spleen. The drug and siRNA were successfully administered in cancer cells with NLCs. Gene silencing and cell death were observed in lung tumor cells (Taratula et al. 2013).

Payne and his co-workers encapsulated all-trans retinoic acid in SLNs using emulsification–ultrasonication method. The developed formulation was evaluated on immunomodulatory A549 cells, which declined pro-inflammatory IL-6 and IL-8 levels indicating a promising approach for local immunomodulation in chronic obstructive pulmonary disease. The A459 cells were evaluated for human mesenchymal stem cells containing hydrogel formulation which resulted in an increase in IL-6 and IL-8 levels indicating pro-inflammatory effect. The combination of SLN based all-trans retinoic acid and human mesenchymal stem cells exhibited potential anti-inflammatory activity (Payne et al. 2019).

Various nanoformulations used in inhalation therapy of respiratory diseases are presented in Table 20.1.

20.5 Liposomes in Respiratory Diseases

Liposomes are colloid-based drug delivery systems composed of a lipid layer with an aqueous center. Therefore, they are suitable for encapsulating lipophilic and hydrophilic drugs and are suitable for pulmonary drug delivery via inhalation for localized drug delivery allowing prolonged action of drug with decreased toxicity (Chellappan et al. 2018; Ng et al. 2018). Such a delivery system improves the pharmacokinetics of drugs especially the poor water-soluble anti-cancer drugs such as paclitaxel (Kiparissides and

Table 20.1 Types of nanoformulations used as inhalation therapy for the treatment of respiratory diseases

S. No.	Type of nanoformulation	Composition of nanoformulation	Drug	Diseases	References
1.	Nanoparticles	Lactose	Salbutamol	Broncho-obstructive conditions	Bhavna et al. (2009)
		Gelatin	Rifampicin	Tuberculosis	Saraogi et al. (2010)
2.	Dendrimers	PEGylated poly-lysine	Doxorubicin	Cancer	Kaminskas et al. (2014)
3.	Fullerenes	Water-soluble C60 fullerenes	C60	Inhibition of allergic response	Iga et al. (2007)
4.	Polymer-drug conjugates	Poly(ethylene glycol)–poly (propylene oxide)–poly(ethylene glycol) triblock co-polymer	Meropenem derivatives	Pulmonary infection including those caused by *Pseudomonas aeruginosa*	Ong et al. (2014)
5.	Polymer-protein conjugate	Polyethyleneimine	mRNA	Diseases due to insufficient or defective production of proteins	Geiger et al. (2015)
6.	Silica nanoparticles	Silica	Radionuclides, fluorescent molecules, oligonucleotides, etc.	Imaging and treatment of various lung diseases	Bradbury et al. (2014)
7.	Quantum dots	Nanocrystals made to fluoresce when stimulated by light	–	Imaging of lung cancer	Iga et al. (2007)
8.	Liposomes	Dilauroylphosphatidylcholine	9-Nitro-20-camptothecin	Lung carcinoma	Verschraegen et al. (2004)
		Dipalmitoylphosphatidylcholine	Cisplatin	Osteosarcoma malignancies of lung	Chou et al. (2013)

Kammona 2008). However, liposomes are less stable and have a small shelf life so surface modification with ligands is being carried out. This leads to increased stability, shelf life, adhesion, and permeability. Different polymers used to improve adhesion and target specificity are polyethylene glycol (PEG), chitosan, Carbopol, hyaluronic acid, etc. (Dua et al. 2019; Mehta et al. 2019). Liposomes can be cationic for gene delivery and anionic for targeting alveolar macrophages. Several studies have shown that liposomes can be used as antimicrobial and antidiabetic agent in gene therapy. FDA has also approved liposomal drug delivery of Amikacin by Insmed for nebulization (Zylberberg and Matosevic 2016).

Frankenberger et al. investigated the role of liposomal methyl predniosolone (MP) in lipopolysaccharide-mediated pro-inflammatory tumor necrosis factor (TNF) and anti-inflammatory interleukin-10 (IL-10) in aleveolar macrophages (AM). This liposomal-mediated drug increased IL-10 production and reduced TNF after exposure to macrophages. It was concluded that liposomes can be used for localized delivery of glucocorticoids with less side effects (Frankenberger et al. 2005). Chono et al. demonstrated the uptake of mannosylated liposomes in comparison to nonmannosylated liposomes in rat alveolar macrophages post intratracheal administration (Chono et al. 2007). Further, Joshi and Misra observed the delivery of ketofin fumerate as a liposomal dry powder in rat lungs for stabilizing mast cells against asthma inflammatory response (Joshi and Misra 2003). Alvarez et al. reported liposomal entrapment of *Dermatophagoide spteronyssius* vaccine against asthma. It has been reported to prevent worsening of asthma by reducing the inflammatory response (Alvarez et al. 2002). Liposomal formulation of Cisplatin is in clinical trial phase I for successful drug targeting with prolonged exposure and minimal side effects (Wittgen et al. 2007). Pulmaquin™ is dual liposomal ciprofloxacin used in *Pseudomonas aeruginosa* infections with noncystic fibrosis bronchiectasis. It shows sustained drug release with minimal side effect (Serisier et al. 2013).

Khademi et al. reported the use of cationic liposomes as adjuvants, with enhanced potency for various tuberculosis subunit vaccines with an increased therapeutic effect by inducing memory to the immune system (Schmidt et al. 2016). Further, it has been reported that cationic liposomes combined with De-O-acylated lipooligosaccharides can improve the effectiveness as for targeting Th1 type immune cells in tuberculosis. Nkanga et al. studied crude soybean lecithin liposomes comprising isoniazid. These liposomes are effective in pulmonary delivery in treating tuberculosis (Nkanga et al. 2017).

20.6 Dendrimers and Micelles in Respiratory Diseases

In the advancement of formulation techniques, a new class of substance has become significantly useful, in overcoming several drug delivery issues in formulation development. These are called dendrimers. Being unique in their primary architecture, these compounds have typical molecular properties that help in the design and development of nanodrugs and nanoformulations. Lately, these substances have gained much attention, especially, in terms of research and development of newer and effective carrier systems (Dufès et al. 2005).

Dendrimers primarily have defined structures which are versatile in delivering drugs. These materials are rapidly emerging due to their high acceptability and robustness. They also have good functionality. There are two major mechanisms by which dendrimers exert their activity; firstly, by entrapping high molecular weight substances, and secondly, by conjugating. Most of the substances that are conjugated are hydrophilic and hydrophobic materials. The potentiality of dendrimers in entrapment is accomplished by a host to guest participation. Deliveries of a range of several entities are made possible with the employment of dendrimers, especially because of their unique structure (Madaan et al. 2014). Lately, more and more newer drug carriers are being designed with the help of dendrimers, which are turning to be promising therapeutic substances in several biomedical applications.

Dendrimers have unique and specific properties. Being profusely branched and organized uniquely, these three-dimensional molecules have considerably lower polydispersity ratio. *Dendron* means *tree*, which resembles the extremely branched structure of the dendrimers. Each new branch is termed as "generation." These are sometimes referred to as *layers* (Tomalia et al. 1985). Dendrimers are being extensively used in nanomedicine. The entire structure conforms to a cascading pattern, with an inner core moiety. The adjacent layers contain functional groups.

Therapeutic substances that have formulation drawbacks primarily in terms of their pharmacokinetic profiles or their pharmacodynamic profiles can improve such parameters with the help of dendrimers. In addition, formulations that incorporate low molecular weight substances in them can also be effectively formulated with dendrimers. Low molecular weight moieties are also known to have developed with the incorporation of such dendrimer polymers. Various biological fluids can also be analyzed and used in the diagnosis of markers, as dendrimers can be conjugated with several types of antibodies and image enhancement markers (Bai et al. 2006). Due to their applications, now these substances are being widely employed and used in the field of pharmaceutical sciences. In addition to the above, dendrimers can also be used as bioavailability enhancers and as agents that modify the release of the drug.

There are several types of dendrimers that are being tested and used in the delivery of nanosubstance and drugs. The most common ones are the polyamidoamine (PAMAM) types. These are followed by poly-propylene imine (PPI) and polyether hydroxylamine (PEHAM). Some other less common types are poly-esteramine (PEA), poly-L-lysine, melamine, and polyglycerol types. Most of these dendritic types are tested for their drug delivery properties (Wolinsky and Grinstaff 2008).

There are several advantages that are possessed by the dendrimers in terms of a typical drug carrier system. These substances have relatively higher water solubility (Duncan and Izzo 2005; Soto-Castro et al. 2012). In addition, they also possess biocompatibility and polyvalency. Moreover, they also have accurate molecular weights (Tomalia 2005; Patton et al. 2006).

There are several advantages and applications of dendrimers. Patri et al. reported the delivery of monoclonal antibodies by using prostate-specific membrane antigen (PSMA) (Patri et al. 2004; Wu et al. 2006). The results were significant in the delivery of the antibodies to prostate tumors. In a similar mechanism, several researchers have succeeded in delivering methotrexate to brain tumor tissues (Shukla et al. 2008). This showed that dendrimers can be used for drug delivery to tumors.

20.7 Dendrimers for Pulmonary Delivery

Dendrimers are also effective in delivering drugs to the lungs and the respiratory system. Shuhua Bai and colleagues have reported the use of dendrimers in the pulmonary delivery of enoxaparin, which eventually had resulted in the prevention of thrombotic events in blood vessels (Bai et al. 2007).

Calu-3, primary alveolar cell lines were studied for their successful intracellular uptake mechanisms using the PAMAM type of dendrimers. In addition, ex vivo studies were also performed using perfused rat lungs. Both the methods were successfully tested by the absence of aggregation with the fluid in the lungs (Morris et al. 2017). The results were promising in terms of target delivery to the lungs.

An in vitro model of the pulmonary epithelium was tested to study the effect of PEGylation when these were conjugated with PAMAM type of dendrimers. The findings showed that there was an increase in the PEG surface density when apical transport increased. This was also observed in in vivo models (Bharatwaj et al. 2015).

Enhancement in the bioavailability of several peptides and hormonal proteins like insulin, calcitonin, and other protein drugs was evaluated in rats. PAMAM types of dendrimers were employed in the study. Various layers or generations were used in addition during the study. The effects in the presence and in the absence of dendrimers were the focus of the study (Dong et al. 2011). The findings show that the dendrimers significantly enhanced the absorption in the lungs for the test substances. It was also observed that the effects were also dependent on the generations of the dendrimers.

20.8 Dendrimers in Respiratory Disorders

One of the most commonly used drugs for asthma is methylprednisolone. It is an important drug that belongs to the class of corticosteroid. The drug primarily reduces inflammation that is associated with asthma. A study was done to evaluate the enhancement in the airway delivery using the methylprednisolone-PAMAM dendrimer conjugate. The study was performed in an animal model of lung inflammation (Inapagolla et al. 2010). The results were determined based on the accumulation of eosinophils in the lungs. Ovalbumin was the allergen used in the experiment. The findings showed that the dendrimers produced a significantly higher positive effect in treating the exacerbations of lung inflammation.

In another study, PAMAM-type dendrimers were used to study the lung delivery of the drug beclomethasone. These dendrimers were tested as nanocarriers targeted toward lung delivery of this drug. In addition, several generations were also employed in the study. Beclomethasone is reported to have poor solubility (Nasr et al. 2014). The observations from the study revealed that dendrimers significantly increased the delivery of the drug to the lung mucosa.

Chronic inflammatory conditions like asthma and COPD is reported to be treated with the help of targeted drug or RNA delivery to the lung endothelium. Small interfering RNAs (siRNAs) were used in the study which were conjugated with dendrimers that were modified chemically. A specific substitution process was adopted where the free amines on the dendrimers were exchanged for alkyl chains (Khan et al. 2015). The most promising materials were used in the study to target the pulmonary endothelium. The findings were significant. In another study, it is reported that phosphorus-based dendrimers having, one of the compounds namely, pyrrolidinium or morpholinium were chosen for enhanced biocompatibility. A Dendrimer complex containing the former substance was reported to be having more significant complexation. The findings suggest that phosphorus-based dendrimers could play a major role in the pulmonary delivery of drugs and moieties (Adam et al. 2017).

Several studies have been reported for the delivery of drug material for cystic fibrosis. PAMAM-based dendrimers have been widely used for cystic fibrosis condition (Brockman et al. 2017). In another study, it was reported that PAMAM dendrimers decreased infection and enhanced improvement.

Several functionally different and potent drugs targeting cancer cells combined together in a delivery module have shown to be a potent way of targeting lung cancers. Nevertheless, a powerful and effective drug carrier is the primary requisite for this. Dendrimers can be used efficiently in this regard to conjugate anticancer drug moieties that can be delivered to the site of cancer cells. This combinatorial drug delivery is shown to be positive in several cancer therapies (Amreddy et al. 2018).

In another study, camptothecin was studied with conjugated dendrimers as delivery carriers. It is reported by Morgan and colleagues that camptothecin was successfully delivered to the cancer cells (Morgan et al. 2003). In addition, it is reported that melamine-based dendrimers were employed to solubilize methotrexate. This in addition also reduced the toxicity of the drug (Neerman et al. 2004).

20.9 Microparticles/Microspheres and Microemulsion in Respiratory Diseases

Chronic respiratory diseases, such as asthma, COPD, cystic fibrosis, silicosis, and pulmonary artery hypertension are the main source of morbidity and mortality around the world (Chellappan et al. 2017; Islam et al. 2017). This is principally a direct result of the maturing populace and expanding pervasiveness of cigarette smoking comprehensively. In this way, it is essential for an effective drug delivery system to convey the remedial moiety to the objective site at the correct time and in an appropriate amount especially with different chronic respiratory diseases, for example, asthma where a prompt therapeutic action is required (Kaur 2017; Jasinski et al. 2017; Madni et al. 2017). Most of the conventional dosage forms have different constraints, for example, portion dumping, nonfocused on impacts, and multiple administration of medication prompting lesser patient consistence, which lead to the development and trends of novel drug delivery systems where nanotechnology is one of the key role players. The field of nanotechnology is where a drug molecule is incorporated into the nanosystems that give pharmacotherapy a different dimension and focus on a cellular approach to drug transport which is much needed for the majority of chronic respiratory conditions (Taguchi et al. 2017; Yu et al. 2017).

Biological properties of nanotransporters like polymers, liposomes, and micelles can be changed and controlled as per the necessity in this manner making them profoundly proficient for pharmacological and therapeutic purposes (Mehta 2016; Momtazi-Borojeni et al. 2017). Improvement of nanocarriers has numerous points of interest, including productive conveyance and accumulation of medication in the affected area even with the physiological condition of compromised vascularization. Moreover, exploratory discoveries have demonstrated that nanotransporters display increasingly efficient tissue penetration thus bringing about expanded tissue explicit activity of medication contrasted with the regular drug administration routes (Abdelaziz et al. 2018; Cryer and Thorley 2019). Despite the fact that utilization of the nanotransporter system is heavily debated inside the respiratory research network, this system offers progressively proficient medication conveyance systems in pulmonary disorders. Accordingly, for characterizing novel drug delivery mechanisms in the time of modern medical science, nanoparticles offer an appealing idea for use in respiratory system (Abdelaziz et al. 2018; Mehta et al. 2018; Cryer and Thorley 2019; Li et al. 2019; Thakur et al. 2019). This is mainly due to the relatively standardised utilization of the drug within the alveolar surface marked with nanocarriers with enhanced dissolvability and delayed release. Such properties further reduce the recurrence of medication and enhance patient compliance with the least side effects (Hatamipour et al. 2018; Hema et al. 2018; Ihrie and Bonner 2018).

20.10 Miscellaneous: Mucoadhesive Drug Delivery

20.10.1 Mucoadhesive Nanoparticles

The purpose of developing mucoadhesive drug delivery systems is to prolong and intensify the contact between delivery carrier and the mucous apical pole, inducing active transport of macromolecular biopharmaceuticals across the biological barriers (Lehr 2000; Smola et al. 2008). Accumulation and retention of particles in the lungs due to the adhesion can lead to enhanced and sustained therapeutic effects and therefore decrease the dosing frequency. This may lead to better patient compliance in chronic lung disease conditions since many of the commercially available inhalation therapeutics need to be used at least twice a day (Weber et al. 2014). The adhesion of nanoparticles to the mucus membrane can be due to the nonspecific forces (van der Waals forces, hydrogen bonding, electrostatic or hydrophobic interactions). Cationic surface charge nanoparticles play an important role in increasing their retention in the mucus membrane (Savla and Minko 2013). A major limitation of mucoadhesive drug delivery systems is their nonspecific adhesion with respect to the substrate, undefined mucoadhesive time, and local side effects. In spite of these limitations, the modulation of epithelial permeability and inhibition of proteolytic enzymes can be achieved by mucoadhesive polymers.

Lectins are nonimmunological glycoproteins that have the capacity to recognize receptor-like structures of the cell membrane and bind to glycoproteins exposed at the epithelial cell surface (Lehr 2000; Smola et al. 2008). Respirable aerosol of a lectin-functionalized liposomal carrier has been reported by Abu-Dahab et al. Cholesterol enhanced the stability of the liposomes during nebulization and upon incubation with pulmonary surfactant preparation. The synthesized liposomes were able to bind to human alveolar cells (A549 and primary cells) (Abu-Dahab et al. 2001).

Amore et al. synthesized fluticasone propionate-loaded solid lipid microparticles using chitosan and alginate and evaluated to access the biocompatibility and effectiveness in controlling senescence and inflammatory processes in cigarette smoke extracts. The synthesized microparticles were found to be more effective than fluticasone propionate alone in controlling oxidative stress in lung inflammation, including ERK1/2 pathway activation and cigarette smoke extract-induced survivin expression (Amore et al. 2017). Chitosan IFN–γ-pDNA nanoparticles reduced the airway hyper-responsiveness and allergen-induced airway inflammation in the BALB/c mouse model of allergic airway disease (Kumar et al. 2003). In a study, *M. tuberculosis*-infected guinea pigs were treated with sodium alginate-chitosan-based nanoparticles containing antitubercular drugs for a period of 15 days. At the end of the study, no *M. tuberculosis* bacteria were observed in the infected lungs treated with mucoadhesive nanoparticles (Zahoor et al. 2005).

Lee et al. found the improved theophylline delivery from thiolated chitosan nanoparticles in ovalbumin-sensitized BALB/c mice model of allergic asthma. The intranasal delivery of nanoparticles increased the anti-inflammatory effects of theophylline compared to pure theophylline (Lee et al. 2006). Chitosan-coated polylactic-co-glycolic acid nanoparticles synthesized by a multiple emulsion solvent evaporation technique may open up a new avenue for efficacious treatment of lung-fungal infection. Tc-99m-labeled nanoparticles had better pulmonary retention for a longer period. A significant improvement in the pharmacokinetic profile of voriconazole was found in chitosan-coated nanoparticles (Paul et al. 2018). Heparin- containing nanoparticles of chitosan and hyaluronic acid have shown promising results in the management of asthma in rat models (Oyarzun-Ampuero et al. 2009).

Successful co-delivery of pemetrexed (a synthetic chemotherapeutic agent) and resveratrol (herbal cancer chemo preventive) has been reported from lyotropic liquid crystalline nanoparticles prepared by the hydrotrope method for effective management of lung cancer. Cetyl trimethyl ammonium bromide was used to increase the encapsulation of pemetrexed by hydrophobic ion pairing. The results demonstrated a concentration- and time-dependent cytotoxicity profile against A549 lung cancer cells. Nanoparticle-administered mice models, with urethane- induced lung cancer, demonstrated promising results in tumor growth inhibition via inhibition of angiogenesis and induction of apoptosis (Abdelaziz et al. 2019).

Wheat germ agglutinin-coated lectin-functionalized poly(lactide-co-glycolide) (PLGA)-based bioadhesive nanoparticles (350–400 nm) have been reported by a two-step carbodiimide procedure to deliver antitubercular drugs. The in vivo performance of the synthesized nanoparticles was studied in guinea pigs through the oral/aerosol route. Following administration of coated nanoparticles to the animal models, the plasma drug concentration was maintained for 6–7 days for rifampicin and 13–14 days for isoniazid and pyrazinamide. The results of mycobacterial colony forming units revealed that three doses of lectin-coated nanoparticles, after every 14 days interval, were as much effective as 45 dosages of pure drug solution (Sharma et al. 2004). Tureli et al. found that the ciprofloxacin-loaded PLGA nanoparticles synthesized by microjet reactor nanoprecipitation method are safe and effective against *Pseudomonas aeruginosa* infections in cystic fibrosis lungs. The outcomes of cytotoxicity study in Calu-3 HTB-55 bronchial epithelial cell line (model for healthy lungs) and CFBE41o⁻ cystic fibrosis-derived bronchial epithelial cell line (model for diseased lungs) suggested that the nanoparticles are well tolerated by the epithelial cells and showed low cytotoxic potential (Tureli et al. 2017). Surface-conjugated PLGA nanoparticles of chitosan have shown efficient targeted delivery and improved oral bioavailability of itraconazole to clear lung infections in *Cryptococcus neoformans*-infected mouse models (Tang et al. 2018). Chitosan-coated (molecular weight 90–150 kDa) PLGA nanoparticles sustained the release of tobramycin over a period of 2 days. The mucoadhesive nanoparticles, prepared by a solvent-evaporation method, had chitosan concentration-dependent activity against *P. aeruginosa* (PA01 strain) (Al-Nemrawi et al. 2018). Inhaled chitosan-coated, PLGA nanoparticles exhibited a sustained release profile of tacrolimus with a lesser dose and side effects in the treatment of bleomycin-induced pulmonary fibrosis (Lee et al. 2016). The study conducted by Zou et al. explored the potential of PLGA nanoparticles as a nonviral vector for lung cancer gene therapy. The PLGA nanoparticles were prepared using Carbopol 940 and Pluronic. Carbopol-stabilized PLGA nanoparticles demonstrated higher transfection efficiency in A549 cells compared to Pluronic-stabilized nanoparticles or naked DNA (Zou et al. 2009).

Targeted drug delivery using nanoformulations via the inhalation route has become an important drug delivery system through the pulmonary route for the treatment of a number of respiratory diseases like COPD, asthma, lung infection, etc. This route allows rapid deposition of the drug in the lungs with decreased side effects compared to other routes of drug administration. The nanoparticles are being used to reduce side effects and toxicity of drugs, but recently, it has been realized that carrier systems themselves may impose risks to the patient (Nassimi et al. 2010).

The kinds of hazards that are introduced by using nanoparticles for drug delivery are beyond those posed by conventional hazards imposed by chemicals in classical delivery matrices. The toxicology of particulate matter differs from toxicology of substances as the composing chemical(s) may or may not be soluble in biological matrices, thus influencing greatly the potential exposure of various internal organs. This may vary from a rather high local exposure in the lungs and a low or neglectable exposure for other organ systems after inhalation. For nanoparticles the situation is different as their size opens the potential for crossing the various biological barriers within the body. In addition, the nanosize also allows for access into the cell and various cellular compartments including the nucleus. A multitude of substances are currently under investigation for the preparation of nanoparticles for drug delivery, varying from biological substances like albumin, gelatine, and phospholipids for liposomes, and more substances of a chemical nature like various polymers and solid metal containing nanoparticles (De Jong and Borm 2008).

20.11 Conclusion

Nanocarrier systems have been found to provide the advantage of sustained-drug release in the lung tissue resulting in improved patient compliance by reducing dosing frequency. In the present review, the potential benefits of nanomedicines in pulmonary diseases have been summarized. Nanotechnology has been observed to be a potentially beneficial approach for the diagnosis and treatment of pulmonary diseases. Various studies have demonstrated promising advancements, efficacy, and safety of NPs for use in pulmonary diseases. However, significant challenges are still there in making nanotherapeutic approaches fully functional in clinical practice. Further studies are required to be done focusing majorly on determining the mechanisms of action of NPs in the treatment of chronic pulmonary diseases and improving their chemical structure to develop the desired nanomedicine or nanotherapeutics.

References

Abdelaziz HM, Gaber M, Abd-Elwakil MM, Mabrouk MT, Elgohary MM, Kamel NM, Elzoghby AO (2018) Inhalable particulate drug delivery systems for lung cancer therapy: nanoparticles, microparticles, nanocomposites and nanoaggregates. J Control Release 269:374–392

Abdelaziz HM, Elzoghby AO, Helmy MW, Samaha MW, Fang JY, Freag MS (2019) Liquid crystalline assembly for potential combinatorial chemo–herbal drug delivery to lung cancer cells. Int J Nanomedicine 14:499–507

Abu-Dahab R, Schäfer UF, Lehr CM (2001) Lectin-functionalized liposomes for pulmonary drug delivery: effect of nebulization on stability and bioadhesion. Eur J Pharm Sci 14(1):37–46

Adam B, Nicolas T, Ilaria A, Anais C, Camilla F, Claudine D, Elias F (2017) Anti-inflammatory effect of anti-TNF-α SiRNA cationic phosphorus dendrimer nanocomplexes administered intranasally in a murine acute lung injury model. Biomacromolecules 18(8):2379–2388

Agustí A, Celli B (2017) Natural history of COPD: gaps and opportunities. ERJ Open Res 3(4):1–10

Al-Nemrawi N, Alshraiedeh NA, Zayed A, Altaani B (2018) Low molecular weight chitosan-coated PLGA nanoparticles for pulmonary delivery of tobramycin for cystic fibrosis. Pharmaceuticals (Basel) 11(1):28

Alvarez MJ, Echechipía S, García B, Tabar AI, Martín S, Rico P, Olaguibel JM (2002) Liposome-entrapped D. pteronyssinus vaccination in mild asthma patients: effect of 1-year double-blind, placebo-controlled trial on inflammation, bronchial hyper-responsiveness and immediate and late bronchial responses to the allergen. Clin Exp Allergy 32(11):1574–1582

Amore E, Ferraro M, Manca ML, Gjomarkaj M, Giammona G, Pace E, Bondì ML (2017) Mucoadhesive solid lipid microparticles for controlled release of a corticosteroid in the chronic obstructive pulmonary disease treatment. Nanomedicine 12(19):2287–2302

Amreddy N, Babu A, Panneerselvam J, Srivastava A, Muralidharan R, Chen A, Ramesh R (2018) Chemo-biologic combinatorial drug delivery using folate receptor-targeted dendrimer nanoparticles for lung cancer treatment. Nanomedicine 14(2):373–384

Asher I, Pearce N (2014) Global burden of asthma among children. Int J Tuberc Lung Dis 18(11):1269–1278

Bai S, Thomas C, Rawat A, Ahsan F (2006) Recent progress in dendrimer-based nanocarriers. Crit Rev Ther Drug Carrier Syst 23(6):437–495

Bai S, Thomas S, Ahsan F (2007) Dendrimers as a carrier for pulmonary delivery of enoxaparin, a low-molecular weight heparin. J Pharm Sci 96(8):2090–2106

Barnes PJ (2003) New concepts in chronic obstructive pulmonary disease. Annu Rev Med 54(1):113–129

Barnes PJ (2011) C4 Drugs for the treatment of airway disease. In: Principles of immunopharmacology. Springer, Basel, Switzerland. pp 321–357

Bateman ED, Hurd SS, Barnes PJ, Bousquet J, Drazen JM, Fitz Gerald JM, Zar HJ (2008) Global strategy for asthma management and prevention: GINA executive summary. Eur Respir J 31(1):143–178

Beloqui A, Solinís MÁ, Rodríguez-Gascón A, Almeida AJ, Préat V (2016) Nanostructured lipid carriers: promising drug delivery systems for future clinics. Nanomedicine 12(1):143–161

Bharatwaj B, Mohammad AK, Dimovski R, Cassio FL, Bazito RC, Conti D, da Rocha SRP (2015) Dendrimer nanocarriers for transport modulation across models of the pulmonary epithelium. Mol Pharm 12(3):826–838

Bhavna AFJ, Mittal G, Jain GK, Malhotra G, Khar RK, Bhatnagar A (2009) Nano-salbutamol dry powder inhalation: a new approach for treating broncho-constrictive conditions. Eur J Pharm Biopharm 71(2):282–291

Bradbury M, Wiesner U, Penate MO, Burns A, Lewis J, Larson S, Quinn T. Multimodal silica-based nanoparticles. Google Patents. 2014.

Brockman SM, Bodas M, Silverberg D, Sharma A, Vij N (2017) Dendrimer-based selective autophagy-induction rescues F508-CFTR and inhibits Pseudomonas aeruginosa infection in cystic fibrosis. PLoS One 12(9):e0184793–e0184799

Celli BR, Mac Nee W (2004) Standards for the diagnosis and treatment of patients with COPD: a summary of the ATS/ERS position paper. Eur Respir J 23(6):932–946

Chellappan DK, Hansbro PM, Dua K, Hsu A, Gupta G, Ng ZY, Panneerselvam J (2017) Vesicular systems containing curcumin and their applications in respiratory disorders - a mini review. Pharm Nanotechnol 5(4):250–254

Chellappan DK, Ng ZY, Wong JY, Hsu A, Wark P, Hansbro N, Dua K (2018) Immunological axis of curcumin-loaded vesicular drug delivery systems. Future Med Chem 10(8):839–844

Chennakesavulu S, Mishra A, Sudheer A, Sowmya C, Suryaprakash Reddy C, Bhargava E (2018) Pulmonary delivery of liposomal dry powder inhaler formulation for effective treatment of idiopathic pulmonary fibrosis. Asian J Pharm Sci 13(1):91–100

Chono S, Tanino T, Seki T, Morimoto K (2007) Uptake characteristics of liposomes by rat alveolar macrophages: influence of particle size and surface mannose modification. J Pharm Pharmacol 59(1):75–80

Chou AJ, Gupta R, Bell MD, Riewe KO, Meyers PA, Gorlick R (2013) Inhaled lipid cisplatin (ILC) in the treatment of patients with relapsed/progressive osteosarcoma metastatic to the lung. Pediatr Blood Cancer 60:580–586

Cruz AA (2007) Global surveillance, prevention and control of chronic respiratory diseases: a comprehensive approach. World Health Organization

Cryer AM, Thorley AJ (2019) Nanotechnology in the diagnosis and treatment of lung cancer. Pharmacol Ther 198:189–205

De Jong WH, Borm PJA (2008) Drug delivery and nanoparticles: applications and hazards. Int J Nanomedicine 3(2):133–149

Dong Z, Hamid KA, Gao Y, Lin Y, Katsumi H, Sakane T, Yamamoto A (2011) Polyamidoamine dendrimers can improve the pulmonary absorption of insulin and calcitonin in rats. J Pharm Sci 100(5):1866–1878

Dozor AJ (2010) The role of oxidative stress in the pathogenesis and treatment of asthma. Ann N Y Acad Sci 1203(1):133–137

Dua K, Rapalli VK, Shukla SD, Singhvi G, Shastri MD, Chellappan DK, Gupta G (2018) Multi-drug resistant Mycobacterium tuberculosis and oxidative stress complexity: emerging need for novel drug delivery approaches. Biomed Pharmacother 107:1218–1229

Dua K, Malyla V, Singhvi G, Wadhwa R, Krishna RV, Shukla SD, Hansbro PM (2019) Increasing complexity and interactions of oxidative stress in chronic respiratory diseases: an emerging need for novel drug delivery systems. Chem Biol Interact 299:168–178

Dufès C, Uchegbu IF, Schätzlein AG (2005) Dendrimers in gene delivery. Adv Drug Deliv Rev 57(15):2177–2202

Duncan R, Izzo L (2005) Dendrimer biocompatibility and toxicity. Adv Drug Deliv Rev 57(15):2215–2237

Frankenberger M, Häussinger K, Ziegler-Heitbrock L (2005) Liposomal methylprednisolone differentially regulates the expression of TNF and IL-10 in human alveolar macrophages. Int Immunopharmacol 5(2):289–299

Geiger J, Aneja MK, Rudolph C. Pulmonary delivery of messenger RNA. Google Patents. 2015.

Girdhar V, Patil S, Banerjee S, Singhvi G (2018) Nanocarriers for drug delivery: mini review. Curr Nanomed 8(2):88–99

GOLD. Global strategy for the diagnosis, management and prevention of COPD, Global initiative for chronic obstructive lung disease (GOLD) 2018. Retrieved from https://goldcoped.org/. Accessed 10 Mar 2019.

Guarascio AJ, Ray SM, Finch CK, Self TH (2013) The clinical and economic burden of chronic obstructive pulmonary disease in the USA. Clinicoecon Outcomes Res 5:235–245

Hamman JH, Enslin GM, Kotzé AF (2005) Oral delivery of peptide drugs. BioDrugs 19(3):165–177

Han Y, Zhang P, Chen Y, Sun J, Kong F (2014) Co-delivery of plasmid DNA and doxorubicin by solid lipid nanoparticles for lung cancer therapy. Int J Mol Med 34(1):191–196

Hatamipour M, Ramezani M, Tabassi SAS, Johnston TP, Ramezani M, Sahebkar A (2018) Demethoxycurcumin: a naturally occurring curcumin analogue with antitumor properties. J Cell Physiol 233(12):9247–9260

Hema S, Thambiraj S, Shankaran DR (2018) Nanoformulations for targeted drug delivery to prostate cancer: an overview. J Nanosci Nanotechnol 18(8):5171–5191

Hickey S (2014) Understanding the impact of inhaler technique on asthma and COPD. Nurse Prescribing 12(10):492–496

Iga AM, Robertson JH, Winslet MC, Seifalian AM (2007) Clinical potential of quantum dots. J Biomed Biotechnol (10):76087–76097

Ihrie MD, Bonner JC (2018) The toxicology of engineered nanomaterials in asthma. Curr Environ Health Rep 5(1):100–109

Inapagolla R, Raja Guru B, Kurtoglu YE, Gao X, Lieh-Lai M, Bassett DJP, Rangaramanujam K (2010) *In vivo* efficacy of dendrimer-methylprednisolone conjugate formulation for the treatment of lung inflammation. Int J Pharm 399:140–147

Islam N, Abbas M, Rahman S (2017) Neuropathic pain and lung delivery of nanoparticulate drugs: an emerging novel therapeutic strategy. CNS Neurol Disord Drug Targets 16(3):303–310

Islan Germán A, Tornello PC, Abraham GA, Duran N, Castro GR (2016) Smart lipid nanoparticles containing levofloxacin and DNase for lung delivery. Design and characterization. Colloids Surf B: Biointerfaces 143:168–176

Jasinski D, Haque F, Binzel DW, Guo P (2017) Advancement of the emerging field of RNA nanotechnology. ACS Nano 11(2):1142–1164

Joshi M, Misra A (2001) Dry powder inhalation of liposomal ketotifen fumarate: formulation and characterization. Int J Pharm 223(1–2):15–27

Joshi M, Misra A (2003) Disposition kinetics of ketotifen from liposomal dry powder for inhalation in rat lung. Clin Exp Pharmacol Physiol 30(3):153–156

Kaminskas LM, McLeodVM RGM, Kelly BD, Haynes JM, Williamson M, Thienthong N, Owen DJ, Porter CJ (2014) Pulmonary administration of a doxorubicin-conjugated dendrimer enhances drug exposure to lung metastases and improves cancer therapy. J Control Release 183:18–26

Kaur SS (2017) Pulmonary drug delivery system: newer patents. Pharm Pat Anal 6(5):225–244

Kc R, Shukla SD, Gautam SS, Hansbro PM, O'Toole RF (2018) The role of environmental exposure to non-cigarette smoke in lung disease. Clin Transl Med 7(1):39–45

Khan OF, Zaia EW, Jhunjhunwala S, Xue W, Cai W, Yun DS, Anderson DG (2015) Dendrimer-inspired nanomaterials for the *in vivo* delivery of siRNA to lung vasculature. Nanotechnol Lett 15(5):3008–3016

Khosa A, Reddi S, Saha RN (2018) Nanostructured lipid carriers for site-specific drug delivery. Biomed Pharmacother 103:598–613

Kiparissides C, Kammona O (2008) Nanotechnology advances in controlled drug delivery systems. Phys Status Solidi C 5(12):3828–3833

Koo HK, Vasilescu DM, Booth S, Hsieh A, Katsamenis OL, Fishbane N, Hackett TL (2018) Small airways disease in mild and moderate chronic obstructive pulmonary disease: a cross-sectional study. Lancet Respir Med 6(8):591–602

Kumar M, Kong X, Behera AK, Hellermann GR, Lockey RF, Mohapatra SS (2003) Chitosan IFN-gamma-pDNA nanoparticle (CIN) therapy for allergic asthma. Genet Vaccin Ther 1(1):3

Kuzmov A, Minko T (2015) Nanotechnology approaches for inhalation treatment of lung diseases. J Control Release 219(10):500–518

Lee DW, Shirley SA, Lockey RF, Mohapatra SS (2006) Thiolated chitosan nanoparticles enhance anti-inflammatory effects of intranasally delivered theophylline. Respir Res 7(1):112

Lee C, Seo J, Hwang HS, Thao LQ, Lee S, Lee ES, Youn YS (2016) Treatment of bleomycin-induced pulmonary fibrosis by inhaled tacrolimus-loaded chitosan-coated poly (lactic-co-glycolic acid) nanoparticles. Biomed Pharmacother 78:226–233

Lehr CM (2000) Lectin-mediated drug delivery: the second generation of bioadhesives. J Control Release 65(1–2):19–29

Li B, Zhang X, Dong Y (2019) Nanoscale platforms for messenger RNA delivery. Wiley Interdiscip Rev Nanomed Nanobiotechnol 11(2):e1530–e1536

Loira-Pastoriza C, Todoroff J, Vanbever R (2014) Delivery strategies for sustained drug release in the lungs. Adv Drug Deliv Rev 75:81–91

Madaan K, Kumar S, Poonia N, Lather V, Pandita D (2014) Dendrimers in drug delivery and targeting: drug-dendrimer interactions and toxicity issues. J Pharm Bioallied Sci 6(3):139–150

Madni A, Batool A, Noreen S, Maqbool I, Rehman F, Kashif PM, Raza A (2017) Novel nanoparticulate systems for lung cancer therapy: an updated review. J Drug Target 25(6):499–512

Makled S, Nafee N, Boraie N (2017) Nebulized solid lipid nanoparticles for the potential treatment of pulmonary hypertension *via* targeted delivery of phosphodiesterase-5-inhibitor. Int J Pharm 517(1–2):312–321

Maretti E, Costantino L, Rustichelli C, Leo E, Croce MA, Buttini F, Iannuccelli V (2017) Surface engineering of solid lipid nanoparticle assemblies by methyl α-d-mannopyranoside for the active targeting to macrophages in anti-tuberculosis inhalation therapy. Int J Pharm 528(1–2):440–451

Mehta P (2016) Dry powder inhalers: a focus on advancements in novel drug delivery systems. J Drug Deliv 2016:8290963–8290968

Mehta P, Bothiraja C, Mahadik K, Kadam S, Pawar A (2018) Phytoconstituent based dry powder inhalers as biomedicine for the management of pulmonary diseases. Biomed Pharmacother 108:828–837

Mehta M, Deeksha, Sharma N, Vyas M, Khurana N, Maurya PK, Satija S (2019) Interactions with the macrophages: an emerging targeted approach using novel drug delivery systems in respiratory diseases. Chem Biol Interact 304:10–19

Momtazi-Borojeni AA, Esmaeili SA, Abdollahi E, Sahebkar A (2017) A review on the pharmacology and toxicology of steviol glycosides extracted from *stevia rebaudiana*. Curr Pharm Des 23(11):1616–1622

Moreno-Sastre M, Pastor M, Esquisabel A, Sans E, Viñas M, Fleischer A, Pedraz JL (2016) Pulmonary delivery of tobramycin-loaded nanostructured lipid carriers for *pseudomonas aeruginosa* infections associated with cystic fibrosis. Int J Pharm 498(1–2):263–273

Morgan MT, Carnahan MA, Immoos CE, Ribeiro AA, Finkelstein S (2003) Dendritic molecular capsules for hydrophobic compounds. J Am Chem Soc 125:15485–15489

Morris C, Aljayyoussi G, Mansour O, Griffiths P, Gumbleton M (2017) Endocytic uptake, transport and macromolecular interactions of anionic PAMAM dendrimers within lung tissue. Pharm Res 34(12):2517–2531

Mosmann TR, Coffman RL (1989) TH1 and TH2 cells: different patterns of lymphokine secretion lead to different functional properties. Annu Rev Immunol 7:145–173

Nasr M, Najlah M, D'Emanuele A, Elhissi A (2014) PAMAM dendrimers as aerosol drug nanocarriers for pulmonary delivery via nebulization. Int J Pharm 461(1–2):242–250

Nassimi M, Schleh C, Lauenstein HD, Hussein R, Hoymann HG, Koch W, Pohlmann G, Krug N, Sewald K, Rittinghausen S, Braun A, Müller-Goymann C (2010) A toxicological evaluation of inhaled solid lipid nanoparticles used as a potential drug delivery system for the lung. Eur J Pharm Biopharm 75(2):107–116

National asthma education and prevention program, third expert panel on the diagnosis and management of asthma. Expert panel report 3: guidelines for the diagnosis and management of asthma. Bethesda: National heart, lung, and blood institute (US); 2007 Aug. Section 2, Definition, pathophysiology and pathogenesis of asthma, and natural history of asthma. Retrieved from: https://www.ncbi.nlm.nih.gov/books/NBK7223/

Neerman MF, Chen HT, Parrish AR, Simanek EE (2004) Reduction of drug toxicity using dendrimers based on melamine. Mol Pharmacol 1:390–393

Newman SP (2017) Drug delivery to the lungs: challenges and opportunities. Ther Deliv 8(8):647–661

Ng ZY, Wong JY, Panneerselvam J, Madheswaran T, Kumar P, Pillay V, Chellappan DK (2018) Assessing the potential of liposomes loaded with curcumin as a therapeutic intervention in asthma. Colloids Surf B: Biointerfaces 172:51–59

Nkanga CI, Krause RW, Noundou XS, Walker RB (2017) Preparation and characterization of isoniazid-loaded crude soybean lecithin liposomes. Int J Pharm 526(1–2):466–473

Ong WZ, Nowak PW, Kim J, Enlow EM, Bourassa J, CUY, Popov A, Chen H. Meropenem derivatives and uses thereof. Google Patents, 2014.

Oyarzun-Ampuero FA, Brea J, Loza MI, Torres D, Alonso MJ (2009) Chitosan-hyaluronic acid nanoparticles loaded with heparin for the treatment of asthma. Int J Pharm 381(2):122–129

Pahal P, Sharma S. Emphysema. [Updated 2019 Feb 23]. In: StatPearls [Internet]. Treasure Island: StatPearls Publishing. 2019. Retrieved from: https://www.ncbi.nlm.nih.gov/books/NBK482217/

Paranjpe M, Müller-Goymann CC (2014) Nanoparticle-mediated pulmonary drug delivery: a review. Int J Mol Sci 15(4):5852–5873

Parasaram V, Nosoudi N, LeClair RJ, Binks A, Vyavahare N (2016) Targeted drug delivery to emphysematous lungs: inhibition of MMPs by doxycycline loaded nanoparticles. Pulm Pharmacol Ther 39:64–71

Patri AK, Myc A, Beals J, Thomas TP, Bander NH, Baker JR Jr (2004) Synthesis and *in vitro* testing of J591 antibody-dendrimer conjugates for targeted prostate cancer therapy. Bioconjug Chem 15(6):1174–1181

Patton DL, Cosgrove Sweeney YT, McCarthy TD, Hillier SL (2006) Preclinical safety and efficacy assessments of dendrimer-based (SPL 7013) microbicide gel formulations in a nonhuman primate model. Antimicrob Agents Chemother 50(5):1696–1700

Paul P, Sengupta S, Mukherjee B, Shaw TK, Gaonkar RH, Debnath MC (2018) Chitosan-coated nanoparticles enhanced lung pharmacokinetic profile of voriconazole upon pulmonary delivery in mice. Nanomedicine 13(5):501–520

Pavord ID, Beasley R, Agusti A, Anderson GP, Bel E, Brusselle G, Bush A (2018) After asthma: redefining airways diseases. Lancet 391(10118):350–400

Payne CM, Burke LP, Cavanagh B, O'Toole D, Cryan SA, Kelly HM (2019) Evaluation of the immunomodulatory effects of all-trans retinoic acid solid lipid nanoparticles and human mesenchymal stem cells in an A549 epithelial cell line model. Pharm Res 36(4):50–56

Rosière R, Van Woensel M, Gelbcke M, Mathieu V, Hecq J, Mathivet T, Wauthoz N (2018) New folate-grafted chitosan derivative to improve delivery of paclitaxel-loaded solid lipid nanoparticles for lung tumor therapy by inhalation. Mol Pharmacol 15(3):899–910

Ruge CA, Kirch J, Lehr C-M (2013) Pulmonary drug delivery: from generating aerosols to overcoming biological barriers—therapeutic possibilities and technological challenges. Lancet Respir Med 1(5):402–413

Sahib MN, Darwis Y, Peh KK, Abdulameer SA, Tan YT (2011) Rehydrated sterically stabilized phospholipid nanomicelles of budesonide for nebulization: physicochemical characterization and *in vitro*, *in vivo* evaluations. Int J Nanomedicine 6:2351–2356

Sapey E, Stockley RA (2006) COPD exacerbations 2: aetiology. Thorax 61(3):250–258

Saraogi GK, Gupta P, Gupta UD, Jain NK, Agrawal GP (2010) Gelatin nanocarriers as potential vectors for effective management of tuberculosis. Int J Pharm 385(1–2):143–149

Savla R, Minko T (2013) Nanotechnology approaches for inhalation treatment of fibrosis. J Drug Target 21(10):914–925

Schmidt ST, Foged C, Korsholm KS, Rades T, Christensen D (2016) Liposome-based adjuvants for subunit vaccines: formulation strategies for subunit antigens and immunostimulators. Pharmaceutics 8(1):7–12

Serisier DJ, Bilton D, De Soyza A, Thompson PJ, Kolbe J, Greville HW, Gonda I (2013) Inhaled, dual release liposomal ciprofloxacin in non-cystic fibrosis bronchiectasis (ORBIT-2): a randomised, double-blind, placebo-controlled trial. Thorax 68(9):812–817

Sharma A, Sharma S, Khuller GK (2004) Lectin-functionalized poly (lactide-co-glycolide) nanoparticles as oral/aerosolized antitubercular drug carriers for treatment of tuberculosis. J Antimicrob Chemother 54(4):761–766

Shukla R, Thomas TP, Desai AM, Kotlyar A, Park SJ, Baker JR (2008) HER2 specific delivery of methotrexate by dendrimer conjugated anti-HER2 mAb. Nanotechnology 19(29):295102–295109

Simpson JL, Scott R, Boyle MJ, Gibson PG (2006) Inflammatory subtypes in asthma: assessment and identification using induced sputum. Respirology (Carlton, Vic) 11(1):54–61

Singhvi G, Banerjee S, Khosa A (2018) Lyotropic liquid crystal nanoparticles: a novel improved lipidic drug delivery system. In: Inorganic materials as smart nanocarriers for drug delivery, 1st edn, William Andrew, Norwich, New York. pp 471–517

Smola M, Vandamme T, Sokolowski A (2008) Nanocarriers as pulmonary drug delivery systems to treat and to diagnose respiratory and non-respiratory diseases. Int J Nanomedicine 3(1):1–6

Soto-Castro D, Cruz-Morales JA, Ramírez Apan MT, Guadarrama P (2012) Solubilization and anticancer-activity enhancement of methotrexate by novel dendrimeric nanodevices synthesized in one-step reaction. Bioorg Chem 41–42:13–21

Taguchi K, Yamasaki K, Sakai H, Maruyama T, Otagiri M (2017) The use of hemoglobin vesicles for delivering medicinal gas for the treatment of intractable disorders. J Pharm Sci 106(9):2392–2400

Tang Y, Wu S, Lin J, Cheng L, Zhou J, Xie J, Liao G (2018) Nanoparticles targeted against cryptococcal pneumonia by interactions between chitosan and its peptide ligand. Nanotechnol Lett 18(10):6207–6213

Taratula O, Kuzmov A, Shah M, Garbuzenko OB, Minko T (2013) Nanostructured lipid carriers as multifunctional nanomedicine platform for pulmonary co-delivery of anticancer drugs and SiRNA. J Control Release 171(3):349–357

Thakur S, Singh B, Mishra V, Yadav N, Giri N, Sharma P, Garg LK (2019) Bilayer tablet based chronotherapeutics in the management of nocturnal asthma: an overview. Recent Pat Drug Deliv Formul 1:1–10

TO PG. Global initiative for chronic obstructive lung. 2018.

Tomalia DA (2005) Birth of a new macromolecular architecture: dendrimers as quantized building blocks for nanoscale synthetic polymer chemistry. Prog Polym Sci 30:294–324

Tomalia DA, Baker H, Dewald J, Hall M, Kallos G, Martin S, Smith P (1985) A new class of polymers: starburst-dendritic macromolecules. Polym J 17:117–132

Tureli NG, Torge A, Juntke J, Schwarz BC, Schneider-Daum N, Türeli AE, Schneider M (2017) Ciprofloxacin-loaded PLGA nanoparticles against cystic fibrosis P. aeruginosa lung infections. Eur J Pharm Biopharm 117:363–371 van Rijt SH, Bein T, Meiners S (2014) Medical nanoparticles for next generation drug delivery to the lungs. Eur Respir J 44:765–774

Verschraegen CF, Gilbert BE, Loyer E, Huaringa A, Walsh G, Newman RA, Knight V (2004) Clinical evaluation of the delivery and safety of aerosolized liposomal 9-nitro-20(s)-camptothecin in patients with advanced pulmonary malignancies. Clin Cancer Res 10:2319–2326

Vieira ACC, Chaves LL, Pinheiro S, Pinto S, Pinheiro M, Lima SC, Reis S (2018) Mucoadhesive chitosan-coated solid lipid nanoparticles for better management of tuberculosis. Int J Pharm 536(1):478–485

Weber S, Zimmer A, Pardeike (2014) Solid lipid nanoparticles (SLN) and nanostructured lipid carriers (NLC) for pulmonary application: a review of the state of the art. Eur J Pharm Biopharm 86(1):7–22

Wenzel SE, Schwartz LB, Langmack EL, Halliday JL, Trudeau JB, Gibbs RL, Chu HW (1999) Evidence that severe asthma can be divided pathologically into two inflammatory subtypes with distinct physiologic and clinical characteristics. Am J Respir Crit Care Med 160(3):1001–1008

Winkler J, Hochhaus G, Derendorf H (2004) How the lung handles drugs: pharmacokinetics and pharmacodynamics of inhaled corticosteroids. Proc Am Thorac Soc 1(4):356–363

Wittgen BP, Kunst PW, van der Born K, van Wijk AW, Perkins W, Pilkiewicz FG, Postmus PE (2007) Phase I study of aerosolized SLIT cisplatin in the treatment of patients with carcinoma of the lung. Clin Cancer Res 13(8):2414–2421

Wolinsky JB, Grinstaff MW (2008) Therapeutic and diagnostic applications of dendrimers for cancer treatment. Adv Drug Deliv Rev 60(9):1037–1055

Wu G, Barth RF, Yang W, Kawabata S, Zhang L, Green-Church K (2006) Targeted delivery of methotrexate to epidermal growth factor receptor-positive brain tumors by means of cetuximab (IMC-C225) dendrimer bioconjugates. Mol Cancer Ther 5(1):52–59

Yu HP, Aljuffali IA, Fang JY (2017) Injectable drug-loaded nanocarriers for lung cancer treatments. Curr Pharm Des 23(3):481–494

Zahoor A, Sharma S, Khuller GK (2005) Inhalable alginate nanoparticles as antitubercular drug carriers against experimental tuberculosis. Int J Antimicrob Agents 26:298–303

Zou W, Liu C, Chen Z, Zhang N (2009) Studies on bioadhesive PLGA nanoparticles: a promising gene delivery system for efficient gene therapy to lung cancer. Int J Pharm 370(1–2):187–195

Zylberberg C, Matosevic S (2016) Pharmaceutical liposomal drug delivery: a review of new delivery systems and a look at the regulatory landscape. Drug Deliv 23(9):3319–3329

21 Nanoweapons Against Tuberculosis

Josef Jampílek and Katarína Kráľová

Abstract

The emerging resistance of *Mycobacterium tuberculosis* and other so-called nontuberculous mycobacteria to clinically used drugs, including second- and third-choice drugs, and the development of cross-resistant or multidrug-resistant strains are alarming. An increase in the number of these infections and the occurrence of nontuberculous opportunistic species are caused by the general immunosuppression of patients, and this fact makes these diseases extremely serious. In spite of the mentioned, the discovery and development of new drugs for systemic administration has not been a priority, as it is a relatively long and risky procedure. Thus, the preparation of nanoparticles/nanoformulations of clinically used drugs can be an approach of first choice. In general, nanomaterials represent a noteworthy alternative for treatment and mitigation of infections caused by resistant pathogens, which are unlikely to develop resistance to nanomaterials. In contrast to conventional drugs, nanomaterials exert efficiency through various mechanisms; in addition to the drug activity itself, they show "intrinsic effects," such as damaging the membrane morphology, disruption of transmembrane energy metabolism and the membrane electron transport chain, generation of reactive oxygen species, etc. In addition, the application of nanoformulations enhances the bioavailability of active substances and enables targeted delivery and controlled release. This contribution provides an exhaustive overview of the investigated nano-based formulations of antimycobacterially effective drugs, such as isoniazid, ethambutol, rifampicin, and bedaquiline. These nanoformulations increase biological potency, as they can ensure fixed-dose drug combinations or nanoencapsulation of drugs with biologically active matrices. In addition, the route of administration can be modified; thus, nano-based drug delivery systems demonstrate significant potential reducing the dosing frequency and shortening the time of treatment. Brief attention is also given to new nanoformulated antituberculosis vaccines. Future prospects of the application of nanotechnology in the treatment of tuberculosis are briefly outlined.

J. Jampílek (✉)
Regional Centre of Advanced Technologies and Materials, Faculty of Science, Palacky University, Olomouc, Czech Republic

Institute of Neuroimmunology, Slovak Academy of Sciences, Bratislava, Slovakia

K. Kráľová
Institute of Chemistry, Faculty of Natural Sciences, Comenius University, Bratislava, Slovakia

S. Talegaonkar, M. Rai (eds.), *Nanoformulations in Human Health*,
https://doi.org/10.1007/978-3-030-41858-8_21

Keywords

Antimycobacterial drugs · Controlled release · Mycobacteria · Nanoformulations · Nanoparticles · Targeted delivery · Tuberculosis · Vaccines

21.1 Introduction

In spite of the great efforts of scientists and physicians supported by WHO, tuberculosis (TB) still ranks among the leading causes of death worldwide; in fact, it is one of the top ten causes of death. After a decrease in TB incidence since the 1950s due to the introduction of new antitubercular agents to clinical practice, morbidity and mortality have risen again since the 1980s; TB has again become a major bacterial cause of worldwide mortality, and thus it remains a serious global problem. Globally, there is an estimate that 10.0 million people have newly developed TB disease, and TB caused an estimated 1.6 million deaths in 2017. This number has been increasing since 2009, in which 5.7 million new cases were reported. Drug-resistant TB continues to be a great health crisis. Globally, 3.5% of new TB cases and 18% of previously treated cases have multidrug-resistant TB (MDR-TB). More than half of previously treated cases are in countries of the former Soviet Union, India, and China. Among the cases of MDR-TB in 2017, 8.5% were estimated to be extensively drug-resistant TB (XDR-TB). About 1.7 billion people, 23% of the world's population, are estimated to have a latent TB infection and are thus at risk of developing active TB disease during their lifetime (WHO 2018).

TB is an infectious disease caused by bacteria from the species *Mycobacterium tuberculosis*, which attacks humans and animals. They usually affect the lungs, but they can also damage other parts of the body. The infection is spread through the air, when a person with an active form of TB coughs, sneezes, or otherwise expands his saliva through the air. Most infections are asymptomatic and latent; approx. one in ten diseases turns into active TB, which, when left untreated, causes death in more than 50% of cases. The most typical symptom is chronic cough with bloody sputum (coughing up or spouting blood), fever, night sweats, and weight loss. The infection of other organs is characterized by a wide range of symptoms. Diagnosis is made by microbiological examination of the sputum or tissue samples taken, tuberculin test, radiology (chest X-ray), or blood tests. Prevention consists of screening and vaccination, predominantly with Bacillus Calmette–Guérin (BCG); BCG vaccination is used for prevention of TB (Herchline and Amorosa 2018; Tuberculosis 2019).

M. tuberculosis was discovered and described on March 24, 1882, by Robert Koch, who was awarded the Nobel Prize for Physiology and Medicine for this discovery in 1905. The chances of eradication of TB ended with the emergence of resistant types in the 1980s, as mentioned above. In 2010, after 20 years, a new species of bacterium belonging to the *M. tuberculosis* complex (together with *M. bovis*, *M. africanum*, *M. canetti*, and *M. microti*) (van Soolingen et al. 1997), *M. mungi*, was discovered (Gagneux 2017). In addition, with the increasing immunocompromised population, the initially nonpathogenic mycobacterial strains (e.g., *M. avium*, *M. kansasii*, *M. xenopi*, *M. intracellulare*, *M. malmoense*, *M. celatum*, *M. goodii*, *M. immunogenum*, *M. simiae*, *M. scrofulaceum*, *M. abscessus*, *M. fortuitum*, *M. chelonae*, *M. smegmatis*, *M. mageritense*, *M. wolinskyi*, *M. genavense*, etc.), so-called atypical or nontuberculous mycobacteria (NTM), have been now recognized as significant human pathogens. Due to suppressed immunity, these strains cause difficult-to-treat or incurable diseases, such as pulmonary disease, lymphadenitis, skin and soft tissue disease, and gastrointestinal and skeletal infections that result in significant morbidity (Ioachimescu and Tomford 2015; Koh 2017).

However, the major causative agent of TB is *M. tuberculosis*, which is a small aerobic rod-shaped bacterium with extremely slow division. It is highly (obligatory) aerobic and needs high levels of oxygen. In general, mycobacteria are characterized by a specific cell wall composition. A high content of lipids, especially mycolic acid, is typical for them in the cell wall, causing a "wax coat on the cell surface" and conferring exceptional properties on the bacterium. Although not stained with Gram stain, they are Gram-positive bacteria. *M. tuberculosis* is genetically variable; differences in the phenotype (biogeographic occurrence) of individual isolated strains can be found. These variations affect the strain resistance and transmission dynamics in treatment-resistant strains (Liu et al. 1996; Druszczynska et al. 2017; Ghazaei 2018; Herchline and Amorosa 2018; Tuberculosis 2019). As mentioned above, the following resistant forms (strains, isolates) can be distinguished (Velayati et al. 2013; Palomino and Martin 2014; WHO 2018; Tuberculosis 2019):

- MDR-TB: resistant against two of the most effective antitubercular first-line drugs, isoniazid and rifampicin
- XDR-TB: resistant to fluoroquinolones and at least one of the injectable second-line drugs (amikacin, capreomycin, kanamycin)
- TDR-TB (totally drug-resistant TB): resistant to the first- and the second-line drugs (isoniazid, rifampicin, streptomycin, ethambutol, pyrazinamide, ethionamide, *para*-aminosalicylic acid, cycloserine, ofloxacin, amikacin, ciprofloxacin, capreomycin, kanamycin)

Treatment is long term, controlled to prevent resistance, and costly. A combination of at least three drugs in a single morning dose is used. Constitutional treatment (initial phase) is usually limited to 2–3 months. Further treatment (continuation phase) is performed on an outpatient basis daily or intermittently for 3–4 months. The minimum treatment period for bacteriologically verified nonresistant TB is 6 months. Clinically used drugs can be divided into lines according to susceptibility (see Table 21.1 and Figs. 21.1, 21.2, 21.3, 21.4, and 21.5) and efficacy as follows (Lemke et al. 2012; de Oliveira et al. 2018; Jampílek 2018; Herchline and Amorosa 2018; Tuberculosis 2019):

Table 21.1 Classification of clinically used antituberculosis drugs

Peroral first line	Isoniazid, rifampicin, rifabutin, pyrazinamide, ethambutol
Parenteral second line	Kanamycin, amikacin, capreomycin, streptomycin, viomycin
Fluoroquinolones	Ofloxacin, levofloxacin, ciprofloxacin, moxifloxacin, gatifloxacin, gemifloxacin
Peroral second line	Cycloserine, terizidone, ethionamide, prothionamide, *para*-aminosalicylic acid
MDR-TB treatment	Amoxicillin/clavulanate, imipenem, clarithromycin, clofazimine, thioacetazone, linezolid, high doses of isoniazid, bedaquiline, delamanid

- Bactericidal – kill dividing bacteria (e.g., rifampicin, streptomycin)
- Bacteriostatic – inhibit the proliferation of bacteria (e.g., isoniazid, pyrazinamide, ethambutol)
- Sterilizing – kill/inhibit the proliferation of so-called persistors (e.g., pyrazinamide, rifampicin)

The increasing resistance refers to the urgency to design and discover antituberculosis agents with a new/innovative mode of action, i.e., to design new entities from new chemical classes influencing new targets (or to design new multitarget agents) (Cieslik et al. 2015; de Oliveira et al. 2018; Goněc et al. 2013, 2016; Imramovský et al. 2007, 2009; Jampílek 2018; Kos et al. 2015a, 2015b; Malík et al. 2018; Pavić et al. 2018; Pospíšilová et al. 2018). On the other hand, the R&D procedure of agents with a new mode of action is relatively long and risky; therefore, many companies and researchers are focused on the preparation of nanoparticles (NPs)/nanoformulations of the existing drugs, because nanomaterials demonstrate antibacterial efficiency through an intrinsic mechanism of action of the drugs reinforced by the effectivity caused by the

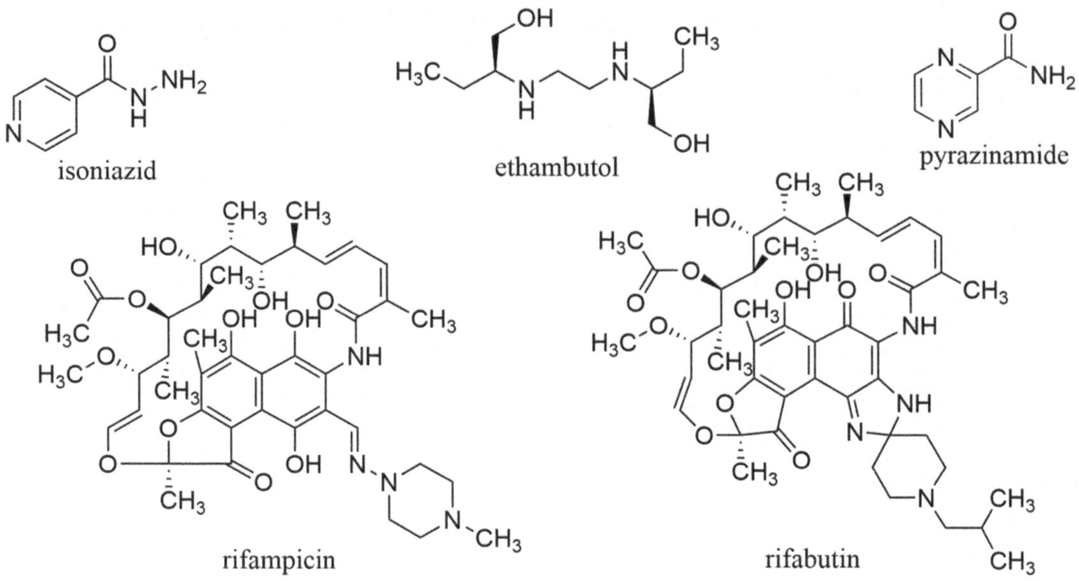

Fig. 21.1 Structures of the chosen peroral first-line drugs

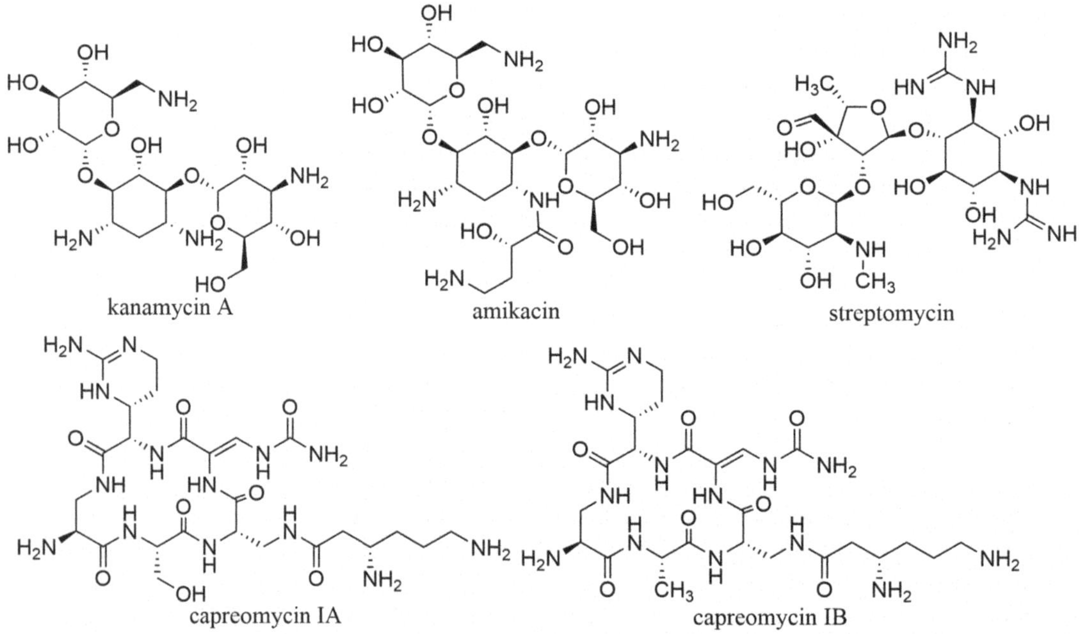

Fig. 21.2 Structures of the chosen parenteral second-line drugs

nanoscale size of drug particles. In addition, the application of nanoformulations enhances the bioavailability of active substances, can modify the route of administration, and can use fixed-dose drug combinations or antibacterial active matrices (Jampílek 2018; Jampílek and Kráľová 2017, 2018, 2019a, 2019b; Banerjee et al. 2020; Gomez et al. 2019; Kashyap et al. 2019; Rebitski et al. 2019).

This contribution provides an exhaustive overview of the investigated nano-based formulations of antimycobacterially effective drugs, such as isoniazid, ethambutol, rifampicin, and bedaquiline. These nanoformulations increase

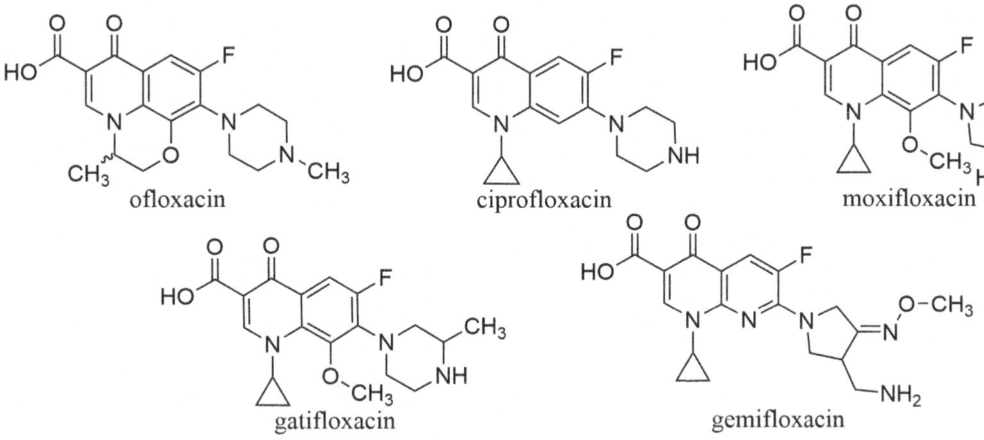

Fig. 21.3 Structures of the chosen fluoroquinolones

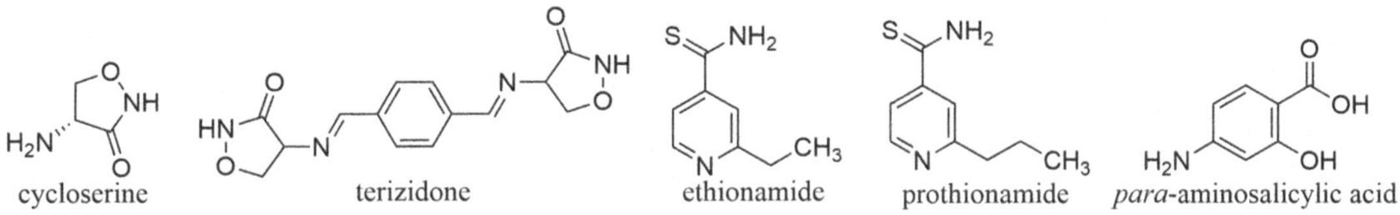

Fig. 21.4 Structures of the chosen peroral second-line drugs

biological potency, as they can ensure fixed-dose drug combinations or nanoencapsulation of drugs with biologically active matrices. In addition, the route of administration can be modified; thus, nano-based drug delivery systems demonstrate significant potential reducing the dosing frequency and shortening the time of treatment. Brief attention is also paid to new nanoformulated antituberculosis vaccines.

21.2 Isoniazid

Isoniazid (INH) is a synthetic antitubercular drug that is in fact a prodrug that has to be activated by bacterial catalase-peroxidase (KatG), which produces an acyl radical reacting with NADH to form a nicotinoyl-NAD complex that binds to enoyl-acyl reductase (InhA) and causes disruption of mycolic acid synthesis and thus inhibition of cell wall formation. INH acts bacteriostatically at low doses, but at high doses bactericidally (Isoniazid 2019).

INH- and rifabutin-loaded chitosan (CS) provided an effective inhalation antitubercular formulation for lung delivery that was able to inhibit bacterial growth by 96% (Cunha et al. 2019). CS microparticles (MPs) loaded with polyvinylpyrrolidone (PVP)/polyitaconic acid NPs with encapsulated INH fabricated using spray-drying technique that were composed of CS:INH-loaded NPs, free INH in the ratio 1:1:1, showed zeta-potential values of +22.6 mV, released the drug predominantly through a diffusion-controlled mechanism, and exhibited 63-fold higher antibacterial activity against *M. tuberculosis* than INH solution, which was due to their positively charged surface enabling more facile binding to the bacterial cell surface as well as the cellular penetration activity of NPs (Omar et al. 2018). INH-loaded CS/carbon nanotubes with a diameter of 150–250 nm and with a considerably prolonged release time of INH showed reduced cytotoxicity and inflammation compared to the free drug without affecting its biological function. Moreover, in a constructed animal model of tuberculous ulcer, they promoted the healing of TB ulcers and notably reduced the number of $CD3^+$ and $CD4^+$ T cells suggesting their potential to be used in the treatment of secondary wound healing of bone TB (Chen et al. 2019).

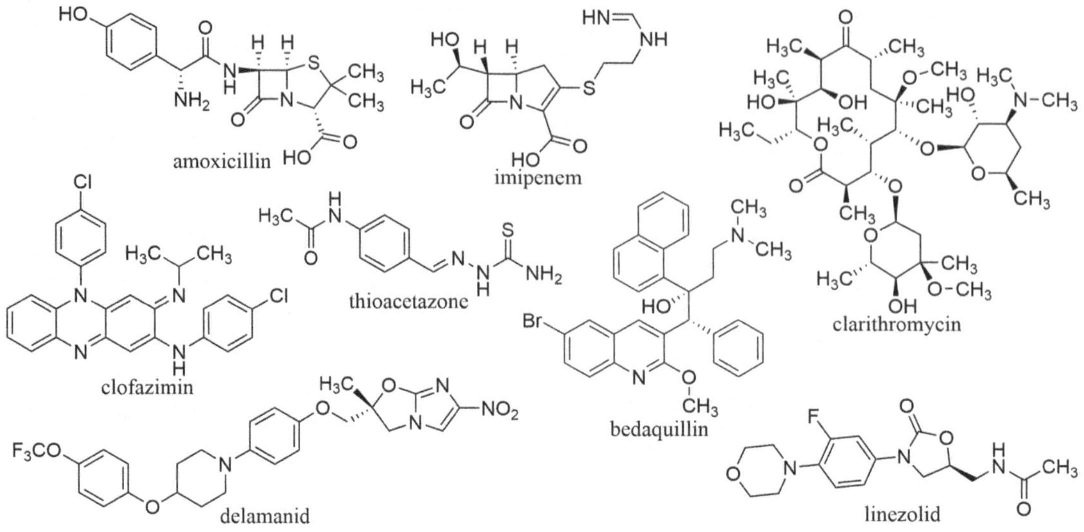

Fig. 21.5 Structures of the chosen drugs used for the treatment of MDR-TB

Solid lipid nanoparticles (SLNPs) for ocular delivery of INH showing extended drug release and enhanced ocular bioavailability and in vivo acute and repeat dose safety were reported by Singh et al. (2019).

A novel liposome-in-hydrogel system consisting of *N*′-dodecanoylisonicotinohydrazide loaded liposomes incorporated into a poly(lactic-co-glycolic acid) (PLGA)-polyethylene glycol (PEG)-PLGA hydrogel designed by Liu et al. (2019) showed thermo-responsive and self-healing properties, and after localized injection, it was able to maintain effective INH concentration by rapid drug release into synovial fluid, followed by a steady-state drug release lasting for several days suggesting promising potential of this nanoformulation for localized treatment of bone TB. Liposomes with encapsulated INH conjugated to Zn(II) phthalocyanine through hydrazone bonding fabricated by film hydration method with a particle size of ca. 506 nm, zeta potential of −55 mV, and 72% encapsulation efficiency (EE) showed pH-dependent behavior and released 22 and 100% INH in media with pH of 7.4 and 4.4, respectively, suggesting that using pH-labile linkages for the conjugation of the drug to phthalocyanines liposomal formulation showing controlled drug release could be prepared (Nkanga and Krause 2018).

Nanoconstructed polymeric micelles consisting of PEG-polylactic acid (PLA) di-block-copolymer conjugated to INH and loaded with rifampicin with particle size of 187.9 ± 2.68 nm and zeta potential of −8.15 ± 1.24 mV showed ca. eightfold reduction in the minimum inhibitory concentration (MIC) value compared to free drugs, being highly effective against sensitive *M. tuberculosis* strains (Rani et al. 2018).

INH loaded in optimized NPs of polymeric pH-sensitive nanogels fabricated using γ-radiation (50 kGy) induced polymerization of itaconic acid (IA) in aqueous solution of the template polymer (PVP) used at ratio PVP:IA = 30:70 exhibited eightfold lower MIC values against *M. tuberculosis* than INH solution, the drug release from the preparation being governed predominantly by the diffusion mechanism (Omar et al. 2017). Inhalation powder of lung-targeted genipin-cross-linked deacetylated CS/INH/rifampicin nanogel particles exhibited extended antibacterial activity due to long-term release of both drugs and a simple pulmonary dose of this formulation resulted in a therapeutic drug concentration in lungs (40–60%) and other organs (<5%) for 24 h (Wu et al. 2018). Fe_3O_4/hyperbranched polyester modified with (2-dodecen-1-yl)succinic anhydride/INH NPs showing magnetic properties, high drug-loading capacity, and EE and pH-responsive diffusion-controlled drug release with release rate being higher in an acidic buffer was reported as nanoformulation suitable for the treatment of TB (Lu et al. 2018). INH-filled Fe_2O_3 hollow nanospheres with a diameter <30 nm and 48 wt% INH-load that were functionalized with dextran showed powerful activity against *M. tuberculosis* and *M. tuberculosis*-infected macrophages (Leidinger et al. 2015).

Mesoporous bioactive glass/metal-organic framework scaffolds with macropores of ca. 400 μm and compressive strength of 3–7 MPa exhibiting good biocompatibility and apatite forming ability in vitro that were fabricated by 3D printing were able to control INH release rate and pH microenvironment due to the degradation of metal-organic framework, and these scaffolds could be used for treating osteoarticular TB (Pei et al. 2018). Carazo et al. (2019) described recently that self-assembling nanohybrids prepared from halloysite nanotubes and INH with an average diameter of 90 nm demonstrated good biocompatibility and enhanced permeability through Caco-2 cellular membranes.

21.3 Rifampicin

Rifampicin (RIF) is a semisynthetic ansamycin antibiotic produced from *Streptomyces mediterranei* with a broad antibacterial spectrum caused by inhibition of DNA-dependent RNA polymerase, thus suppressing RNA synthesis (Rifampicin 2019).

RIF-loaded SLNPs with an average diameter of 456 ± 11 nm and 84.12% EE showing drug loading of 15.68 ± 1.52% were characterized by long-term stability and could withstand various gastrointestinal tract media (Chokshi et al. 2018). Lipid NP formulations (SLNPs and nanostructured lipid carriers (NLCs)) encapsulating both INH and RIF prolonged encapsulated RIF release and improved its chemical stability in the presence of INH in a simulated gastric acidic environment, and in vitro cell culture studies showed their well-quantifiable uptake in a human alveolar macrophage cell line (Banerjee et al. 2018). Maretti et al. (2016) prepared RIF-loaded SLNP assemblies using the melt emulsifying technique followed by freeze-drying, whereby quick-freezing combined with a certain grade of sample dilution before the prefreezing step without the use of cryoprotectants exhibited the most favorable impact on powder respirability and the respirable fraction achieved >50%. Using the melt emulsifying technique, Maretti et al. (2017) fabricated SLNPs from biocompatible lipid components (cholesteryl myristate combined with palmitic acid or tripalmitin) in the presence of methyl α-D-mannopyranoside as the targeting moiety that after loading with RIF were found to be suitable for alveolar macrophage passive targeting and were able to maintain the required drug concentration within SLNPs along the respiratory tract before macrophage internalization. RIF-loaded SLNPs surface-decorated with novel mannose derivatives (conjugates of 2,3,4,6-tetra-*O*-acetyl-1-(2-aminoethyl)-α-D-mannose with carboxylic acids (C_8, C_{12}, C_{14}, and C_{16}) were able to more efficiently enter the macrophages (ca. 80%) than free RIF (ca. 20%) and nonfunctionalized SLNPs (ca. 40%) and caused a decrease of RIF intracellular concentration by 40% due to the saturated mannose receptors of J774 cells. Fine particle fraction of poor cohesive powder fabricated using these NPs represented ca. 30–50% and showed good respirability with the perspective to be used in anti-TB inhaled therapy (Maretti et al. 2019). Mannosylated NLC loaded with RIF with particle size ca. 315 nm and drug EE >90% showing pH-sensitive RIF release exhibited strong uptake by bone marrow-derived macrophages and efficiently decreased the intracellular growth of mycobacteria (Vieira et al. 2017). Mannosylated SLNPs encapsulating RIF with particle sizes ranging from 160 to 250 nm and drug EE ca. 75% showing improved internalization in macrophages were reported to be suitable for the selective delivery of RIF to macrophages (Vieira et al. 2018a). RIF loaded CS-coated SLNPs with a size of ca. 245–344 nm, a zeta potential of +40 mV, and >90% EE showed higher in vitro mucoadesive properties and higher permeability in alveolar epithelial cells A549 than uncoated

SLNPs suggesting their potential to be used for safe and efficient management of TB (Vieira et al. 2018b).

Using soy lecithin and low-molecular-weight CS, a lipopolysaccharide polyelectrolyte complex encapsulated RIF was prepared with mean particle size of 151.6 nm, zeta potential of +33.0 mV, and 64.25% EE showing a sustained release profile, and in ex vivo permeability studies, twofold increase in RIF permeability within 8 h was observed (Sumaila et al. 2019). RIF-loaded polymer-glycerosomes (vesicles composed of phospholipids, glycerol, and water), which were combined with trimethyl chitosan chloride or with sodium hyaluronate reduced the in vitro drug toxicity on A549 cells and showed improved efficacy against *Staphylococcus aureus* than the pure drug, and their intratracheal administration to rats resulted in improved RIF accumulation in lungs. Moreover, the aptitude of these vesicles to be nebulized was always higher than that of drug dispersion (Melis et al. 2016).

RIF-loaded nanolipid polymer composites fabricated by a microemulsion-spray-dry technique with particle sizes ranging from 382.5 to 561.8 nm, zeta potential from −32.5 to −26.5 mV, and drug EE 61.25–73.14% exhibiting an initial burst release of RIF followed by a controlled RIF release profile were designed by Mulla et al. (2017).

As a promising tool for the controlled delivery of RIF or other antitubercular drugs, wheat germ agglutinin conjugated SLNPs were reported as well (Pooja et al. 2015).

RIF-loaded alginate cellulose nanocrystal hybrid NPs with a particle size of 100 nm achieved using sonication exhibited pH-dependent swelling and a sustained in vitro drug release (Thomas et al. 2018a). Zinc-alginate beads with entrapped RIF showing a pH-dependent swelling behavior exhibited sustained drug release that was more prominent in pH 7.4 than 1.2 and showed good antibacterial activity (Thomas et al. 2018b). RIF-loaded Zn^{2+} ion cross-linked sodium alginate-g-allylamine-mannose polymer NPs (<300 nm) exhibited strong antimicrobial activities against *M. tuberculosis* and evaluation of the alveolar macrophage targeting via cellular uptake by A549 cells showed that Zn^{2+} concentration of the NPs increased the intracellular concentration of RIF and enhanced the antitubercular efficiency (Praphakar et al. 2017a). Sodium alginate coated with CS and Tween 80 NPs used as nanocarrier for co-delivery of RIF and ascorbic acid with mean particle size of 324.0 ± 40.7 nm, zeta potential of −28.52 ± 0.47 mV, and hydrophilic surface showed considerably higher antibacterial activity against nine clinical strains of *M. tuberculosis* than the free drug, whereby solid pellets easily redispersible after lyophilization and suitable for treatment of pulmonary TB infection could be prepared by the addition of sucrose (1% w/v) to the suspension of NPs (Scolari et al. 2019).

RIF encapsulated in octanoyl CS NPs prepared by the double emulsion solvent evaporation technique without cross-linking with an average hydrodynamic diameter of 253 ± 19.06 nm and EE of 64.86 ± 7.73% showed sustained release over 72 hours, the formulation was stable for >2 months, and due to superb aerosolization properties, it could be used for pulmonary delivery of drugs (Petkar et al. 2018). Phosphorylated low molecular weight κ-carrageenan-CS NPs fabricated by emulsification technique, followed by ionic gelation technique, in which both RIF and INH were loaded in an amorphous form, showed an initial burst release of drugs followed by regular prolonged releases and were reported to be suitable for antituberculosis multidrug delivery (Praphakar et al. 2017b, 2019). Biodegradable magnetic iron oxide NP cross-linked PEG hybrid CS gel beads loaded with RIF (70.20 ± 3.50 nm) and dual responsive to pH and the magnetic field showed higher RIF releasing efficacy at pH = 5.0 (maximum efficiency of 71.00 ± 0.87%), whereby this efficacy could be modified by altering the external magnetic field and the weight percentage of PEG (Kesavan et al. 2018). Both RIF and rifabutin-loaded CS MPs with mass median aerodynamic diameter ca. 5 μm and fine particle fractions of 21.46–29.97% showed sustained in vitro drug release in simulated lung fluid of pH 7.4 (12 h for RIF and 96 h for RFB), the MPs were internalized within the human macrophage cell line in vitro, and their administration did not show local adverse effects in Sprague Dawley rats (Pai et al. 2016). INH- and RIF-loaded spray-dried inhalable CS NPs with a mean shape of 230 ± 4.5 nm were found to be more effective against the mycobacterium than free drugs, and until 24 h post nebulization, both drugs were detected in lungs, liver, spleen, and kidney suggesting that the formulation could be used for effective treatment of TB (Garg et al. 2016).

Synthesis and characterization of acetylated amylose and development of inclusion complexes with RIF showing a mean size of 70–100 nm were described by Ribeiro et al. (2017).

Antibiotics such as RIF, ciprofloxacin, and erythromycin loaded into nanocarriers prepared from β-cyclodextrin (β-CD) grafted with D-mannose or D-glucose were reported to show antibacterial activity against *Escherichia coli*, *Pseudomonas aeruginosa*, *Acinetobacter*, and *S. aureus*, including methicillin-resistant strains, and they can potentiate the activity of these antibiotics, especially against multidrug-resistant bacteria (Li et al. 2016). The evaluation of the effectiveness of powders prepared from highly branched cyclic dextrin in the pulmonary delivery of a single-dosage form of INH and RIF showed that they had higher emitted dose and fine-particle fractions than formulations fabricated with lactose, maltose, sucrose, β-CD, and methyl β-CD as well as the highest drug content suggesting that highly branched cyclic dextrin used as an excipient is suitable for a single-dosage preparation of INH and RIF (Kadota et al. 2017). RIF and levofloxacin complexed with CD and conjugated to curdlan NPs showed sustained release of both the drugs over a prolonged period of time. They killed more than 95% of *M. smegmatis* within the macrophages (Basha et al. 2019).

RIF loaded 1,3-β-glucan functionalized PLGA NPs enhanced the intracellular pharmacokinetics of RIF in THP-1 derived macrophages causing at least a ten-fold increase in the uptake of RIF (Tukulula et al. 2018).

RIF-loaded *N*-(2-hydroxypropyl) methacrylamide–PLGA NPs with a mean particle size of 260.3 ± 2.21 nm and a zeta potential of −6.63 ± 1.28 mV showed sustained drug release and ca. fourfold higher antibacterial activity against sensitive *M. tuberculosis* strain than the free RIF (Rani et al. 2019). Matryoshka-type gastroresistant formulation of RIF-loaded PLGA NPs with methacrylic acid–ethyl acrylate coating, which could release RIF under simulated intestinal conditions, however, due to coating being protected from degradation under simulated gastric conditions, exhibited a sustained drug release and was found to be more effective in elimination of *M. tuberculosis* when applying against infected macrophages than the free drug (Andreu et al. 2019). Nonspherical RIF-loaded PLGA MPs for inhalation fabricated using L-leucine and L-aspartic acid (which were added in aqueous phase) were prepared using a spray-dryer via emulsion. The fine particle fraction (<4.7 μm) of MPs obtained with a leucine concentration of 0.2% (w/v) achieved 6.9-fold higher value compared to conventional MPs (43.4 ± 5.7% vs. 6.3 ± 4.0%), whereby the phagocytic ratio of alveolar macrophages (rat alveolar macrophage derived NR8383 cells) observed with MPs prepared in the presence of leucine was considerably higher and the RIF concentration in alveolar macrophages reached 0.34 ± 0.16 μg/mL (Takeuchi et al. 2018). PLGA NPs loaded with RIF and INH benzhydrazone (showing 15-fold higher drug loading in PLGA NPs than INH) exhibited slow and sustained release over a period of 1 month and more effectively inhibited *M. tuberculosis* H37Rv strain than free drugs. RIF loaded in PLGA NPs consistently inhibited the growth at 70% MIC of pure RIF (1 μg/mL), while INH benzhydrazone loaded PLGA NPs as well as pure INH benzhydrazone showed inhibition at MIC equivalent to the MIC of INH (0.1 μg/mL) (Hakkimane et al. 2018). RIF, INH, and pyrazinamide-loaded branched PLGA–PEG based copolymer NPs were designed by Gajendiran et al. (2019) for the controlled release of the drugs. This formulation demonstrated sustained release of RIF for 840 h, INH for 72 h, and pyrazinamide for 720 h.

Smooth, sphere-like INH- and RIF-loaded bovine serum albumin NPs with a mean diameter of 60.5 ± 4.6 nm and 87.8% and 98.0% EE for

INH and RIF, respectively, exhibited slow and sustained drug release resulting in 97% INH cumulative release in 6 days and full release of RIF in 5 days (Ge et al. 2018a). Intravenous administration of INH- and RIF-loaded bovine serum albumin NPs in rabbits was found to maintain effective blood plasma concentrations of both drugs for an extended period of time, and nanoformulations showed also good and sustained in vitro release effects (Ge et al. 2018b).

Rifampicin (RIF) NP surface functionalized with a tuftsin-modified peptide exhibited a controlled drug release profile; they were not cytotoxic and were pronouncedly more internalized by macrophages due to selective recognition of receptors located on infected alveolar macrophages than nonfunctionalized RIF NPs, being twofold more effective against *M. tuberculosis* than free RIF (Carneiro et al. 2019).

RIF-loaded porous polycaprolactone (PCL) microspheres prepared by oil-in-oil emulsion solvent evaporation method showing a porous structure, particle diameters from 50.54 to 57.34 μm, and an EE up to 61.86% at drug-loading content of 1.51% exhibited controlled release (80% of the drug released after 10 days) and antibacterial activity against *S. aureus* (Mei et al. 2018). Spherical RIF-loaded CS-graft-PCL/ferulic acid (FA) polymer micelles with a mean size of 100–210 nm were found to release RIF and FA at pH 5.3 much faster than at pH 7.4 because swelling of the micelles at lower pH values connected with the rapid degradation of ester and amide bonds present in the micelles, and this nanoformulation successfully entered into A549 cell lines (Praphakar et al. 2017c). Mucoadhesive guar gum hydrogel interconnected CS-g-PCL micelles loaded with RIF showed antibacterial activity against *Klebsiella pneumoniae* and *S. aureus* and excellent activity against THP-1 cells causing apoptosis in a time-dependent manner, suggesting their potential to be used for the intracellular alveolar macrophage treatment (Yuan et al. 2019).

Methoxy-PEG-b-PCL NPs loaded with RIF with particle sizes 20–110 nm were efficiently taken up by macrophages and depending on polymer blocks' molecular weights showed the cell uptake half-lives to be 2.4–21 min and the degradation half-lives from 51.6 min to ca. 20 h after the internalization. Moreover, using a zebrafish model of TB, these NPs were notably more potent compared to free RIP (Trousil et al. 2019). RIF encapsulated within nanopolymersomes prepared using di- and tri-block PEG-PCL copolymers enhanced the apparent RIF aqueous solubility and promoted drug accumulation in macrophages (RAW 264.7) compared to RIF solution (Moretton et al. 2015). Norbornene (NOR)-PEG-INH and NOR-PEG-RIF copolymers containing encapsulated INH and RIF in NOR exhibited antibacterial activity against H37Rv strain of *M. tuberculosis* with MIC values of 0.05 μg/mL and 0.5 μg/mL, respectively, and low drug dosages of drugs in NOR nanocarrier showed activity comparable with free INH and RIF (Kumarasingam et al. 2018).

Mucoadhesive RIF-Gantrez™ AN-119 NPs hydrophobized with ethyl cellulose with a mean particle size of 400–450 nm when administered intraduodenally in rats showed higher Peyer's patch uptake and an increased lung/plasma RIF ratio indicating lymph-mediated lung targeting. Moreover, a significantly higher lung/liver ratio observed with these NPs suggested lower hepatic exposure (Bachhav et al. 2018).

Biodegradable amino acid-based poly(ester amide) NPs with encapsulated RIF showed higher antibacterial activity of RIF against *M. smegmatis* than free RIF and cellular uptake in NR8383 cells suggesting their potential application in treating TB (Praphakar et al. 2016).

RIF incorporated to solidified self-nanoemulsifying drug delivery system demonstrated immediate release (85% of RIF within 15 min) and improved pharmacokinetic profiles in comparison with RIF suspension (Hussain et al. 2019).

Citric acid-coated magnetite NPs in conjunction with either IHN or RIF showing a mean diameter of 9 nm were uptaken by *M. smegmatis*, and they enhanced the membrane permeability by promoting a higher influx of drugs into the cells and ensured a twofold higher intracellular RIF concentration compared with that of free drugs (Padwal et al. 2015). Magnetically targeted co-delivery of hydrophilic (INH) and hydrophobic (RIF) antitubercular drugs loaded in hollow mesoporous ferrite NPs was reported as a delivery system with enhanced chemotherapeutic effect (Xu et al. 2018).

Moradi et al. (2018) simultaneously loaded RIF and INH into graphene oxide (GO) and the drug-loaded nanocarriers were coated with biopolymers (CS and gum tragacanth) achieving diameters of 120–130 nm. This formulation released 93% of INH after 60 h, and 88% of RIF after 72 h, whereby the co-loaded nanocarriers exhibited the same efficacy against *M. tuberculosis* as pure drugs in their MIC concentrations.

21.4 Pyrazinamide

Pyrazinamide (PZA) is a prodrug that is converted by pyrazinamidase to the active form of pyrazinoic acid that inhibits the effect of fatty acid synthase (FAS)-I and FAS-II enzymes that synthesize short-chain mycolic acids (FAS-I) and longer-chain mycolic acids (FAS II). Another unspecific effect is caused by accumulation of pyrazinoic acid, which reduces the intracellular pH resulting in inactivation of enzymes. PZA acts bactericidally on dormant strains and thus accelerates TB treatment (Pyrazinamide 2019).

Karmakar et al. (2018) incorporated PZA in NLC fabricated using hydrogenated soy phosphatidylcholine, tristearin, and oleic acid and surface modified by PEG 2000 (contributing to the enhancement of their steric stability due to introduction of additional layer representing a preventative barrier toward the expulsion of surface accumulated drug). This nanoformulation showing improved EE and drug loading exhibited a sustained release profile.

Following a single nebulization of SLNPs incorporating RIF, INH, and PZA that were prepared by the emulsion solvent diffusion technique, to guinea pigs the therapeutic drug concentrations were maintained in the plasma for 5 days and in the organs (lungs, liver, and spleen) for 7 days, while free drugs were cleared within 1 or 2 days, and nanoformulations showed a sevenfold higher mean residence time and drug bioavailability. Moreover, nebulization of drug-loaded SLNPs to infected guinea pigs on every 7th day indicated that no tubercle bacilli were detected in the lungs/spleen after seven doses of treatment, while for an equivalent therapeutic benefit, 46 daily doses of orally administered free drugs were necessary (Pandey and Khuller 2005).

Alginate NPs encapsulating INH, RIF, PZA, and ethambutol fabricated by controlled cation-induced gelification of alginate with a mean particle size of 235.5 nm and high EE (70–90% for INH and PZA, 80–90% for RIF and 88–95% for ethambutol) showed pronouncedly higher bioavailabilities compared to free drugs. This was reflected in the fact that after administration of the encapsulated drugs the drug levels exceeding MIC_{90} were observed in organs until day 15, while upon free drug administration, the drug levels >MIC_{90} were estimated only up to day 1 (Ahmad et al. 2006).

Using Taguchi method the optimized PZA-loaded PLGA NPs were prepared by the double emulsion method showing particle size approx. 170 nm, zeta potential of about −1 mV, 7–8% EE, and a drug loading of 3.1% (Pham et al. 2015). PEGylated PLGA NPs encapsulating RIF, moxifloxacin, and PZA fabricated using the water-in-oil-in-water double emulsification method with poly(vinyl alcohol) (PVA) as a stabilizer were reported to be suitable to target the niche of *M. tuberculosis*, and their application in the therapy could reduce the drug dosing frequency or increase the dosing interval (Adesina et al. 2015). Just three oral doses of PLGA NPs encapsulating ethambutol in combination with PLGA NPs encapsulating RIF + INZ + PZA to *M. tuberculosis* H37Rv infected mice administered on every 10th day resulted in undetectable bacilli in the organs replacing 28 conventional doses of free drugs suggesting that the therapy using a four-drug combination could shorten the duration of TB chemotherapy and reduce the dosing frequency (Pandey et al. 2006). The chemotherapeutic efficacy in *M. tuberculosis* H37Rv-infected guinea pigs at the subtherapeutic dose was reported also for PLGA NPs loaded with antitubercular drugs RIF, INH, and PZA (Sharma et al. 2004a), and wheat germ agglutinin-coated PLGA NPs were recommended as oral/aerosolized carriers of RIF, INH, and PZA for treatment of TB (Sharma et al. 2004b).

High therapeutic efficacy of PZA liposomes prepared using dipalmitoyl phosphatidyl choline and cholesterol at a ratio of 7:2, injected twice weekly to mice infected by *M. tuberculosis*, was reported by El-Ridy et al. (2007).

Nanocomposites of natural silk sericin grafted over the maleate gellan gum surface and CS, which were loaded with RIF and PZA, exhibited sustained release of 79% RF and 82% PZA for 120 h at pH 4.0 and showed improved antimycobacterial activity and rapid delivery of drugs at TB-infected macrophage, whereby the nanoformulation was effectively internalized into the bacterial cells and MH-S cells and release of both drugs inside the cells resulted in the damage of the cell membrane (Mehnath et al. 2019). Multidrug delivery system consisting of CS-g-(cetyl alcohol-maleic anhydride-PZA) polymeric micelles with incorporated RIF and entrapped AgNPs on micelles exhibited controlled release behavior and was able to enhance the biocompatibility and cytotoxic effect on the cells reflected in reduced cell viability and higher cell apoptosis, and it could be considered as a candidate for immediate therapeutic effects for alveolar macrophages (Praphakar et al. 2018).

RIF, PZA, and INH encapsulated within the hydrophobic core of micelles (singly or in dual combination) formed by self-assembly of PVP-PCL diblock copolymers with varying chain lengths showing sizes from 150 to 205 nm and the critical micelle concentration (CMC) in order 1–10 μM released the drugs in vitro (phosphate-buffered saline (PBS) solution at 37 °C) in a sustained manner following the order INH > PZA > RIF (Veeren et al. 2013).

Spherical PZA loaded polymeric (Eudragit® RS-100) NPs prepared by simultaneous double-emulsion (w/o/w) solvent evaporation/diffusion technique with particle sizes ranging from 45.51 to 300.4 nm and drug EE of 80.9% exhibited after early burst release a controlled release over a period of 24 h and they were found to be effectively uptaken by alveolar macrophages (Varma et al. 2015).

Inhalation technology allows the delivery of the drug to lesions rapidly and without first-pass toxicity. Toxicity of PZA does not enable to increase sufficiently the dose at administration per os. However, using the inhalation with pyrazinoic acid, which would acidify pulmonary lesions, as an adjunct therapy, the enhancement of the bactericidal activity of the orally administered PZA could be observed. Considering that most resistance arises in the pncA gene that converts PZA to pyrazinoic acid, the above treatment could act on most PZA-resistant strains (Mitchison and Fourie 2010). Addition of L-leucine and using an ethanolic solvent positively affected the physicochemical properties and aerodynamic behavior of nano spray-dried PZA-L-leucine powders; the best aerosolization performance was observed with the co-spray dried PZA with 20% L-leucine in a 10% ethanol feed solvent (Kaewjan and Srichana 2016).

21.5 Ethambutol

Ethambutol (EMB) is a synthetic antitubercular agent inhibiting arabinosyl transferases, i.e., the bacterial cell wall complex production is inhibited and thus increases cell wall permeability. In addition, it inhibits RNA synthesis and decreases replication. EMB exhibits side effects and cellular toxicity (Ethambutol 2019). The comparison of an untreated and EMB-treated *M. smegmatis* mc(2)155 using proteomic analysis showed that among 22 identified proteins 16 were over-expressed and 6 under-expressed, whereby these proteins predominantly affected energy metabolism as well as synthesis and modification of macromolecules (Jiang et al. 2011).

In experimental *M. avium* infection in mice, the chemotherapeutic effects of weekly administered PLGA NPs containing encapsulated antitubercular drugs with negative zeta potential and particle sizes 227.3 ± 16.4 nm for rifabutin, 334.35 ± 11.7 nm for azithromycin, and 509.85 ± 20.5 nm for EMB showing sustained release of drugs inside the plasma and organs were found to be equivalent to daily administered free drugs (Grewal et al. 2018).

Ahmad et al. (2015) designed a dimple-shaped CS carrier for delivering EMB dihydrochloride from a dry powder inhaler to the lungs, in which spherical CS carriers had a dimpled surface. This provided shallow cavities to which the drug was bound and the mass median aerodynamic diameter of the drug ranged from 2.3 to 2.7 μm, with the fine particle fractions (aerosolized particles <4.4 μm) representing 32–42% of the nominal dose. Encapsulation of EMB HCl in nisosomes prepared by the thin-film hydration method resulted in controlled drug release and the formulation was able to deliver more drugs to mice lungs for a prolonged period of time resulting in decreased bacterial counts in lung homogenates (El-Ridy et al. 2015).

Spherical EMB NPs prepared by double-emulsion solvent evaporation method using PCL polymer and PVA emulsifier with particle sizes 280–300 nm labeled with ^{99m}Tc were reported to be applicable for both imaging and therapy of TB, because almost 18% of the NPs were uptaken by the lungs in male C57Bl/6 mice infected with *Mycobacterium bovis* BCG (Neto et al. 2019).

Nemati et al. (2019) fabricated biocompatible nontoxic dry powder inhaler formulations by spray-drying of EMB-loaded SLNs with and without mannitol showing particle size <100 nm and > 98% EE, which could be used for the direct pulmonary treatment of TB.

Nanoformulation of EMB with multifunctional GO and magnetic NPs exhibited sustained release in PBS solution at two physiological pH (7.4 and 4.8) and antibacterial activity against *M. smegmatis* with the effective MIC of 2.1 μg/mL, while this nanoformulation was not toxic to eukaryotic 3T3 cells (Saifullah et al. 2017a). The nanodelivery formulation composed of EMB loaded on GO showed high biocompatibility with mouse fibroblast cells and good antimycobacterial activity against *M. smegmatis* with an effective MIC of 0.72 μg/mL. However, ETB-GO inhibited *M. smegmatis* biofilm formation at effective concentration 1.496 μg/mL, which is higher than the MIC of the planktonic bacterial cells (0.39 μg/mL) suggesting that the slow release of the drug is not effective against a biofilm colony (Saifullah et al. 2017b).

21.6 Other Antitubercular Used Drugs

21.6.1 Drugs of Natural Origin: Antibiotics

Cycloserine (D-4-aminoisoxazolidin-3-on) is an antibiotic produced by *Streptomyces garyphalus*. It is a cyclic serinamide that inhibits L-alanine racemase (generates D-alanine from L-alanine) and D-alanylalanine synthetase that incorporates D-alanine into the pentapeptide that is needed for peptidoglycan synthesis, thus blocking cell wall synthesis (Cycloserine 2019). Poly(butyl cyanoacrylate) nanocapsules prepared by interfacial polymerization of miniemulsions, which were loaded with D-cycloserine, showed EE in the range of 39–51% and an in vitro initial burst release of the drug followed by a slow release. It could be mentioned that the relevant physicochemical and technological properties of prepared nanocapsules were pronouncedly affected by the external oil phase used (Musumeci et al. 2011).

Kanamycin is a bacteriocidal aminoglycoside antibiotic isolated from the bacterium *Streptomyces kanamyceticus*. Kanamycin is most commonly used in the form of kanamycin sulfate (KAS), and it is administered in parenteral form. KAS is a *M. tuberculosis* protein synthesis inhibitor (irreversibly binds to 30S-subunit of ribosome and 16S rRNA) with a very short plasma half-life of 2.5 h, and high doses of this drug needed to reach the therapeutic levels in the plasma result in serious nephrotoxicity/ototoxicity (Kanamycin 2019). KAS-loaded PLGA vitamin E TPGS (D-α-*tocopherol* polyethylene glycol succinate) MPs and NPs showed sustained drug release up to 10 and 13 days, respectively, in PBS at pH 7.4, whereby the $AUC_{0\text{-inf}}$ value of nanoscale formulation estimated in the in vivo pharmacokinetic test in Wistar rats was approx. 1.62-fold higher than that of microscale formulation. Using nanoscale formulation also a 1.20-fold increase in the KAS uptake through the alveolar macrophage was observed as well (Mustafa et al. 2016). KAS-PLGA-TPGS NPs surface modified by affixation of PEG and adsorption of water-soluble CS to the particle surface showing a zeta potential of +3.61 mV exhibited pronounced prolongation in blood circulation, reduced protein binding, and considerable prolongation of blood circulation half-life resulting in reduced kidney sequestration compared to the unmodified KAS-PLGA-TPGS NPs suggesting that such nanoformulation could reduce the frequency of KAS dosing, and thus decrease the incidence of nephrotoxicity/ototoxicity (Mustafa et al. 2017a). Conjugation of KAS with AuNPs resulted also in a notable reduction of its MIC values against bacterial strains of *E. coli* DH5α, *Micrococcus luteus*, and *S. aureus* compared to its free form (Saha et al. 2007).

Amikacin (AMK) is a semi-synthetic aminoglycoside antibiotic that is derived from above-mentioned kanamycin (Amikacin 2019). Spherical AMK-loaded PLGA NPs showing a particle size of 260.3 ± 2.05 nm, a zeta potential of −12.9 ± 1.12 mV, and drug content of 40.10 ± 1.87 μg/mg prepared by double emulsion solvent evaporation exhibited biphasic release pattern, improved permeation across intestinal epithelium due to the uptake of NPs by Peyer's patches of intestinal epithelium, and endocytic uptake via enterocytes as well as antibacterial activity against *P. aeruginosa*, *K. pneumoniae*, and *E. coli* (Fatima et al. 2018, 2019). Atyabi et al. (2009) prepared thiolated CS NPs as an oral delivery system for AMK. In AMK loaded NPs (mean size of 280 nm), which were prepared by gelation using tripolyphosphate, the formation of disulfide bond was obtained by a time-dependent oxidation process and the formulation showed antibacterial activity against *P. aeruginosa* and *Staphylococcus*.

Loading of AMK, lipid solubility of which was improved by hydrophobic ion pairing with sodium myristyl sulfate, into self-emulsifying delivery systems resulted in up to twofold higher drug amounts permeating through the cystic fibrosis mucus compared with control, and the formulation exhibited sustained release of AMK (Hetenyi et al. 2018). Investigation of AMK-loaded liposomes surface-modified by adsorption of PEG 4000, Tween 80, poloxamer 407, and gelatin showed that highest serum levels in mice were obtained with administration of the PEG- and Tween 80-modified liposomes, while gelatin-modified liposomes increased the AMK concentration in the liver from 36 to 66 mg/kg suggesting that surface modification of liposomes effectively altered the organ distribution of compounds. Moreover, 14% of α-2-macroglobulin was adsorbed on the gelatin liposomes (Bucke et al. 1998).

AMK loaded in cholesterol SLNPs and administered through pulmonary route to male rats by Microsprayer® resulted in higher drug concentration in lungs than kidneys suggesting that such formulation applied for pulmonary delivery could reduce the side effects of the drug in kidneys, while sustained drug release from formulation enables to prolong the drug dosing intervals (Varshosaz et al. 2013). AMK-loaded SLNPs, which were lyophilized using cryoprotectants in order to increase their stability, showed twofold lower MIC and MBC values compared to the free drug suggesting that fewer doses of this formulation could be efficient in the treatment of the infection with less adverse effects and more safety. Zeta potential of lyophilized particles was increased to +17 mV from +4 mV before lyophilization and storage of particles at a higher temperature resulted in accelerated drug release (Ghaffari et al. 2011).

Capreomycin (CPM) is a cyclic peptide antibiotic produced by *Streptomyces capreolus* that inhibits protein synthesis by binding to the 70S ribosomal unit (Capreomycin 2019). CPM-Pd and ofloxacin-Pd loaded PLA MPs were fabricated by spray-drying of noncolloidal particle dispersions in acetonitrile PLA solution in fast-drying regime, and it was found that morphology of feedstock particles predominantly determined the MPs morphology and it could be considered as a major parameter influencing final MP properties (Giovagnoli et al. 2014). CPM combined in solution with hydrophobic counterions like oleate, linoleate, and linolenate resulted in hydrophobic ion-pairs that were spray-dried, and it was found that application of mini as well as nano spray-dryer was suitable to maintain a high ion-paired content in the case of CPM oleate, while for CPM linoleate and linolenate the mini spray-dryer was the most appropriate. The antibacterial efficacy of CPM oleate and linoleate against *M. tuberculosis* was comparable with that of CPM sulfate, while that of CPM linolenate was lower. Considering the lowest toxic potential for CPM oleate, this compound is the most promising to be used as supergenerics in pulmonary TB treatment (Schoubben et al. 2013). Poly(ethyl cyanoacrylate) NPs loaded with CPM sulfate were designed and investigated as well (Zhaparova et al. 2012). In vitro studies of CPM sulfate release from poly(ethyl cyanoacrylate) NPs performed also by Burkeev et al. (2013) confirmed the potential of this formulation in treatment of TB. pH-responsive polymeric nanocapsules were fabricated by Loiko et al. (2013) using the reversible addition-fragmentation chain transfer–based vesicle templating approach in the presence of CPM sulfate. The most stable hollow latex particles were obtained with the monomer composition of *N,N*-(dimethylamino) ethyl methacrylate/methyl methacrylate (1:1) used for the formation of the polymeric shells, and the EE of the drug reached approx. 70%. The relatively fast drug release from these nanocapsules at pH 6.5 could be slowed by using a thicker polymer shell.

Rifapentine (RFP) is an ansamycin antibiotic that similar to RIF specifically interacts with bacterial RNA polymerase (Rifapentine 2019). RFP highly binds (98%) to plasma proteins resulting in low concentrations in the lungs at oral administration. These limitations could be overcome by inhalation of crystalline RFP; however, the delivery of crystalline RFP particles in BALB/c mice by intratracheal insufflation at a dose of 20 mg/kg caused a transient neutrophil-associated inflammatory response in the lungs that resolved over 7 days suggesting that the applied dose for pulmonary delivery of RFP could be limited to once a week at a dose $\leq$20 mg/kg (Parumasivam et al. 2017). RFP-linezolid-loaded PLGA MPs prepared using the oil-in-water emulsion solvent evaporation method showing a particle size of 27.38 ± 1.28 μm and an EE of 55.53 ± 0.78 and 16.87 ± 0.47% for RFP and linezolid, respectively, released 21.37 ± 0.68% RFP in 3 days and 43.56 ± 2.54% linezolid in 1 day followed by a sustained release phase when the drugs were retained on the surface of bronchial mucosa of canines for 20 days, suggesting that MPs loaded with multiple anti-TB drugs could be used in the bronchoscopic interventional therapy of cavitary pulmonary TB (Huang et al. 2017).

Rifabutin (RFB) is another ansamycin antibiotics with the same mode of action as abovementioned. RFB is used for the treatment of TB infections as well as *M. avium* complex (MAC) infection in immunocompromised and/or HIV patients (Rifabutin 2019). RFB encapsulated in glyceryl monostearate NPs (of 345 ± 17.96 nm) fabricated by the solvent diffusion evaporation method showed sustained drug release in simulated intestinal fluid (pH 6.8) up to 48 h and PBS (pH 7.4) up to 7 days, and following a single oral administration of these SLNPs, the therapeutic drug concentrations in plasma and in the tissues (lungs, liver, and spleen) were maintained for 4 and 7 days, respectively. The fivefold higher oral bioavailability of RFB from SLNPs than that observed with the administration of free RFB suggested that using this formulation could result in a decreased dose and dosing frequency for successful management of MAC infection (Nirbhavane et al. 2017). The RFB-loaded SLNPs, which were included in spherical microspheres using excipients like mannitol and trehalose through a spray-drying technique, achieved the tested organs 15 and 30 min post pulmonary administration in vivo and exhibited enhanced activity against *M. tuberculosis* infection in a murine model of infection with a *M. tuberculosis* strain H37Rv (Gaspar et al. 2017).

β-Glucan particles (GP) prepared from yeast cells by acidic and alkaline extraction spray dried prior to RFB loading and sealing of GP pores with calcium alginate hydrogel showing particle sizes in the range from 2.9 to 6.1 μm (>75% if particles were below 3.5 μm), an EE of 81.46 ± 4.9%, and drug loading approx. 40.5 ± 1.9% exhibited a sustained release via diffusion and were phagocytosed by macrophage(s) within 5 min (Upadhyay et al. 2017). Exposure of glucan MPs loaded with RFB NPs was found to augment a robust innate immune response including the induction of reactive oxygen and nitrogen species, autophagy, and apoptosis within *M. tuberculosis*-infected J774 macrophage cells, and in a test performed in murine macrophage, this formulation showed approx. 2.5-fold higher efficiency than free RFB (Upadhyay et al. 2019). Spray-dried konjac glucomannan MPs developed to provide direct lung delivery of a combination of RFB and INH by inhalation, in which the drugs were associated to MPs with efficiencies of 88–104%, were designed by Guerreiro et al. (2019). Cunha et al. (2018) fabricated inhalable fucoidan MPs associating simultaneously INH (97%) and RFB (95%) and showing adequate aerodynamic properties for pulmonary delivery with a mass median aerodynamic diameter of 3.6–3.9 μm that could be captured by macrophages in a dose-dependent manner. These MPs are able to activate the target cells, which were reflected in effective inhibition of mycobacterial growth in vitro.

21.6.2 Drugs of Synthetic Origin

Ofloxacin (OFX) is a "cidal" synthetic antibacterial chemotherapeutic agent from the class of fluoroquinolones (the second generation) inhibiting DNA gyrase (bacterial toposiomerase II) and toposiomerase IV, i.e., suppresses DNA replication (Ofloxacin 2019). Wu et al. (2014) investigated the effect of hyaluronic acid (HA) and polylysine as internal phase additives on the efficiency of PLGA microspheres to encapsulate hydrophilic OFX and found that microspheres with HA inside showed higher drug loading amounts than those with polylysin inside, whereby increasing both polyelectrolytes in the internal phase burst release could be observed, the release rate of the microspheres with polylysin being faster. The in vitro uptake of OFX from OFX-loaded glutaraldehyde-cross-linked CS microspheres prepared using a water-in-oil emulsification method with a particle size of 1–6 μm and drug content of 27% (w/w) to alveolar macrophages (NR8383) was markedly improved compared to free drug, which was reflected in >3.5-fold greater cellular OFX concentrations at 4 and 24 h after the application suggesting potential of such formulation for pulmonary inhalation (Park et al. 2013). Investigation of respirable OFX MPs and NPs and multifunctional antibiotic particles with or without lung surfactant 1,2-dipalmitoyl-sn-glycero-3-phosphocholine (DPPC) for targeted dry powder inhalation delivery as a pulmonary nanomedicine showed that residual partial crystallinity influenced aerosol dispersion of OFX and most of the compositions of OFX-DPPC inhalation powders (Duan et al. 2013). Liposomal formulations encapsulating RIF and OFX with particle size of 160.6 nm showing EE of 66.89 ± 10.9% and 40.61 ± 8.7% for RIF and OFX, respectively, and superb antimycobacterial activity that were characterized with notable colloidal stability up to 120 days were reported as an effective theranostic agent against mycobacterial infections in the mouse model (Kaul et al. 2016). Nanosystem $MnFe_2O_4$ with surface modified by CS prolonged the release of OFX in a controlled manner sustained for a period of 3 days. Thus this formulation can be used for intestinal targeted drug delivery through oral administration by avoiding the drug release in the highly acidic gastric fluid region of the stomach (Taavoni-Gilan 2019).

Levofloxacin (LOFX) is the optically active L-isomer of OFX (Levofloxacin 2019). Lopez-Lopez et al. (2019) reported that the emulsion-solvent evaporation method using dichloromethane as organic solvent is the best method for fabrication of LOFX loaded PLGA NPs exhibiting slow drug release. However, the antibacterial activity of these NPs against *Enterococcus faecalis* CECT 481, *S. aureus* ATCC 27697, *E. coli* CECT 101, and *P. aeruginosa* ATCC 27853 was approximately half of that corresponding to the pure drug, while for *Mycobacterium phlei* CECT 3009 and *K. pneumoniae* CECT 143, the antibacterial efficiency of the pure LOFX was approx. fourfold higher. NPs of fluoroquinolone antibiotics prepared using oil-in-water (o/w) microemulsion formulation comprising *N*-butyl acetate/Tween 80/ethanol/water exhibited high drug loadings (4.20 wt% LOFX, 3.16 wt% CPX, 2.53 wt% MOX, 1.36 wt% gatifloxacin, and 0.70 wt% OFX), whereby the drugs were accumulated at the interface layer of the micelle, which can support controlled release of the drug during systemic circulation. Moreover, lyophilized LOFX showed long-term stability, amorphous morphology, and improved dissolution rate (Saleem et al. 2018). Floating liquid crystalline molecularly imprinted polymer coated carbon nanotubes for LOFX delivery were reported by Zhang et al. (2018). LOFX loaded CS NPs converted into the sol-gel system to enhance the corneal residence time for ocular delivery were designed by Ameeduzzafar et al. (2018). PVA composite nanofibers containing conjugated LOFX-CS enabled minimizing the burst release behavior and achieving sustained release of the drug (Jalvandi et al. 2017). An overview of lipid-based nanosized delivery systems for fluoroquinolones was presented by Furneri et al. (2017). Improvement of LOFX antibacterial activity by conjugation with AuNPs was described as well (Bagga et al. 2017).

Ciprofloxacin (CPX) belongs also to the second generation of fluoroquinolones (Ciprofloxacin 2019). CPX has limited aqueous solubility that was significantly increased by Aytac et al. (2019) who complexed CPX into hydroxypropyl-β-CDs with a diameter of 90 nm. Optimized lipid-polymer hybrid NPs (LPNPs) loaded with both INH and CPX hydrochloride fabricated by the double-emulsification solvent evaporation method showed particle sizes 111.81 ± 1.2 and 172.23 ± 2.31 nm, respectively, and they exhibited sustained and controlled release at lower pH and addition of PLGA in LPNPs as the polymeric core resulted in a stable product. The spray-dried powder of drug-loaded LPNPs produced nanoaggregates showing suitable morphology, density, flowability, and reconstitutibility for inhaled drug delivery and reached maximum internalization efficiency in vivo (Bhardwaj et al. 2016a). 4-Aminophenyl-α-D-mannopyranoside was used as a surface functionalized ligand for fabrication of ligand-anchored pH-sensitive liposomes prepared by thin film hydration for the combined delivery of INH and CPX HCl. The liposomes exhibited slow release at alkaline pH (58–64%) as compared to macrophage pH (81–87%) and achieved a much higher concentration in the alveolar macrophage compared to conventional pH-sensitive liposomes suggesting that they could be used for the targeted drug therapy in pulmonary TB (Bhardwaj et al. 2016b). CPX loaded poly(isobutyl cyanoacrylate) NPs were found to be more potent against MAC in human macrophages than the free drug (Fawaz et al. 1998). Encapsulated CPX nanocrystals in liposomes consisting of sucrose, magnesium stearate, and isoleucine showed controlled drug release and were suitable for delivery of CPX by inhalation as an aerosol (Khatib et al. 2019) similar to CPX-loaded polymeric nanomicelles (Farhangi et al. 2019).

The NO-releasing CPX 2-methoxy-4-(3-[4′-(nitrooxy)butoxy]-3-oxo-1-propenyl]phenyl ester exhibited significant antimicrobial activity against both extracellular and intracellular *M. tuberculosis* H37Rv strains also at low-nanomolar concentrations when the unaltered CPX was ineffective, which might both shorten the time of the chemotherapy and reduce the rise of drug-resistant strains. However, it could be mentioned that *M. tuberculosis* is able to evoke a response to combat the toxic effect of NO, and the effect of NO-releasing drugs in vivo may be reduced in the presence of NO scavengers and reductants (Ciccone et al. 2003).

Gatifloxacin (GTX) is a member of the 4th generation of fluoroquinolones (Gatifloxacin 2019). Its NPs were prepared by nanoprecipitation using PLGA 502 and Tween 80 or Labrafil as surface modifiers, and using rhodamine-loaded PLGA nanoparticles prepared with and without the surface modifiers, in vivo blood–brain barrier transport in male Wistar rats was evaluated. The formulation prepared with Tween 80 showing an EE of 28.2%, a particle size of 176.5 nm, and a zeta-potential of −20.1 mV could be considered as a promising drug delivery system to treat cerebral TB (Marcianes et al. 2017). GTX incorporated into PLGA NPs showed increased half-life and mean residence time as well as $AUC_{0\to 36}$ in blood plasma (Blynskaya et al. 2011). Abouelmagd et al. (2019) prepared tannic acid complexes with GTX that proved to be a suitable carrier for pH-sensitive delivery of water-soluble drugs.

Gemifloxacin represents another member of the fourth-generation fluoroquinolones with the same mode of action (Gemifloxacin 2019). Layered zinc hydroxide-gemifloxacin, an inorganic–organic nanohybrid with successfully intercalated drug into the layered zinc hydroxide interlayer showing also more thermal stability than pure gemifloxacin exhibited remarkably faster drug release rate at pH 7.4 than its composite with CS (Nabipour et al. 2016).

Moxifloxacin (MOX) is also a synthetic fluoroquinolone chemotherapeutic agent of the fourth generation showing rapid clearance (24 h) from the body, and therefore treatment with repetitive doses is necessary that may cause hepatotoxicity and acquisition of MOX resistant-TB (Moxifloxacin 2019). By affixation of PEG to MOX-PLGA NPs and adsorption of water-soluble CS to the particle surface, surface-modified NPs were fabricated characterized by controlled delivery and circulating in the bloodstream for an extended period of time, reduced protein binding and showing reduced liver sequestration of the drug compared with MOX-PLGA NPs without surface modification. Moreover, sustained release behavior of the surface-modified NPs could indicate reduction of dosing frequency (Mustafa et al. 2017b). Biodegradable antibacterial microspheres, in which both RIF and MOX were loaded into PLGA by the w/o/w double emulsion solvent evaporation technique showing an average particle size of 16.62 μm and a drug EE of 33.25% (MOX) and 49.0% (RIF), respectively, showed enhanced antibacterial activity against *S. aureus* by effectively inhibiting antibacterial biofilm formation and could be used for local drug delivery in treating osteomyelitis (Qiao et al. 2019). The drug conjugates of INH and MOX prepared using hydrolyzable linkers, chloroacetyl chloride, and succinyl chloride, which were encapsulated in PLGA NPs, could be useful for the synergistic treatment of TB to combat multiple drug resistance (MDR) exhibited by mycobacterium species (Moin et al. 2016). Combination of MOX-, ethionamide-, and econazole-loaded PLGA NPs tested in a MDR-TB infected mouse model was able to decrease the congestion in the lungs to 50%, and chemotherapy of MDR-TB-infected mice with weekly doses of these three drug nanoformulations resulted in the clearance of bacilli from lungs and spleen (Vemuri et al. 2016). As a promising formulation for effective management of ocular infections, MOX-loaded PLA/PCL hybrid polymeric matrix showing antibacterial activity against *E. coli*, *P. aeruginosa*, and *Staphylococcus* was described as well (Hezma and Rajeh 2018).

Hyaluronic-acid-modified lipid-polymer hybrid NPs encapsulating MOX displaying excellent ocular tolerance and showing considerable enhancement of the mean residence time and area under the curve ($AUC_{0\text{-}6h}$) in an in vivo precorneal retention study in rabbits compared to values observed with the commercial product could be used as an ocular drug delivery system for prolonged precorneal retention, better corneal permeability, and enhanced ocular bioavailability (Liu et al. 2018). Nanosuspension of MOX-loaded gelatin NPs with a particle size of 175 ± 1.11 nm and a zeta potential of +24 ± 0.12 mV showed higher in vivo antibacterial activity against *S. aureus* than the commercial market product MoxiGram® in the test performed on the corneal eye surface of rabbits, and using cup-plate method, its better antimicrobial activity against *Bacillus subtilis* was estimated as well (Mahor et al. 2016). CS microspheres for intrapulmonary administration of MOX designed by Ventura et al. (2008) with particle sizes 2.5–6.0 μm (suitable for inhalation) showed prolonged MOX release after a pronounced burst release, and using in vitro bronchial epithelium model consisting of a monolayer of Calu-3 human bronchial epithelial cells mounted on Franz diffusion cells, it was shown that the microspheres effectively retarded the absorption of MOX within 6 h compared to free drug. MOX conjugates with hydroxypropyl cellulose (self-assembling into nanowires with diameters of ca. 30 nm and hydroxyethyl cellulose-MOX conjugates (self-assembling into

NPs of 150–350 nm) exhibited sustained drug release and their administration in rabbits resulted in considerably higher MOX plasma half-life over 24 h as well as improved drug bioavailability (Abbas et al. 2016).

MOX-loaded liposomes fabricated using the lipid film hydration method with a mean particle size of 60.5 ± 0.72 nm and a drug EE of 92.24 ± 0.24% were reported to offer a satisfactory aqueous humor release profile after intracameral application to rabbits (Ferreira et al. 2018). MOX-loaded nanoliposomes coated with 4-aminophenyl-α-D-manno-pyranoside showed high antitubercular activity as well as increased macrophage uptake (Hamed et al. 2019).

Mesoporous SiO_2 NPs functionalized with pH-sensitive nanovalves (consisting of a stalk covalently attached to the pore entrances of SiO_2 NPs and a cap molecule, CD, which interacts with the organic moiety of the stalk through hydrophobic–hydrophobic interaction and traps the cargo inside the pores) loaded with MOX were found to be highly effective in killing *Francisella tularensis* in infected macrophages, and in a mouse model of lethal pneumonic tularemia they were able to kill *F. tularensis* more than an equivalent amount of free drug (Li et al. 2015). MOX-loaded mesoporous SiO_2 NPs functionalized with disulfide snap-tops selectively releasing the drug intracellularly in response to the redox potential could kill *F. tularensis* in macrophages in a dose-dependent fashion, and in a mouse model of lethal pneumonic tularemia, they prevented weight loss, illness, and death of animals and strongly reduced *F. tularensis* in the lungs, liver, and spleen, being pronouncedly more efficient than the free drug (Lee et al. 2016).

Ethionamide (ETH) is a thioamide of isonicotinic acid. It is a prodrug activated by ethionamide monooxygenase (EthA). The active drug then binds to NAD^+ to form an adduct that inhibits InhA in the same manner as INH, i.e., disrupts mycolic acid synthesis, which leads to inhibition of cell wall formation. ETH is characterized by poor aqueous solubility and strong tendency to crystallize and due to its low therapeutic index treatment with this drug is associated with severe toxic side effects (Ethionamide 2019). Vale et al. (2012) reported that by loading ETH into thermally carbonized porous silicon MPs the solubility and permeability of ETH was significantly improved, while toxicity of this formulation against HepG2, Caco-2, and RAW macrophage cells was pronouncedly lower than that of free ETH. Carboxylic acid functionalized thermally hydrocarbonized porous SiNPs conjugated with ETH showed stronger antimicrobial activity against *M. tuberculosis* strain H37Rv than free ETH, which could be connected with the weakening of the bacterial cell wall that improves conjugate-penetration. Using such ETH-conjugated NPs in the treatment of MDR-TB, reducing dosing frequency of the drug could be achieved (Vale et al. 2017).

ETH-loaded PLGA NPs with particle size of 286 ± 26 nm, zeta-potential of −13 ± 2.5 mV, and 35.2 ± 3.1% EE, when administered orally to mice, exhibited sustained release of ETH for 6 days in the plasma compared to 6 h estimated for free drug, and pronounced improvement in pharmacokinetic parameters and ETH was detected in the lung, liver, and spleen for up to 5–7 days suggesting that using such nanoformulation reducing dosing frequency of ETH in treatment of MDR TB could be obtained (Kumar et al. 2011a). ETH-loaded PLGA NPs fabricated by a solvent evaporation method, in which the drug was encapsulated in crystalline form, showed sustained in vitro release up to 15 days; their per oral administration to mice was not accompanied with toxic effects, and the bodyweight of animals was practically not affected (Kumar et al. 2011b).

In ETH-loaded CS alginate NPs stabilized with carrageenan fabricated using simple inotropic gelation with a mean particle size of 300 nm and showing controlled release over 96 h, the carrageenan improved the stability of NPs during formulation process as well as the entrapment of ETH in the NPs, whereby pronounced antimycobacterial activity of ETH-loaded NPs against H37Ra mycobacterium strain was estimated (Abdelghany et al. 2017).

Niosomes loaded with both cycloserine (hydrophilic) and ETH (lipophilic) showing a particle size of 137.4 nm and EE >70%, which were characterized by sustained release up to 3 days, exhibited greater antibacterial activity against *M. smegmatis* than the free drug combination (Kulkarni et al. 2019).

It was found that "booster" molecules could greatly increase the ETH antimycobacterial efficacy, and therefore Costa-Gouveia et al. (2017) co-encapsulated ETH and its booster BDM41906 (5,5,5-trifluoro-1-[4-(3-thiazol-2-yl-[1,2,4]oxadiazol-5-yl)-piperidin-1-yl]-pentan-1-one) in biodegradable polymeric NPs enabling to overcome the tendency of ETH to crystallize and the limited water solubility of the booster. The NPs fabricated from the cross-linked poly(2-hydroxy-1,3-propylenedioxy) polycyclodextrin polymer were found to show the best physicochemical properties for the simultaneous delivery of [ETH:booster] pair in the lungs and administration of NP suspension directly into mouse lungs using a Microsprayer®. The NP suspension administered directly into mouse lungs using a Microsprayer® resulted in 3-log decrease of the pulmonary mycobacterial load after six administrations compared to untreated mice. NPs of a co-drug of ETH and a new drug BDM43266 (4-(2-methyl-1,3-thiazol-4-yl)-*N*-(3,3,3-trifluoropropyl)benzamide) prepared using glutaric linker with particle size ca. 200 nm, administered intranasally, significantly reduced the population of *M. tuberculosis* in the mouse lungs (Pastor et al. 2019).

Prothionamide (PTH) is a homologue of ETH with the same mechanism of action and properties specified for the treatment of MDR-TB (Prothionamide 2019). Dry powder inhaler prepared by freeze-drying of CS-coated PTH showed sustained release up to 96.91% in 24 h following the initial burst release, and administration of a single dose of this nanoformulation to Wistar rats was able to maintain the drug concentration exceeding MIC for more than 12 h and increased the PTH residency in the lung tissues for more than 24 h (Debnath et al. 2018).

Perchlozone© (4-thioureido-iminomethylpyridinium perchlorate) is an antitubercular drug derived from thioacetazone (Thioacetazone 2019), developed, and therefore marketed only by the Russian Federation. Similar to a pattern drug, it is a prodrug activated by ethionamide monooxygenase (EthA). It inhibits FAS-II dehydratase, i.e., interferes with mycolic acid synthesis, and thus inhibits the generation of mycobacterial cell wall. It shows a narrow therapeutic spectrum, high hepatotoxicity, and fast drug resistance (Gopal and Dick 2015). It was shown that when Perchlozone© encapsulated in PLA-based MPs and NPs (particle sizes 1100 and 170 nm, respectively), which were modified with single-chain camel immunoglobulin G (IgG) for targeting, was injected intraperitoneally and intravenously into the mice with experimental TB, the MPs and NPs were internalized by phagocytic macrophages and transported to inner organs attacked by TB, better survival and lower degree of lung manifestations were observed with IG-modified NPs (Churilov et al. 2018).

para-Aminosalicylic acid (PAS) is a bacteriostatic antituberculotic drug inhibiting folic acid synthesis by binding to pteridine synthetase. In addition, it inhibits the synthesis of mycobactin, a component of mycobacterial cell wall (*para*-Aminosalicylic acid 2019). MPs prepared by spray-drying from ethanol/water solvent systems using ammonium carbonate as a pore-forming agent at application of low inlet temperatures resulted in a novel solid of stoichiometry PAS/ammonia/water, 2:1:0.5 (at higher temperatures pure PAS was obtained), and spray-dried PAS powders could be used for pulmonary delivery (Gad et al. 2012). GO air-dried hydrogel fabricated by lyophilization of the hydrogel prepared using GO and PAS in solution phase exhibited effective antimicrobial activity and in vitro cytotoxicity against *S. aureus* and *E. coli*, respectively and more invasive characteristics in *M. tuberculosis* H37Rv than the equivalent amount of pure PAS (More et al. 2019). The nanoscale formulation based on PAS and zinc-layered hydroxide (ZLH) prepared using zinc nitrate salt as a precursor showed fourfold higher efficiency of PAS against *M. tuberculosis* (MIC 1.40 μg/mL) than the free PAS (MIC 5.0 μg/mL); it was biocompatible with human normal lung cells MRC-5 and mouse fibroblast cells-3T3 and showed sustained release of PAS in a human body-simulated PBS solution at pH values of 7.4 and 4.8 (Saifullah et al. 2014a). Good biocompatibility of the PAS-ZLH nanocomposites against normal human MRC-5 lung cells and sustained release of PAS from such nanocomposites were reported previously as well (Saifullah et al. 2013, 2014b).

Clofazimine (CFZ) inhibits mycobacterial growth and binds to mycobacterial DNA, which leads to disruption of the cell cycle and killing of the bacterium. It binds to bacterial potassium transporters, thereby inhibiting their function. CFZ is the main drug for the treatment of leprosis (caused by *Mycobacterium leprae*) (Clofazimine 2019). Chen et al. (2018) used acetophenone as the chaperone for CFZ enabling loading of a high amount of CFZ into the mesoporous SiO_2 NPs as well as contributing to pronouncedly (2300-fold) higher CFZ release from the mesoporous SiO_2 NPs in an aqueous biorelevant environment compared with SiO_2 NPs without acetophenone treatment, whereby the optimized nanoformulation effectively inhibited *M. tuberculosis* in vitro. By loading CFZ into nanoporous SiO_2 particles, the amorphous state of CLZ was stabilized, and up to 20-fold increase of the drug solubility in simulated gastric fluid and markedly improved permeation through model intestinal cell layer was observed, reaching efficacious antimicrobial concentrations in TB-infected macrophages (Valetti et al. 2017a). Using antitubercular drug CFZ, it was shown that label-free fluorescent mesoporous SiO_2 MPs and NPs prepared by controlled thermal decomposition of carboamino groups linked on the surface could be applied as lipophilic multifunctional drug carriers enabling monitoring of drug release in biological environments by means of fluorescence lifetime and could be of interest in the field of theranostics (Valetti et al. 2017b).

By loading of CFZ into oligomeric carrier sulfobutylether-β-CDs prepared by cross-linking β-CD with epichlorohydrin followed by sulfonation in a strongly alkaline aqueous medium NPs with particle sizes 20–60 nm were prepared to show IC_{50} values <100 nM against *Staphylococcus epidermidis*, including clinical isolates of *S. epidermidis* (some displaying MDR) (Wankar et al. 2018).

PLGA NPs of CFZ and dapsone (antileprotics), drugs used in combination in therapy against various *Mycobacterium* species, showing a positive zeta potential of +27.4 mV released 82% dapsone and 68% CFZ and exhibited notably improved in vivo efficacy against *M. tuberculosis* H37Rv strain in infected small animal model reflected in stronger reduction of bacterial loads in the lungs from log10 of CFU/g to 2.7 ± 0.34 compared to administration of solution of drugs and diseased control (4.9 ± 0.21 and 6.8 ± 0.23, respectively) (Li et al. 2017).

Linezolid (LZD) is the first drug from the class of oxazolidinones, selective inhibitors of bacterial protein synthesis by binding to 23S ribosomal RNA of the 50S subunit. Thus, it prevents the formation of a functional 70S initiation complex (Linezolid 2019). LZD-loaded Eudragit® RS 100 polymeric NPs prepared by double emulsion solvent evaporation method showing particle sizes 47–119 nm, zeta potential ranging from −32 to −41 mV, and EE of 75.56–80.42% were reported to be suitable for effective drug delivery against MDR TB (Shaji and Kumbhar 2019). Nanoemulsion formulation of LZD exhibited higher antibacterial activity against *Staphylococcus* and lower cytotoxicity compared to free LZD with minimum biofilm inhibitory concentration of 73.68% (Mohamed et al. 2018). Parisi et al. (2014) synthesized oxazolidin-2-one derivatives (simplified analogs of Linezolid) showing moderate antimicrobial activity against *E. coli* and *S. cerevisiae* (MIC 16 μg/mL), the activity of which was significantly increased (MIC <4 μg/mL) after incorporation into lecithin-based nanoemulsion, poly(*N*-vinylpyrrolidone)methacrylic acid grafted copolymer, and spherical polymeric NPs, whereby these nanoformulations could be used to overcome cellular penetration constraints.

Bedaquiline (BDQ), a bactericidal diarylquinoline antimycobacterial chemotherapeutic agent, is an adenosine triphosphate (ATP) synthase inhibitor (binds to c subunit), which is an essential enzyme for the generation of energy in mycobacterial cells. It was approved only for the combination treatment of MDR-TB by FDA on December 28, 2012. However, treatment with BDQ is usually accompanied with nausea and it causes cardiac arrhythmias. Therefore this drug is not recommended for children and pregnant or lactating women, and its use could be restricted to patients with MDR-TB or more complex drug resistance who cannot otherwise be treated with a minimum of three effective drugs (Field 2015; Fox and Menzies 2013; Bedaquiline 2019).

By mixing of freeze-dried CS NPs of BDQ prepared using ionic gelation method with lactose preblend, a respirable powder was fabricated (optimized particle size of 109.7 ± 9.3 nm with a zeta potential of 36 ± 2.1 mV). The prepared formulation was able to efficiently deliver BDQ into the lungs and based on the in vitro and in vivo toxicity studies showed better safety profile than conventional dry powder inhaler formulation and oral solution (Rawal et al. 2018). De Matteis et al. (2018) achieved high encapsulation efficiency and drug loading values by encpsulating BDQ in lipid NPs and CS-based nanocapsules, and the nanoformulations were found to exhibit in vitro antibacterial activity against *M. tuberculosis* and superb compatibility of both carriers with animal cells.

Ritsema et al. (2018) encapsulated hydrophobic BDQ and hydrophilic vancomycin into different PEGylated polymeric NPs based on aliphatic polyesters prepared from diblock copolymers, in which PEG block was attached to an aliphatic polyester block (PLGA, poly(lactic-co-hydroxymethyl glycolic acid) or poly(lactic-co-benzyloxymethyl glycolic acid). In the formulations almost complete encapsulation of BDQ and approx. 30% for vancomycin, independent of the polymer type, was achieved, whereby a predominantly diffusion-controlled release of BDQ from all formulations was observed, while vancomycin was released by a combination of diffusion and polymer degradation showing the fastest release from the most hydrophilic polymer.

21.7 Metal-Based Antitubercular Nanoformulations

Sarkar et al. (2015) investigated the effects of bare AgNP (20 and 110 nm) and surface-modified AgNPs with citrate or PVP capping on cellular toxicity and innate immune responses against *M. tuberculosis* by human monocyte-derived macrophages (MDM) and found that AgNP exposure can potentially impair *M. tuberculosis*-induced activation of Toll-like receptor (TLR) signaling in MDM reflected by the suppression of target gene expression downstream of TLR pathway. To the suppression of the *M. tuberculosis*-induced host response in the presence of AgNPs could contribute also stress-induced Hsp72 protein-mediated inhibition of the activation of the nuclear factor NF-κB pathway. The suppressive effect on *M. tuberculosis*-induced immune responses was predominantly connected with the physicochemical properties of the AgNPs and not with Ag^+ ions released from the NPs (Sarkar et al. 2015). Using in vitro and ex vivo THP-1 infection model, it was shown that AgNPs fabricated by chemical route were more efficient in inhibition of active and dormant stage mycobacterial growth than the biogenic AgNPs. AgNPs showed more specificity toward mycobacteria (selectivity index 11–23) than toward other pathogenic bacteria suggesting that they have the potential to be used in treatment of TB (Singh et al. 2015). Larimer et al. (2014) cultivated *M. smegmatis* strain mc(2)155 in AgNP-enriched agar, and small bacterial population that survived was re-exposed to AgNPs and $AgNO_3$. It was found that after only a single exposure, mutant *M. smegmatis* populations were resistant to AgNPs and $AgNO_3$. Moreover, MIC values of INH for these Ag resistant mutants were fourfold higher than those for the mc(2)155 strain, while core resistance was not conferred to other toxic metal ions, and the mutants had lower resistance to $CuSO_4$ and $ZnSO_4$ than the mc(2)155 strain. Uraskulova and Gujsan (2017) studied the effectiveness of the application of AgNPs for the treatment of TB of the upper respiratory tract using nanoscale silver preparations, Argovit-C and Vitargol. The bactericidal activity of 3% Argovit-C solution reached 100% with respect to the medically-resistant mycobacteria at both maximum and minimum concentrations of IHN and the preparation showed also therapeutic effectiveness in a clinical study. Consequently, the researchers recommended the inhalation of the 3.3% Argovit-C solution twice daily for 10 minutes during 2 months for the local treatment of laryngeal TB. AgNPs inhibited not only the reference strains of *M. tuberculosis* and *M. bovis* but also the MDR strain of *M. tuberculosis* showing MICs of 1, 4, and 16 μg/mL. On the other hand, the estimated MIC values for clinical isolates of *M. bovis* and *M. tuberculosis* were 4–32 and 1–16 μg/mL, respectively, and an in vitro chemotherapeutic effect of AgNPs against *Mycobacterium* spp. was observed as well (Selim et al. 2018).

Bimetallic Au-Ag NPs green synthesized using medicinal plant extracts (*Barleria prionitis*, *Plumbago zeylanica*, or *Syzygium cumini*) inhibited *M. tuberculosis* and *M. bovis* BCG in both active and dormant stages showing MIC <2.56 μg/mL and were more potent as AgNPs. At tenfold MIC concentration of 30 μg/mL, they exhibited up to 45% cytotoxicity after 48 h, whereby the best specificity and selectivity to kill mycobacteria showed AgNPs synthesized using *S. cumini* (Singh et al. 2016). Gupta et al. (2018) designed a bis(pyrrolide-imine) Au(III) chelate showing ability to inhibit a panel of diverse *M. tuberculosis* and *M. abscessus* clinical isolates. This Au(III) chelate exhibited potent activity against bacterial topoisomerase 1A (Topo1) enzymes but not gyrase because it was demonstrated that it lacked cross-resistance with fluoroquinolones that target the mycobacterial gyrase.

Biosynthesized AgNPs and ZnNPs with particle sizes 40 and 60 nm, respectively, effectively inhibited multidrug-resistant pathogens. AgNPs were effective against drug-resistant clinical isolates of MRSA, VRE, ESBL, MDR, and *P. aeruginosa* with MIC in the range of 1.25–5 mg/mL, while ZnNPs specifically inhibited Gram-positive bacteria like *S. aureus*, including its drug-resistant variant MRSA. Moreover, both AgNPs and ZnNPs were effective against *M. tuberculosis* and its MDR strain with an MIC of 1.25 mg/mL and showed synergistic action in combination with gentamicin (Punjabi et al. 2018). Jafari et al. (2016, 2017) investigated the bactericidal impact of Ag, ZnO, and mixed AgZnO colloidal NPs on *M. tuberculosis* H37Rv phagocytized by THP-1 cell lines and found that NPs applied at a ratio 2(Ag):8(ZnO) and 8(Ag):2(ZnO) did not have any antitubercular effects on phagocytized H37Rv *M. tuberculosis*, while 0.663 ppm of 5(Ag):5(ZnO) had the ability to kill *M. tuberculosis* H37 Rv similar to 40 ppm of RIF, whereby phagocytized H37Rv *M. tuberculosis* into the THP-1 had died without any toxicity effects against THP-1 and MRC-5 cell lines.

Spherical ZnO NPs synthesized using leaf extract of *Limonia acidissima* L. as a reducing and capping agent with particle sizes ranging from 12 to 53 nm were found to control the growth of *M. tuberculosis* at 12.5 μg/mL suggesting that ZnO NPs could be used as a medicinal ingredient for treatment of TB (Taranath and Patil 2016). Inhibition of *M. tuberculosis* H37Ra strain at concentrations as low as 12.5 μg/mL showed also ZnO NPs prepared by solution combustion synthesis using lemon juice as biofuel (Gopala Krishna et al. 2017).

Zeolitic imidazolate framework-8 (ZIF-8) showing uniform cube-like morphologies with a diameter ca. 400 nm, which were after calcination transformed into hollow nanocages with porous shells consisted of interconnected NPs with diameters ranging from 20 to 40 nm, inhibited the growth of *M. tuberculosis*, whereby the estimated MIC of 12.5 μg/mL was comparable with that of the commercial organic medicines. Low crystal quality, high surface defect level, and rich surface functional groups on ZnO nanocage contributed to its more easy adsorption on the cell membrane as well as to the release of Zn^{2+} ions from the ZnO lattice and formation of ROS resulted in the damage of bacterial DNA and finally in the apoptosis of mycobacterial cells (Cui et al. 2018).

Sato et al. (2017) prepared NLCs loaded with Cu(II) complexes, namely $CuCl_2(INH)_2]\cdot H_2O$ (Cu-1), $[Cu(NCS)_2(INH)_2]\cdot 5H_2O$ (Cu-2), and $[Cu(NCO)_2(INH)_2]\cdot 4H_2O$ (Cu-3) showing enhanced antibacterial activity against *M. tuberculosis* compared to free Cu(II) complexes. The

MIC values of nanoformulations containing Cu(II) complexes were 1.87, 2.31, and 1.96 μg/mL for Cu-1, Cu-2, and Cu-3, respectively compared to 103.63, 63.26, and 80.71 μg/mL estimated for free Cu(II) complexes suggesting that incorporation into NLCs caused ca. 55-, 27-, and 41-fold enhancement of antibacterial activity.

Nanofomulation of Ga(III) encapsulated in folate-or mannose-conjugated block copolymers showed sustained Ga(III) release for 15 days, facilitated phagosome maturation, and significantly inhibited *M. tuberculosis* growth in human monocyte-derived macrophages (Choi et al. 2017a). Ga(III) NPs were found pronouncedly to inhibit the replication of both HIV and *M. tuberculosis*, their addition to mononuclear phagocytes already infected with *M. tuberculosis* or HIV was able to considerably reduce these infections, and macrophages that were coinfected with HIV and *M. tuberculosis* and loaded with GaNPs reduced the levels of interleukin-6 (IL-6) and IL-8 secretion for up to 15 days after drug loading suggesting that delivery of GaNPs to macrophages could be utilized as a potent long-acting approach for suppressing HIV and *M. tuberculosis* coinfection of macrophages in vitro (Choi et al. 2017b). Similar results related to prolonged-acting, multitargeting GaNPs strongly inhibiting the growth of both HIV and mycobacteria in coinfected human macrophages were reported also by Narayanasamy et al. (2015).

21.8 Conclusion

As mentioned above, TB has again become a very serious global disease. The rate of development of new drugs and their approval by authorities for use in patients is not sufficient compared to the rates, at which various types of resistance in *M. tuberculosis* develop, or the "devastation" of human population immunity and associated risks of the occurrence of new mycobacterial opportunistic pathogens continue. Thus, the current trend is to reuse old drugs, but they have to be formulated in nanosized particles to ensure their effectiveness and potency, which can provide an overall increase in bioavailability, improved stability, controlled release, targeted distribution to affected tissues, and an additive or synergistic increase of their potency due to the physical effects of the nanoparticles and/or the combination of different antitubercular effective agents, especially against MDR strains. In addition, better bioavailability of drugs from these nanoformulations allows a lower frequency of administration of a drug to a patient, i.e., higher compliance. Of course, the development of nanoformulations of antitubercular drugs is much faster in delivering particular results on the drug market (due to a simpler approval procedure); thus it can be hoped that the fight against TB using various nanoformulations/nanocomposites/nanosystems will be successful. On the other hand, although the original drugs have been approved, their nanonization or incorporation into nanoformulations will give them different physicochemical properties, which should lead to a deep investigation of their toxicological profile in relation to normal human cells in order to avoid various undesirable processes and thus eliminate risks and nonspecific factors associated with the administration of nanodrugs in general for organs and tissues.

Acknowledgments This study was supported by the Ministry of Education of the Czech Republic (LO1305), Palacký University in Olomouc (IGA_PrF_2020_023) and by the Slovak Research and Development Agency (APVV-0516-12 and APVV-14-0547).

References

Abbas NS, Amin M, Hussain MA, Edgar KJ, Tahir MN, Tremel W (2016) Extended release and enhanced bioavailability of moxifloxacin conjugated with hydrophilic cellulose ethers. Carbohydr Polym 136:1297–1306

Abdelghany S, Alkhawaldeh M, AlKhatib HS (2017) Carrageenan-stabilized chitosan alginate nanoparticles loaded with ethionamide for the treatment of tuberculosis. J Drug Deliv Sci Technol 39:442–449

Abouelmagd SA, Abd Ellah NH, Amen O, Abdelmoez A, Mohamed NG (2019) Self-assembled tannic acid complexes for pH-responsive delivery of antibiotics: role of drug-carrier interactions. Int J Pharm 562:76–85

Adesina SK, Ezeonyebuchi U, Akala EO (2015) The effect of formulation variables on drug loading of antitubercular drugs in nanoparticle formulations. Mater Res Express 2:095403

Ahmad Z, Pandey R, Sharma S, Khuller GK (2006) Pharmacokinetic and pharmacodynamic behaviour of antitubercular drugs encapsulated in alginate nanoparticles at two doses. Int J Antimicrob Agents 27:409–416

Ahmad MI, Ungphaiboon S, Srichana T (2015) The development of dimple-shaped chitosan carrier for ethambutol dihydrochloride dry powder inhaler. Drug Dev Ind Pharm 41:791–800

Ameeduzzafar ISS, Bukhari SNA, Ahmad J, Ali A (2018) Formulation and optimization of levofloxacin loaded chitosan nanoparticle for ocular delivery: in-vitro characterization, ocular tolerance and antibacterial activity. Int J Biol Macromol 108:650–659

Amikacin (2019) DrugBank. Canadian Institutes of Health Research, Canada. https://www.drugbank.ca/drugs/DB00479

Andreu V, Larrea A, Rodriguez-Fernandez P, Alfaro S, Gracia B, Lucia A, Uson L, Gomez AC, Mendoza G, Lacoma A, Dominguez J, Prat C, Sebastian V, Ainsa JA, Arruebo M (2019) Matryoshka-type gastro-resistant microparticles for the oral treatment of *Mycobacterium tuberculosis*. Nanomedicine 14:707

Atyabi F, Talaie F, Dinarvand R (2009) Thiolated chitosan nanoparticles as an oral delivery system for amikacin: in vitro and ex vivo evaluations. J Nanosci Nanotechnol 9:4593–4603

Aytac Z, Ipek S, Erol I, Durgun E, Uyar T (2019) Fast-dissolving electrospun gelatin nanofibers encapsulating ciprofloxacin/cyclodextrin inclusion complex. Colloids Surf B: Biointerfaces 178:129–136

Bachhav SS, Dighe VD, Devarajan PV (2018) Exploring Peyer's patch uptake as a strategy for targeted lung delivery of polymeric rifampicin nanoparticles. Mol Pharm 15:4434–4445

Bagga P, Siddiqui HH, Akhtar J, Mahmood T, Zahera M, Khan MS (2017) Gold nanoparticles conjugated levofloxacin: for improved antibacterial activity over levofloxacin alone. Curr Drug Deliv 14:1114–1119

Banerjee S, Roy S, Bhaumik KN, Kshetrapal P, Pillai J (2018) Comparative study of oral lipid nanoparticle formulations (LNFs) for chemical stabilization of antitubercular drugs: physicochemical and cellular evaluation. Artif Cells Nanomed Biotechnol 46:S540–S558

Banerjee S, Roy S, Bhaumik KN, Pillai J (2020) Mechanisms of the effectiveness of lipid nanoparticle formulations loaded with anti-tubercular drugs combinations toward overcoming drug bioavailability in tuberculosis. J Drug Targeting 28:55–69

Basha RY, Kumar TSS, Doble M (2019) Dual delivery of tuberculosis drugs via cyclodextrin conjugated curdlan nanoparticles to infected macrophages. Carbohydr Polym 218:53–62

Bedaquiline (2019) DrugBank. Canadian Institutes of Health Research, Canada. https://www.drugbank.ca/drugs/DB08903

Bhardwaj A, Mehta S, Yadav S, Singh SK, Grobler A, Goyal AK, Mehta A (2016a) Pulmonary delivery of antitubercular drugs using spray-dried lipid-polymer hybrid nanoparticles. Artif Cells Nanomed Biotechnol 44:1544–1555

Bhardwaj A, Grobler A, Rath G, Goyal AK, Jain AK, Mehta A (2016b) Pulmonary delivery of antitubercular drugs using ligand anchored pH sensitive liposomes for the treatment of pulmonary tuberculosis. Curr Drug Deliv 13:909–922

Blynskaya EV, Alekseev KV, Kondakov SE, Alyautdin RN, Balaban'yan VY (2011) Preparation and evaluation of bioavailability of gatifloxacine-loaded nanoparticles. Mosc Univ Chem Bull 66:129–132

Bucke WE, Leitzke S, Diederichs JE, Borner K, Hahn H, Ehlers S, Muller RH (1998) Surface-modified amikacin-liposomes: organ distribution and interaction with plasma proteins. J Drug Target 5:99–108

Burkeev MZ, Zhaparova LZ, Tazhbaev EM, Zhumagalieva TS, Ali SI, van Herk AM (2013) In vitro studies of capreomycin sulfate release from polyethylcyanoacrylate nanoparticles. Pharm Chem J 47:154–156

Capreomycin (2019) DrugBank. Canadian Institutes of Health Research, Canada. https://www.drugbank.ca/drugs/DB00314

Carazo E, Sandri G, Cerezo P, Lanni C, Ferrari F, Bonferoni C, Viseras C, Aguzzi C (2019) Halloysite nanotubes as tools to improve the actual challenge of fixed doses combinations in tuberculosis treatment. J Biomed Mater Res A 107:1513–1521

Carneiro SP, Carvalho KV, de Oliveira Aguiar Soares RD, Carneiro CM, de Andrade MHG, Duarte RS, Dos Santos ODH (2019) Functionalized rifampicin-loaded nanostructured lipid carriers enhance macrophages uptake and antimycobacterial activity. Colloids Surf B: Biointerfaces 175:306–313

Chen W, Cheng CA, Lee BY, Clemens DL, Huang WY, Horwitz MA, Zink JI (2018) Facile strategy enabling both high loading and high release amounts of the water-insoluble drug clofazimine using mesoporous silica nanoparticles. ACS Appl Mater Interfaces 10:31870–31881

Chen GQ, Wu YL, Yu DP, Li RB, Luo WY, Ma GF, Zhang C (2019) Isoniazid-loaded chitosan/carbon nanotubes microspheres promote secondary wound healing of bone tuberculosis. J Biomater Appl 33:989–996

Choi SR, Britigan BE, Moran DM, Narayanasamy P (2017a) Gallium nanoparticles facilitate phagosome maturation and inhibit growth of virulent *Mycobacterium tuberculosis* in macrophages. PLoS One 12:e0177987

Choi SR, Britigan BE, Narayanasamy P (2017b) Ga(III) nanoparticles inhibit growth of both *Mycobacterium tuberculosis* and HIV and release of interleukin-6 (IL-6) and IL-8 in coinfected macrophages. Antimicrob Agents Chemother 61:e02505–e02516

Chokshi NV, Khatri HN, Patel MM (2018) Formulation, optimization, and characterization of rifampicin-loaded solid lipid nanoparticles for the treatment of tuberculosis. Drug Dev Ind Pharm 44:1975–1989

Churilov L, Korzhikov-Vlakh V, Sinitsyna E, Polyakov D, Darashkevich O, Poida M, Platonova G, Vinogradova

T, Utekhin V, Zabolotnykh N, Zinserling V, Yablonsky P, Urtti A, Tennikova T (2018) Enhanced delivery of 4-thioureidoiminomethylpyridinium perchlorate in tuberculosis models with IgG functionalized poly(lactic acid)-based particles. Pharmaceutics 11:2

Ciccone R, Mariani F, Cavone A, Persichini T, Venturini G, Ongini E, Colizzi V, Colasanti M (2003) Inhibitory effect of NO-releasing ciprofloxacin (NCX 976) on *Mycobacterium tuberculosis* survival. Antimicrob Agents Chemother 47:2299–2302

Cieslik W, Spaczyńska E, Malarz K, Tabak D, Nevin E, O'Mahony J, Coffey A, Mrozek-Wilczkiewicz A, Jampílek J, Musioł R (2015) Investigation of the antimycobacterial activity of 8-hydroxyquinoline. Med Chem 11(8):771–779

Ciprofloxacin (2019) DrugBank. Canadian Institutes of Health Research, Canada. https://www.drugbank.ca/drugs/DB00537

Clofazimine (2019) DrugBank. Canadian Institutes of Health Research, Canada. https://www.drugbank.ca/drugs/DB00845

Costa-Gouveia J, Pancani E, Jouny S, Machelart A, Delorme V, Salzano G, Iantomasi R, Piveteau C, Queval CJ, Song OR, Flipo M, Deprez B, Saint-André JP, Hureaux J, Majlessi L, Willand N, Baulard A, Brodin P, Gref R (2017) Combination therapy for tuberculosis treatment: pulmonary administration of ethionamide and booster co-loaded nanoparticles. Sci Rep 7:5390

Cui JW, Wang L, Han YQ, Liu WG, Li ZY, Guo Z, Hu YS, Chang Z, Yuan QP, Wang JS (2018) ZnO nano-cages derived from ZIF-8 with enhanced anti mycobacterium-tuberculosis activities. J Alloys Compd 766:619–625

Cunha L, Rodrigues S, da Costa AMR, Faleiro ML, Buttini F, Grenha A (2018) Inhalable fucoidan microparticles combining two antitubercular drugs with potential application in pulmonary tuberculosis therapy. Polymers 10:636

Cunha L, Rodrigues S, da Costa AMR, Faleiro L, Buttini F, Grenha A (2019) Inhalable chitosan microparticles for simultaneous delivery of isoniazid and rifabutin in lung tuberculosis treatment. Drug Dev Ind Pharm 45(8):1313–1320

Cycloserine (2019) DrugBank. Canadian Institutes of Health Research, Canada. https://www.drugbank.ca/drugs/DB00260

de Oliveira VJ, Ishiki HM, Scotti MT, Scotti L (2018) Multi-target antitubercular drugs. Curr Top Med Chem 18(9):750–758

De Matteis L, Jary D, Lucia A, Garcia-Embid S, Serrano-Sevilla I, Perez D, Ainsa JA, Navarro FP, de la Fuente JM (2018) New active formulations against *M. tuberculosis*: Bedaquiline encapsulation in lipid nanoparticles and chitosan nanocapsules. Chem Eng J 340:181–191

Debnath SK, Saisivam S, Debanth M, Omri A (2018) Development and evaluation of chitosan nanoparticles based dry powder inhalation formulations of Prothionamide. PLoS One 13:e0190976

Druszczynska M, Kowalski K, Wawrocki S, Fol M (2017) Diversity and functionality of mycobacterial mycolic acids in relation to host-pathogen interactions. Curr Med Chem 24(38):4267–4278

Duan JH, Vogt FG, Li XJ, Hayes D, Mansour HM (2013) Design, characterization, and aerosolization of organic solution advanced spray-dried moxifloxacin and ofloxacin dipalmitoylphosphatidylcholine (DPPC) microparticulate/nanoparticulate powders for pulmonary inhalation aerosol delivery. Int J Nanomedicine 8:3489–3505

El-Ridy MS, Mostafa DM, Shehab A, Nasr EA, El-Alim SA (2007) Biological evaluation of pyrazinamide liposomes for treatment of *Mycobacterium tuberculosis*. Int J Pharm 330:82–88

El-Ridy MS, Yehia SA, Kassem MA, Mostafa DM, Nasr EA, Asfour MH (2015) Niosomal encapsulation of ethambutol hydrochloride for increasing its efficacy and safety. Drug Deliv 22:21–36

Ethambutol (2019) DrugBank. Canadian Institutes of Health Research, Canada. https://www.drugbank.ca/drugs/DB00330

Ethionamide (2019) DrugBank. Canadian Institutes of Health Research, Canada. https://www.drugbank.ca/drugs/DB00609

Farhangi M, Mahboubi A, Kobarfard F, Vatanara A, Mortazavi SA (2019) Optimization of a dry powder inhaler of ciprofloxacin-loaded polymeric nanomicelles by spray drying process. Pharm Dev Technol 24:584–592

Fatima S, Iqbal Z, Panda AK, Samim M, Talegaonkar S, Ahmad FJ (2018) Polymeric nanoparticles as a platform for permeability enhancement of class III drug amikacin. Colloids Surf B: Biointerfaces 169:206–213

Fatima S, Panda AK, Talegaonkar S, Iqbal Z, Ahmad FJ (2019) Optimization and designing of amikacin-loaded poly(D,L-lactide-co-glycolide) nanoparticles for effective and sustained drug delivery. J Pharm Bioallied Sci 11:83–95

Fawaz F, Bonini F, Maugein J, Lagueny AM (1998) Ciprofloxacin loaded polyisobutylcyanoacrylate nanoparticles: pharmacokinetics and in vitro antimicrobial activity. Int J Pharm 168:255–259

Ferreira KSA, dos Santos BMA, Lucena NP, Ferraz MS, Carvalho RDF, Duarte AP, Magalhaes NSS, Lira RPC (2018) Ocular delivery of moxifloxacin-loaded liposomes. Arq Bras Oftalmol 81:510–513

Field SK (2015) Bedaquiline for the treatment of multidrug-resistant tuberculosis: great promise or disappointment? Ther Adv Chron Dis 6:170–184

Fox GJ, Menzies D (2013) A review of the evidence for using bedaquiline (TMC207) to treat multi-drug resistant tuberculosis. Infect Dis Ther 2:123–144

Furneri PM, Fuochi V, Pignatello R (2017) Lipid-based nanosized delivery systems for fluoroquinolones: a review. Curr Pharm Des 23:6696–6704

Gad S, Tajber L, Corrigan OI, Healy AM (2012) Preparation and characterisation of novel spray-dried nano-structured *para*-aminosalicylic acid particulates for pulmonary delivery: impact of ammonium carbonate on morphology, chemical composition and solid state. J Pharm Pharmacol 64:1264–1274

Gagneux S (2017) Strain variation in the *Mycobacterium tuberculosis* complex: its role in biology, epidemiology and control. Springer International Publishing AG, Cham

Gajendiran M, Jo H, Kim K, Balasubramanian S (2019) In vitro controlled release of tuberculosis drugs by amphiphilic branched copolymer nanoparticles. J Ind Eng Chem 77:181–188

Garg T, Rath G, Goyal AK (2016) Inhalable chitosan nanoparticles as antitubercular drug carriers for an effective treatment of tuberculosis. Artif Cells Nanomed Biotechnol 44:997–1001

Gaspar DP, Gaspar MM, Eleuterio CV, Grenha A, Blanco M, Goncalves LMD, Taboada P, Almeida AJ, Remunan-Lopez C (2017) Microencapsulated solid lipid nanoparticles as a hybrid platform for pulmonary antibiotic delivery. Mol Pharm 14:2977–2990

Gatifloxacin (2019) DrugBank. Canadian Institutes of Health Research, Canada. https://www.drugbank.ca/drugs/DB01044

Ge ZH, Ma R, Xu GX, Chen Z, Zhang DF, Wang Q, Hei L, Ma W (2018a) Development and in vitro release of isoniazid and rifampicin-loaded bovine serum albumin nanoparticles. Med Sci Monit 24:473–478

Ge ZH, Ma R, Xu GX, Bai J, Liang SM, Chen Z, Wang Q, Ma W (2018b) Pharmacokinetics of isoniazid and rifampicin-loaded bovine serum albumin nanoparticles in rabbits. Lat Am J Pharm 37:1938–1944

Gemifloxacin (2019) DrugBank. Canadian Institutes of Health Research, Canada. https://www.drugbank.ca/drugs/DB01155

Ghaffari S, Varshosaz J, Saadat A, Atyabi F (2011) Stability and antimicrobial effect of amikacin-loaded solid lipid nanoparticles. Int J Nanomedicine 6:35–43

Ghazaei C (2018) *Mycobacterium tuberculosis* and lipids: insights into molecular mechanisms from persistence to virulence. J Res Med Sci 23:63

Giovagnoli S, Palazzo F, Di Michele A, Schoubben A, Blasi P, Ricci M (2014) The influence of feedstock and process variables on the encapsulation of drug suspensions by spray-drying in fast drying regime: the case of novel antitubercular drug-palladium complex containing polymeric microparticles. J Pharm Sci 103:1255–1268

Gomez AG, Syed S, Marshall K, Hosseinidoust Z (2019) Liposomal nanovesicles for efficient encapsulation of staphylococcal antibiotics. ACS OMEGA 4:10866–10876

Goněc T, Kos J, Zadražilová I, Peško M, Keltošová S, Tengler J, Bobál P, Kollár P, Čížek A, Kráľová K, Jampílek J (2013) Antimycobacterial and herbicidal activity of ring-substituted 1-hydroxynaphthalene-2-carboxanilides. Bioorg Med Chem 21(21):6531–6541

Goněc T, Pospíšilová Š, Kauerová T, Kos J, Doháňošová J, Oravec M, Kollár P, Coffey A, Liptaj T, Čížek A, Jampílek J (2016) *N*-alkoxyphenylhydroxynaphthalenecarboxamides and their antimycobacterial activity. Molecules 21(8):1068

Gopal P, Dick T (2015) The new tuberculosis drug Perchlozone® shows cross-resistance with thiacetazone. Int J Antimicrob Agents 45(4):430–433

Grewal TK, Majeed S, Sharma S (2018) Therapeutic implications of nano-encapsulated rifabutin, azithromycin & ethambutol against experimental *Mycobacterium avium* infection in mice. Indian J Med Res 147:594–602

Guerreiro F, Pontes JF, da Costa AMR, Grenha A (2019) Spray-drying of konjac glucomannan to produce microparticles for an application as antitubercular drug carriers. Powder Technol 342:246–252

Gupta R, Felix CR, Akerman MP, Akerman KJ, Slabber CA, Wang WJ, Adams J, Shaw LN, Tse-Dinh YC, Munro OQ, Rohde KH (2018) Evidence for inhibition of topoisomerase 1A by gold(III) macrocycles and chelates targeting *Mycobacterium tuberculosis* and *Mycobacterium abscessus*. Antimicrob Agents Chemother 62:e01696–e01717

Gopala Krishna P, Paduvarahalli Ananthaswamy P, Trivedi P, Chaturvedi V, Bhangi Mutta N, Sannaiah A, Erra A, Yadavalli T (2017) Antitubercular activity of ZnO nanoparticles prepared by solution combustion synthesis using lemon juice as bio-fuel. Mater Sci Eng C Mater Biol Appl 75:1026–1033

Hakkimane SS, Shenoy VP, Gaonkar SL, Bairy I, Guru BR (2018) Antimycobacterial susceptibility evaluation of rifampicin and isoniazid benz-hydrazone in biodegradable polymeric nanoparticles against *Mycobacterium tuberculosis* H37Rv strain. Int J Nanomedicine 13:4303–4318

Hamed A, Osman R, Al-Jamal KT, Hoayel SM, Geneidi AS (2019) Enhanced antitubercular activity, alveolar deposition and macrophages uptake of mannosylated stable nanoliposomes. J Drug Deliv Sci Technol 51:513–523

Herchline TE, Amorosa JK (2018) Tuberculosis (TB). Medscape. https://www.emedicine.medscape.com/article/230802-overview

Hetenyi G, Griesser J, Fontana S, Gutierrez AM, Ellemunter H, Niedermayr K, Szabo P, Bernkop-Schnuerch A (2018) Amikacin-containing self-emulsifying delivery systems via pulmonary administration for treatment of bacteria infections of cystic fibrosis patients. Nanomedicine 13:717–732

Hezma AM, Rajeh A (2018) Spectroscopic and drug delivery studies of moxifloxacin loaded polylactic acid/polycaprolacton polymeric matrix for medical application. Res J Pharm, Biol Chem Sci 8:1163–1170

Huang JY, Chen Z, Li Y, Li L, Zhang GY (2017) Rifapentine-linezolid-loaded PLGA microspheres for interventional therapy of cavitary pulmonary tuberculosis: preparation and in vitro characterization. Drug Des Devel Ther 11:585–592

Hussain A, Shakeel F, Singh SK, Alsarra IA, Faruk A, Alanazi FK, Christoper GVP (2019) Solidified SNEDDS for the oral delivery of rifampicin: evaluation, proof of concept, in vivo kinetics, and in silico GastroPlus™ simulation. Int J Pharm 566:203–217

Imramovský A, Polanc S, Vinšová J, Kočevar M, Jampílek J, Rečková Z, Kaustová J (2007) A new modification of antitubercular active molecules. Bioorg Med Chem 15(7):2551–2559

Imramovský A, Vinšová J, Monreal-Férriz J, Doležal R, Jampílek J, Kaustová J, Kunc F (2009) New antituberculotics originated from salicylanilides with promising in vitro activity against atypical mycobacterial strains. Bioorg Med Chem 17(10):3572–3579

Ioachimescu OC, Tomford JW (2015) Nontuberculous mycobacterial disorders. In: Carey W (ed) Disease management project. Cleveland Clinic—Centre for Continuing Education, Cleveland. http://www.clevelandclinicmeded.com/medicalpubs/diseasemanagement/infectious-disease/nontuberculous-mycobacterial-disorders/Default.htm

Isoniazid (2019) DrugBank. Canadian Institutes of Health Research, Canada. https://www.drugbank.ca/drugs/DB00951

Jafari AR, Mosavi T, Mosavari N, Majid A, Movahedzade F, Tebyaniyan M, Kamalzadeh M, Dehgan M, Jafari S, Arastoo S (2016) Mixed metal oxide nanoparticles inhibit growth of *Mycobacterium tuberculosis* into THP-1 cells. Int J Mycobacteriol 5:S181–S183

Jafari A, Mosavari N, Movahedzadeh F, Nodooshan SJ, Safarkar R, Moro R, Kamalzadeh M, Majidpour A, Boustanshenas M, Mosavi T (2017) Bactericidal impact of Ag, ZnO and mixed AgZnO colloidal nanoparticles on H37Rv *Mycobacterium tuberculosis* phagocytized by THP-1 cell lines. Microb Pathog 110:335–344

Jalvandi J, White M, Gao Y, Truong YB, Padhye R, Kyratzis IL (2017) Polyvinyl alcohol composite nanofibres containing conjugated levofloxacin-chitosan for controlled drug release. Mat Sci Eng C Mat Biol Appl 73:440–446

Jampílek J (2018) Design and discovery of new antibacterial agents: advances perspectives, challenges. Curr Med Chem 25(38):4972–5006

Jampílek J, Kráľová K (2017) Nano-antimicrobials: activity, benefits and weaknesses. In: Ficai A, Grumezescu AM (eds) Nanostructures for antimicrobial therapy. Elsevier, Amsterdam, pp 23–54

Jampílek J, Kráľová K (2018) Application of nanobioformulations for controlled release and targeted biodistribution of drugs. In: Sharma AK, Keservani RK, Kesharwani RK (eds) Nanobiomaterials: applications in drug delivery. CRC Press, Warentown, pp 131–208

Jampílek J, Kráľová K (2019a) Nanotechnology based formulations for drug targeting to central nervous system. In: Keservani RK, Sharma AK (eds) Nanoparticulate drug delivery systems. Apple Academic Press & CRC Press, Warentown, pp 151–220

Jampílek J, Kráľová K (2019b) Natural biopolymeric nanoformulations for brain drug delivery. In: Keservani RK, Sharma AK, Kesharwani RK (eds) Nanocarriers for brain targetting: principles and applications. Apple Academic Press & CRC Press, Warentown, pp 131–203

Jiang T, Zhan YY, Sun MZ, Liu SQ, Zang SZ, Ma YF, Xin Y (2011) The novel responses of ethambutol against *Mycobacterium smegmatis* mc(2)155 revealed by proteomics analysis. Curr Microbiol 62:341–345

Kadota K, Senda A, Tagishi H, Ayorinde JO, Tozuka Y (2017) Evaluation of highly branched cyclic dextrin in inhalable particles of combined antibiotics for the pulmonary delivery of anti-tuberculosis drugs. Int J Pharm 517:8–18

Kaewjan K, Srichana T (2016) Nano spray-dried pyrazinamide-L-leucine dry powders, physical properties and feasibility used as dry powder aerosols. Pharm Dev Technol 21:68–75

Kanamycin (2019) DrugBank. Canadian Institutes of Health Research, Canada. https://www.drugbank.ca/drugs/DB01172

Karmakar G, Nahak P, Guha P, Roy B, Nath RK, Panda AK (2018) Role of PEG 2000 in the surface modification and physicochemical characteristics of pyrazinamide loaded nanostructured lipid carriers. J Chem Sci 130:UNSP 42

Kashyap G, Ameta G, Ameta C, Ameta R, Punjabi PB (2019) Synthesis and characterization of polyaniline-drug conjugates as effective antituberculosis agents. Bioorg Med Chem Lett 29:1363–1369

Kaul A, Chaturvedi S, Attri A, Kalra M, Mishra AK (2016) Targeted theranostic liposomes: rifampicin and ofloxacin loaded pegylated liposomes for theranostic application in mycobacterial infections. RSC Adv 6:28919–28926

Kesavan MP, Ayyanaar S, Vijayakumar V, Raja JD, Annaraj J, Sakthipandi K, Rajesh J (2018) Magnetic iron oxide nanoparticles (MIONs) cross-linked natural polymer-based hybrid gel beads: controlled nano anti-TB drug delivery application. J Biomed Mater Res A 106:1039–1050

Khatib I, Khanal D, Ruan J, Cipolla D, Dayton F, Blanchar JD, Chan HK (2019) Ciprofloxacin nanocrystals liposomal powders for controlled drug release via inhalation. Int J Pharm 566:641–651

Koh WJ (2017) Nontuberculous mycobacteria – overview. Microbiol Spectr 5(1). https://doi.org/10.1128/microbiolspec.TNMI7-0024-2016

Kos J, Nevin E, Šoral M, Kushkevych I, Goněc T, Bobál P, Kollár P, Coffey A, O'Mahony J, Liptaj T, Kráľová K, Jampílek J (2015a) Synthesis and antimycobacterial properties of ring-substituted 6-hydroxynaphthalene-2-carboxanilides. Bioorg Med Chem 23(9):2035–2043

Kos J, Zadražilová I, Nevin E, Šoral M, Goněc T, Kollár P, Oravec M, Coffey A, O'Mahony J, Liptaj T, Kráľová K, Jampílek J (2015b) Ring-substituted 8-hydroxyqui noline-2-carboxanilides as potential antimycobacterial agents. Bioorg Med Chem 23(15):4188–4196

Kulkarni P, Rawtani D, Barot T (2019) Formulation and optimization of long acting dual niosomes using Box-Behnken experimental design method for combinative delivery of Ethionamide and D-cycloserine in

Tuberculosis treatment. Colloids Surf A Physicochem Eng Asp 565:131–142

Kumar G, Sharma S, Shafiq N, Pandhi P, Khuller GK, Malhotra S (2011a) Pharmacokinetics and tissue distribution studies of orally administered nanoparticles encapsulated ethionamide used as potential drug delivery system in management of multi-drug resistant tuberculosis. Drug Deliv 18:65–73

Kumar G, Malhotra S, Shafiq N, Pandhi P, Khuller GK, Sharma S (2011b) In vitro physicochemical characterization and short term in vivo tolerability study of ethionamide loaded PLGA nanoparticles: potentially effective agent for multidrug resistant tuberculosis. J Microencapsul 28:717–728

Kumarasingam K, Vincent M, Mane SR, Shunmugam R, Sivakumar S, Devi KRU (2018) Enhancing antimycobacterial activity of isoniazid and rifampicin incorporated norbornene nanoparticles. Int J Mycobacteriol 7:84–88

Larimer C, Islam MS, Ojha A, Nettleship I (2014) Mutation of environmental mycobacteria to resist silver nanoparticles also confers resistance to a common antibiotic. Biometals 27:695–702

Lee BY, Li ZL, Clemens DL, Dillon BJ, Hwang AA, Zink JI, Horwitz MA (2016) Redox-triggered release of moxifloxacin from mesoporous silica nanoparticles functionalized with disulfide snap-tops enhances efficacy against pneumonic tularemia in mice. Small 12:3690–3702

Leidinger P, Treptow J, Hagens K, Eich J, Zehethofer N, Schwudke D, Oehlmann W, Luensdorf H, Goldmann O, Schaible UE, Dittmar KEJ, Feldmann C (2015) Isoniazid@Fe_2O_3 nanocontainers and their antibacterial effect on tuberculosis mycobacteria. Angew Chem Int Ed 54:12597–12601

Lemke TL, Williams DA, Roche VF, Zito SW (2012) Antimycobacterial agents. In: Foye's principles of medicinal chemistry, 7th edn. Wolters Kluwer Health & Lippincott Williams & Wilkins, Baltimore, pp 1175–1198

Levofloxacin (2019) DrugBank. Canadian Institutes of Health Research, Canada. https://www.drugbank.ca/drugs/DB01137

Li ZL, Clemens DL, Lee BY, Dillon BJ, Horwitz MA, Zink JI (2015) Mesoporous silica nanoparticles with pH-sensitive nanovalves for delivery of moxifloxacin provide improved treatment of lethal pneumonic tularemia. ACS Nano 9:10778–10789

Li M, Neoh KG, Xu LQ, Yuan L, Leong DT, Kang ET, Chua KL, Hsu LY (2016) Sugar-grafted cyclodextrin nanocarrier as a "Trojan horse" for potentiating antibiotic activity. Pharm Res 33:1161–1174

Li HZ, Ma SH, Zhang HM, Liu JM, Wu YX, Cao PQ, Gao X (2017) Nano carrier mediated co-delivery of dapsone and clofazimine for improved therapeutic efficacy against tuberculosis in rats. Biomed Res India 28:1284–1289

Linezolid (2019) DrugBank. Canadian Institutes of Health Research, Canada. https://www.drugbank.ca/drugs/DB00601

Liu J, Barry ICE, Besra GS, Nikaido H (1996) Mycolic acid structure determines the fluidity of the mycobacterial cell wall. J Biol Chem 271:29545–29551

Liu D, Lian YF, Fang QY, Liu L, Zhang JD, Li J (2018) Hyaluronic-acid-modified lipid-polymer hybrid nanoparticles as an efficient ocular delivery platform for moxifloxacin hydrochloride. Int J Biol Macromol 116:1026–1036

Liu P, Guo BB, Wang SF, Ding JS, Zhou WH (2019) A thermo-responsive and self-healing liposome-in-hydrogel system as an antitubercular drug carrier for localized bone tuberculosis therapy. Int J Pharm 558:101–109

Loiko OP, van Herk AM, Ali SI, Burkeev MZ, Tazhbayev YM, Zhaparova LZ (2013) Controlled release of Capreomycin sulfate from pH-responsive nanocapsules. E-Polymers 13:189–202

Lopez-Lopez M, Fernandez-Delgado A, Moya ML, Blanco-Arevalo D, Carrera C, de la Haba RR, Ventosa A, Bernal E, Lopez-Cornejo P (2019) Optimized preparation of levofloxacin loaded polymeric nanoparticles. Pharmaceutics 11:57

Lu TT, Wu Y, Zhao CL, Su F, Liu JE, Ma ZY, Han QR (2018) One-step fabrication and characterization of Fe_3O_4/HBPE-DDSA/INH nanoparticles with controlled drug release for treatment of tuberculosis. Mat Sci Eng C Mat Biol Appl 93:838–845

Mahor A, Prajapati SK, Verma A, Gupta R, Iyer AK, Kesharwani P (2016) Moxifloxacin loaded gelatin nanoparticles for ocular delivery: formulation and in-vitro, in-vivo evaluation. J Colloid Interface Sci 483:132–138

Malík I, Csöllei J, Solovič I, Pospíšilová Š, Michnová H, Jampílek J, Čížek A, Kapustíková I, Čurillová J, Pecháčová M, Stolaříková J, Pecher D, Oravec M (2018) Dibasic derivatives of phenylcarbamic acid against mycobacterial strains: old drugs and new tricks? Molecules 23(10):2493

Marcianes P, Negro S, Garcia-Garcia L, Montejo C, Barcia E, Fernandez-Carballido A (2017) Surface-modified gatifloxacin nanoparticles with potential for treating central nervous system tuberculosis. Int J Nanomedicine 12:1959–1968

Maretti E, Rustichelli C, Romagnoli M, Balducci AG, Buttini F, Sacchetti F, Leo E, Iannuccelli V (2016) Solid lipid nanoparticle assemblies (SLNas) for an anti-TB inhalation treatment-A design of experiments approach to investigate the influence of pre-freezing conditions on the powder respirability. Int J Pharm 511:669–679

Maretti E, Costantino L, Rustichelli C, Leo E, Croce MA, Buttini F, Truzzi E, Iannuccelli V (2017) Surface engineering of solid lipid nanoparticle assemblies by methyl α-D-mannopyranoside for the active targeting to macrophages in anti-tuberculosis inhalation therapy. Int J Pharm 528:440–451

Maretti E, Costantino L, Buttini F, Rustichelli C, Leo E, Truzzi E, Iannuccelli V (2019) Newly synthesized surfactants for surface mannosylation of respirable

SLN assemblies to target macrophages in tuberculosis therapy. Drug Deliv Transl Res 9:298–310

Mehnath S, Sithika MAA, Arjama M, Rajan M, Praphakar RA, Jeyaraj M (2019) Sericin-chitosan doped maleate gellan gum nanocomposites for effective cell damage in *Mycobacterium tuberculosis*. Int J Biol Macromol 122:174–184

Mei QJ, Luo PP, Zuo Y, Li JD, Zou Q, Li YB, Jiang DM, Wang YN (2018) Formulation and in vitro characterization of rifampicin-loaded porous poly(ε-caprolactone) microspheres for sustained skeletal delivery. Drug Des Devel Ther 12:1533–1544

Melis V, Manca ML, Bullita E, Tamburini E, Castangia I, Cardia MC, Valenti D, Fadda AM, Peris JE, Manconi M (2016) Inhalable polymer-glycerosomes as safe and effective carriers for rifampicin delivery to the lungs. Colloids Surf B: Biointerfaces 143:301–308

Mitchison DA, Fourie PB (2010) The near future: improving the activity of rifamycins and pyrazinamide. Tubeculosis 90:177–181

Mohamed MA, Nasr M, Elkhatib WF, Eltayeb WN (2018) In vitro evaluation of antimicrobial activity and cytotoxicity of different nanobiotics targeting multidrug resistant and biofilm forming *Staphylococci*. Biomed Res Int 2018:7658238

Moin A, Raizaday A, Hussain T, Nagshubha B (2016) Development and optimization of dual drugs (isoniazid and noxifloxacin) loaded functional PLGA nanoparticles for the synergistic treatment of tuberculosis. Curr Drug Deliv 13:1034–1052

Moradi S, Taran M, Mohajeri P, Sadrjavadi K, Sarrami F, Karton A, Shahlaei M (2018) Study of dual encapsulation possibility of hydrophobic and hydrophilic drugs into a nanocarrier based on bio-polymer coated graphene oxide using density functional theory, molecular dynamics simulation and experimental methods. J Mol Liq 262:204–217

More MP, Chitalkar RV, Bhadane MS, Dhole SD, Patil AG, Patil PO, Deshmukh PK (2019) Development of graphene-drug nanoparticle based supramolecular self assembled pH sensitive hydrogel as potential carrier for targeting MDR tuberculosis. Mater Technol 34:324–335

Moretton MA, Cagel M, Bernabeu E, Gonzalez L, Chiappetta DA (2015) Nanopolymersomes as potential carriers for rifampicin pulmonary delivery. Colloids Surf B: Biointerfaces 136:1017–1025

Moxifloxacin (2019) DrugBank. Canadian Institutes of Health Research, Canada. https://www.drugbank.ca/drugs/DB00218

Mulla JAS, Mabrouk M, Choonara YE, Kumar P, Chejara DR, du Toit LC, Pillay V (2017) Development of respirable rifampicin-loaded nano-lipomer composites by microemulsion-spray drying for pulmonary delivery. J Drug Deliv Sci Technol 41:13–19

Mustafa S, Devi VK, Pai RS (2016) Comparative study of kanamycin sulphate microparticles and nanoparticles for intramuscular administration: preparation in vitro release and preliminary in vivo evaluation. J Microencapsul 33:679–688

Mustafa S, Devi VK, Pai RS (2017a) Kanamycin sulphate loaded PLGA-vitamin-E-TPGS long circulating nanoparticles using combined coating of PEG and water-soluble chitosan. J Drug Deliv 2017:1253294

Mustafa S, Devi VK, Pai RS (2017b) Effect of PEG and water-soluble chitosan coating on moxifloxacin-loaded PLGA long-circulating nanoparticles. Drug Deliv Transl Res 7:27–36

Musumeci T, Ventura CA, Carbone C, Pignatello R, Puglisi G (2011) Effects of external phase on D-cycloserine loaded W/O nanocapsules prepared by the interfacial polymerization method. Eur J Med Chem 46:2828–2834

Nabipour H, Sadr MH, Soltani B (2016) Synthesis, identification and in vitro drug release of layered zinc hydroxide-gemifloxacin nanohybrids. J Incl Phenom Macrocycl Chem 85:261–269

Narayanasamy P, Switzer BL, Britigan BE (2015) Prolonged-acting, multi-targeting gallium nanoparticles potently inhibit growth of both HIV and mycobacteria in co-infected human macrophages. Sci Rep 5:8824

Nemati E, Mokhtarzadeh A, Panahi-Azar V, Mohammadi A, Hamishehkar H, Mesgari-Abbasi M, Dolatabadi JEN, de la Guardia M (2019) Ethambutol-loaded solid lipid nanoparticles as dry powder inhalable formulation for tuberculosis therapy. AAPS PharmSciTech 20:120

Neto EH, Pinto SR, Portilho FL, da Costa MD, Pereira JX, Nigro F, Ricci E, Candea ALP, Henriques MDMD, Santos-Oliveira R (2019) Development and biological evaluation of a new nanotheranostic for tuberculosis. Drug Deliv Transl Res 9:97–105

Nirbhavane P, Vemuri N, Kumar N, Khuller GK (2017) Lipid nanocarrier-mediated drug delivery system to enhance the oral bioavailability of rifabutin. AAPS PharmSciTech 18:829–837

Nkanga CI, Krause RWM (2018) Conjugation of isoniazid to a zinc phthalocyanine via hydrazone linkage for pH-dependent liposomal controlled release. Appl Nanosci 8:1313–1323

Ofloxacin (2019) DrugBank. Canadian Institutes of Health Research, Canada. https://www.drugbank.ca/drugs/DB01165

Omar SM, Maziad NA, El-Tantawy NM (2017) Design of isoniazid smart nanogel by gamma radiation-induced template polymerization for biomedical application. Pharm Res 34:1872–1885

Omar SM, Maziad NA, El-Tantawy NM (2018) Pulmonary delivery of isoniazid in nanogel-loaded chitosan hybrid microparticles for inhalation. J Aerosol Med Pulm Drug Deliv 32:78

para-Aminosalicylic acid (2019) DrugBank. Canadian Institutes of Health Research, Canada. https://www.drugbank.ca/drugs/DB00233

Padwal P, Bandyopadhyaya R, Mehra S (2015) Biocompatible citric acid-coated iron oxide nanoparticles to enhance the activity of first-line anti-TB drugs in *Mycobacterium smegmatis*. J Chem Technol Biotechnol 90:1773–1781

Pai RV, Jain RR, Bannalikar AS, Menon MD (2016) Development and evaluation of chitosan microparticles based dry powder inhalation formulations of rifampicin and rifabutin. J Aerosol Med Pulm Drug Deliv 29:179–195

Palomino JC, Martin A (2014) Drug resistance mechanisms in *Mycobacterium tuberculosis*. Antibiotics 3(3):317–340

Pandey R, Khuller GK (2005) Solid lipid particle-based inhalable sustained drug delivery system against experimental tuberculosis. Tuberculosis 85:227–234

Pandey R, Sharma S, Khuller GK (2006) Chemotherapeutic efficacy of nanoparticle encapsulated antitubercular drugs. Drug Deliv 13:287–294

Parisi OI, Fiorillo M, Caruso A, Cappello AR, Saturnino C, Puoci F, Panno A, Dolce V, El-Kashef H, Sinicropi MS (2014) Enhanced cellular uptake by "pharmaceutically oriented devices" of new simplified analogs of Linezolid with antimicrobial activity. Int J Pharm 461:163–170

Park JH, Jin HE, Kim DD, Chung SJ, Shim WS, Shim CK (2013) Chitosan microspheres as an alveolar macrophage delivery system of ofloxacin via pulmonary inhalation. Int J Pharm 441:562–569

Parumasivam T, Ashhurst AS, Nagalingam G, Britton WJ, Chan HK (2017) Inhalation of respirable crystalline rifapentine particles induces pulmonary inflammation. Mol Pharm 14:328–335

Pastor A, Machelart A, Li X, Willand N, Baulard A, Brodin P, Gref R, Desmaele D (2019) A novel codrug made of the combination of ethionamide and its potentiating booster: synthesis, self-assembly into nanoparticles and antimycobacterial evaluation. Org Biomol Chem 17:5129–5137

Pavić K, Perković I, Pospíšilová Š, Machado M, Fontinha D, Prudêncio M, Jampílek J, Coffey A, Endersen L, Rimac H, Zorc B (2018) Primaquine hybrids as promising antimycobacterial and antimalarial agents. Eur J Med Chem 143:769–779

Pei P, Tian ZF, Zhu YF (2018) 3D printed mesoporous bioactive glass/metal-organic framework scaffolds with antitubercular drug delivery. Microporous Mesoporous Mater 272:24–30

Petkar KC, Chavhan S, Kunda N, Saleem I, Somavarapu S, Taylor KMG, Sawant KK (2018) Development of novel octanoyl chitosan nanoparticles for improved rifampicin pulmonary delivery: optimization by factorial design. AAPS PharmSciTech 19:1758–1772

Pham DD, Fattal E, Tsapis N (2015) Pyrazinamide-loaded poly(lactide-co-glycolide) nanoparticles: optimization by experimental design. J Drug Deliv Sci Technol 30(Part B):384–390

Pooja D, Tunki L, Kulhari H, Reddy BB, Sistla R (2015) Characterization, biorecognitive activity and stability of WGA grafted lipid nanostructures for the controlled delivery of Rifampicin. Chem Phys Lipids 193:11–17

Pospíšilová Š, Kos J, Michnová H, Kapustíková I, Strharský T, Oravec M, Móricz ÁM, Bakonyi J, Kauerová T, Kollár P, Čížek A, Jampílek J (2018) Synthesis and spectrum of biological activities of novel *N*-arylcinnamamides. Int J Mol Sci 19(8):2318

Praphakar RA, Munusamy MA, Sadasivuni KK, Rajan M (2016) Targeted delivery of rifampicin to tuberculosis-infected macrophages: design, in-vitro, and in-vivo performance of rifampicin-loaded poly(ester amide)s nanocarriers. Int J Pharm 513:628–635

Praphakar RA, Munusamy MA, Alarfaj AA, Kumar SS, Rajan M (2017a) Zn^{2+} cross-linked sodium alginate-g-allylamine-mannose polymeric carrier of rifampicin for macrophage targeting tuberculosis nanotherapy. New J Chem 41:11324–11334

Praphakar RA, Alarfaj AA, Munusamy MA, Dusthackeer VNA, Subbiah SK, Rajan M (2017b) Phosphorylated κ-carrageenan-facilitated chitosan nanovehicle for sustainable anti-tuberculosis multi drug delivery. ChemistrySelect 2:7100–7107

Praphakar RA, Munusamy MA, Rajan M (2017c) Development of extended-voyaging anti-oxidant linked amphiphilic polymeric nanomicelles for anti-tuberculosis drug delivery. Int J Pharm 524:168–177

Praphakar RA, Jeyaraj M, Ahmed M, Kumar SS, Rajan M (2018) Silver nanoparticle functionalized CS-g-(CA-MA-PZA) carrier for sustainable anti-tuberculosis drug delivery. Int J Biol Macromol B 118:1627–1638

Praphakar RA, Sumathra M, Ebenezer RS, Vignesh S, Shakila H, Rajan M (2019) Fabrication of bioactive rifampicin loaded κ-Car-MA-INH/Nano hydroxyapatite composite for tuberculosis osteomyelitis infected tissue regeneration. Int J Pharm 565:543–556

Prothionamide (2019) DrugBank. Canadian Institutes of Health Research, Canada. https://www.drugbank.ca/drugs/DB12667

Punjabi K, Mehta S, Chavan R, Chitalia V, Deogharkar D, Deshpande S (2018) Efficiency of biosynthesized silver and zinc nanoparticles against multi-drug resistant pathogens. Front Microbiol 9:2207

Pyrazinamide (2019) DrugBank. Canadian Institutes of Health Research, Canada. https://www.drugbank.ca/drugs/DB00339

Qiao ZW, Yuan Z, Zhang WP, Wei DH, Hu NM (2019) Preparation, in vitro release and antibacterial activity evaluation of rifampicin and moxifloxacin-loaded poly(D,L-lactide-co-glycolide) microspheres. Artif Cells Nanomed Biotechnol 47:790–798

Rani S, Gothwal A, Khan I, Pachouri PK, Bhaskar N, Gupta UD, Chauhan DS, Gupta U (2018) Smartly engineered PEGylated di-block nanopolymeric micelles: duo delivery of isoniazid and rifampicin against *Mycobacterium tuberculosis*. AAPS PharmSciTech 19:3237–3248

Rani S, Gothwal A, Pandey PK, Chauhan DS, Pachouri PK, Gupta UD, Gupta U (2019) HPMA-PLGA based nanoparticles for effective in vitro delivery of rifampicin. Pharm Res 36:UNSP 19

Rawal T, Patel S, Butani S (2018) Chitosan nanoparticles as a promising approach for pulmonary delivery of bedaquiline. Eur J Pharm Sci 124:273–287

Rebitski EP, Souza GP, Santana SAA, Pergher SBC, Alcantara ACS (2019) Bionanocomposites based on

cationic and anionic layered clays as controlled release devices of amoxicillin. Appl Clay Sci 173:35–45
Ribeiro AC, Rocha A, Soares RMD, Fonseca LP, da Silveira NP (2017) Synthesis and characterization of acetylated amylose and development of inclusion complexes with rifampicin. Carbohydr Polym 157:267–274
Rifabutin (2019) DrugBank. Canadian Institutes of Health Research, Canada. https://www.drugbank.ca/drugs/DB00615
Rifampicin (2019) DrugBank. Canadian Institutes of Health Research, Canada. https://www.drugbank.ca/drugs/DB01045
Rifapentine (2019) DrugBank. Canadian Institutes of Health Research, Canada. https://www.drugbank.ca/drugs/DB01201
Ritsema JAS, Herschberg EMA, Borgos SE, Lovmo C, Schmid R, Te Welscher YM, Storm G, van Nostrum CF (2018) Relationship between polarities of antibiotic and polymer matrix on nanoparticle formulations based on aliphatic polyesters. Int J Pharm 548:730–739
Saha B, Bhattacharya J, Mukherjee A, Ghosh AK, Santra CR, Dasgupta AK, Karmakar P (2007) In vitro structural and functional evaluation of gold nanoparticles conjugated antibiotics. Nanoscale Res Lett 2:614–622
Saifullah B, Arulselvan P, El Zowalaty ME, Fakurazi S, Webster TJ, Geilich B, Hussein MZ (2014a) Development of a highly biocompatible antituberculosis nanodelivery formulation based on *para*-aminosalicylic acid-zinc layered hydroxide nanocomposites. Sci World J 2014:401460
Saifullah B, El Zowalaty ME, Arulselvan P, Fakurazi S, Webster TJ, Geilich BM, Hussein MZ (2014b) Antimycobacterial, antimicrobial, and biocompatibility properties of *para*-aminosalicylic acid with zinc layered hydroxide and Zn/Al layered double hydroxide nanocomposites. Drug Des Devel Ther 8:1029–1036
Saifullah B, Maitra A, Chrzastek A, Naeemullah B, Fakurazi S, Bhakta S, Hussein MZ (2017a) Nanoformulation of ethambutol with multifunctional graphene oxide and magnetic nanoparticles retains its anti-tubercular activity with prospects of improving chemotherapeutic efficacy. Molecules 22:1697
Saifullah B, Chrzastek A, Maitra A, Naeemullah B, Fakurazi S, Bhakta S, Hussein MZ (2017b) Novel anti-tuberculosis nanodelivery formulation of ethambutol with graphene oxide. Molecules 22:1560
Saifullah B, Hussein MZ, Hussein-Al-Ali SH, Arulselvan P, Fakurazi S (2013) Sustained release formulation of an anti-tuberculosis drug based on para-amino salicylic acid-zinc layered hydroxide nanocomposite. Chem Cent J 7:72
Saleem MA, Nazar MF, Yameen B, Khan AM, Hussain SZ, Khalid MR (2018) Structural insights into the microemulsion-mediated formation of fluoroquinolone nanoantibiotics. ChemistrySelect 3:11616–11621
Sarkar S, Leo BF, Carranza C, Chen S, Rivas-Santiago C, Porter AE, Ryan MP, Gow A, Chung KF, Tetley T, Zhang J, Georgopoulos PG, Ohman-Strickland PA, Schwander S (2015) Modulation of human macrophage responses to mycobacterium tuberculosis by silver nanoparticles of different size and surface modification. Plos ONE 10:e0143077
Sato MR, Oshiro JA, Machado RTA, de Souza PC, Campos DL, Pavan FR, da Silva PB, Chorilli M (2017) Nanostructured lipid carriers for incorporation of copper(II) complexes to be used against *Mycobacterium tuberculosis*. Drug Des Devel Ther 11:909–920
Schoubben A, Blasi P, Marenzoni ML, Barberini L, Giovagnoli S, Cirotto C, Ricci M (2013) Capreomycin supergenerics for pulmonary tuberculosis in vitro, and in vivo characterization. Eur J Pharm Biopharm 83:388–395
Scolari IR, Paez PL, Sanchez-Borzone ME, Granero GE (2019) Promising chitosan-coated alginate-Tween 80 nanoparticles as rifampicin coadministered ascorbic acid delivery carrier against *Mycobacterium tuberculosis*. AAPS PharmSciTech 20:67
Selim A, Elhaig MM, Taha SA, Nasr EA (2018) Antibacterial activity of silver nanoparticles against field and reference strains of *Mycobacterium tuberculosis*, *Mycobacterium bovis* and multiple-drug-resistant tuberculosis strains Rev Sci Tech 37:823–830
Shaji J, Kumbhar M (2019) Formulation and characterization of linezolid loaded Eudragit RS 100 polymeric nanoparticles. Int J Pharma Sci Res 10:1944–1952
Sharma A, Pandey R, Sharma S, Khuller GK (2004a) Chemotherapeutic efficacy of poly(D/L-lactide-co-glycolide) nanoparticle encapsulated antitubercular drugs at sub-therapeutic dose against experimental tuberculosis. Int J Antimicrob Agents 24:599–604
Sharma A, Sharma S, Khuller GK (2004b) Lectin-functionalized poly(lactide-co-glycolide) nanoparticles as oral/aerosolized antitubercular drug carriers for treatment of tuberculosis. J Antimicrob Chemother 54:761–766
Singh M, Guzman-Aranguez A, Hussain A, Srinivas CS, Kaur IP (2019) Solid lipid nanoparticles for ocular delivery of isoniazid: evaluation, proof of concept and in vivo safety & kinetics. Nanomedicine 14:465–491
Singh R, Nawale LU, Arkile M, Shedbalkar UU, Wadhwani SA, Sarkar D, Chopade BA (2015) Chemical and biological metal nanoparticles as antimycobacterial agents: a comparative study. Int J Antimicrob Agents 46:183–188
Singh R, Nawale L, Arkile M, Wadhwani S, Shedbalkar U, Chopade S, Sarkar D, Chopade BA (2016) Phytogenic silver, gold, and bimetallic nanoparticles as novel antitubercular agents. Int J Nanomedicine 11:1889–1897
Sumaila M, Ramburrun P, Kumar P, Choonara YE, Pillay V (2019) Lipopolysaccharide polyelectrolyte complex for oral delivery of an anti-tubercular drug. AAPS PharmSciTech 20:107
Taavoni-Gilan A (2019) Chemical synthesis of $MnFe_2O_4$/chitosan nanocomposites for controlled release of ofloxacin drug. J Chin Chem Soc 66:600–607

Takeuchi I, Taniguchi Y, Tamura Y, Ochiai K, Makino K (2018) Effects of L-leucine on PLGA microparticles for pulmonary administration prepared using spray drying: fine particle fraction and phagocytotic ratio of alveolar macrophages. Colloids Surf A Physicochem Eng Asp 537:411–417

Taranath TC, Patil B (2016) *Limonia acidissima* L. leaf mediated synthesis of zinc oxide nanoparticles: a potent tool against *Mycobacterium tuberculosis*. Int J Mycobacteriol 5:197–204

Thioacetazone (2019) DrugBank. Canadian Institutes of Health Research, Canada. https://www.drugbank.ca/drugs/DB12829

Thomas D, Latha MS, Thomas KK (2018a) Synthesis and in vitro evaluation of alginate-cellulose nanocrystal hybrid nanoparticles for the controlled oral delivery of rifampicin. J Drug Deliv Sci Technol 46:392–399

Thomas D, Latha MS, Thomas KK (2018b) Zinc-alginate beads for the controlled release of rifampicin. Orient J Chem 34:428–433

Trousil J, Syrova Z, Dal NJK, Rak D, Konefal R, Pavlova E, Matejkova J, Cmarko D, Kubickova P, Pavlis O, Urbanek T, Sedlak M, Fenaroli F, Raska I, Stepanek P, Hruby M (2019) Rifampicin nanoformulation enhances treatment of tuberculosis in zebrafish. Biomacromolecules 20:1798–1815

Tuberculosis (2019) Mayo Foundation for Medical Education and Research. Mayo Clinic, USA. https://www.mayoclinic.org/diseases-conditions/tuberculosis/symptoms-causes/syc-20351250

Tukulula M, Gouveia L, Paixao P, Hayeshi R, Naicker B, Dube A (2018) Functionalization of PLGA nanoparticles with 1,3-β-glucan enhances the intracellular pharmacokinetics of rifampicin in macrophages. Pharm Res 35:UNSP 111

Upadhyay TK, Fatima N, Sharma D, Saravanakumar V, Sharma R (2017) Preparation and characterization of β-glucan particles containing a payload of nano-embedded rifabutin for enhanced targeted delivery to macrophages. EXCLI J 16:210–228

Upadhyay TK, Fatima N, Sharma A, Sharma D, Sharma R (2019) Nano-Rifabutin entrapment within glucan microparticles enhances protection against intracellular *Mycobacterium tuberculosis*. Artif Cells Nanomed Biotechnol 47:427–435

Uraskulova BB, Gujsan AO (2017) The clinical and bacteriological study of the effectiveness of the application of silver nanoparticle for the treatment of tuberculosis. Vestn Otorinolaringol 2017:54–57

van Soolingen D, Hoogenboezem T, de Haas PEW, Hermans PWM, Koedam MA, Teppema KS, Brennan PJ, Besra GS, Portaels F, Top J, Schouls LM, van Embden JDA (1997) A novel pathogenic taxon of the *Mycobacterium tuberculosis* complex, Canetti: characterization of an exceptional isolate from Africa. Int J Syst Bacteriol 47(4):1236–1245

Vale N, Makila E, Salonen J, Gomes P, Hirvonen J, Santos HA (2012) New times, new trends for ethionamide: in vitro evaluation of drug-loaded thermally carbonized porous silicon microparticles. Eur J Pharm Biopharm 81:314–323

Vale N, Correia A, Silva S, Figueiredo P, Makila E, Salonen J, Hirvonen J, Pedrosa J, Santos HA, Fraga A (2017) Preparation and biological evaluation of ethionamide-mesoporous silicon nanoparticles against *Mycobacterium tuberculosis*. Bioorg Med Chem Lett 27:403–405

Valetti S, Xia X, Costa-Gouveia J, Brodin P, Bernet-Camard MF, Andersson M, Feiler A (2017a) Clofazimine encapsulation in nanoporous silica particles for the oral treatment of antibiotic-resistant *Mycobacterium tuberculosis* infections. Nanomedicine 12:831–844

Valetti S, Wankar J, Ericson MB, Feiler A, Manet I (2017b) Mesoporous silica particles as a lipophilic drug vehicle investigated by fluorescence lifetime imaging. J Mater Chem B 5:3201–3211

Varma JNR, Kumar TS, Prasanthi B, Ratna JV (2015) Formulation and characterization of pyrazinamide polymeric nanoparticles for pulmonary tuberculosis: efficiency for alveolar macrophage targeting. Indian J Pharm Sci 77:258–266

Varshosaz J, Ghaffari S, Mirshojaei SF, Jafarian A, Atyabi F, Kobarfard F, Azarmi S (2013) Biodistribution of amikacin solid lipid nanoparticles after pulmonary delivery. Biomed Res Int 2013:136859

Veeren A, Bhaw-Luximon A, Jhurry D (2013) Polyvinylpyrrolidone-polycaprolactone block copolymer micelles as nanocarriers of anti-TB drugs. Eur Polym J 49:3034–3045

Velayati AA, Farnia P, Masjedi MR (2013) The totally drug resistant tuberculosis (TDR-TB). Int J Clin Exp Med 6(4):307–309

Vemuri N, Khuller GK, Prabhakar T, Pal N, Gupta P, Gupta U (2016) Nanoformulations of moxifloxacin, econazole and ethionamide as novel treatment regimens against MDR TB – an experimental study. Curr Nanosci 12:110–117

Ventura CA, Tommasini S, Crupi E, Giannone I, Cardile V, Musumeci T, Puglisi G (2008) Chitosan microspheres for intrapulmonary administration of moxifloxacin: interaction with biomembrane models and in vitro permeation studies. Eur J Pharm Biopharm 68:235–244

Vieira ACC, Magalhaes J, Rocha S, Cardoso MS, Santos SG, Borges M, Pinheiro M, Reis S (2017) Targeted macrophages delivery of rifampicin-loaded lipid nanoparticles to improve tuberculosis treatment. Nanomedicine 12:2721–2736

Vieira ACC, Chaves LL, Pinheiro M, Lima SAC, Ferreira D, Sarmento B, Reis S (2018a) Mannosylated solid lipid nanoparticles for the selective delivery of rifampicin to macrophages. Artif Cells Nanomed Biotechnol 46:S653–S663

Vieira ACC, Chaves LL, Pinheiro S, Pinto S, Pinheiro M, Lima SC, Ferreira D, Sarmento B, Reis S (2018b) Mucoadhesive chitosan-coated solid lipid nanoparticles for better management of tuberculosis. Int J Pharm 536:478–485

Wankar J, Bonvicini F, Benkovics G, Marassi V, Malanga M, Fenyvesi E, Gentilomi GA, Reschiglian P, Roda B, Manet I (2018) Widening the therapeutic perspectives of clofazimine by its loading in sulfobutylether β-cyclodextrin nanocarriers: Nanomolar IC_{50} values against MDR *S. epidermidis*. Mol Pharm 15:3823–3836

WHO (2018) Global Tuberculosis Report 2018, World Health Organization. WHO Press, Geneva

Wu G, Chen L, Li H, Deng CL, Chen XF (2014) Comparing microspheres with different internal phase of polyelectrolyte as local drug delivery system for bone tuberculosis therapy. Biomed Res Int 2014:297808

Wu T, Liao WP, Wang W, Zhou J, Tan WG, Xiang WB, Zhang JL, Guo LN, Chen T, Ma D, Yu WY, Cai X (2018) Genipin-crosslinked carboxymethyl chitosan nanogel for lung-targeted delivery of isoniazid and rifampin. Carbohydr Polym 197:403–413

Xu C, Yu SC, Liu LL, Wu XP, Dai HL (2018) Magnetically targeted co-delivery of hydrophilic and hydrophobic drugs with hollow mesoporou ferrite nanoparticles. RSC Adv 8:15326–15335

Yuan XZ, Praphakar RA, Munusamy MA, Alarfaj AA, Kumar SS, Rajan M (2019) Mucoadhesive guargum hydrogel inter-connected chitosan-g-polycaprolactone micelles for rifampicin delivery. Carbohydr Polym 206:1–10

Zhang LP, Tan XX, Huang YP, Liu ZS (2018) Floating liquid crystalline molecularly imprinted polymer coated carbon nanotubes for levofloxacin delivery. Eur J Pharm Biopharm 127:150–158

Zhaparova LZ, Tazhbayev YM, Burkeev MZ, Kazhmuratova AT, Zhumagaliyeva TS, Ali SI, van Herk AM (2012) Synthesis and characterization of polyethyl cyanoacrylate nanoparticles loaded with capreomycin sulfate. Pharm Chem J 46:6–9

22 Magnetic Nanoparticle Nanoformulations for Alternative Therapy of Cancer by Magnetic/Superparamagnetic Hyperthermia

Costică Caizer, Cristina Dehelean, Dorina Elena Coricovac, Isabela Simona Caizer, and Codruta Şoica

Abstract

Superparamagnetic hyperthermia, obtained by increasing the temperature to 42–43 °C in tumor tissue where magnetic nanoparticles are found, as a result of superparamagnetic relaxation, following the application of an external alternating magnetic field at a frequency of hundreds of kiloherz, is an alternative method that is noninvasive and apparently lacking toxicity and that has real potential as a cancer therapy. However, magnetic nanoparticles used as thermal mediators play a very important role in the efficacy of the method in the irreversible destruction of tumors. The NPs must meet a number of physical and magnetic characteristics in order to obtain the maximum hyperthermal effect, but also a reduced or even lack of toxicity on healthy cells. This chapter presents just this aspect of biocompatibility/cytotoxicity and nanoformulations of magnetic nanoparticles for their use in superparamagnetic hyperthermia. We will consider the recent nanoformulations that could be used successfully in superparamagnetic hyperthermia, tested in vitro and in vivo, as well as current trends in dual therapy, thermochemotherapy, or thermoradiotherapy.

Keywords

Magnetic IONPs · Nanoformulations · Toxicity · Superparamagnetic hyperthermia · Cancer therapy

C. Caizer (✉)
West University of Timisoara, Faculty of Physics, Timisoara, Romania
e-mail: costica.caizer@e-uvt.ro

C. Dehelean · D. E. Coricovac
"Victor Babes" University of Medicine and Pharmacy, Faculty of Pharmacy, Department of Toxicology and Drug Industry, Timisoara, Romania

I. S. Caizer
"Victor Babes" University of Medicine and Pharmacy, Faculty of Medicine, Timisoara, Romania

C. Şoica
"Victor Babes" University of Medicine and Pharmacy, Faculty of Pharmacy, Timisoara, Romania

Nomenclature

AMF	Alternating magnetic field
B16-F10	Murine melanoma cell line
Bio-MNP	Biocompatible magnetic nanoparticle
Bio-SPMNP	Biocompatible superparamagnetic nanoparticle
BHK-21	Baby hamster kidney cells
CKD	Chronic kidney disease
CT-26	Colorectal cancer cells
DOX	Doxorubicin

S. Talegaonkar, M. Rai (eds.), *Nanoformulations in Human Health*,
https://doi.org/10.1007/978-3-030-41858-8_22

DCFDA	2′,7′–dichlorofluorescin diacetate
DMSA	Dimercaptosuccinic acid
FDA	Food and Drug Administration
G4@IONPs	Fourth-generation dendrimer-coated iron oxide nanoparticles
HaCaT	Human immortalized keratinocytes
HDF1	Human fibroblast cell line
HER2	Human epidermal growth factor receptor
HIV	Human immunodeficiency virus
hsp70	Heat shock protein gene
IONP	Iron oxide nanoparticle
LDH	Lactate dehydrogenase assay
LSMO	Dextran-coated $La_{0.75}Sr_{0.25}MnO_3$
M059K	Glioblastoma cells
MCF-7	Human breast carcinoma cell line
MCLs	Magnetic cationic liposomes
MDA-MB-231	Human breast cancer cell line
MEO_2MA	2-(2-methoxyethoxy)ethyl methacrylate
MFH	Magnetic fluid hyperthermia
MG-63	Bone-cancer cell line
MHT	Magnetic hyperthermia
MLs	Magnetic liposomes
MION	Magnetic iron oxide nanoparticle
MNP	Magnetic nanoparticle
MRI	Magnetic resonance imaging
MTT	3-(4,5-dimethylthiazol-2-yl)-2,5-diphenyltetrazolium bromide
NP	Nanoparticle
OEGMA	Oligo(ethylene glycol) methacrylate
PEG	Polyethylene glycol
PEG-PLA	Poly(ethylene glycol)-poly(lactide)
PEI	Polyethylenimine
PTT	Photothermal therapy
RES	Reticuloendothelial system
RG-2	Rat glioma cells
SAR	Specific absorption rate
SLP	Specific loss power
SPMHT	Superparamagnetic hyperthermia
SPION	Superparamagnetic iron oxide nanoparticle
SPMNP	Superparamagnetic nanoparticle
T-9	Rat glioma cells
U251	Human glioma cells
XTT	2,3-bis-(2-methoxy-4-nitro-5-sulfophenyl)-2H-tetrazolium-5-carboxanilide

22.1 Introduction

In alternative therapies against tumors, one of the most promising methods at the present time is superparamagnetic hyperthermia (SPMHT) (Rosensweig 2002; Ito et al. 2003; Matsuoka et al. 2004; Jordan et al. 2006; Johannsen et al. 2007; Hou et al. 2009; Kobayashi 2011; Caizer 2013, 2014; Wang et al. 2017). This method was recently introduced in cancer therapy and is based on increasing the temperature of magnetic nanoparticles (MNPs) dispersed in a tumor to around 42–43 °C, noninvasively, as a result of superparamagnetic relaxation in the alternative magnetic field at a frequency of 10^2 kHz (Rosensweig 2002). Many studies have been conducted on magnetic hyperthermia (MHT) with MNPs and superparamagnetic nanoparticles (SPMNPs), as well as in vitro and in vivo studies (Ito et al. 2004; Gazeau et al. 2008; Hu et al. 2012; Alphandéry et al. 2013; Caizer et al. 2013; Di Corato et al. 2015; Caizer 2017; Kandasamy et al. 2018a, b; Yan et al. 2018; Zhou et al. 2018; Tian et al. 2019), which show the feasibility of the method in the destruction of tumor cells.

However, studies on MHT with nanoparticles (NPs) having superparamagnetic behavior in the external magnetic field, called SPMHT, have shown that this is more effective than MHT (Pavel et al. 2008; Pavel and Stancu 2009; Caizer et al. 2010). This is due, first of all, to the specific loss power (SLP), which is greater than that of common NPs, which leads to more efficient heating and a higher specific absorption rate (SAR).

Secondly, in the case of SPMNPs, they are smaller in size, usually in a range of approx. 5–20 nm, than those used in common MHT, where NPs are larger (>20 nm), which implies at least two advantages: (i) reduced toxicity and (ii) easier entry of NPs into cells, which makes it the most efficient method, by destroying cells from the inside (intracellular therapy).

In the case of large NPs used in MHT, besides the two aspects mentioned previously, which become disadvantages, in this case, there is another major disadvantage: high magnetic fields must be used to obtain the loss power necessary in hyperthermia. This is because the power dissipated in this case is obtained as a result of the magnetization with hysteresis (hysteresis loop) of the large NPs, the power being proportional to the surface area of the hysteresis loop. High loss power is equivalent to obtaining a large hysteresis loop, and this can only be achieved in high fields. However, the use of high magnetic fields (*H*) raises major difficulties in terms of both obtaining their application at high frequencies (*f*) and their use in human body therapy, where the known admissible dose should not be exceeded, e.g., $Hf < 5 \times 10^9$ Am^{-1}Hz (Hergt and Dutz 2007).

After achieving the maximum efficiency of 100% in the destruction of tumors, besides the use of SPMHT in antitumor therapy, with the physical and magnetic aspects of optimizing the method, another very important issue is the nanoformulation of MNPs with various biochemical agents, so as to obtain the most suitable biocompatible NPs for this type of therapy, without toxicity.

A search in the PubMed database on the keywords "iron oxide nanoparticles" led to a considerable number of published articles – over 14,600, with the earliest mentioning iron oxide NPs used in biomedicine (magnetoresponsive indomethacin NPs) dating from 1988 (Malaiya and Vyas 1988), which indicates that this type of NP is ranked among the first NPs studied for biomedical applications. The interest in iron oxide NPs (IONPs) as effective tools in the medical and pharmaceutical domains is still elevated since from the 1January until 31 July 2019 over 800 studies were published that included the words "iron oxide nanoparticles" (source: PubMed database). The distinct features of IONPs, like superparamagnetism, high colloidal stability, and low toxicity, make these NPs attractive for multiple uses, particularly in the biomedical field: MHT, magnetic resonance imaging (MRI) as contrast mediators, targeted drug delivery systems, gene therapy, magnetic cell splitting, tissue repair, cancer treatment, and so forth (Laffon et al. 2018; Hataminia et al. 2019). It worth mentioning that beyond the many advantages of IONPs, the widespread use of these NPs has raised serious concerns in terms of potential toxicity, causing researchers to devote considerable attention to the appraisal of NPs' safety profiles (according to the PubMed database, over 1500 published articles investigated IONP toxicity).

Several fundamental physical, chemical, and biological properties should be present for NPs to be considered appropriate for use in clinical practice: (i) charge: the optimal charge of NPs for in vivo applications, including tumor targeting, is near neutral or weakly negative; (ii) zeta potential – establishes a solution's stability – NPs <100 nm possess a negative net potential, whereas NPs >100 nm present a positive potential; (iii) coating (as polyethylene glycol (PEG), oleate or oleic acid, dextran, chitosan, dimercaptosuccinic acid (DMSA), poly(L-lactic acid), citrate, silica, starch): dictates the circulation half-time of NPs by interfering with the recognition and elimination of intravenously administered NPs via the reticuloendothelial system (RES); (iv) size: IONPs 10–100 nm in size are recommended for intravenous use, while NPs >200 nm and <10 nm are seized by the spleen or discarded by renal clearance; (v) shape: influences the cellular uptake of NPs by macrophages (the spherical shape is internalized faster compared to other shapes); and (vi) functional targeting: assures strong binding to target cells and prolonged contact/retention in target area (Belanova et al. 2018; Durymanov et al. 2015; Arami et al. 2015).

This chapter presents an overview of the latest data concerning the nanoformulations of magnetic IONPs with a focus on their applications in MHT/SPMHT as an alternative cancer therapy by describing the main mechanisms of action and the therapeutic potential of this technique. Moreover, the fundamental physical and magnetic issues regarding MHT and SPMHT and the in vitro and in vivo fate of magnetic IONPs after their administration in terms of toxicity are also presented and discussed.

22.2 Magnetic Nanoparticles in Alternative Cancer Therapy by Superparamagnetic Hyperthermia

MNPs that are used in MHT or SPMHT are generally ferrimagnetic (FiM), due to both the possibility of their magnetization in high-frequency fields (Valenzuela 1994) and their low toxicity compared to ferromagnetic (FM) NPs. Although the FM NPs have a magnetic moment per particle larger than those of the FiM (Cullity and Graham 2009), due to the parallel orientation and the same orientation of the atomic (or ionic) magnetic moments (Fig. 22.1a) compared to the opposite and unequal orientation of magnetic moments in the case of FiM (Fig. 22.1b), which would be beneficial in MHT, they are not yet used. However, it is not excluded that such NPs as iron (Rosensweig 2002) or their alloys (e.g. iron-platinum (Fe-Pt)) (Habib et al. 2008) may be successfully used in the near future, and even more efficiently, in MHT or SPMHT. Now with modern nanobiotechnology these FM NPs can be made perfectly biocompatible and nontoxic for nanometric sizes, which would be a great advantage in hyperthermia.

22.2.1 Magnetic Behavior in Static Magnetic Field

The magnetization $\vec{M}$, which macroscopically characterizes a material from a magnetic point of view, is given by the vector sum of the atomic (or ionic) magnetic moments $\vec{\mu}_{\mathrm{m}}$ per unit volume V,

$$\vec{M} = \frac{\sum_i \vec{\mu}_{\mathrm{m},i}}{V} \tag{22.1}$$

or

$$\vec{M} = \frac{d\vec{\mu}}{dV} \tag{22.2}$$

respectively, in the case of a continuous distribution of magnetic moments.

For a magnetic domain with uniaxial symmetry (Fig. 22.2a) having volume V where the magnetization is uniform and stable, and equal to the spontaneous magnetization (or saturation) $\vec{M}_{\mathrm{s}}$ of the material, the magnetic moment of the domain will be

$$\mu_{\mathrm{md}} = \int_{(V)} M_{\mathrm{s}} dV \tag{22.3}$$

In the case of NPs that are not too large, e.g., <20–25 nm for soft FiM NPs, they are generally of a single domain, so that in the case of spherical approximation (Fig. 22.2b) the magnetic moment of the NP is

$$m_{\mathrm{NP}} = M_{\mathrm{s}} V_{\mathrm{NP}} \tag{22.4}$$

and

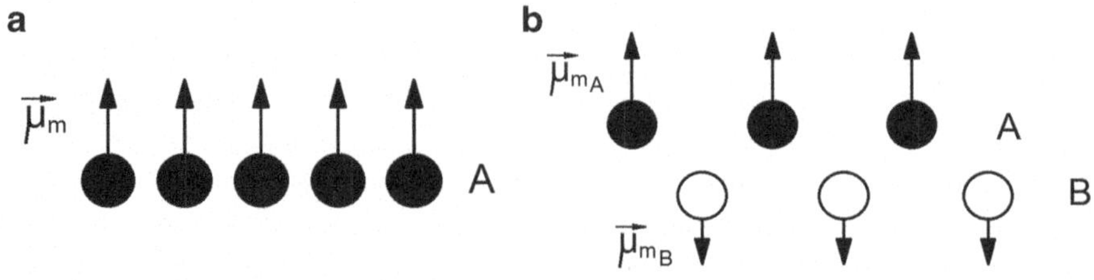

Fig. 22.1 Schematic representation of orientation of ionic magnetic moments in NPs with (**a**) ferromagnetic and (**b**) ferrimagnetic structure

Fig. 22.2 (**a**) Magnetic domain and (**b**) spherical NP for uniaxial crystalline symmetry; e.m.a. is the easy magnetization axis

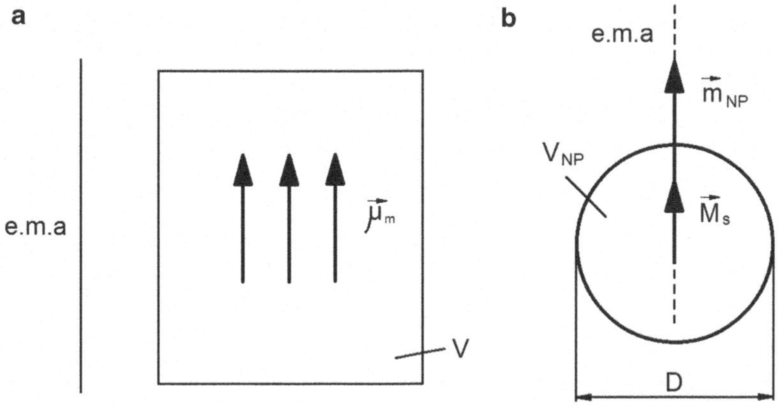

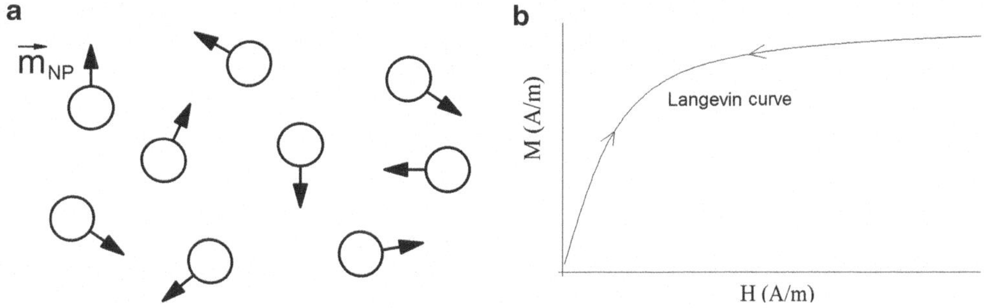

Fig. 22.3 (**a**) SPMNP system and (**b**) their magnetization in external static magnetic field

$$m_{NP} = \frac{\pi D^3}{6} M_s \quad (22.5)$$

where D is the magnetic diameter of the NP.

In an external magnetic field of intensity H (Caizer 2016), a system of single-domain NPs with magnetic moments m_{NP} (Eq. (22.4)) oriented in all directions at room temperature (Fig. 22.3a) will tend to orient in the direction of the applied magnetic field. The magnetization of the NP system takes place according to a Langevin law, just like the magnetization of a paramagnetic atomic system (Jacobs and Bean 1963):

$$M = n m_{NP} \left(\coth \frac{\mu_0 m_{NP} H}{k_B T} - \frac{k_B T}{\mu_0 m_{NP} H} \right) \quad (22.6)$$

where $n m_{NP}$ is the saturation magnetization M_{sat} of the NP system and

$$L = \left(\coth \frac{\mu_0 m_{NP} H}{k_B T} - \frac{k_B T}{\mu_0 m_{NP} H} \right) \quad (22.7)$$

is a Langevin function with $\xi = \mu_0 m_{NP} H / k_B T$ argument. In Eq. (22.6) n is NP concentration, μ_0 is the permeability of a vacuum, and k_B is Boltzmann's constant. Therefore, this behavior in the magnetic field of NPs is called superparamagnetic behavior (Bean and Livingston 1959), being specific to MNPs made up of many atoms (ions) with magnetic moments (e.g., even more than 10^5 atoms/ions in a magnetic domain), compared to the paramagnetic behavior of individual atoms/ions.

When the magnetic field increases from zero to the maximum value corresponding to the magnetic saturation, the magnetization of the SPMNP system increases according to the Langevin function (Fig. 22.3b), the saturation magnetization being a constant. At the decrease of the magnetic field from the saturation value to zero, the magnetization of the system returns to zero on the same curve (arrows on curve in Fig. 22.3b).

In conclusion, in this case the hysteresis loop is missing, a loop that exists in the case of large NPs, generally >25–30 nm for soft FiM NPs.

For low-magnetization fields, when the condition $\xi \ll 1$ is met, developing the Langevin function in series for a small argument, the magnetization of the NP system will be

$$M = \frac{\mu_0 n m_{NP}^2 H}{3k_B T} \quad (22.8)$$

According to Eq. (22.8), in this case the variation of the magnetization of the NP system with the applied field is linear, at a constant temperature.

For high magnetic fields, when $\xi \to \infty$, the Langevin function (Eq. (22.7)) takes the value 1 ($L \to 1$), and the magnetization of the NP system in this case will be

$$M = nm_{NP} \quad (22.9)$$

or

$$M = M_{sat} \quad (22.10)$$

respectively.

According to Eqs. (22.5) and (22.9), at a fixed concentration, the saturation magnetization of a NP system depends on the size of the NPs (by diameter D), M_s being a material characteristic.

22.2.2 Magnetic Behavior in External Alternating Magnetic Field. Superparamagnetic Relaxation

In an alternative magnetic field with low frequency (quasi-static), at room temperature, the magnetization and magnetic behavior of the SPMNP system will greatly depend on the amplitude of the magnetic field, as illustrated in Fig. 22.4, for three practical cases, two limits (a) and (c) and one intermediate (b).

Case (a) corresponds to a situation where the amplitude of the external alternative magnetic field is small (or very small) (H <), so that the magnetization of the NPs is in the linear area of the Langevin function (Eq. (22.8), Fig. 22.3b). Case (c) is the one corresponding to the very large amplitude of the external alternative magnetic field (H >>) (corresponding to the magnetic saturation). And case (b) corresponds to the situation when the magnetic field amplitude is moderate (but not very large), so that the magnetization deviates from the linear variation, following a Langevin-type curve.

In SPMHT, cases (a) and (b) are of interest, with case (c) being excluded due to the very large magnetic field, which is practically unusable.

In contrast, in MHT, where large NPs are used, it even case (c) would be of interest since there a hysteresis loop is followed as wide as possible, and this can be done in large or very large magnetic fields to obtain the hyperthermic effect being promoted.

As the frequency of the alternating magnetic field (AMF) increases, the magnetization can no longer immediately follow the variation of the magnetic field, and a delay in the time of the magnetization with respect to the field takes place, a phenomenon known as magnetic relaxation. At higher frequencies (kHz – MHz) the time delay is greater. As a result of this delay, there is dissipation (loss) of energy, which leads to the heating of the NPs.

In the Debye model it is shown that the complex components of magnetic susceptibility ($\chi = M/H$) $\chi = \chi' + \chi''$ are

$$\chi' = \frac{\chi_0}{1+(\omega\tau)^2} \quad (22.11)$$

and

$$\chi'' = \chi_0 \frac{\omega\tau}{1+(\omega\tau)^2} \quad (22.12)$$

where χ_0 is the static magnetic susceptibility, $\omega = 2\pi f$, where f is the frequency of the AMF, and τ is the relaxation time.

The magnetic relaxation time in the case of NPs dispersed in a fluid generally has two components (Néel 1949; Brown 1963), determined by the rotation of the magnetic moment inside the NP (Néel) and the rotation of the NP in fluid (Brown), under the action of the AMF. However, in the case of SPMHT, when the NPs are fixed in

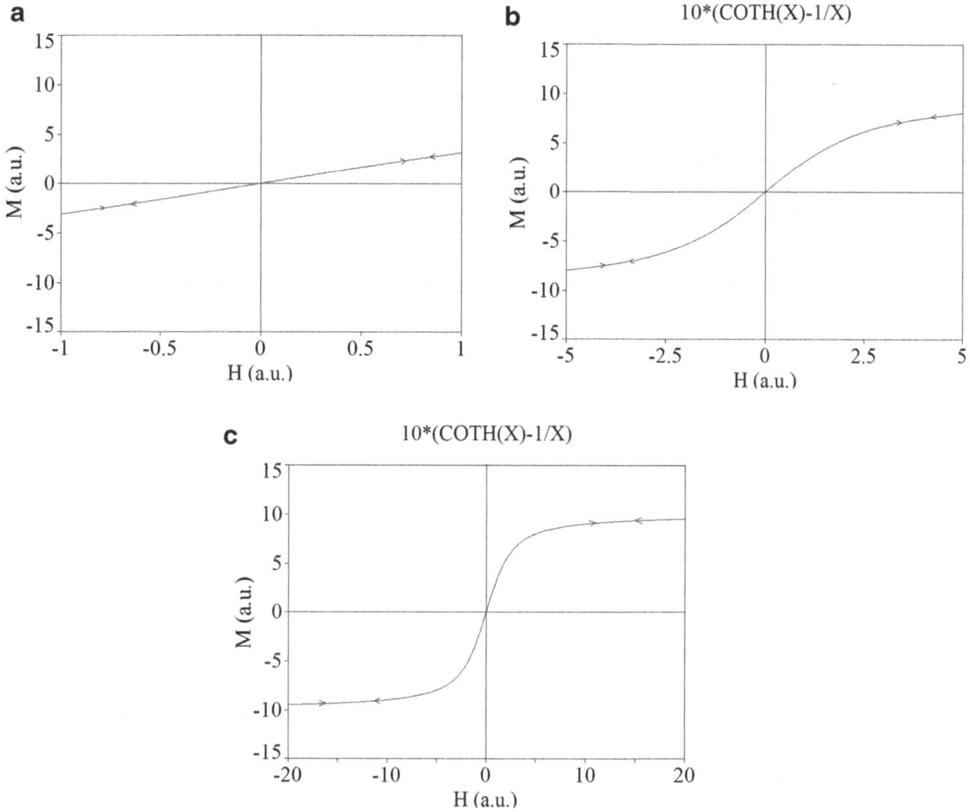

Fig. 22.4 Variation in magnetization of SPMNP system with intensity of quasi-static alternative magnetic field; (**a**) for low magnetic field (H <), (**b**) moderate magnetic field (H >), and (**c**) high magnetic field (H >>)

the tumor (tissue), only the Néel-type relaxation occurs, so that the relaxation time in this case will be

$$\tau = \tau_N = \tau_0 \exp\left(\frac{KV_{NP}}{k_B T}\right) \qquad (22.13)$$

where K is the magnetic anisotropy constant and τ_0 is a time constant that usually has the value 10^{-9} s (Back et al. 1998).

In a magnetic field of small amplitude, the static magnetic susceptibility χ_0 can be approximated by the Langevin relation

$$\chi_0 = \frac{3\chi_i}{\xi}\left(\coth\xi - \frac{1}{\xi}\right) \qquad (22.14)$$

where χ_i is the initial magnetic susceptibility and ξ the Langevin parameter

$$\xi = \frac{\mu_0 m_{NP} H}{k_B T} \qquad (22.15)$$

given by the ratio of the magnetic moment energy of the NP in the magnetic field H and the thermal energy at temperature T.

22.2.3 Specific Loss Power and Heating Rate

In an AMF with amplitude H and frequency f, the loss power is given by the equation (Rosensweig 2002)

$$P = \pi\mu_0\chi'' f H^2 \qquad (22.16)$$

Thus, in the case of NPs with superparamagnetic behavior in an AMF with frequency f and amplitude H, the dissipated power can be determined by considering the component χ'' of the complex magnetic susceptibility of the NP system, given by Eq. (22.12), where τ and χ_0 are given by Eqs. (22.13) and (22.14). At the same time, in the case of MHT experiments, in order to not have a dependence of the power dissipated by the nature of the material, the SLP will be considered: P/ρ, where ρ is the density of material.

In adiabatic conditions it is possible to evaluate the increase of the ΔT temperature of a system in a time interval Δt from the application of an AMF, using the formula

$$\Delta T = \frac{P}{\rho c}\Delta t \quad (22.17)$$

or heating rate (speed) T/t, where c is the specific heat. This formula is very important in SPMHT experiments since it allows for the quantitative estimation of the time necessary to reach a temperature of 42–43 °C, which is required in hyperthermia, as a function of other parameters that are in the SLP formula (Eq. (22.16)), respectively, in the magnetic susceptibilities χ'' (Eq. (22.12)) and χ_0 (Eq. (22.14)), and the practical parameters of the external applied magnetic field: H and f.

Figure 22.5 shows a concrete case in which the SLP was determined for magnetite NPs (Fe_3O_4), which are suitable for SPMHT. Power was calculated computationally in three dimensions depending on the frequency of the magnetic field f and the diameter D of monodisperse NPs for a usual magnetic field H of 10 kA/m (Caizer 2014). The data used in the computed calculation are shown in Table 22.1.

The obtained diagram makes it possible to accurately determine the diameter of the NPs (D_0) to be used in SPMHT, corresponding to the maximum dissipated power. Thus, for a diameter of approx. 15 nm is obtained the time temperature dependence in Fig. 22.6 at the same amplitude of the magnetic field and frequency of $f = 150$ kHz.

The result shows, under the specified conditions, that the necessary temperature can be reached in the hyperthermia of tumors of 42–43 °C (hyperthermic temperature) at an interval of 80 s. This time is a very good one without posing a danger of exposure to therapy that will be too long, which can affect healthy tissues.

Figure 22.7 shows an increase of temperature for 30 minutes in MHT by applying AMF with the parameters $H = 21.0$ kAm^{-1} and $f = 340$ kHz, in the experimental case of hydrophilic graphene-based yolk-shell MNPs functionalized with copolymer Pluronic F-127 (GYSMNP@PF127) conjugated with the drug doxorubicin (DOX) (Rodrigues et al. 2018). For this nanosystem the optimum temperature in hyperthermia is reached for 10–15 minutes.

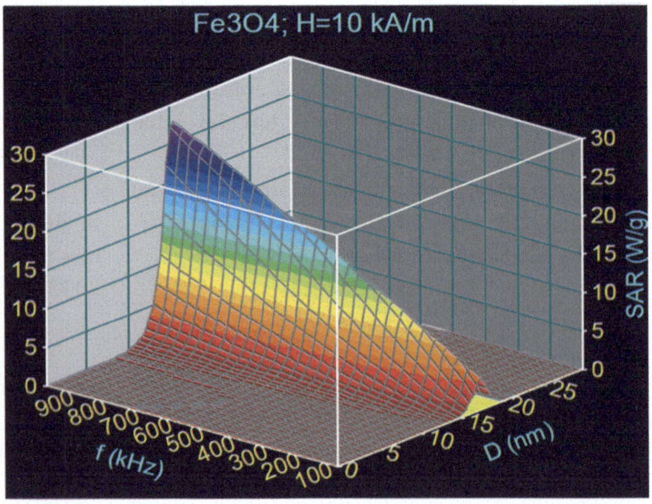

Fig. 22.5 3D diagram of SAR in case of Fe_3O_4 NPs (Caizer 2014). (CCL 2014, IOP Publishing. Reproduced by permission of CCL-IOP Publishing.)

Table 22.1 Characteristic observables of NPs and alternating magnetic field parameters (Caizer 2014)

Sample	M_s (kA/m)	K (kJ/m^3)	ρ (g/cm^3)	ε	f (kHz)	H (kA/m)
Fe_3O_4	477	11	5.24	0.017	150	10

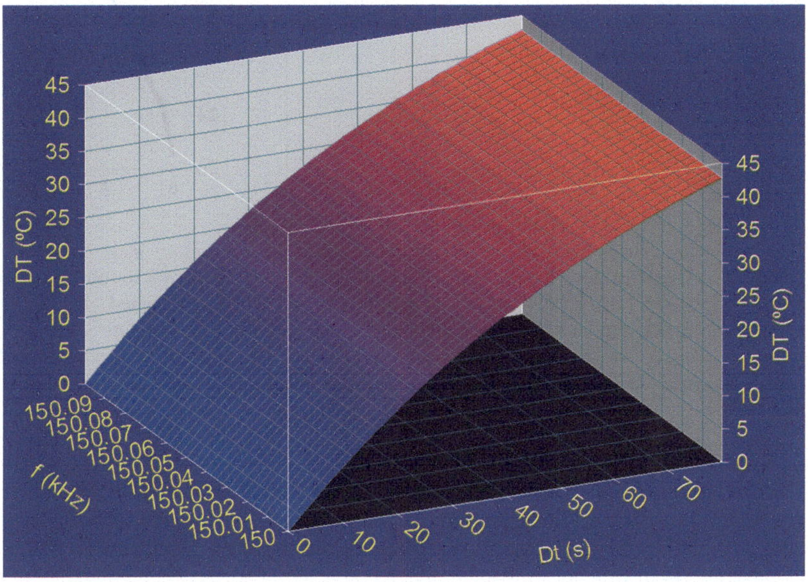

Fig. 22.6 Temperature increase in Δt time interval for optimal diameter $D_0 = 15$ nm of Fe_3O_4 SPMNPs in the case of SPMHT with parameters $H = 10$ kHz, $f = 150$ kHz (the result will be published by Caizer (2019))

22.3 Magnetic Nanoparticle Nanoformulations. Biocompatibility

MNPs exhibit highly interesting in vivo applications based on their intrinsic magnetic and superparamagnetic properties that enable them to be used in the diagnosis and treatment of malignant pathologies (Williams 2017). Their use requires parenteral administration, intravenous or local, which poses several challenges, mainly in terms of formulation and biocompatibility (Chen et al. 2012). Design maps can be developed to rationally apply hypothermic treatments and choose the most appropriate administration route depending on the intrinsic properties and biodistribution abilities of the NPs (Cervadoro et al. 2013).

A key step in magnetic nanoformulation is the achievement of physical stability of the dispersed NPs. A second aspect is NP biocompatibility, which requires the implementation of effective ways to make NPs unrecognizable by the immune system and expand their biological lifetime.

An important issue is the homogeneous distribution of MNPs at the tumor level, which makes it possible to achieve a uniform and well-controlled temperature pattern without hot spots or unheated tumor regions; a potential solution might involve multipoint injections directly at the tumor level, but overall the practical difficulties are overwhelming (Dutz and Hergt 2014; Kudr et al. 2017).

Systemic administration raises other challenges, such as efficient concentrations at the tumor level and the avoidance of clearance by the immune system. So far, several solutions have been adopted, in particular coating with various organic layers (i.e., synthesis of core-shell nanohybrids) and antibody binding (Ito et al. 2005).

The in situ preparation of functionalized MNPs with short-chain molecules containing carboxylic groups was reported by Kandasamy et al. in 2016 and 2018 (Kandasamy et al. 2016, 2018a, b). MNPs can be subjected to further chemical or biological conjugation without additional surface functionalization (Kandasamy et al. 2016); they showed good biocompatibility

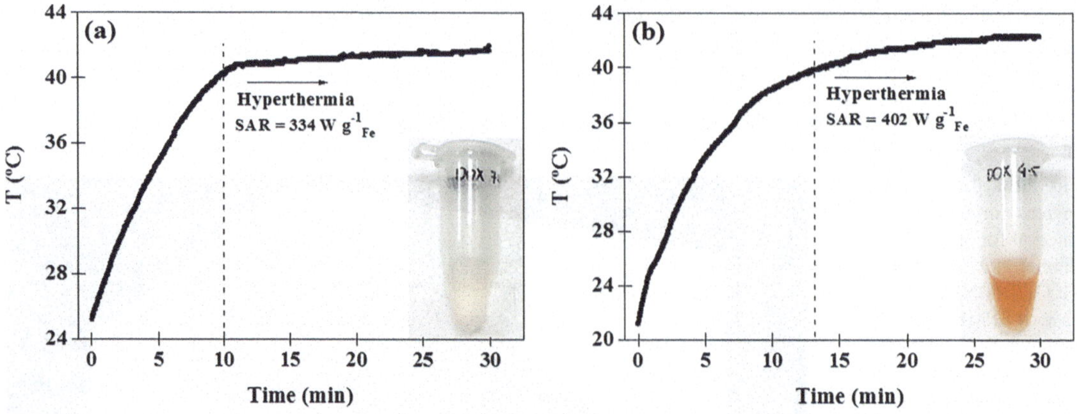

Fig. 22.7 Magnetically induced thermal response curve of GYSMNP@PF127-DOX (3.0 mg GYSMNP-DOX mL^{-1}) for dual pH- and thermal-responsive drug delivery: (**a**) dispersed in phosphate buffer at 7.4 to mimic physiological microenvironment and (**b**) dispersed in phosphate buffer at 4.5 to mimic tumor microenvironment. Samples were subjected to an AMF (f = 340 kHz and H = 21.0 kAm^{-1}) for 30 minutes. Inset shows drug-containing supernatant resulting from each hyperthermia experiment (Rodrigues et al. 2018)

and high magnetization and were thoroughly investigated in terms of heating responses and efficacies using a wide range of AMFs and dispersion media (Kandasamy et al. 2018a, b). Spherically shaped superparamagnetic iron oxide nanoparticles (SPIONs) exhibited stronger and faster hyperthermia effects than commercially available ferrofluids and provided higher killing efficiency toward MCF-7 breast tumor cells.

Multifunctionalized MNPs were synthesized by Aires et al. in 2015 by using bovine serum albumin as coating to improve the colloidal stability and magnetic response (Aires et al. 2015). Albumin induces hemocompatibility, delays clearance by the immune system, and deters the adsorption of other proteins; in addition, it allows for the attachment of anticancer drugs, thereby providing the opportunity to combine hyperthermia with drug delivery in the treatment of cancer.

Tagged dextran-coated MNPs containing ferric oxide were synthesized by conjugating the specific antihuman epidermal growth factor receptor (HER2) aptamer to the surface of the NPs (Pala et al. 2014). Using fluorescence microscopy, the authors were able to prove the high specificity of the tagged NPs toward the overexpressing HER2 receptor human adenocarcinoma SK-BR3 cells; also, a significantly lower dose of tagged NPs versus nontagged ones was needed to achieve similar effects of hyperthermia, thereby reducing the occurrence of side effects.

Stable, biocompatible, and easily dispersible MNPs were synthesized by coating magnetite NPs with a temperature- and pH-responsive polymer, poly(2-(dimethylamino)ethyl methacrylate); their heating capacity was investigated, revealing higher SARs than bare MNPs (Reyes-Ortega et al. 2017), thereby enabling the therapeutic use of hyperthermia. Other pH and temperature dual responsive polymer-modified SPIONs were synthesized using glutamic acid and N-isopropylacrylamide as co-monomers; carboxymethyl cellulose-induced SPION water solubility while folic acid served as the tagging agent (Patra et al. 2015). When interacted with an external magnetic field, the modified SPIONs showed very fast and efficient temperature increase, thus exhibiting promising solutions for cancer treatment and diagnosis.

Polyethylenimine (PEI), oleic acid, and Pluronic F-127 were used by Tomitaka et al. in 2012 as coating materials for Fe_3O_4 NPs in order to prevent NP aggregation and to enable their enhanced permeability and retention effects (Tomitaka et al. 2012a). The three coating materials possess various properties that make them suitable for biomedical applications in cancer treatment: (1) PEI is a water-soluble polymer bearing amine groups able to facilitate the binding and transport of nucleic acids; (2) oleic acid facilitates the surface covalent binding of tumor-targeting antibodies; and (3) Pluronic F-127 provides biocompatibility and, consequently, a longer biological lifetime due to its structural similarity with polyethylene glycols. Out of the three coating materials, Pluronic F-127 was selected by the authors as being suitable for the preparation of MNPs that could act as a heat source for hyperthermia; the main reason behind this decision was the fact that Pluronic-coated NPs exhibited heat dissipation in an independent manner from the viscosity of the surrounding environment (Tomitaka et al. 2012b). The NPs thus obtained were further subjected to in vitro studies using HeLa ovarian cancer cell cultures; while no cytotoxicity was recorded, the hyperthermia treatment significantly reduced cell viability by mediating apoptosis through the mitochondrial pathway.

Oleic acid coating was used for the synthesis of biocompatible colloidal suspension of IONPs with magnetic properties, which revealed a lack of toxicity both in vitro and in vivo (Coricovac et al. 2017).

Usually, the most common MNPs are based on ferrite or iron oxide due to their intrinsic magnetic properties; however, in some cases, such as bone malignant pathologies, special NPs that are able to ensure bone substitution as well as hyperthermia must be designed (Li et al. 2018). A biocompatible magnetic biomaterial containing Fe^{3+} and Ni^{2+} (2:1) cosubstituted hydroxyapatite NPs was obtained and evaluated in terms of physicochemical stability, biocompatibility, and hyperthermia potential (Karunamoorthi et al. 2013). The studies revealed significant hyperthermia properties and a low level of toxicity, probably due to the incorporation of cytotoxic groups of the magnetic phase into the biocompatible phases represented by hydroxyapatite and tricalcium phosphate.

Clustered superparamegnetic particles were obtained to prevent the leakage of SPIONs from the capillaries of healthy tissues and to increase their relaxivity and SAR (Hayashi et al. 2013). The clusters were decorated with folic acid and polyethylene glycol in order to promote a high tumor concentration; both clustering and surface decoration were conducted via thiol-ene click reaction. The modified SPION nanoclusters accumulated at a high level at a tumor site, facilitating enhanced MRI contrast; also, the application of an AMF led to a higher tumor temperature compared to the surrounding tissues, in the end significantly reducing tumor volume and meaningfully improving survival time for the experimental mice.

Gadolinium-doped dextran-coated magnetite NPs were investigated as potential theranostic agents due to their ability to enhance MRI contrast as well as to act as hyperthermia mediators (Palihawadana-Arachchige et al. 2017). Despite the fact that gadolinium may reduce magnetization, thereby hampering hyperthermia efficiency, the authors revealed that by selecting the proper composition of Gd-doped Fe_3O_4 NPs one may achieve higher SARs; however, future studies are needed to achieve the theranostic use of Gd-doped Fe_3O_4 NPs as both diagnostic and therapeutic agents.

Magnesium-doped iron oxide SPIONs were designed and synthesized to achieve efficient hyperthermia to completely eliminate tumor tissue (Jang et al. 2017); in addition to being highly biocompatible, magnesium was selected as doping material due to the fact that magnetically induced heating power can be effectively controlled by adjusting the concentration and distribution of Mg^{2+} cations within SPIONs. In vitro and in vivo hyperthermia studies demonstrated SPIONs' great ability to destroy cancer cells due to their significant heating power within the biologically safe range of AMFs.

Gold-coated SPIONs with suitable physicochemical and biological properties revealed a four- to fivefold increase in released heat compared to bare SPIONs under a low-frequency oscillating magnetic field (Mohammad et al.

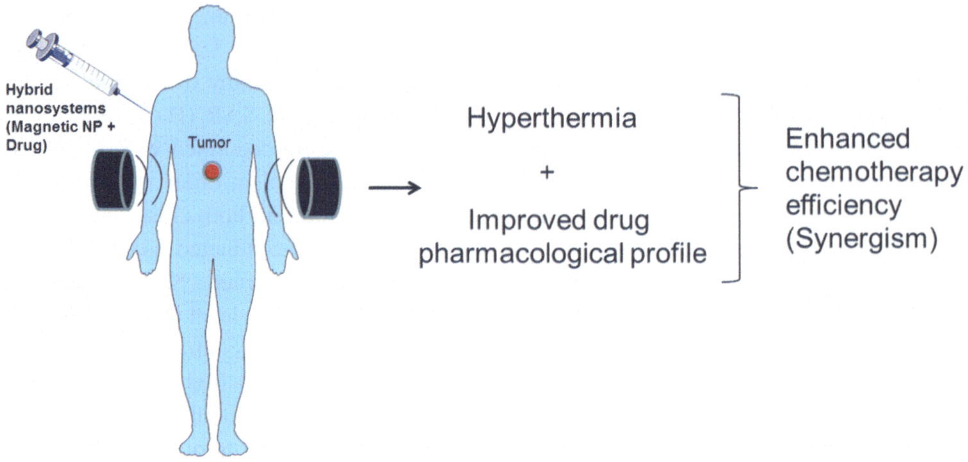

Fig. 22.8 Thermo-chemosensitization through the use of hybrid nanosystems. (The image contains elements from Servier Medical Art)

2010). In vitro studies have shown that in the absence of an external magnetic field, gold-coated SPIONs do not act as cytotoxic agents on cancer cells.

The most recent approach in the field of magneto-nanoformulations is the design of hybrid nanosystems (Fig. 22.8), which associate MNPs used either for diagnostic or treatment purposes with anticancer drugs that thus benefit from an improved pharmacological profile; this particular approach has become known as thermo-chemosensitization, that is, the enhancement of chemotherapy efficiency through simultaneous hyperthermia; studies have revealed that MHT induces higher concentrations of anticancer drugs at the tumor level, probably due to the hyperthermia effect on tumor vasculature as well as an increased drug cytotoxicity by mechanisms not yet fully understood (Hervault and Thanh 2014). Overall, one might classify the combined effect of thermo-chemotherapy as synergistic, in particular when mild hyperthermia is applied; in addition, the potential occurrence of treatment-induced secondary cancers is significantly lower (Hervault and Thanh 2014).

An excellent review concerning the diagnosis, targeting, and treatment of prostate cancer by means of MNPs was published in 2017 by Chowdhury et al.; the review concludes that modified MNPs that combine targeted drug delivery with MHT might represent potential future theranostic solutions for prostate cancer. Most importantly, these theranostic nanoformulations might allow the monitorization of disease progression while the treatment is ongoing based on the "see-and-treat" principle (Chowdhury et al. 2017).

The scientific literature mentions three main nanoformulations for the combined use of MNPs and anticancer drugs: liposomes, micelles, and polymer nanoformulations. Several such nanoformulations and their main characteristics are given in Table 22.2.

22.3.1 Liposomes

Liposomes are spherical nanovesicles that exhibit an aqueous core and a lipophilic outer bilayer and currently represent a very popular option for drug delivery due to several practical reasons: (1) the possibility of entrapping both hydrophilic and hydrophobic drugs in either core or outer layer, (2) improved drug pharmacokinetic and toxicological profiles, and (3) high possibility of fine surface tuning for optimized pharmacological properties (Alavi et al. 2017).

Magnetoliposomes represent an attractive possibility for allowing a combined chemother-

Table 22.2 Magnetic nanoformulations

Magnetic nanoparticles	Organic coating component	Experimental records	Reference
Liposomes			
Iron oxide	Oleic acid, phospholipid bilayer	Excellent targeting ability, thermosensitivity, high responsiveness to alternating magnetic field, and laser processing simultaneously improved tumor cell killing effects; real-time monitoring of cancer progression through fluorescence and MRI	Guo et al. (2018)
Iron oxide	Phospholipid bilayer	Cell damage depends on bulk temperature and duration of treatment, but mainly on cell type and thermal energy/cell during magnetic hyperthermia treatment	Engelmann et al. (2018)
Iron oxide	Citric acid, phospholipid bilayer	Targeted delivery, controlled drug release; significant tumor regression	Babincová et al. (2018)
Manganese ferrite nanoparticles ($MnFe_2O_4$)	Phospholipid bilayer	High encapsulation efficiency superparamagnetic behavior; simultaneous use as nanocarriers and hyperthermia agents	Rodrigues et al. (2017)
Cobalt ferrite nanoparticles	Oleic acid, phospholipid bilayer	Drug release through modification of membrane state; controlled drug release	Nappini et al. (2011)
Polymer nanoformulations			
Iron oxide	Pluronic F-127	Short-term, tumor-specific, hyperthermic treatment; long-term sustained drug delivery	Wang et al. (2013)
Iron oxide	Carboxymethylcellulose	Simultaneous use as nanocarriers and hyperthermia agents	Carvallho et al. (2019)
Iron oxide	Poly-N-isopropyl-acrylamide	Controlled synergistic tumor destruction through drug release and hyperthermia	Chang et al. (2014)
Cobalt ferrite nanoparticles	Poly(maleic anhydride-*alt*-1-octadecene)	High specific absorption rate	Nam et al. (2018)
Cobalt-doped ferrite nanoparticles	Human ferritin protein, poly(ethylene glycol)	Enhanced magnetic anisotropy and hyperthermic efficiency compared to undoped sample	Fantechi et al. (2014)
Micelles			
Mn-Zn-ferrite nanoparticles	2-(2-methoxyethoxy)ethyl methacrylate (MEO_2MA) and oligo(ethylene glycol) methacrylate (OEGMA)	Temporospatial synchronism of thermochemotherapy; synergistic effect, enhanced tumor cell sensitivity, reduced side effects	Li et al. (2018)
Iron oxide	Poly(ethylene glycol)-poly(lactide) (PEG-PLA)	Higher effectiveness compared to either hyperthermia or chemotherapy alone	Kim et al. (2015)
Iron oxide	Poly(N-isopropylacrylamide-co-acrylamide)-block-poly(ε-caprolactone)	Responsiveness to magnetic heating at physiologically relevant temperatures; significant MRI contrast enhancement abilities	Kim et al. (2013)
Iron oxide	Amphipatic chitosan	Intracellular responsive delivery and thermotherapy; complete regression of primary breast tumor without inducing secondary progression	Manigandan et al. (2018)
Iron oxide	Polystyrenegraft-poly(2-vinylpyridine) copolymer poly(acrylic acid)-block-poly(2-hydroxyethyl acrylate) double-hydrophilic block copolymer	Significant decrease in cell viability depending on incubation concentration and exposure time to alternating magnetic field, dual-dose effect	Nguyen (2018)

apy and MHT and provide biocompatibility and transport facilities for loaded chemotherapeutics without adding systemic toxicity (Gogoi et al. 2014).

Phosphatidylcholine liposomes containing maghemite NPs were obtained using a thin-film hydration method and tested in vitro on healthy and tumor colon cell lines as well as on blood cell lines for biocompatibility (Lorente et al. 2018). That study revealed high cellular uptake with mitochondria accumulation, in particular in cancer cells; also, the application of an external magnetic field induced cell migration, supporting the use of magnetoliposomes for biomedical purposes. The controlled release of the encapsulated drug through MHT is an important aspect when designing magnetoliposomes; the drug encapsulation efficiency seems to depend on the amount of MNPs (Ferreira et al. 2016).

Thermosensitive magnetic nanovesicles were prepared using a biphasic suspension of dextran-coated $La_{0.75}Sr_{0.25}MnO_3$ (LSMO) and Fe_3O_4 NPs at a ratio of 10:1, where the combination of the two inorganic nanomaterials provides the possibility of self-controlled hyperthermia, while the nanovesicular formulation enables the loading of anticancer drugs, such as paclitaxel (Gogoi et al. 2014). The biphasic nanohybrid formulation induced a synergistic cytotoxic effect during in vitro studies on MCF-7 breast cancer cells. In terms of biocompatibility, in vitro and in vivo studies revealed the absence of adverse effects while the therapeutic efficacy was preserved (Gogoi et al. 2017).

Two newly designed types of magnetoliposomes containing magnesium ferrite NPs were tested as nanocarriers for curcumin, revealing that the drug can be preferentially directed toward the tumor site, where it will be released through membrane cell fusion; the simultaneous application of MHT is possible, allowing a dual cancer therapy (Cardoso et al. 2018).

22.3.2 Polymer Nanoformulations

Polymer nanoformulations encompass a huge variety of components and gained their place in the biomedical field mainly due to important design flexibility in terms of polymer choice (biodegradable or nonbiodegradable polymers), functionalization, and synthetic approaches (via direct polymerization or use of preformed polymers) (Banik et al. 2015).

A polymer nanoformulation embedding both MNPs and anticancer drugs was designed by Balasubramanian et al. in 2014. It consists of two anticancer drugs, curcumin and 5-fluorouracil, and MNPs encapsulated in poly(D,L-lactic-co-glycolic acid) and functionalized with two cancer tagging agents (Balasubramanian et al. 2014); synergistic strong and fast citotoxic activity was recorded upon applying MHT on MCF-7 and G-1 cancer cells.

A copolymer of methyl methacrylate/ethylene glycol dimethacrylate/hydroxyl ethyl methacrylate was used as polymer envelope for the simultaneous embedding of magnetite particles and gemcitabine in order to provide a multifunctional platform for the hyperthermia-triggered release of the anticancer drug (Iglesias et al. 2018). The application of an AMF induced MHT at 43 °C for precise time intervals, which substantially improved the drug-release rate, reaching 100% release in less than 4 hours.

22.3.3 Micelles

Micelles are nanoformulations synthesized by the spontaneous assembly of surfactant molecules in an aqueous environment, exhibiting a hydrophobic core, which may accommodate lipophilic drugs, and a hydrophillic outer layer provided by the surfactant polar groups (Hervault and Thanh 2014). Thermosensitive micelles can be obtained through the use of a thermoresponsive polymer that can be grafted either on the polar head or the nonpolar tail (Hervault and Thanh 2014).

Block copolymer micelles incorporating hydrophobically modified MNPs were designed by Glover et al. in order to evaluate the hyperthermia efficacy as well as thermally enhanced drug release; the incorporated MNPs were able to preserve their heating properties, reaching hyperthermia conditions after 5 minutes and triggering drug release (Glover et al. 2013).

Hybrid gold/IONPs were embedded in block copolymer micelles for the purpose of combined hyperthermia and chemotherapy as well as optical imaging (Kim et al. 2009). The inorganic core-shell NPs were self-assembled within the polymer hydrophobic polymer core, which contained block copolymers of poly(N-isopropylacrylamide-co-acrylamide)-block-poly(-caprolactone); these NPs combine the advantages of gold and MNPs while the micelle structure provides water solubility, bioavailability for the loaded components, reduced aggregation, and improved stability in an aqueous biological environment.

22.4 In Vitro and In Vivo Viability/Cytotoxicity of Magnetic Nanoparticle Nanoformulations

22.4.1 Magnetic Hyperthermia

Emerging strategies are required in the oncology domain since conventional therapies (chemotherapy, radiotherapy, and surgery) are invasive techniques with numerous side effects (e.g., myelosuppression, cardiotoxicity, neurotoxicity, peripheral neuropathy, damage to surrounding tissues), and, according to the latest studies, IONPs with superparamagnetic properties represent an alternative with great potential (LeBrun and Zhu 2018; Dulińska-Litewka et al. 2019). Their superparamagnetic potential, together with their increased stability in biological media, biocompatibility, low toxicity, biodegradability, long retention time, capacity to agglomerate under a magnetic field, and accessibility for functionalization, place these NPs among the most studied NPs for biological applications (Vallabani and Singh 2018).

The most currently studied clinical applications of IONPs, particularly in the field of tumorigenesis, are MHT, MRI as contrast agent, and controlled/targeted drug delivery (Dulińska-Litewka et al. 2019), subjects that will be further discussed in what follows.

22.4.1.1 IONP Application as a Contrast Agent in Magnetic Resonance Imaging

MRI is a noninvasive technique that is used to visualize the anatomy of different organs (brain, liver, heart) and to detect the presence of different injuries (like cancer lesions) (Vallabani and Singh 2018; Dulińska-Litewka et al. 2019). A wide palette of contrast agents with magnetic properties has been developed in recent years (e.g., gadolinium, quantum dots with paramagnetic micelles, liposomes), and increased attention has focused on iron oxides with superparamagnetic properties, which proved highly efficacious as contrast agents applied in MRI detection. A magnetic IONP authorized by the U.S. Food and Drug Administration (FDA) as therapy to combat the iron deficit associated with chronic kidney disease (CKD) is ferumoxytol (Feraheme). Besides the therapeutic role of ferumoxytol, this compound also proved to be effective as an imaging tool for labeling stem cells for in vivo monitorization or as a noninvasive method to supervise preclinical and clinical experiments that involve stem cell therapies (Castaneda et al. 2011; Vallabani and Singh 2018). The superparamagnetic behavior and large magnetic moment of IONPs allow them to serve as an agent that produces negative contrast (a type – T2 contrast agent). One of the drawbacks associated with these iron NPs is a dark signal that was detected in T2 images, a signal that is responsible for difficulties in identifying areas of interest. A method to overcome this drawback consists in coating IONPs with citrate, which led to efficient NPs with both positive and negative contrast qualities (Vallabani and Singh 2018).

22.4.1.2 IONPs' Application as Biosensors

IONPs functionalized as nanozymes represent novel nanotechnology-based tools with applicability to biomedicine. This type of NP preserves the natural biological properties of enzymes (e.g., superoxide dismutase, oxidases, peroxidases) and in addition comes with multiple benefits, such as augmented stability at different pH and temperature levels, a reduction in synthesis costs, and plural uses as a single platform. The enzyme-like features of nanozymes have expanded the areas of application in the biomedical field: biomarkers for cancer diagnostics (several enzymes are reliable markers for different illnesses, including cancer) and the development of biosensors that can quantify the levels of cholesterol, glucose, urea, and oxygenated water, molecules with key roles in cellular metabolic processes (Gawande et al. 2016; Vallabani and Singh 2018).

22.4.1.3 IONPs' Application in Photothermal Therapy

The intrinsic properties of IONPs make them suitable tools for both magnetic and photothermal applications. This dual character of IONPs was highlighted by Espinosa et al., who tested the response of iron nanocubes (formulated as an aqueous suspension) to AMF and near-infrared laser irradiation exposure, which consisted of a significant augmentation of heating effects (two- to fivefold) compared to a magnetic field alone. This procedure proved highly efficient both in vitro (triggered cancer cell apoptosis) and in vivo (tumor regression) (Espinosa et al. 2016). Another example of IONPs designed for photothermal cancer therapy was proposed by Chen et al.: crystallized IONPs functionalized with polysiloxane-containing copolymer that possesses an antibiofouling capacity. Intravenous administration of these NPs following laser irradiation resulted in complete tumor regression with no relapse (Chen et al. 2014).

22.4.1.4 IONPs' Application as Drug Carriers

The multifunctional properties of IONPs were tailored to improve their efficacy as drug carriers for therapies of different illnesses (mainly cancer). A method to augment the effectiveness of breast cancer therapy (chemo- and radiotherapy) was proposed by PirayeshIslamianet al. The method involved testing doxorubicin conjugated with superparamagnetic mesoporous hydroxyapatite nanocomposites and deoxy-D-glucose (PirayeshIslamian et al. 2017; Vallabani and Singh 2018). A recent study conducted by Ye and coauthors proved that Fe_3O_4 NPs improved the antitumor effect of cryoablation in MCF-7 cells by impairing the capacity of intracellular ice formation during the freezing process (Ye et al. 2017).

22.4.1.5 Magnetic Hyperthermia

The term *hyperthermia* has a Greek origin and refers to the generation of heat in high concentration, heat that the body fails to dissipate by thermoregulation (Gkanas 2013; LeBrun and Zhu 2018). According to the medical oncology definition, *hyperthermia* describes a therapeutic approach by which an established region of interest is subjected to an increase in temperature above 40 °C (Perigo et al. 2015) for an extended period of time (Spirou et al. 2018; LeBrun and Zhu 2018). The beneficial effects of rising body temperature in treating illnesses and fighting infection have been known since 1866, when clinicians used different bacteria or other infectious agents to treat syphilis, gonorrhea, epilepsy, and even tumors (face sarcoma and melanoma) by inducing high fever over 40 °C (Bierman 1942; LeBrun and Zhu 2018; Spirou et al. 2018). In recent years, hyperthermia has evolved from an approach involving raising whole-body temperature (using thermal chambers and blankets) (Perigo et al. 2015) to localized hyperthermia that acts by heating a certain region by means of optimized external devices (microwave radiation, implanted electrodes, ultrasounds, and laser irradiation) (Moros et al. 2015); side effects are minimal (LeBrun and Zhu 2018). Moreover, a considerable number of preclinical and clinical studies have been performed (even randomized clinical trials) to verify the outcome of hyperthermia coupled with radiotherapy/chemotherapy for different cancer treatments; this strategy being has no additional adverse effects and offers an improved therapeutic effect (De Haas-Kock et al. 2009; Lutgens et al. 2010; Chang et al. 2018).

Depending on the temperature values applied to achieve hyperthermia within the target cells/

tissues, this process can be classified into diathermia (37–41 °C), a method used to treat/relieve arthritis symptoms, moderate hyperthermia (41–46 °C), which induces protein denaturation and aggregation, DNA crosslinking, which leads to apoptosis as the endpoint, and thermal ablation (46–50 °C), which triggers extensive necrosis, coagulation, and carbonization (Gkanas 2013; Hilger et al. 2005; LeBrun and Zhu 2018). Another term that is used to describe hyperthermia is mild hyperthermia, which refers to temperatures up to 42 °C (Spirou et al. 2018). The methods used to clinically induce local hyperthermia have been improved over time and include radiofrequency, ultrasound, microwave, and laser ablation (a method that is used to treat superficial skin cancers); however, some drawbacks were noted: (i) inefficient as stand-alone therapies, (ii) invasive because it involves inserting one or more probes, (iii) causes thermal injuries to surrounding healthy tissue, and (iv) reduced control and confinement of heat to tumor area (LeBrun and Zhu 2018).

The elevated temperatures that are characteristic of hyperthermia have been associated with several detrimental effects in cells/tissues (several differences have been described between normal and tumor cells due to the acidic microenvironment of tumor cells, but no disparities between intrinsic thermosensitivity were recorded), including cell death via complex molecular pathways (protein and DNA denaturation, impaired mitochondria, interference with intracellular transport, changes in cytoskeleton, alterations of plasma and subcellular organelle membranes, sequential loss of enzyme functions), augmented perfusion within tumors, increased concentration of chemotherapeutic drugs and higher oxygen concentrations leading to a greater response of tumors to radiotherapy, and enhanced immune response of immune cytotoxic cells against tumor cells.

The degree of in vitro cytotoxicity induced by hyperthermia is dependent on temperature and exposure time (Chang et al. 2018; Spirou et al. 2018; LeBrun and Zhu 2018). A relevant aspect to note is the possibility of cells that escape death after hyperthermia to develop thermotolerance due to some major classes of proteins (heat shock proteins) and enzymes that repair the damage and transform these cells into resistant ones (Richter et al. 2010; Chang et al. 2018).

Since hyperthermia is not effective as a single therapy, several studies proposed its use as complementary treatment in combination with radio- and chemotherapy, this combination becoming the subject of several randomized clinical trials that are currently in progress and of others that are finished (Chang et al. 2018). Hyperthermia proved to be a potent radiosensitizer via protein denaturation and inactivation of the proteins responsible for DNA repair, thus suppressing the repair of DNA damage triggered by radiotherapy and augmenting the death of tumor cells (Kampinga and Dikomey 2001; Chang et al. 2018; Spirou et al. 2018). Hyperthermic therapy acts synergistically with different chemotherapeutic agents as cisplatin, cyclophosphamide, and bleomycin, whereas in the case of doxorubicin, 5-fluorouracil, and vincristine, no significant effects were observed. The mechanistic pathways involved in the sensitization of cancer cells to chemotherapeutic agents consist of augmented tumor blood circulation and enhanced vascular permeability, which increases drug concentration at a target site (Song et al. 2005; Chang et al. 2018).

Beyond the multiple advantages and applications of hyperthermia, some inconveniences were asserted, such as a lack of specificity against tumor cells (both healthy and cancer cells are sensitive to heat), inducement of burns in healthy tissues surrounding targeted cancerous tissues, difficulty of reaching an accurate temperature for promoting cytotoxic effects (43 °C for rodent cells and 43.5 °C for human cell lines) at target sites and the occurrence of overheating, unreliable localization, and a narrowed penetration of heat and development of thermotolerance (Moros et al. 2015; Chang et al. 2018; Spirou et al. 2018).

An updated version of hyperthermia, with augmented therapeutic effects and negligible adverse effects, is represented by MHT. MHT is a phenomenon that describes the ability of MNPs to produce heat in the presence of a suitable AMF via hysteresis energy loss and Néel or Brown relaxation (Moros et al. 2015). The first reference of this technique for cancer treatment dates from 1957, and between then and now notable progress was recorded in this field, MHT being assessed, at present, in preclinical and clinical trials as adjuvant therapy for different tumors (Moros et al. 2015).

Compared to hyperthermia, MHT brings notable advantages, including offering targeted delivery by tailoring NP surfaces to specific bioactive molecules, providing a controlled temperature increment by means of remote-switchable instruments represented by NPs (Moros et al. 2015), making deeper penetration into tissues by applying an AMF, administering MNPs in different concentrations and for longer durations within the target sites being available for multiple treatment sessions, enhancing heating capacity determined by nanosized magnetic particles, controlling the size and morphology of NPs (by augmenting their biocompatibility and reducing the adsorption of blood proteins – biocorona), and offering multiple drug delivery routes because it is a minimally invasive technique (Perigo et al. 2015; Gkanas 2013; Chang et al. 2016). The disparities in terms of clinical efficiency between hyperthermia and MHT are illustrated in Fig. 22.9.

An ideal magnetic material for MHT is represented by magnetic IONPs (10–100 nm), based on the following considerations: iron is an inorganic element naturally found in organisms that is involved in key cellular processes, has high biocompatibility because it is recycled within organisms via metabolic pathways, superparamagnetic properties, and low toxicity (human body tolerates a dose of 5 mg/kg body mass); another very important aspect is that magnetite and maghemite are activated by AMFs (Perigo et al. 2015; Zahedi-Tabar et al. 2019; Spirou et al. 2018). The magnetic properties of IONPs stem from the existence of iron ions with different valences in their crystal structure; these unpaired ions have oppositely aligned magnetic moments, leading to strong magnetization (Chang et al. 2018).

The application of AMFs stimulates IONPs to produce heat by two mechanisms: hysteresis loss and relaxational losses (Chang et al. 2018; LeBrun and Zhu 2018; Mahmoudi et al. 2018). Hysteresis losses in bulk take place in large IONPs that present multiple magnetic domains in their structure (Chang et al. 2018; LeBrun and Zhu 2018). The heat that results after AMF appli-

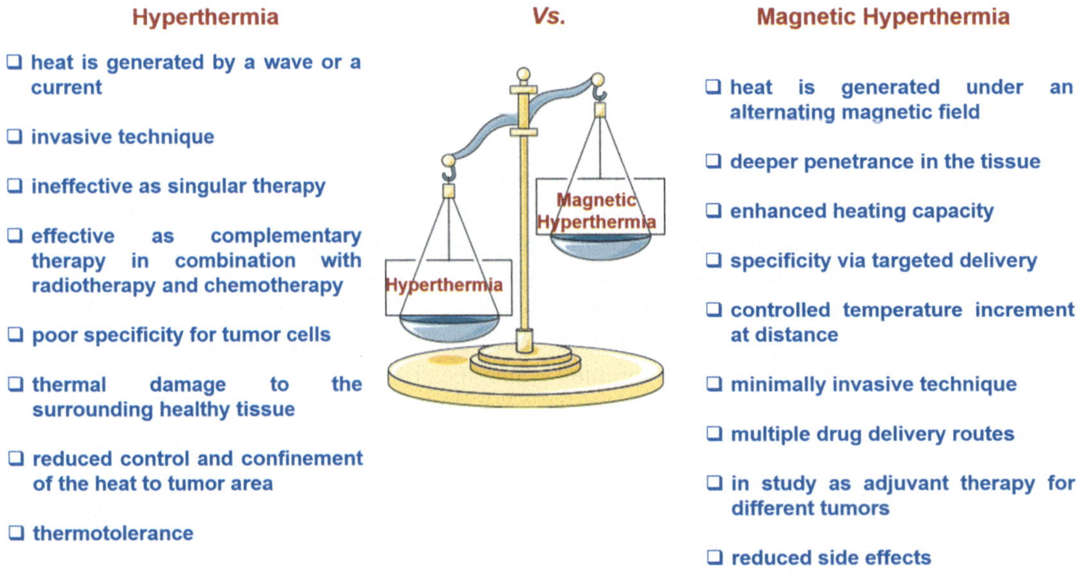

Fig. 22.9 Comparison between hyperthermia and MHT in terms of therapeutic potential

cation represents a difference in energy owing to the alignment of the magnetic moments of the NPs with the direction of the magnetic field (Kirschning et al. 2012; Chang et al. 2018; LeBrun and Zhu 2018). A decrease in IONP size is directly correlated with the reduction of the number of magnetic domains, with a single magnetic domain remaining at a threshold size (Houlding and Rebrov 2012; Chang et al. 2018).

The heat produced via relaxational losses occurs in superparamagnetic, single-domain NPs with sizes less than 25 nm. Two types of relaxation losses have been described: Néel and Brown relaxations (Chang et al. 2018; LeBrun and Zhu 2018). Néel relaxation can be defined as rapid changes that occur in a particle's magnetic moment when it is exposed to an AMF, an alignment that is contrary to the particle's crystalline structure, resulting in heat production. Brownian relaxation consists in frictional heat resulting from the physical rotation of particles within a supporting medium when the particles attempt to realign themselves with a changing magnetic field (Suto et al. 2009; Suriyanto et al. 2017; Ruta et al. 2015; Chang et al. 2018).

MNPs for MHT can be administered intravenously (the NPs are coated with a drug or carrier proteins and targeted for cancer cells) or direct intratumoral injections, a more invasive method with multiple advantages (Chang et al. 2018; LeBrun and Zhu 2018; Dulińska-Litewka et al. 2019; Mahmoudi et al. 2018). Other routes of delivery for the MNPs have also been also described as intraperitoneal (for ovarian, pancreatic, and gastric cancers), intra-arterial (liver cancers), and intracavitary (Chang et al. 2018).

MHT using magnetic IONP efficiency in treating cancer was tested in various models, including in in vitro and in vivo studies. An overview of these models is presented in Table 22.3.

MHT was officially introduced in clinical practice in 2011 for the treatment of glioblastoma in combination with conventional therapies (Dulińska-Litewka et al. 2019). Recent studies proved the use of MHT as a method to treat cancer under different approaches: (i) in combination with brachytherapy for prostate cancer, (ii) to stimulate the immune response in a murine melanoma model, (iii) in combination with radio frequency to treat gastrointestinal diseases (Crohn disease, colitis ulcerosa, and cancer), (iv) in therapy for patients diagnosed with HIV (Dulińska-Litewka et al. 2019).

Besides the numerous advantages and biomedical applications of MHT, this method also has several limitations: it has not been used in a clinical setting for any type of cancer, it makes it difficul to control the deposition of NPs at target sites, NPs are nonuniformly dispersed within tumors/tissues of interest, and it makes it difficult to estimate the proper thermal dose by predicting the temperature-time history (LeBrun and Zhu 2018).

22.4.2 Toxicity Assessment of IONPs

According to the ISO standard, the term *nanoparticle* refers to particles that possess one, two, or three external dimensions in a nanoscale range of 1–100 nm, dimensions that allow them to interact at a cellular (10–100 nm), subcellular (20–250 nm), genetic (10–100 nm), and even protein level (3–50 nm) (Markides et al. 2012).

The use of IONPs for biomedical purposes could be considered a double-edged sword since, on the one hand, IONPs possess multiple advantages (MRI-based clinical applications, targeted carriers due to their susceptibility to manipulation by an external magnetic field, promising therapy for tumor cells via MHT, reduced side effects of conventional drugs), but, on the other hand, their small dimensions facilitate their ability to cross different biological membranes in organisms, leading to unexpected noxious effects (Laffon et al. 2018; Nyström and Fadeel 2012).

In light of several recent studies (Yang et al. 2017; Laffon et al. 2018) that revealed the toxicity of IONPs both in vitro and in vivo, it has become essential to design a strategy for the evaluation of NPs' toxicological profile by understanding the mechanism of action and the molecular processes involved.

The ability of IONPs to enter cells and accumulate in different cellular organs as lysosomes,

Table 22.3 Applications of MHT using IONPs

Magnetic iron oxide bionanoparticle type	In vitro/in vivo studies	Toxicity endpoints induced by magnetic hyperthermia	Reference
Magnetic cationic liposomes – MCLs	T-9 rat glioma cells	Increased uptake of positively charged MCLs by glioma cells; a significant reduction of cell viability was reached at 43 °C after 40 minutes of magnetic irradiation	Shinkai et al. (1996)
Polyethylene glycol-based magnetic hydrogel nanocomposites	M059K glioblastoma cells	Selective cell death of glioblastoma cells by applying thermoablative temperatures (60–63 °C)	Meenach et al. (2010)
Iron oxide MNPs – nanomagnetic fluid	U251 human glioma cells	A dose-dependent inhibition of human glioma cell proliferation and presence of chromatin condensation, cytoplasmic vacuoles, and apoptotic bodies	Xu et al. (2017)
Monodisperse magnetic iron nanoparticles	B16-F10 – murine melanoma cell line	Mild magnetic hyperthermia did not impair melanoma cell viability but upregulated *hsp70* (heat shock protein) gene expression, a protein with key roles in sensibilization of cells to radiotherapy/chemotherapy	Moros et al. (2015)
Citric acid-coated zinc-doped magnetite nanoparticles ($Zn_{0.4}Fe_{2.6}O_4$)	Bone-cancer cell line – MG 63	Significant cell death after mild (42 °C) and extreme (47 °C) magnetic hyperthermia; in addition, even mild hyperthermia triggered differentiation of MG-63 cells to a more mature phenotype with a decreased capacity for self-renewal by upregulating alkaline phosphatase (ALP) expression, an early marker of osteogenesis	Moise et al. (2018)
Iron oxide magnetic nanoparticles	DA3, MCF-7, and HeLa	Significant cell death via apoptosis in all cell lines; the most sensitive cell line was MCF-7 (viability % < 3.5%)	Gkanas (2013)
Polycarboxylic iron oxide nanoparticles conjugated with doxorubicin	Human breast cancer cell lines – MCF-7 and MDA-MB-231	Targeted cytotoxicity in breast cancer cells, MCF-7 and MDA-MB-231, by promoting apoptosis and lesser noxious effects on normal human mammary epithelial cells, MCF 10A	Catalano (2018)
Fourth-generation dendrimer-coated iron oxide nanoparticles – G4@IONPs	Human breast cancer cell line (MCF-7) and human fibroblast cell line (HDF1)	A significantly reduced viability of MCF-7 cells (36.7% viable cells), whereas HDF1 cells (63.5% viable cells) were less sensitive to magnetic hyperthermia	Salimi et al. (2018)
Human-like collagen protein-coated MNPs	Baby hamster kidney BHK-21 cells	No toxic effects on cell viability, suitable for magnetic hyperthermia experiments	Chang et al. (2016)
Magnetite nanoparticles	Muscle tissue from cow	Thermoablation (87 °C) induced tissue alterations characterized by light-brown discoloration, pyknotic cell nuclei and degenerated myofibrils	Hilger et al. (2000)
Iron oxide MNPs – nanomagnetic fluid	Nude male mice inoculated with U251 human glioma cells	Dose-dependent inhibition of tumor development; tumors with hemorrhage and necrosis	Xu et al. (2017)
Magnetic fluid hyperthermia (MFH), combined with external radiation	Dunning model of prostate cancer using Copenhagen rats	Reduced tumor growth after magnetic hyperthermia and radiation	Johannsen et al. (2006)

(continued)

Table 22.3 (continued)

Magnetic iron oxide bionanoparticle type	In vitro/in vivo studies	Toxicity endpoints induced by magnetic hyperthermia	Reference
Biocompatible superparamagnetic nanoparticles	Rat malignant glioma using RG-2 cells in Fisher rats	A single intratumoral injection with magnetic fluid followed by two thermotherapy treatments determined a prolongation of rat survival; histopathological evaluation indicated large areas of necrosis next to particle deposits, tumor cells with a decreased proliferation rate, and reactive astrogliosis adjacent to tumor	Jordan et al. (2006)
Magnetic fluid hyperthermia	C3H mouse with induced mammary carcinoma	Dextran magnetite magnetic fluid administered intratumorally and exposed to an alternative magnetic field led to decrease in tumor volume and widespread tumor necrosis	Jordan et al. (1997)
Magnetic iron oxide nanoparticles (MIONs)	Squamous cell carcinoma	Intravenously administered MIONs under the effect of an AMF heated the tumor cells until ablation temperature, 60 °C, with no toxic effects for healthy surrounding tissue	Huang and Hainfeld (2013)
Porphyrin-coated MIONs	Melanoma	Intratumoral injection of MIONS followed by three short 10-minute AMF exposures decreased murine B16-F10 melanoma tumor volume; intravenous injection followed by three consecutive days of AMF exposure also proved efficient at decreasing tumor volume	Balivada et al. (2010)
MIONs conjugated to ChL6, an antibody that targets tumor-associated antigen L6	Breast cancer	Intravenously administered magnetic nanoparticles followed by magnetic hyperthermia induced tumor growth delay in a mouse model of breast cancer using HBT3477 xenografts	DeNardo et al. (2007)
Magnetic hydroxyapatite nanoparticles	Colorectal cancer cells (CT-26 cell line) implanted in mice	Tumor growth skrinkage was induced by magnetic hydroxyapatite nanoparticles exposed to AMF	LeBrun and Zhu (2018)
Ferrofluid	PC3 tumors in mice	A reduction of tumor volume with areas of necrosis in center of tumor and apoptosis events in periphery	LeBrun and Zhu (2018)

mitochondria, phagosomes, and vesicles (Catalano 2017) could be responsible for the noxious effects associated with IONP exposure. The main in vitro toxicity endpoints described for IONPs are decreased viability, oxidative stress, DNA damage, mitochondrial alterations, alterations in cell morphology and cell motility, cell membrane disruption, effects that are dependent on multiple factors such as cell type, IONP size, and concentration used, the capping agent, and the exposure time (Laffon et al. 2018; Liu et al. 2014).

The in vitro impact of IONPs has been studied intensively in recent years, but the results obtained were somewhat contradictory, with some studies affirming that IONPs are biocompatible and nontoxic at low concentrations (<100 μg/mL) (Kunzmann et al. 2011) and others reporting noxious effects even at these low doses (Laffon et al. 2018). No cell viability decrease was recorded following IONP exposure in human T lymphocytes, monocytes, primary rat astrocytes and neurons, human macrophages and amniotic fluid cells, murine microglial cells, fibroblasts, and macrophages (Laffon et al. 2018). A significant decrease in normal cell viability depending on concentration and exposure time was recorded in alveolar epithelial A459 cells after Fe_2O_3 exposure, in rat astrocytes treated with aminosilane- or starch-coated magnetite, and in human T lymphocytes exposed to IONPs coated with carboxyl or amine groups (Laffon et al. 2018).

In one of our previous studies, it was proved that magnetite and maghemite NPs double-

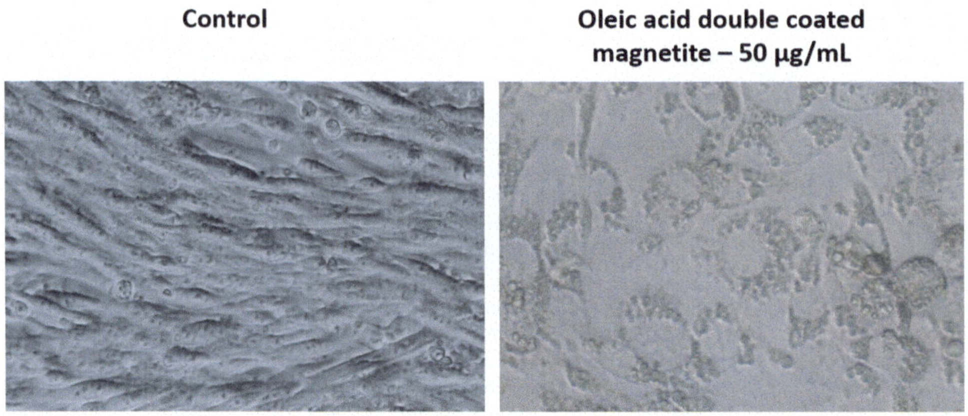

Fig. 22.10 HaCaT cell aspect after treatment with magnetite double coated with oleic acid for 24 hours, 50 µg/mL

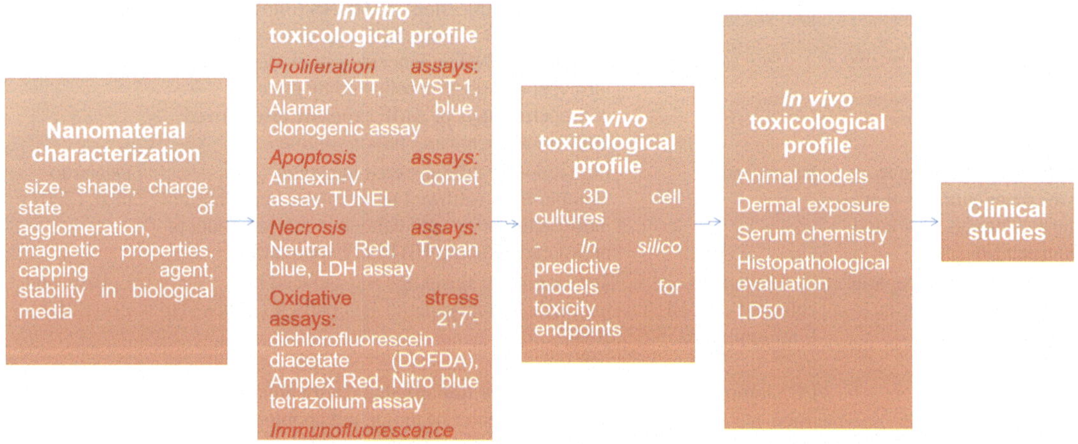

Fig. 22.11 Schematic representation of steps involved in assessment of NP toxicological profile

coated with oleic acid are nontoxic for human immortalized keratinocytes, HaCaT, at concentrations of 25 µg/mL after 24-hour stimulation. Moreover, the NPs had a stimulatory effect on cell migration and proliferation assessed by means of a scratch assay (Coricovac et al. 2017). In a more recent study, our group showed that a higher concentration (50 µg/mL) of magnetite double coated with oleic acid induced a significant decrease in HaCaT cell viability, whereas uncoated NPs had no impact on this parameter. In addition, the decreased viability was accompanied by the presence of a special phenomenon – enucleation characterized by the presence of holes within the cells as the nucleus was drawn out (Fig. 22.10) (Moacă et al. 2019).

Since engineered NPs are being applied more and more widely, it is essential to determine the fate of these NPs after their administration by investigating their safety/hazard potential. In this regard, intense discussions have been held among specialized groups to define a strategy for the evaluation of nanomaterial-induced hazards (Nyström and Fadeel 2012; Landsiedel et al. 2017). A schematic protocol to assess NPs' toxicological profile is presented in Fig. 22.11.

22.5 Conclusions

Magnetic IONPs are among the first and most studied NPs for clinical use and remain important due to their multiple biomedical applications and to the associated challenges, the topic being always of interest. Though considerable progress has been made in the field of MHT and SPMHT, which uses biocompatible magnetic IONPs, further investigations are still required to overcome the present limitations. Better ways of assessing the toxicity of these NPs since studies that have done so following chronic/long-term exposure are rather scarce.

The key to successful cancer therapy by MHT and, recently, SPMHT, for the complete destruction of tumors, depends on four essential factors: (i) finding the most suitable SPION MNPs for MHT, (ii) establishing the appropriate nanoformulations of MNPs to achieve very good biocompatibility and eliminate toxicity to healthy tissues surrounding tumors, (iii) using high-efficacy SPMHT instead of MHT, and (iv) establishing adequate in vivo protocols for the application of SPMHT in different types of cancer in order to obtain the maximum efficiency in the destruction of tumor cells.

Issue (ii) and, partially, issue (iii) were presented and discussed in this chapter. For issue (iv), more data will be needed in future research in order to be able to outline a steps toward a thorough investigation into the efficacy of the method in cancer therapy and its application to humans in preclinical and clinical settings.

References

Aires A, Ocampo SM, Cabrera D, Cueva L, de la Salas G, Teran FJ, Cortajarena AL (2015) BSA-coated magnetic nanoparticles for improved therapeutic properties. J Mater Chem B 3(30):6239–6247

Alavi M, Karimi N, Safaei M (2017) Application of various types of liposomes in drug delivery systems. Adv Pharm Bull 7(1):3–9

Alphandéry E, Chebbi I, Guyot F, Durand-Dubief M (2013) Use of bacterial magnetosomes in the magnetic hyperthermia treatment of tumours: a review. Int J Hyperth 29:801–809

Arami H, Khandhar A, Liggitt D, Krishnan KM (2015) In vivo delivery, pharmacokinetics, biodistribution and toxicity of iron oxide nanoparticles. Chem Soc Rev 44:8576–8607

Babincová N, Sourivong P, Babinec P, Bergemann C, Babincová M, Durdík Š (2018) Applications of magnetoliposomes with encapsulated doxorubicin for integrated chemotherapy and hyperthermia of rat C6 glioma. Z Naturforsch C J Biosci 73(7–8):265–271

Back CH, Weller D, Heidmann J, Mauri D, Guarisco D, Garwin EL, Siegmann HC (1998) Magnetization reversal in ultrashort magnetic field pulses. Phys Rev Lett 81:3251–3254

Balasubramanian S, Girija AR, Nagaoka Y, Iwai S, Suzuki M, Kizhikkilot V, Yoshida Y, Maekawa T, Nair SD (2014) Curcumin and 5-fluorouracil-loaded, folate- and transferrin-decorated polymeric magnetic nanoformulation: a synergistic cancer therapeutic approach, accelerated by magnetic hyperthermia. Int J Nanomedicine 9:437–459

Balivada S, Rachakatla RS, Wang H, Samarakoon TN, Dani RK, Pyle M, Kroh FO, Walker B, Leaym X, Koper OB, Tamura M, Chikan V, Bossmann SH, Troyer DL (2010) A/C magnetic hyperthermia of melanoma mediated by iron(0)/iron oxide core/shell magnetic nanoparticles: a mouse study. BMC Cancer 10:119

Banik BL, Fattahi P, Brown JL (2015) Polymeric nanoparticles: the future of nanomedicine. Wiley Interdiscip Rev Nanomed Nanobiotechnol 8(2):271–299

Bean CP, Livingston LD (1959) Superparamagnetism. J Appl Phys 30:S120–S129

Belanova AA, Gavalas N, Makarenko YM, Belousova MM, Soldatov AV, Zolotukhin PV (2018) Physicochemical properties of magnetic nanoparticles: implications for biomedical applications in vitro and in vivo. Oncol Res Treat 41(3):139–143

Bierman W (1942) The history of fever therapy in the treatment of disease. Bull N Y Acad Med 18(1):65–75

Brown WF (1963) Thermal fluctuations of a single-domain particle. Phys Rev 130:1677–1686

Caizer C (2013) SPMHT with biocompatible SPIONs for destroy the cancer cells. The 8th international conference Fine Particle Magnetism (ICFPM-2013). 24–27 June, Perpignan

Caizer C (2014) Computational study on superparamagnetic hyperthermia with biocompatible SPIONs to destroy the cancer cells. J Phys Conf Ser 521:012015–012014

Caizer C (2016) Nanoparticle size effect on some magnetic properties. In: Aliofkhazraei M (ed) Handbook of nanoparticles. Springer, Switzerland

Caizer C (2017) Magnetic hyperthermia using magnetic metal/oxide nanoparticles with potential in cancer therapy. In: Rai M, Shegokar R (eds) Metal nanoparticles in pharma. Springer, Switzerland

Caizer C (2019) Magnetic/Superparamagnetic Hyperthermia as an Effective Noninvasive Alternative Method for Therapy of Malignant Tumors. In: Rai M,

Jamil B (eds.) Nanotheranostics: Applications and limitations. Springer, Switzerland

Caizer C, Stancu A, Postolache P, Dumitru I, Bodale I, Vlazan P (2010) The magnetic properties of the $Co_\delta Fe_{(3-\delta)}O_4$ surfacted nanoparticles with potential applications in cancer therapy. The 7th international conference on Fine Particle Magnetism (ICFPM-2010). 21–24 June, Uppsala

Caizer C, Soica C, Dehelean C, Radu A, Caizer IS (2013) Study on toxicity of the superparamagnetic nanoparticles on the cells in order to use them in cancer therapy. The 8th international conference Fine Particle Magnetism. 24–27 June, Perpignan

Cardoso BD, Rio ISR, Rodrigues ARO, Fernandes FCT, Almeida BG, Pires A, Pereira AM, Araújo JP, Castanheira EMS, Coutinho PJG (2018) Magnetoliposomes containing magnesium ferrite nanoparticles as nanocarriers for the model drug curcumin. R Soc Open Sci 5:181017

Carvallho SM, Leonel AG, Mansur AA, Carvalho IC, Krambrock K, Mansur HS (2019) Biomater Sci 7:2102–2122

Castaneda RT, Khurana A, Khan R, Daldrup-Link HE (2011) Labeling stem cellswithferumoxytol, an FDA-approvedironoxidenanoparticle. J Vis Exp 57:e3482

Catalano E (2017) In vitro biological validation and cytocompatibility evaluation of hydrogel iron-oxide nanoparticles. AIP Conf Proc 1873:020011

Catalano E (2018) Targeted tumor drug delivery and magnetic hyperthermia for cancer treatment by chemotherapeutic-conjugated magnetic nanoparticles. AIP Conf Proc 1990:020022

Cervadoro A, Giverso C, Pande R, Sarangi S, Preziosi L, Wosik J, Brazdeikis A, Decuzzi P (2013) Design maps for the hyperthermic treatment of tumors with superparamagnetic nanoparticles. PLoS One 8(2):e57332

Chang PEJ, Purushotham S, Rumpel H, Kee IHC, Ng RTH, Chow PKH, Ramanujan RV, Tan CK (2014) Novel dual magnetic drug targeting and hyperthermia therapy in hepatocellular carcinoma with thermosensitive polymer-coated nanoparticles. J Gastrointest Dig Syst 4:198

Chang L, Liu XL, Di Fan D, Miao YQ, Zhang H, Ma HP, Liu QY, Ma P, Xue WM, Luo YE, Fan HM (2016) The efficiency of magnetic hyperthermia and in vivo histocompatibility for human-like collagen protein-coated magnetic nanoparticles. Int J Nanomedicine 11:1175–1185

Chang D, Lim M, Goos JACM, Qiao R, Ng YY, Mansfeld FM, Jackson M, Davis TP, Kavallaris M (2018) Biologically targeted magnetic hyperthermia: potential and limitations. Front Pharmacol 9:831

Chen D, Tang Q, Li X, Zhou X, Zang J, Xue WQ, Xiang JY, Guo CQ (2012) Biocompatibility of magnetic Fe_3O_4 nanoparticles and their cytotoxic effect on MCF-7 cells. Int J Nanomedicine 7:4973–4982

Chen H, Burnett J, Zhang F, Zhang J, Paholaka H (2014) Highly crystallize dironoxide nanoparticles as effective and biodegradable mediators for photothermal cancer therapy. J Mater Chem B 2(7):757–765

Chowdhury P, Roberts AM, Khan S, Hafeez BB, Chauhan SC, Jaggi M, Yallapu MM (2017) Magnetic nanoformulations for prostate cancer. Drug Discov Today 22(8):1233–1241

Coricovac DE, Moacă EA, Pinzaru I, Cîtu C, Soica C, Mihali CV, Păcurariu C, Tutelyan VA, Tsatsakis A, Dehelean CA (2017) Biocompatible colloidal suspensions based on magnetic Iron oxide nanoparticles: synthesis, characterization and toxicological profile. Front Pharmacol 8:154

Cullity BD, Graham CD (2009) Introduction to magnetic materials, second edition. Wiley, Hoboken

De Haas-Kock DF, Buijsen J, Pijls-Johannesma M, Lutgens L, Lammering G, van Mastrigt GA, De Ruysscher DK, Lambin P, van der Zee J (2009) Concomitant hyperthermia and radiation therapy for treating locally advanced rectal cancer. Cochrane Database Syst Rev (3):CD006269

DeNardo SJ, De Nardo GL, Natarajan A, Miers LA, Foreman AR, Gruettner C, Adamson GN, Ivkov R (2007) Thermal dosimetry predictive of efficacy of 111In- ChL6 nanoparticle AMF–induced thermoablative therapy for human breast cancer in mice. J Nucl Med 48:437–444

Di Corato R, Béalle G, Kolosnjaj-Tabi J, Espinosa A, Clément O, Silva A, Ménager C, Wilhelm C (2015) Combining magnetic hyperthermia and photodynamic therapy for tumor ablation with photoresponsive magnetic liposomes. ACS Nano 9:2904–2916

Dulińska-Litewka J, Łazarczyk A, Hałubiec P, Szafrański O, Karnas K, Karewicz A (2019) Superparamagnetic iron oxide nanoparticles-current and prospective medical applications. Materials (Basel) 12(4):617

Durymanov MO, Rosenkranz AA, Sobolev AS (2015) Current approaches for improving intratumoral accumulation and distribution of nanomedicines. Theranostics 5:1007–1020

Dutz S, Hergt R (2014) Magnetic particle hyperthermia - a promising tumour therapy? Nanotechnology 25(45):452001

Engelmann UM, Roeth AA, Eberbeck D, Buhl EM, Neumann UP, Schmitz-Rode T, Slabu I (2018) Combining bulk temperature and nanoheating enables advanced magnetic fluid hyperthermia efficacy on pancreatic tumor cells. Sci Rep 8:13210

Espinosa A, Di Corato R, Kolosnjaj-Tabi J, Flaud P, Pellegrino T, Wilhelm C (2016) Duality of ironoxidenanoparticles in cancer therapy: amplification of heatingefficiencyby magnetic hyperthermia and photothermal bimodal treatment. ACS Nano 10(2):2436–2446

Fantechi E, Innocenti C, Zanardelli M, Fittipaldi M, Falvo E, Carbo M, Shullani V, Di Cesare ML, Ghelardini C, Ferretti AM, Ponti A, Sangregorio C, Ceci P (2014) A smart platform for hyperthermia application in cancer treatment: cobalt-doped ferrite nanoparticles mineralized in human ferritin cages. ACS Nano 8(5):4705–4719

Ferreira RV, Martins TM, Goes AM, Fabris JD, Cavalcante LC, Outon LE, Domingues RZ (2016) Thermosensitive gemcitabine-magnetoliposomes for combined hyperthermia and chemotherapy. Nanotechnology 27(8):085105

Gawande MB, Goswami A, Felpin FX, Asefa T, Huang X, Silva R, Zou X, Zboril R, Varma RS (2016) Cu and Cu-based nanoparticles: synthesis and applications in catalysis. Chem Rev 116:3722–3811

Gazeau F, Lévy M, Wilhelm C (2008) Optimizing magnetic nanoparticle design for nanothermotherapy. Nanomedicine 3:831–844

Gkanas EI (2013) In vitro magnetic hyperthermia response of iron oxide MNP's incorporated in DA3, MCF-7 and HeLa cancer cell lines. Cent Eur J Chem 11:1042–1054

Glover AL, Bennett JB, Pritchett JS, Nikles SM, Nikles DE, Nikles JA, Brazel CS (2013) Magnetic heating of iron oxide nanoparticles and magnetic micelles for cancer therapy. IEEE Trans Magn 49:231–235

Gogoi M, Sarma HD, Bahadur D, Banerjee R (2014) Biphasic magnetic nanoparticles-nanovesicle hybrids for chemotherapy and self-controlled hyperthermia. Nanomedicine 9:955–970

Gogoi M, Jaiswal MK, Sarma HD, Bahadur D, Banerjee R (2017) Biocompatibility and therapeutic evaluation of magnetic liposomes designed for self-controlled cancer hyperthermia and chemotherapy. Integr Biol 9:555–565

Guo Y, Zhang Y, Ma J, Li Q, Li Y, Zhou X, Zhao D, Song H, Chen Q, Zhu X (2018) Light/magnetic hyperthermia triggered drug released from multi-functional thermo-sensitive magnetoliposomes for precise cancer synergetic theranostics. J Control Release 272:145–158

Habib AH, Ondeck CL, Chaudhary P, Bockstaller MR, McHenry ME (2008) Evaluation of iron-cobalt/ferrite core-shell nanoparticles for cancer thermotherapy. J Appl Phys 103:07A307-07A307-3

Hataminia F, Noroozi Z, Mobaleghol EH (2019) Investigation of iron oxide nanoparticle cytotoxicity in relation to kidney cells: a mathematical modeling of data mining. Toxicol In Vitro 59:197–203

Hayashi K, Nakamura M, Sakamoto W, Yogo T, Miki H, Ozaki S, Abe M, Matsumoto T, Ishimura K (2013) Superparamagnetic nanoparticle clusters for cancer theranostics combining magnetic resonance imaging and hyperthermia treatment. Theranostics 3(6):366–376

Hergt R, Dutz S (2007) Magnetic particle hyperthermia – biophysical limitations of a visionary tumour therapy. J Magn Magn Mater 311:187–192

Hervault A, Thanh NT (2014) Magnetic nanoparticle-based therapeutic agents for thermo-chemotherapy treatment of cancer. Nanoscale 6(20):11553–11573

Hilger I, Hergt R, Kaiser WA (2000) Effects of magnetic thermoablation in muscle tissue using iron oxide particles: an in vitro study. Investig Radiol 35(3):170–179

Hilger I, Hergt R, Kaiser WA (2005) Towards breast cancer treatment by magnetic heating. J Magn Magn Mater 293:314–331

Hou CH, Hou SM, Hsueh YS, Lin J, Wu HC, Lin FH (2009) The in vivo performance of biomagnetic hydroxy apatite nanoparticles in cancer hyperthermia therapy. Biomaterials 30:3956–3960

Houlding TK, Rebrov EV (2012) Application of alternative energy forms in catalytic reactor engineering. Green Processes Synth 1:19–31

Hu R, Zhang X, Liu X, Xu B, Yang H, Xia Q, Li L, Chen C, Tang J (2012) Higher temperature improves the efficacy of magnetic fluid hyperthermia for Lewis lung cancer in a mouse model. Thorac Cancer 3:34–39

Huang HS, Hainfeld JF (2013) Intravenous magnetic nanoparticle cancer hyperthermia. Int J Nanomedicine 8:2521–2532

Iglesias GR, Reyes-Ortega F, Checa Fernandez BL, Delgado ÁV (2018) Hyperthermia-triggered gemcitabine release from polymer-coated magnetite nanoparticles. Polymers (Basel) 10(3):269

Ito A, Tanaka K, Honda H, Abe S, Yamaguchi H, Kobayaschi T (2003) Complete regression of mouse mammary carcinoma with a size greater than 15 mm by frequent repeated hyperthermia using magnetite nanoparticles. J Biosci Bioeng 96:364–369

Ito A, Kuga Y, Honda H, Kikkawa H, Horiuchi A, Watanabe Y, Kobayashi T (2004) Magnetite nanoparticle-loaded anti-HER2 immunoliposomes for combination of antibody therapy with hyperthermia. Cancer Lett 212:167–175

Ito A, Shinkai M, Honda H, Kobayashi T (2005) Medical application of functionalized magnetic nanoparticles. J Biosci Bioeng 100(1):1–11

Jacobs IS, Bean CP (1963) Fine particles, thin films and exchange anisotropy. In: Rado GT, Suhl H (eds) Magnetism, vol 3. Academic Press, New York, pp 271–350

Jang J, Lee J, Seon J, Ju E, Kim M, Kim YI, Kim MG, Takemura Y, Arbab AS, Kang KW, Park KH, Paek SH, Bae S (2017) Giant magnetic heat induction of magnesium-doped γ-Fe_2O_3 superparamagnetic nanoparticles for completely killing tumors. Adv Mater 30(6):1704362

Johannsen M, Thiesen B, Gneveckow U, Taymoorian K, Waldöfner N, Scholz R, Deger S, Jung K, Loening SA, Jordan A (2006) Thermotherapy using magnetic nanoparticles combined with external radiation in an orthotopic rat model of prostate cancer. Prostate 66(1):97–104

Johannsen M, Gneveckow U, Thiesen B, Taymoorian K, Cho CH, Waldofner N, Scholz R, Jordan A, Loening SA, Wust P (2007) Thermotherapy of prostate cancer using magnetic nanoparticles: feasibility, imaging, and three-dimensional temperature distribution. Eur Urol 52:1653–1662

Jordan A, Scholz R, Wust P, Fähling H, Krause J, Wlodarczyk W, Sander B, Vogl T, Felix R (1997)

Effects of magnetic fluid hyperthermia (MFH) on C3H mammary carcinoma in vivo. Int J Hyperth 13(6):587

Jordan A, Scholz R, Maier-Hauff K, van Landeghem FK, Waldoefner N, Teichgraeber U, Pinkernelle J, Bruhn H, Neumann F, Thiesen B, von Deimling A, Felix R (2006) The effect of thermotherapy using magnetic nanoparticles on rat malignant glioma. J Neuro-Oncol 78:7–14

Kampinga HH, Dikomey E (2001) Hyperthermic radiosensitization: mode of action and clinical relevance. Int J Radiat Biol 77:399–408

Kandasamy G, Surendran S, Chakrabarty A, Kale SN, Maity D (2016) Facile synthesis of novel hydrophilic and carboxyl-amine functionalized superparamagnetic iron oxide nanoparticles for biomedical applications. RSC Adv 6:99948–99959

Kandasamy G, Sudame A, Bhati P, Chakrabarty A, Maity D (2018a) Systematic investigations on heating effects of carboxyl-amine functionalized superparamagnetic iron oxide nanoparticles (SPIONs) based ferrofluids for in vitro cancer hyperthermia therapy. J Mol Liq 256:224 237

Kandasamy G, Sudame A, Luthra T, Saini K, Maity D (2018b) Functionalized hydrophilic superparamagnetic iron oxide nanoparticles for magnetic fluid hyperthermia application in liver cancer treatment. ACS Omega 3:3991–4005

Karunamoorthi R, Suresh Kumar G, Prasad AI, Vatsa RK, Thamizhavel A, Girija EK (2013) Fabrication of a novel biocompatible magnetic biomaterial with hyperthermia potential. J Am Ceram Soc 97(4):1115–1122

Kim DH, Rozhkova EA, Rajh T, Bader SD, Novosad V (2009) Synthesis of hybrid gold/iron oxide nanoparticles in block copolymer micelles for imaging drug delivery and magnetic hyperthermia. IEEE Trans Magn 45:4821–4824

Kim DH, Vitol EA, Liu J, Balasubramanian S, Gosztola DJ, Cohen EE, Novosad V, Rozhkova EA (2013) Stimuli-responsive magnetic nanomicelles as multifunctional heat and cargo delivery vehicles. Langmuir 29(24):7425–7432

Kim HC, Kim E, Jeong SW, Ha TL, Park SI, Lee SG, Lee SJ, Lee SW (2015) Magnetic nanoparticle-conjugated polymeric micelles for combined hyperthermia and chemotherapy. Nanoscale 7(39):16470–16480

Kirschning A, Kupracz L, Hartwig J (2012) New synthetic opportunities in miniaturized flow reactors with inductive heating. Chem Lett 41:562–570

Kobayashi T (2011) Cancer hyperthermia using magnetic nanoparticles. Biotechnol J 6:1342–1347

Kudr J, Haddad Y, Richtera L, Heger Z, Cernak M, Adam V, Zitka O (2017) Magnetic nanoparticles: from design and synthesis to real world applications. Nanomaterials (Basel) 7(9):243

Kunzmann A, Andersson B, Vogt C, Feliu N, Ye F, Gabrielsson S, Toprak MS, Buerki-Thurnherr T, Laurent S, Vahter M, Krug H, Muhammed M, Scheynius A, Fadeel B (2011) Efficient internalization of silica-coated iron oxide nanoparticles of different sizes by primary human macrophages and dendritic cells. Toxicol Appl Pharmacol 253:81–93

Laffon B, Fernández-Bertólez N, Costa C, Brandão F, Teixeira JP, Pásaro E, Valdiglesias V (2018) Cellular and molecular toxicity of iron oxide nanoparticles. Adv Exp Med Biol 1048:199–213

Landsiedel R, Ma-Hock L, Wiench K, Wohlleben W, Sauer UG (2017) Safety assessment of nano materials using an advanced decision-making framework, the DF4nanoGrouping. J Nanopart Res 19(5):171

LeBrun A, Zhu L (2018) Magnetic nanoparticle hyperthermia in cancer treatment: history, mechanism, imaging-assisted protocol design, and challenges. In: Shrivastava D (ed) Theoryand applications of heat transfer in humans, First Edition. Wiley, pp 631–667

Li M, Bu W, Ren J, Li J, Deng L, Gao M, Gao X, Wang P (2018) Enhanced synergism of thermo-chemotherapy for liver cancer with magnetothermally responsive nanocarriers. Theranostics 8(3):693–709

Liu Y, Xia Q, Liu Y, Zhang S, Cheng F, Zhong Z, Wang L, Li H, Xiao K (2014) Genotoxicity assessment of magnetic iron oxide nanoparticles with different particle sizes and surface coatings. Nanotechnology 25:42510

Lorente C, Cabeza L, Clares B, Ortiz R, Halbaut L, Delgado AV, Perazzoli G, Prados J, Arias JL, Melguizo C (2018) Formulation and in vitro evaluation of magnetoliposomes as a potential nanotool in colorectal cancer therapy. Colloids Surf B: Biointerfaces 171:553–565

Lutgens L, van der Zee J, Pijls-Johannesma M, De Haas-Kock DF, Buijsen J, Mastrigt GA, Lammering G, De Ruysscher DK, Lambin P (2010) Combined use of hyperthermia and radiation therapy for treating locally advanced cervix carcinoma. Cochrane Database Syst Rev (3):CD006377

Mahmoudi K, Bouras A, Bozec D, Ivkov R, Hadjipanayis C (2018) Magnetic hyperthermia therapy for the treatment of glioblastoma: a review of the therapy's history, efficacy and application in humans. Int J Hyperth 34(8):1316–1328

Malaiya A, Vyas SP (1988) Preparation and characterization of indomethacin magnetic nanoparticles. J Microencapsul 5(3):243–253

Manigandan A, Handi V, Sundaramoorthy NS, Dhandapani R, Radhakrishnan J, Sethuraman S, Subramanian A (2018) Responsive nanomicellar theranostic cages for metastatic breast cancer. Bioconjug Chem 29(2):275–286

Markides H, Rotherham M, El Haj AJ (2012) Biocompatibilityand toxicity of magnetic nanoparticles in regenerative medicine. J Nanomater 2012:1–12

Matsuoka F, Shinkai M, Honda H, Kubo T, Sugita T, Kobayashi T (2004) Hyperthermia using magnetite cationic liposomes for hamster osteosarcoma. Biomagn Res Technol 2(3):1–6

Meenach SA, Hilt JZ, Anderson KW (2010) Poly(ethyleneglycol)-based magnetic hydrogel nanocomposites for hyperthermia cancer therapy. Acta Biomater 6:1039–1046

Moacă EA, Farcaş C, Coricovac D, Avram S, Mihali CV, Draghici GA, Loghin F, Păcurariu C, Dehelean C (2019) Oleic acid double coated Fe_3O_4 nanoparticles as anti-melanoma compounds with a complex mechanism of activity-in vitro and in vivo assessment. J Biomed Nanotechnol 15(5):893–909

Mohammad F, Balaji G, Weber A, Uppu RM, Kumar CSSR (2010) Influence of gold nanoshell on hyperthermia of superparamagnetic iron oxide nanoparticles. J Phys Chem C 114(45):19194–19201

Moise S, Byrne JM, El Haj AJ, Telling ND (2018) The potential of magnetic hyperthermia for triggering the differentiation of cancer cells. Nanoscale 10(44):20519–20525

Moros M, Ambrosone A, Stepien G, Fabozzi F, Marchesano V, Castaldi A, Tino A, de la Fuente JM, Tortiglione C (2015) Deciphering intracellular events triggered by mild magnetic hyperthermia in vitro and in vivo. Nanomedicine (Lond) 10(14):2167–2183

Nam PH, Lu LT, Linh PH, Manh DH, Thanh Tam LT, Phuc NX, Phong PT, Lee IJ (2018) Polymer-coated cobalt ferrite nanoparticles: synthesis, characterization, and toxicity for hyperthermia applications. New J Chem 42:14530–14541

Nappini S, Bonini M, Ridi F, Baglioni P (2011) Structure and permeability of magnetoliposomes loaded with hydrophobic magnetic nanoparticles in the presence of a low frequency magnetic field. Soft Matter 7(10):4801

Néel L (1949) Théorie du traînage magnétique des ferromagnétiques en grains fins avec application aux terres cuites. Ann Geophys 5:99–136

Nguyen TT, Mammeri F, Ammar S (2018) Iron oxide and gold based magneto-plasmonic nanostructures for medical applications: A review. Nanomaterials 8:149

Nyström AM, Fadeel B (2012) Safety assessment of nanomaterials: implications for nanomedicine. J Control Release 161(2):403–408

Pala K, Serwotka A, Jeleń F, Jakimowicz P, Otlewski J (2014) Tumor-specific hyperthermia with aptamer-tagged superparamagnetic nanoparticles. Int J Nanomedicine 9:67–76

Palihawadana-Arachchige M, Naik VM, Vaishnava PP, Jena BP, Naik R (2017) Gd-doped superparamagnetic magnetite nanoparticles for potential cancer theranostics. In: Seehra MS (ed) Nanostructured materials - fabrication to applications. Intech Open. https://doi.org/10.5772/intechopen.68219

Patra S, Roy E, Karfa P, Kumar S, Madhuri R, Sharma PK (2015) Dual-responsive polymer coated superparamagnetic nanoparticle for targeted drug delivery and hyperthermia treatment. ACS Appl Mater Interfaces 7(17):9235–9246

Pavel M, Stancu A (2009) Study of the optimum injection sites for a multiple metastases region in cancer therapy by using MFH. IEEE Trans Magn 45:4825–4828

Pavel M, Gradinariu G, Stancu A (2008) Study of the optimum dose of ferromagnetic nanoparticles suitable for cancer therapy using MFH. IEEE Trans Magn 44:3205–3208

Perigo EA, Hemery G, Sandre O, Ortega D, Garaio E, Plazaola F, Teran FJ (2015) Fundamentals and advances in magnetic hyperthermia. Appl Phys Rev 2:1–104

PirayeshIslamian J, Hatamian M, Aval NA, Rashidi MR, Mesbahi A, Mohammadzadeh M, AsghariJafarabadi M (2017) Targeted superparamagnetic nanoparticles coated with 2-deoxy-d-glucose and doxorubicin more sensitize breast cancer cells to ionizing radiation. Breast 33:97–103

Reyes-Ortega F, Delgado ÁV, Schneider EK, Checa Fernández BL, Iglesias GR (2017) Magnetic nanoparticles coated with a thermosensitive polymer with hyperthermia properties. Polymers (Basel) 10(1):10

Richter K, Haslbeck M, Buchner J (2010) The heat shock response: life on the verge of death. Mol Cell 40:253–266

Rodrigues ARO, Almeida BG, Rodrigues JM, Queiroz MJRP, Calhelha RC, Ferreira ICFR, Pires A, Pereira AM, Araújo JP, Coutinho PJG, Castanheira EMS (2017) Magnetoliposomes as carriers for promising antitumor thieno[3,2-b]pyridin-7-arylamines: photophysical and biological studies. RSC Adv 7:15352–15361

Rodrigues R, Baldi G, Doumett S, Garcia-Hevia L, Gallo J, Bañobre-López M, Dražić G, Calhelha R, Ferreira I, Rui Lima R, Gomes H, Silva A (2018) Multifunctional graphene-based magnetic nanocarriers for combined hyperthermia and dual stimuli-responsive drug delivery. Mater Sci Eng C 93:206–217

Rosensweig RE (2002) Heating magnetic fluid with alternating magnetic field. J Magn Magn Mater 252:370–374

Ruta S, Chantrell R, Hovorka O (2015) Unified model of hyperthermia via hysteresis heating in systems of interacting magnetic nanoparticles. Sci Rep 5:9090

Salimi M, Sarkar S, Saber R, Delavari H, Alizadeh AM, Mulder HT (2018) Magnetic hyperthermia of breast cancer cells and MRI relaxometry with dendrimer-coated iron-oxide nanoparticles. Cancer Nanotechnol 9(1):7

Shinkai M, Yanase M, Honda H, Wakabayashi T, Yoshida J, Kobayashi T (1996) Intracellular hyperthermia for cancer using magnetite cationic liposomes: in vitro study. Jpn J Cancer Res 87(11):1179–1183

Song CW, Park HJ, Lee CK, Griffin R (2005) Implications of increased tumor blood flow and oxygenation caused by mild temperature hyperthermia in tumor treatment. Int J Hyperth 21:761–767

Spirou SV, Basini M, Lascialfari A, Sangregorio C, Innocenti C (2018) Magnetic hyperthermia and radiation therapy: radiobiological principles and current practice. Nanomaterials (Basel). 8(6). pii: E401

Suriyanto, Ng EY, Kumar SD (2017) Physical mechanism and modeling of heat generation and transfer in magnetic fluid hyperthermia through Neelian and Brownian relaxation: a review. Biomed Eng Online 16:36

Suto M, Hirota Y, Mamiya H, Fujita A, Kasuya R, Tohji K, Jeyadevan B (2009) Heat dissipation mechanism of magnetite nanoparticles in magnetic fluid hyperthermia. J Magn Magn Mater 321:1493–1496

Tian X, Liu S, Zhu J, Qian Z, Bai L, Pan Y (2019) Biofunctional magnetic hybrid nanomaterials for theranostic applications. Nanotechnology 30:032002 (10pp)

Tomitaka A, Ueda K, Yamada T, Takemura Y (2012a) Heat dissipation and magnetic properties of surface-coated Fe_3O_4 nanoparticles for biomedical applications. J Magn Magn Mater 324(21):3437–3442

Tomitaka A, Yamada T, Takemura Y (2012b) Magnetic nanoparticle hyperthermia using pluronic-coated nanoparticles: an in vitro study. J Nanomaterials 2012:480626, 5 pages

Valenzuela R (1994) Magnetic ceramics. Cambridge University Press, pp 137–142

Vallabani NVS, Singh S (2018) Recent advances and future prospects of iron oxide nanoparticles in biomedicine and diagnostics. 3 Biotech 8(6):279

Wang SY, Liu MC, Kang KA (2013) Magnetic nanoparticles and thermally responsive polymer for targeted hyperthermia and sustained anti-cancer drug delivery. Adv Exp Med Biol 765:315–321

Wang F, Yang Y, Ling Y, Liu J, Cai X, Zhou X, Tang X, Liang B, Chen Y, Chen H, Chen D, Li C, Wang Z, Hu B, Zheng Y (2017) Injectable and thermally contractible hydroxypropyl methyl cellulose/Fe_3O_4 for magnetic hyperthermia ablation of tumors. Biomaterials 128:84e93

Williams HM (2017) The application of magnetic nanoparticles in the treatment and monitoring of cancer and infectious diseases. Biosci Horiz: Int J Stud Research 10:hzx009

Xu H, Zong H, Ma C, Ming X, Shang M, Li K, He X, Cao L (2017) Evaluation of nanomagnetic fluid on malignant glioma cells. Oncol Lett 13:677–680

Yan H, Shang W, Sun X, Zhao L, Wang J, Xiong Z, Yuan J, Zhang R, Huang Q, Wang K, Li B, Tian J, Kang F, Feng SS (2018) "All-in-One" Nanoparticles for trimodality imaging-guided intracellular photo-magnetic hyperthermia therapy under intravenous administration. Adv Funct Mater 28:1705710. (1-12)

Yang Y, Qin Z, Zeng W, Yang T, Cao Y, Mei C, Kuang Y (2017) Toxicity assessment of nanoparticles in various systems and organs. Nanotechnol Rev 6(3):279–289

Ye P, Kong Y, Chen X, Li W, Liu D, Xie Y, Zhou Y, Zou H, Chang Z, Dai H, Kong X, Liu P (2017) Fe_3O_4 nanoparticles and cryoablation enhance ice crystal formation to improve the efficiency of killing breast cancer cells. Oncotarget 8:11389–11399

Zahedi-Tabar Z, Bagheri-Khoulenjani S, Amanpour S, Mirzadeh H (2019) A review on the application of in vitro and in vivo models of cancerous tumors for the study of the hyperthermia effect. Basic Clin Cancer Res 11:71–81

Zhou P, Zhao H, Wang Q, Zhou Z, Wang J, Deng G, Wang X, Liu Q, Yang H, Yang S (2018) Photoacoustic-enabled self-guidance in magnetic hyperthermia Fe@ Fe_3O_4 nanoparticles for theranostics *in vivo*. Adv Healthcare Mater 7:e1701201

Index

S. Talegaonkar, M. Rai (eds.), *Nanoformulations in Human Health*,
https://doi.org/10.1007/978-3-030-41858-8

Q

R

V

W

X

Z

The manufacturer's authorised representative in the EU is Springer
Nature Customer Service Centre GmbH, Europaplatz 3, 69115 Heidelberg,
Germany. If you have any concerns regarding our products, please
contact ProductSafety@springernature.com

Printed and bound by CPI Group (UK) Ltd, Croydon, CR0 4YY
30/09/2026
02225503-0020